The Eye in Infancy

The Eye in Infancy

Sherwin J. Isenberg, M.D.
Professor and Vice-Chairman
Jules Stein Eye Institute
Harbor-UCLA Medical Center
Department of Ophthalmology
UCLA School of Medicine
Los Angeles and Torrance, California

YEAR BOOK MEDICAL PUBLISHERS, INC.
CHICAGO • LONDON • BOCA RATON

1 2 3 4 5 6 7 8 9 0 C R 93 92 91 90 89

Library of Congress
Library of Congress Cataloging-in-Publication Data

The Eye in infancy / [edited by] Sherwin J. Isenberg.
p. cm.
Includes bibliographies and index.
ISBN 0-8151-4805-4
1. Vision disorders in children. 2. Infants—Diseases.
3. Pediatric ophthalmology. I. Isenberg, Sherwin J.
[DNLM: 1. Eye Diseases—in infancy & childhood. WW600 E975]
RE48.2.C5E94 1989
618.92'0977—dc19 88-20868
DNLM/DLC CIP
for Library of Congress

Sponsoring Editor: David K. Marshall
Associate Managing Editor, Manuscript Services: Deborah Thorp
Production Project Manager: Gayle Paprocki
Proofroom Manager: Shirley E. Taylor

CONTRIBUTORS

Leonard Apt, M.D.
Professor of Ophthalmology
Director Emeritus
Division of Pediatric Ophthalmology
Jules Stein Eye Institute
UCLA School of Medicine
Los Angeles, California

Steven M. Archer, M.D.
Assistant Professor
Department of Ophthalmology
Indiana University
Indianapolis, Indiana

George R. Beauchamp, M.D.
Department of Ophthalmology
Cleveland Clinic Foundation
Cleveland, Ohio

J.S. Crawford, M.D.C., F.R.C.S. (C.), D.O.M.S.
Professor and Acting Chairman
Department of Ophthalmology
University of Toronto
Former Head of Eye Department
Hospital for Sick Children
Toronto, Ontario, Canada

Christopher J. Dickens, M.D.
Research Consultant
The Foundation for Glaucoma Research
St. Mary's Hospital
San Francisco, California
Peralta Hospital
Oakland, California

Christine M. Disteche, Ph.D.
Associate Professor of Pathology
University of Washington
University Hospitals
Seattle, Washington

Paul B. Donzis, M.D.
Clinical Instructor
UCLA School of Medicine
Jules Stein Eye Institute
Los Angeles, California

Harry S. Dweck, M.D.
Professor of Pediatrics
Associate Professor of Obstetrics
Director, Regional Neonatal Intensive Care Unit
New York Medical College
Director, Regional Neonatal Intensive Care Unit
Westchester Medical Center
Valhalla, New York

Thomas D. France, M.D.
Professor, University of Wisconsin
Director, Pediatric Ophthalmology & Strabismus
University of Wisconsin Hospital & Clinics
Madison, Wisconsin

David S. Friendly, M.D.
Professor of Ophthalmology
George Washington University
Chairman, Department of Ophthalmology
Childrens Hospital National Medical Center
Washington, D.C.

Anne B. Fulton, M.D.
Associate Professor of Ophthalmology
Harvard Medical School
Senior Associate in Ophthalmology
Children's Hospital
Boston, Massachusetts

Nancy Hamming, M.D.
Assistant Professor of Ophthalmology
Rush-Presbyterian-St. Luke's Hospital
Assistant Clinical Professor Ophthalmology
University of Illinois Eye and Ear Infirmary
Chicago, Illinois

Eugene M. Helveston, M.D.
Professor of Ophthalmology
University of Indiana
Director, Section of Pediatric Ophthalmology
James Whitcomb Riley Hospital for Children
Indianapolis, Indiana

Robert W. Hered, M.D.
Chief, Division of Pediatric Ophthalmology
Nemours Children's Clinic
Jacksonville, Florida

David A. Hiles, M.D.
Clinical Professor of Ophthalmology
University of Pittsburgh
Chief of Ophthalmology
Children's Hospital of Pittsburgh
Pittsburgh, Pennsylvania

Gary N. Holland, M.D.
Assistant Professor of Ophthalmology
Jules Stein Eye Institute
UCLA School of Medicine
Los Angeles, California

H. Dunbar Hoskins, Jr., M.D.
Clinical Professor
Department of Ophthalmology
University of California at San Francisco
San Francisco Medical Center
San Francisco, California

Creig S. Hoyt, M.D.
Professor of Ophthalmology and Pediatrics
Director of Pediatric Ophthalmology
University of California Medical Center at San Francisco
San Francisco, California

Sherwin J. Isenberg, M.D.
Professor and Vice-Chairman
Jules Stein Eye Institute
Harbor-UCLA Medical Center
Department of Ophthalmology
UCLA School of Medicine
Los Angeles and Torrance, California

Jane D. Kivlin, M.D.
Associate Professor of Ophthalmology
Department of Ophthalmology
University of Utah
University of Utah Medical Center
Primary Childrens' Medical Center
Salt Lake City, Utah

David Anson Lee, M.D.
Assistant Professor of Ophthalmology
UCLA School of Medicine
Jules Stein Eye Institute
UCLA School of Medicine
Los Angeles, California

Toni G. Marcy, M.D.
Academic Coordinator
Director, UCLA Intervention Program for Visually Handicapped Children
UCLA Medical Center
Los Angeles, California

Lois J. Martyn, M.D.
Associate Professor of Ophthalmology
Associate Professor in Pediatrics
Temple University School of Medicine
Pediatric Ophthalmologist
St. Christopher's Hospital for Children
Philadelphia, Pennsylvania

Andrew Q. McCormick, B.S., M.D., C.M.
Clinical Associate Professor
Department of Ophthalmology
University of British Columbia
British Columbia's Children's Hospital
Vancouver, British Columbia, Canada

Marilyn B. Mets, M.D.
Assistant Professor of Pediatrics and Ophthalmology
University of Chicago
Pritzker School of Medicine
Division Director
Pediatric Ophthalmology & Ophthalmic Genetics
Chicago, Illinois

Marilyn T. Miller, M.D.
Professor of Clinical Ophthalmology
Director of Pediatric Ophthalmology & Strabismus
University of Illinois at Chicago
Chicago, Illinois

Roberta A. Pagon, M.D.
Associate Professor of Pediatrics
Adjunct Associate Professor of Ophthalmology
University of Washington
Head, Children's Hospital and Medical Center Regional Genetics Clinic
Children's Hospital and Medical Center
Seattle, Washington

Earl A. Palmer, M.D.
Associate Professor of Ophthalmology and Pediatrics
The Oregon Health Sciences University
Director, Elks Children's Eye Clinic
University Hospitals and Clinics
Portland, Oregon

Robert C. Pashby, M.D., F.R.C.S.C.
Assistant Professor
Department of Ophthalmology
University of Toronto
Mount Sinai Hospital
Hospital for Sick Children
Toronto, Ontario, Canada

Dale L. Phelps, M.D.
Associate Professor of Pediatrics and Ophthalmology
University of Rochester
Strong Memorial Hospital
Rochester, New York

Graham E. Quinn, M.D.
Assistant Professor
Department of Ophthalmology
University of Pennsylvania
Children's Hospital of Philadelphia
Philadelphia, Pennsylvania

Venkat Reddy, B.A.
Department of Ophthalmology
University of Chicago
Chicago, Illinois

Richard M. Robb, M.D.
Associate Professor of Ophthalmology
Harvard Medical School
Ophthalmologist-in-Chief
The Children's Hospital
Boston, Massachusetts

Arthur L. Rosenbaum, M.D.
Professor of Ophthalmology
Chief, Division of Pediatric Ophthalmology
Jules Stein Eye Institute
UCLA Medical Center
Los Angeles, California

Jeffrey S. Schwartz, M.D.
Eye Institute of West Florida
Largo Medical Hospital
Largo, Florida

Vrinda Telang, M.D. (deceased)
Assistant Professor-Neonatology
New York Medical College
Westchester Medical Center
Valhalla, New York

Elise Torczynski, M.D.
Professor of Clinical Ophthalmology
Pritzker School of Medicine
University of Chicago
Rush-Presbyterian-St. Luke's Hospital
Cook County Hospitals
Chicago, Illinois

Paul T. Urrea, M.D., M.P.H.
Clinical Instructor
University of Southern California School of Medicine
Division of Ophthalmology
Children's Hospital of Los Angeles
Doheny Eye Institute
Los Angeles, California

Gary A. Varley, M.D.
Department of Ophthalmology
University of Iowa
University of Iowa Hospitals and Clinics
Iowa City, Iowa

Barry A. Weissman, O.D., Ph.D.
Associate Professor of Ophthalmology
Jules Stein Eye Institute
UCLA School of Medicine
Los Angeles, California

FOREWORD

The acquisition of a senior status among your colleagues in a specialty is expected to endow you with a perspective not shared by those more junior. For this reason, I presume, came Dr. Isenberg's invitation for me to write a foreword for this most up-to-date and highly valued text in our subspecialty of pediatric ophthalmology.

From my perspective, I could emphasize for the reader the exponential increase of knowledge in pediatric ophthalmology that occurs with the passing of successive years. But what specialty in medicine is not similarly experiencing the same phenomenon? The fact is that the entire spectrum of science annually continues to accelerate the rate of expansion of its knowledge base.

The specific front of the multifarious knowledge base in pediatric ophthalmology that currently is expanding most rapidly involves the developing visual system that occurs from embryogenesis through infancy. The substance of this book addresses this important front.

My perspective of pediatric ophthalmology coincides with the advent of television; both entered my life at the same time slightly more than 40 years ago. I am unable to estimate the total work force involved in the television industry 40 years ago but I can estimate it for the specialty of pediatric ophthalmology. If more than two ophthalmologists were involved it was not my good fortune to have known them. Early in the era of the development of pediatric ophthalmology some general ophthalmologists maintained an interest and made substantial contributions within isolated areas of the newly evolving subspecialty. Yet, the consensus among ophthalmologists 40 years ago was often expressed as, "Who needs pediatric ophthalmology?" As history unfolded, the passing years soundly answered that question with, "The patient." Now, hundreds of researchers and clinicians exclusively work in this subspecialty. Today, the benefit that comes to the visual systems of many little patients is striking by comparison to its absence 40 years ago.

Pediatric ophthalmology by its nature is a rather pervasive subspecialty, covering a wide area as it cuts across many of the anatomically determined or disease-oriented subspecialties. The magnitude of the field of pediatric ophthalmology is associated with a corresponding large knowledge base that lends itself to be sorted into smaller units. Who, 40 years ago, would have predicted that a 29-chapter book would be written by 39 different authors, restricted in content to knowledge about the eye in infancy. The ophthalmologist wag of 40 years ago would have likely responded, "Which infant's eye, right or left, is the book written for?"

Indeed, it is to the credit of basic and clinical researchers that such a volume of knowledge has built up. But this mass of knowledge can render value to the patient only by authors organizing and relating its pertinent aspects to the person destined to use it. We, who are best able to use it, forever will be grateful to Dr. Isenberg and his many contributors for compiling and presenting this very useful information about the infant's visual system.

MARSHALL M. PARKS, M.D.
Clinical Professor of Ophthalmology
George Washington University Medical Center
Washington, D.C.

FOREWORD

During the past 25 years there has been a remarkable burgeoning of scientific knowledge focusing on the beginning of life. This has included a series of landmark discoveries concerning the human eye.

This volume brings together invaluable information about normal and abnormal development of the eye in fetal life, during the newborn period, and in infancy. Additionally, it provides authoritative information regarding diagnosing and treating the various conditions affecting the eye during these periods. Also included are important aids in accomplishing the difficult task of examining the eye during infancy. *The Eye in Infancy* should prove to be an invaluable resource in our nurseries and offices.

ROSEMARY D. LEAKE, M.D.
Professor of Pediatrics
UCLA School of Medicine
Chief of Neonatal Division
Harbor/UCLA Medical Center
Los Angeles, California

PREFACE

Childbearing ideally would include the meticulous selection of the date and method of conception, care and nurturing during the pregnancy, and a well-planned delivery. In many ways, the development of this book has proceeded along similar lines.

Prior to conception, parents must achieve adulthood themselves. For giving me the tools to practice and teach pediatric ophthalmology in an adult fashion, I must express gratitude to four great teachers of ophthalmology. Dr. Leonard Apt, the first full-time academic pediatric ophthalmologist, has been a role model as a researcher and practitioner of pediatric ophthalmology. Our association has been especially close and personal, and remains so to this day. Dr. Morton Goldberg demonstrated how to apply a combination of clinical sense, keen knowledge of medical literature, and proper research techniques to ophthalmology. Dr. Martin Urist taught me the power of simple observation and how to simultaneously love life and strabismus. Finally, Dr. Marshall M. Parks personifies one who can dedicate the practical aspects of ophthalmic science to the children he loves so much. To each of these great men I owe a debt I can never repay.

For conception to occur, both desire and interest need to be stimulated. (1) The desire was provided by ophthalmologists, pediatricians, and neonatologists. A number of these medical specialists, realizing my interest in research of the infantile eye, asked where a comprehensive book dealing only with the eyes of newborns and infants could be obtained. After reviewing the texts currently available, it became obvious to me that such a book did not exist. It is for those practitioners, as well as researchers of the eyes of babies, that this book is primarily intended. (2) The interest was obtained from the excitement of studying, examining, and treating infants. This interest was fueled by interactions with my dear colleague, Dr. John Heckenlively, and with a splendid team of researchers in neonatology at the Harbor-UCLA Medical Center in Torrance, Calif. Under the leadership of Dr. Rosemary Leake, the nurses of the Perinatal Research Center, including Susan Everett-Chamberlain, Roberta Rich, John Pescetti, Sarah Alvarez, Eileen Goldblatt, Chris Mori, and Artemiza McCullough have been both the stimulus and tool to investigate many new aspects of the infant eye. Dr. S. Eric Wilson, Chairman of the Department of Surgery at Harbor, has provided a working environment that encourages these efforts. At the Jules Stein Eye Institute, the interest would never have been realized without the ongoing encouragement and support of the director and chairman, Dr. Bradley Straatsma, who appreciates the importance of the eyes of babies.

What is conception but an exchange of genetic material? This genetic material reflects all past knowledge regarding the eyes of infants derived from previous investigations. I must thank the numerous researchers who have enlightened us with their inquiries. Among these people are all of the scientists who have contributed to this volume as well as such luminaries as Drs. Gunter K. von Noorden, Davida Teller, John Flynn, Velma Dobson, and many others.

Following conception, one enters the expectant period of pregnancy. During this juncture, I contacted all of the gifted physicians who contributed to this project and encountered universal enthusiasm. I am most grateful to each of these experts who have shared their knowledge and experience in specific areas of infantile ophthalmic interest with us.

During pregnancy, many new tasks are undertaken and life can become very confusing. For her organizational talents, secretarial skills, and unquestioning fidelity to this project, I thank Ms. Jean Shimizu. Without her, this endeavor would not have been as timely or as pleasant. I also thank Ms. Natalie Stone for her unflagging and compassionate devotion to our pediatric patients.

Finally, after a pregnancy delayed by many unforeseen obstacles, the delivery occurs. For this act, I am grateful to Mr. David K. Marshall and his colleagues at Year Book Medical Publishers for their faith in this book and their many excellent suggestions.

Now that the baby has arrived, one should examine it. This book is organized into four sections. The first section presents aspects of the infantile eye that are of common interest to pediatricians and ophthalmologists. These aspects include embryology, physical and visual development, examination techniques, pharmacology, amblyopia, teratology, and the fascinating topic of transient phenomena found in the newborn eye. The second section is a thorough and systematic tome dealing with the diagnosis and treatment of congenital abnormalities of the eyes, eyelids, and orbit that are evident in the first year of life. It is arranged anatomically and is intended to assist those interested in congenital ocular disorders of either a specific or general nature. The third section discusses ocular disorders of infants that are acquired, such as trauma (due to birth or child abuse), infections, and retinopathy of prematurity. The fourth section presents the role of the eye in systemic diseases of infants and the unpleasant but important topic of the blind infant. Not only is the diagnosis discussed, but the importance of how the physician should relate to the patient and his family is emphasized.

As in many new ventures in life, there is often something won and something lost. Although we have witnessed the birth of a new book, something has vanished that can never be regained. That, of course, is time. To my terrific children, Jason, Ethan, Seth, and Kim, I apologize for all the lost evenings and weekends we did not spend together since I began work on this project. To my wife Rina, who outwardly constantly encouraged me while deep inside surely regretted lost family time and companionship, I appreciate her constant support and return her loving devotion.

SHERWIN J. ISENBERG, M.D.

CONTENTS

PART I

General Considerations of the Newborn Eye

1 The Eye of the Newborn: A Neonatologist's Perspective

Vrinda Telang, M.D.†
Harry S. Dweck, M.D.

With advances in perinatal medicine, almost every organ can now be evaluated prior to birth. For example, the lungs and kidneys can be evaluated by analysis of amniotic fluid, the heart can be evaluated by fetal electrocardiography as well as fetal echocardiography, and even the brain can be evaluated by fetal electroencephalography. The eye, however, is one of the major organs whose prenatal assessment remains elusive. Hence the need for careful examination after birth.

The human eye has evolved from a simple organ converting light to energy into a complex visual organ with connections to the brain to process light into useful information. The eye is more sophisticated than the most advanced camera, with the capacity to accurately and rapidly focus objects at various distances in a multitude of colors. It is aptly said that the eye is attached to the head and the head to the body.

As the mirror of the brain, its examination can provide a variety of information about the condition not only of the brain but of the underlying health of the patient.

DEVELOPMENT OF THE EYE

In the embryo, formation of the eye begins at approximately the 22nd day of fetal life (stage 10).[1] During the next 6 to 8 weeks of intrauterine life, the development of the eye is largely completed in the dark environment of the uterus.

The eye develops from both the surface ectoderm and a neuroectodermal evagination of the forebrain, with a contribution from the mesoderm between these two layers. The retina, which is also derived from the neuroectoderm, receives its blood supply from the optic artery (a branch of the ophthalmic artery) and its nerve supply from the optic nerve. The surface ectoderm is the anlage of the lens, whose fibers develop from its nucleus in concentric layers starting at the equator, with continuing deposition of layers throughout life.

The hyaloid system of the tunica vasculosa lentis is a transitory vascular system that invests the lens anteriorly and posteriorly and nourishes many structures of the eye. This system atrophies by 35 weeks of gestation. At

†Deceased.

maturity, the lens has neither a blood nor a nerve supply. The ophthalmoscopic examination of the capsule of the lens epithelium is hence of great value in the accurate assessment of gestational age in prematurely born babies of less than 35 weeks' gestation.

The eyelids are fused until approximately 25 weeks but may remain closed until 32 weeks.[1] Eyelid fusion may not, therefore, be a valid sign of viability in a newborn as previously presumed.

In the newborn, the eye is approximately two thirds of its ultimate size. It grows rapidly during the first year after birth and reaches adult size by adolescence.[1] Myelination begins at birth, perhaps stimulated by exposure to light, and is complete by $2^1/_2$ months of age in a full-term baby.[1]

Some aspects of the progression of maturation (Table 1–1)[2] of vision and the eye are important in the care of newborns. Preterm infants are unable to adequately restrict the amount of light their retina may be exposed to because the pupillary light reflex is not present until 30 weeks of gestation.[2] In the full-term infant, however, the pupils are normally constricted for the first several weeks.

True or protective blinking (in response to an object coming toward the eyes) is not present until 2 to 5 months after full-term birth.[2]

Parents are frequently concerned about strabismus in newborns, but their fears can be allayed since eye movements are not always coordinated in the normal newborn until 3 to 6 months of age.[2] Fixed strabismus, however, should be referred to an ophthalmologist. In some babies, the epicanthal folds of the upper lids obscure the medial corner of the eye, thereby giving the appearance of strabismus (pseudostrabismus). This normal state is easy to confirm if the reflection of a light directed at the eyes appears in the center of each pupil. One can also note the lateral movements of the eyes by rotating the light while holding the baby in the upright position. Doll's eye movements (the eyes lag behind the turning of the head from side to side with the baby in the supine position) are normally present at 2 to 3 months of age when the baby can fixate well.

Parents should be aware that tears are normally not present with crying until 1 to 3 months of age in a full-term infant.

TABLE 1–1.
Maturation of Vision and the Eye*

Description	Age
Pupillary light reaction present	30 wk gestation
Pupillary light reaction well developed	1 mo
Lid closure in response to bright light	30 wk gestation
Blink response to visual threat	2–5 mo
Visual fixation present	Birth
Fixation well developed	2 mo
Conjugate horizontal gaze well developed	Birth
Conjugate vertical gaze well developed	2 mo
Vestibular eye rotations well developed	34 wk gestation
Optokinetic nystagmus well developed	Birth
Visual following well developed	3 mo
Accommodation well developed	4 mo
Visual evoked potential acuity at adult level	6 mo
Grating acuity preferential looking at adult level	2 yr
Snellen letter acuity at adult level	2 yr
End of critical period for monocular visual deprivation	10 yr
Ocular alignment stable	1 mo
Fusional convergence well developed	6 mo
Stereopsis well developed	6 mo
Stereoacuity (Titmus) at adult level	7 yr
Eyeball 70% of adult diameter	Birth
Eyeball 95% of adult diameter	3 yr
Cornea 80% of adult diameter	Birth
Cornea 95% of adult diameter	1 yr
Differentiation of fovea completed	4 mo
Myelination of optic nerve completed	7 mo–2 yr
Iris stromal pigmentation well developed	6 mo

*Modified from Greenwald MJ: Visual development in infancy and childhood. *Pediatr Clin North Am* 1983; 30:977.

VISION IN THE NEWBORN

The visual acuity of a full-term at birth is approximately 20/400.[2] This is attributed to the short diameter of the newborn eye and retinal immaturity, although incomplete myelination of the optic nerve may also be a factor. Visual evoked potentials have been utilized to study the capacity of the newborn to see objects.

To provide for visual stimulation for prematurely born babies cared for in neonatal intensive care units, many programs place mobiles and patterns of faces and geometric designs around the bedsides of infants within their range of visual acuity (Fig 1–1).

Studies using monocular visual deprivation (e.g., eye patching or unilateral eye disease) have revealed that the eye continues to develop synapses in the visual cortex during the first 10 years after birth. The effect of monocular deprivation in children is profound amblyopia in the deprived eye despite normal structural integrity.[2] Hence, unilateral ophthalmic lesions should be treated as early as possible. Bilateral visual deprivation may also produce significant impairment of vision; however, the prognosis for intact vision is better.[2] Adult visual acuity of 20/20 is normally achieved by 2 years of age.[2]

THE EYE AND LIGHT

After birth, the retina is fully exposed to light for the first time. In preterm newborns less than 34 weeks' gestational age, the retina is immature and may be adversely affected by excess light. Animal studies have clearly documented retinal injury with exposure to intense light.[3,4] It is for these reasons that the eyes of newborns receiving phototherapy, whose intensity of light may be 400 ft-c or more, are protected with eyeshields to prevent possible damage to the neonatal retina (Fig 1–2). With the prevalent use of phototherapy, it is important to frequently remove the eyeshields (with the phototherapy lights turned off) for brief periods of time to prevent visual deprivation and to check for corneal abrasions and xerophthalmia.

A recent provocative study[5] has raised questions regarding continuous exposure to ambient light greater than 60 ft-c, a level frequently seen and even exceeded in many neonatal intensive care units. Although this study was not well controlled, the authors suggest that prematurely born babies continually exposed to ambient light of this intensity may have a higher predisposition to retinopathy of prematurity. For the present, however, no definitive recommendations can be made on the basis of this unconfirmed study.

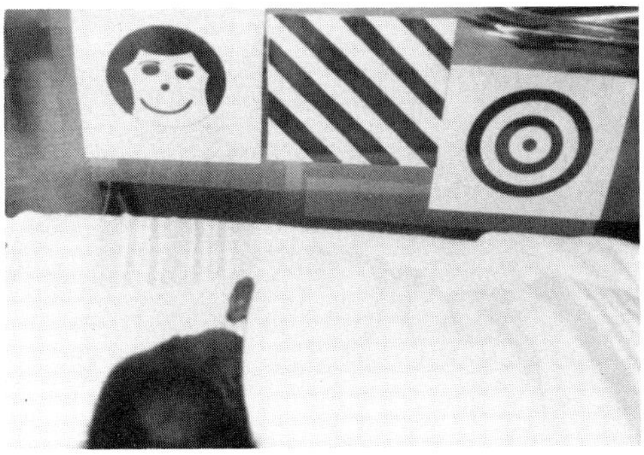

FIG 1–1.
Examples of the types of geometric designs used to provide visual stimulation for growing premature infants.

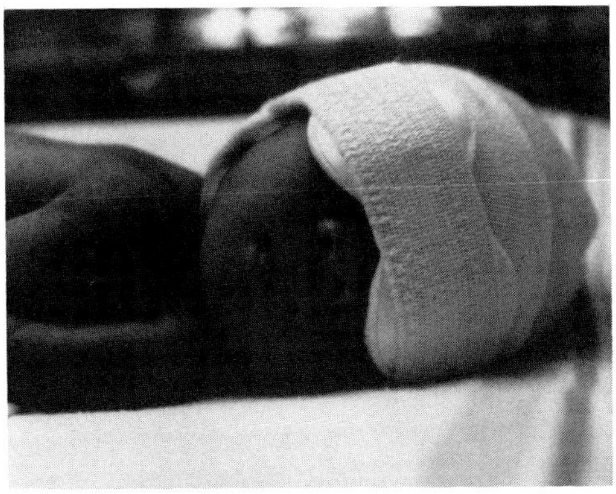

FIG 1–2.
Eyeshield on an infant receiving phototherapy. Note how the nares are not obstructed by the position of the shield.

THE EYE IN RELATION TO GENERAL HEALTH

The eye can be an important source of information regarding the general health status of the newborn. Its examination can be particularly valuable in diagnosing many infectious and metabolic diseases as well as in syndrome identification.

The scleras should be examined for evidence of jaundice. While the scleras of the newborn normally have a bluish tint, a marked blue color is seen in osteogenesis imperfecta and Ehlers-Danlos syndrome.

Absence of the iris of the eye may be familial (as an autosomal dominant); however, in 10% of such infants, it may be associated with an increased incidence of Wilms' tumor.

Ophthalmoscopic examination for a red reflex should be done as part of the initial examination in all newborns. A white reflex is evidence of a retinoblastoma, whereas cataracts may appear as black spots.

The detection of other eye abnormalities including corneal opacities and pupillary abnormalities also requires early ophthalmologic consultation.

Retinopathy of prematurity, a disease common in infants of very low birth weight (<1,500 gm) and newborns receiving supplementary oxygen, is detected only by a thorough funduscopic examination through a well-dilated pupil. It should be performed by an ophthalmologist experienced in examining newborns at risk for this disease. At approximately 6 weeks after birth and again at 3, 6, and 12 months, ophthalmoscopic examination should be done in newborns, especially those born prematurely, who received supplementary oxygen. Those with positive findings may require longer and more frequent examinations.

Attention to the detail of using artificial tears in caring for the sickest babies in the neonatal intensive care unit whose eyes remain open can prevent exposure keratopathy.

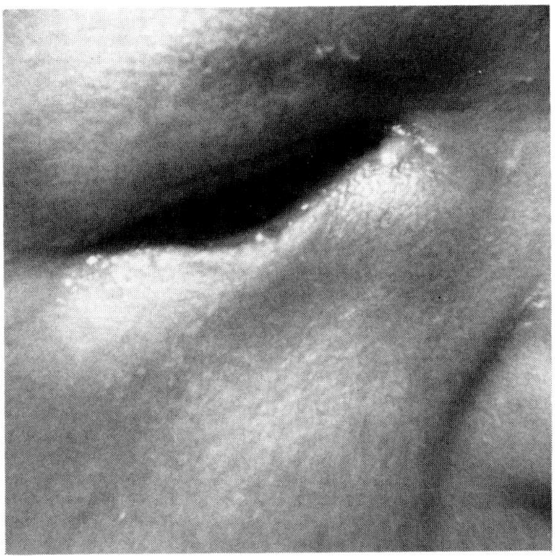

FIG 1–3.
Conjunctivitis and associated dacryocystitis and exudate in a newborn infant.

INFECTIOUS DISEASES

Physicians caring for newborns frequently consult with ophthalmologists for corroborative evidence of intrauterine infections in babies who are small for gestational age and in the presence of congenital malformations that have associated abnormalities of the eye.

Bacterial

Conjunctivitis (Fig 1–3) in the newborn from any etiology warrants a routine culture from a swab of the palpebral conjunctiva since a local infection of the eye in the newborn could lead to a serious systemic infection. If the baby appears ill, systemic cultures (blood, cerebrospinal fluid, and urine) should be obtained and systemic antibiotics administered. If indicated, a Gram stain (for gram-negative diplococci), a Giemsa stain (for *Chlamydia trachomatis*), and appropriate additional cultures should be obtained.

Eye infections with *Neisseria gonorrhoeae* can be frequently accompanied by neonatal sepsis and disseminated disease. The diagnosis can be made easily by anaerobic culture of the eye discharge. The culture swab should be applied immediately at the bedside to the appropriate media including a chocolate agar medium, which should be at room temperature. Treatment, after obtaining systemic cultures, requires systemic penicillin.

Eye prophylaxis has markedly reduced the incidence of this local and systemic disease in newborns. However, chemical conjunctivitis may occur within the first 24 hours after instillation of silver nitrate to prevent gonococcal ophthalmia neonatorum.

Viral

The eye is frequently involved in transplacentally acquired viral infections, particularly cytomegalovirus and rubella. The ophthalmic manifestations in chronic intrauterine viral infections are similar, with diagnostic findings including cataracts, retinal dysplasia, necrotizing chorioretinitis, and viral inclusion bodies. Some viruses may be cultured from the lens of an infected neonatal eye for months or even years after birth.[6]

Evidence of viral infection may be confirmed by isolation of the virus from cultures of nasopharyngeal swabs, blood, buffy coat, or urine. Chronic intrauterine viral infections may be indicated by an elevated serum IgM level from a sample of cord blood from a baby.[7]

While most neonatal viral infections are untreatable, herpes simplex infections can be treated with adenosine arabinoside. The best prognosis for survival is in infants with superficial involvement of the skin, eye, or mouth who are treated early, although significant psychomotor and ocular sequelae can occur.[6,7] The long-term prognosis for patients with central nervous system or eye pathology is extremely guarded.[8]

Fungal

Candida albicans sepsis is an uncommon disease of newborns, though it is seen more frequently in sick preterm babies after prolonged antibiotic therapy for bacterial infections. In babies with disseminated candidiasis, *Candida* endophthalmitis may be detected by finding haziness of the vitreous around fluffy white lesions.[7] If detected early, *Candida* infections can be successfully treated with amphotericin B.

Protozoal

Toxoplasmosis is one of the most common causes of chorioretinitis.[7] The disease is usually acquired in the second trimester of pregnancy and is associated with intrauterine growth retardation and hydrocephalus. Manifestations in the eye include papillitis in addition to chorioretinitis. Diagnosis is confirmed by the Sabin-Feldman dye test or an enzyme-linked immunosorbent assay (ELISA).[7] Treatment is possible with pyrimethamine, but the prognosis for recovery of vision is poor.

THE EYE IN INBORN ERRORS OF METABOLISM

Disorders of metabolism, though rarely detected in the newborn period, can affect the eye. Certain inborn errors of metabolism have frequently associated ocular abnormalities.

Albinism, a disorder of amino acid metabolism, is easily diagnosed upon eye examination by the absence of pigmentation in the iris and retina.

Galactosemia, a disorder of carbohydrate metabolism, should be suspected in all babies with congenital cataract since early intervention with a lactose-free diet can reverse the lenticular accumulation of dulcitol, the offending compound. Maternal diabetes has been implicated as a possible causal factor in optic nerve hypoplasia with sector-type field defects.[9]

The cherry-red spot in the macula of a newborn or young infant is a finding of some of the variants of sphingolipidoses (Niemann-Pick infantile disease and Tay-Sachs disease) and mucolipidoses (GM_1 generalized gangliosidosis and neuraminidase deficiency).

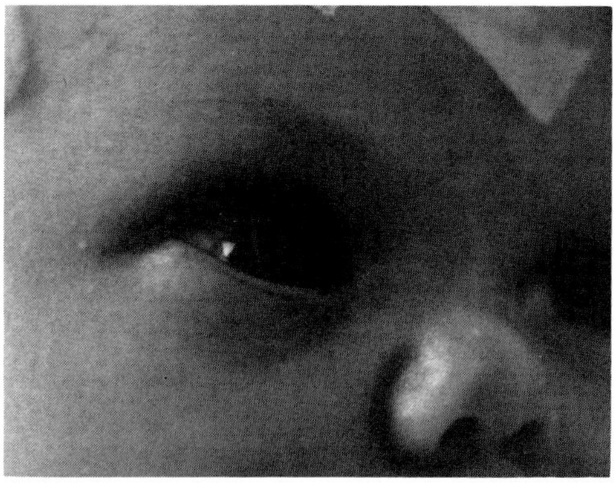

FIG 1–4.
Subconjuctival hemorrhage in the eye of a baby born by spontaneous vaginal delivery.

EFFECT OF LABOR AND DELIVERY

The normal process of vaginal delivery after uncomplicated labor can have profound effects on the eye. The elevated intrauterine pressure can interfere with venous return from the eye and lead to raised intraocular pressures and hemorrhage. Subconjunctival hemorrhages (usually flame or crescent shaped) and hemorrhages peripheral to the iris are commonly seen and resolve within 10 days (Fig 1–4). Retinal hemorrhages may normally be seen in up to 25% of newborns and will usually disappear in 6 to 8 weeks after birth.

In more severe cases, however, the trauma can be more profound in babies with abnormally presenting parts such as face and brow presentations, leading to retrobulbar hemorrhage and buphthalmos. These may require the immediate attention of an ophthalmologist.

The care of the sick newborn frequently requires the skills and talents of experts from multiple disciplines. It is critically important in newborns with diseases of the eye that consultation by the neonatologist with the ophthalmologist be coordinated and each lend their expertise toward improving the quality of life of high-risk infants.

Acknowledgment

The photographs appear through the courtesy of David A. Clark, M.D., which the authors gratefully acknowledge.

REFERENCES

1. Moore KL: *The Developing Human*, ed 3. Philadelphia, WB Saunders Co, 1982.
2. Greenwald MJ: Visual development in infancy and childhood. *Pediatr Clin North Am* 1983; 30:977–993.
3. Noell WK, Walker VS, Kang BS, et al: Retinal damage by light in rats. *Invest Ophthalmol* 1966; 5:450.
4. Messner KH, Maisels MJ, Leure-DuPree AE: Phototoxicity to the new born primate retina. *Invest Ophthalmol Vis Sci* 1978; 17:178.
5. Glass P, Avery GB, Subramanina KN, et al: Effect of bright light in the hospital nursery on the incidence of retinopathy of prematurity. *N Engl J Med* 1985; 313:401.
6. Behrman RE, Vaughan VC III: *Nelson Textbook of Pediatrics*, ed 12. Philadelphia, WB Saunders Co, 1983.
7. Remington JS, Klein JO: *Infectious Diseases of the Fetus and Newborn Infant*, ed 2. Philadelphia, WB Saunders Co, 1983.
8. Avery GB: *Neonatology. Pathophysiology and Management of the Newborn*, ed 3. JB Lippincott Co, 1975.
9. Harley RD: *Pediatric Ophthalmology*, ed 2. Philadelphia, WB Saunders Co, 1983.

2 Normal Development of the Eye and Orbit Before Birth: The Development of the Eye

Elise Torczynski, M.D.

In this chapter, the basic steps in the embryonic and fetal development of the eye are described. Due to size limitations, only the major phases of ocular organogenesis can be described. Many exciting insights obtained through ultrastructural and other technically sophisticated studies must be omitted because of the constraints of space. Indeed, even such a basic subject as vascular development of the eye and orbit receives only the most rudimentary treatment in this chapter because it is such a complex process. Many references are included for those wishing more information.[1–6]

INTRODUCTION

The period of embryogenesis extends from the fertilization of the ova until the rudimentary formation of the central nervous system at about the third week. Little is known of the early stages of ocular development during embryogenesis. Early in development the neural plate is a mass of undifferentiated pluripotent cells. Some evidence suggests that the paraxial mesoderm underlying the neural phase induces a midline font of cells to become eye-forming tissues. From the midline location, the cells move laterally and anteriorly to establish two eye-forming centers[1] (Fig 2–1). During the third week the anterior neural plate is open, and the neural folds are just beginning to emerge and rise above the plane of the plate. The optic primordium, or anlage, first becomes identifiable in the human embryo at about the 22nd day or 7th somite stage of development (Fig 2–2).

At this stage in the embryo, several tissues emerge that have importance for the development of the eyes. The first of these is the ectoderm, which segregates into three regions: laterally as surface ectoderm, at the summit of the neural folds as neural crest cells, and medially in the neural plate as neuroectoderm (Fig 2–3). Beneath the neural plate is the paraxial mesoderm, which not only induces the overlying neuroectoderm to be-

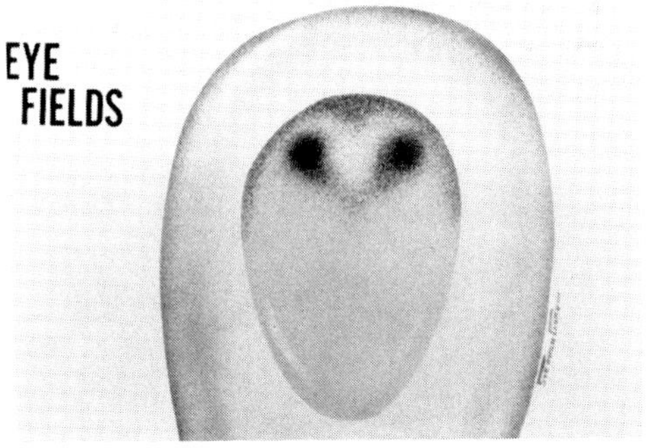

FIG 2–1.
Artist's conception of the eye fields developing from a midline font of cells induced in the open neural plate. Neural folds have not formed. Eye-forming cells move anteriorly and laterally.

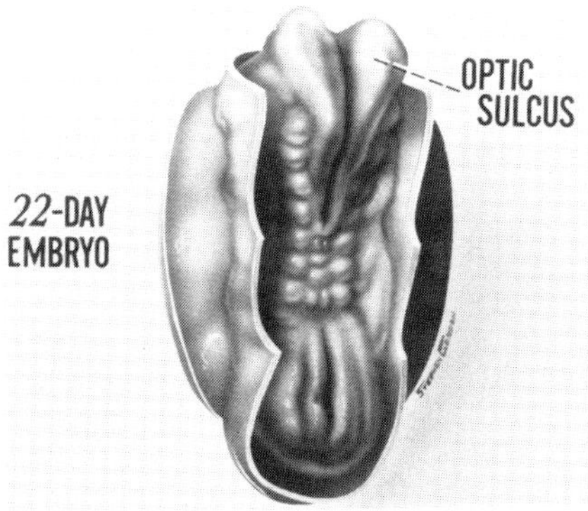

FIG 2–2.
Optic sulcus, or pit, first develops in the lateral aspect of the developing neural folds in the 22-day-old embryo. Somites have formed posteriorly, and the neural tube begins closure in the midregion of the body.

come the ocular primordia but also has a growth-supporting role in early ocular development. Later the vascular endothelium and extraocular muscles emerge from the paraxial mesoderm.

The anterior end of the neural plate expands to form the neural folds, which arise superiorly and outwardly. As folds in the head region are forming, the neural folds in the midbody region are already beginning to close. Several dilatations and constrictions appear in the anterior neural tube as the folds close. These segregate the developing brain into the hindbrain, midbrain, and forebrain. From the forebrain, or prosencephalon, two regions, namely, the telencephalon and diencephalon, develop. It is from the diencephalic region that the ocular analagen and later chiasm develop. In the widest portion of the neural folds, the earliest indication of the ocular sulcus, or pit, is an indentation parallel to the crest of the neural fold (see Fig 2–2). With closure of the neural tube, the sulci continue to indent and form the optic vesicles. The optic vesicles balloon outward as lateral outpouchings at the anterior end of the neural tube and may be seen externally (Fig 2–4). The primary optic vesicles continue to expand and are laterally attached to the brain by the optic stalks by the 24th day. The ectoderm that composes the optic vesicles is continuous through the optic stalks with the ectoderm of the neural tube, which forms the wall of the forebrain.

During the fourth week (5-mm stage) the optic vesicle stimulates the formation of the lenticular placode from the surface ectoderm. The surface cells thicken, elongate, and begin to indent (Fig 2–5). With indentation, invag-

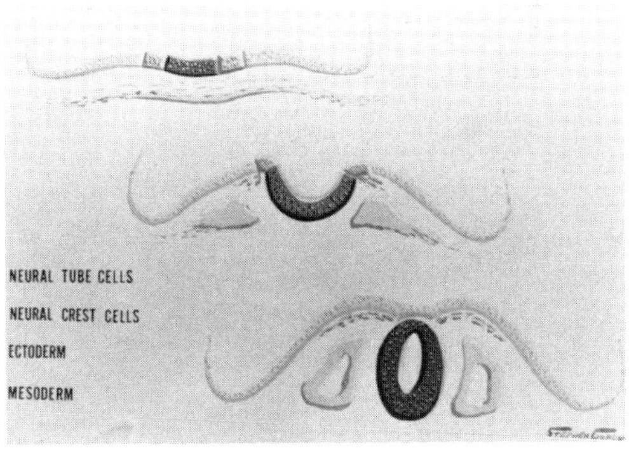

FIG 2–3.
Open neural plate with dark neuroectodermal cells centrally *(top)*. The block of lighter cells adjacent to the neuroectodermal cells represents the neural crest cells. *(middle)*. Notice the early migration of the neural crest cells underneath the surface ectoderm. The surface ectoderm is represented by the lightest cells located most laterally in the *top* and *middle* figures. Beneath the ectoderm is a triangular block of cells that becomes the paraxial mesoderm, which is important for induction of the eye and for its nourishment and growth support. Neural crest cells have migrated completely below the surface ectoderm *(bottom)*. The neural tube has closed.

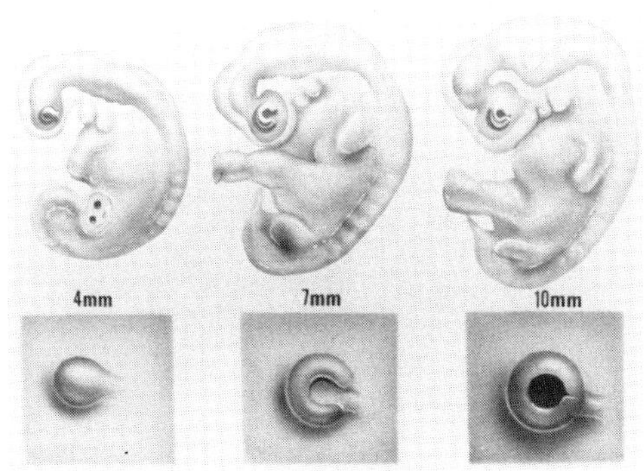

FIG 2–4.
The upper series shows the developing eye in relation to the entire body. Note the poor formation of the head region until the 10-mm stage when extensive folding and constrictions of the neural tube have taken place. The lower sequence shows the development of the optic vesicle, invagination with formation of the optic cup and fetal fissure in the center, and in the lower right the formation of the optic cup with closure of the fetal fissure. Limb buds form in the 10-mm stage of the embryo. (From Torczynski E: Ocular development and congenital anomalies, in Lewis RA (ed): *The Basic and Clinical Science Course,* section 1, *Fundamentals and Principles of Ophthalmology.* San Francisco, American Academy of Ophthalmology, 1988–89. Used with permission.)

ination of both the optic vesicle and the lenticular placode occurs (Fig 2–6). The invagination of the primary optic vesicle forms the optic cup, which initially consists of two layers of cells, the inner one being folded or compressed against the outer layer. The cup is not a complete sphere, but inferiorly and ventrally forms the embryonic or fetal fissure. Through the fissure, mesenchymal and vascular tissues enter the globe, principally the hyaloid artery system posteriorly (Fig 2–7). The embryonic fissure is continuous from the optic stalk to the anterior margin of the optic cup. The fissure extends down the stalk almost to its junction with the central nervous system. The optic cup is composed of an outer layer of cells that remains throughout life as a monolayer of cuboidal cells, the retinal pigment epithelium, and an inner layer of invaginated cells, the neurosensory retina. The original cavity of the optic vesicle remains as a potential space, the subretinal, throughout life. The formation and closure of the embryonic fissure is transitory, formed by invagination during the fifth week (the 4.5-mm stage). It is completely formed and sealed by the 20-mm stage, the end of the seventh week. Closure is complete when the

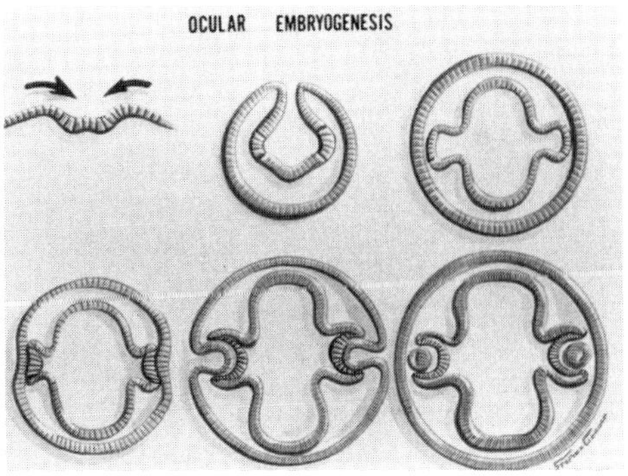

FIG 2–5.
Schema of ocular embryogenesis. Eye fields are slightly thickened areas on the neural plate *(upper right).* The first hint of the neural folds is seen. Neural folds are closing to form the neural tube *(upper middle).* Optic pits begin to evaginate toward the surface ectoderm *(upper right).* The neural tube is closed. The optic pits have evaginated to form optic vesicles that now approach the surface ectoderm. Optic vesicles induce thickening in the surface ectoderm as the lenticular plate *(lower left).* Both the lenticular plate and optic vesicle are just beginning the process of invagination. Invagination of the lens vesicle and optic vesicle is well advanced *(lower middle).* Notice that the lenticular vesicle is pinching off from the surface ectoderm. The lenticular vesicle has totally pinched off from the surface ectoderm, now a smooth surface *(lower right).* The optic vesicle is now the layered optic cup. Embryonic fissure cannot be seen here.

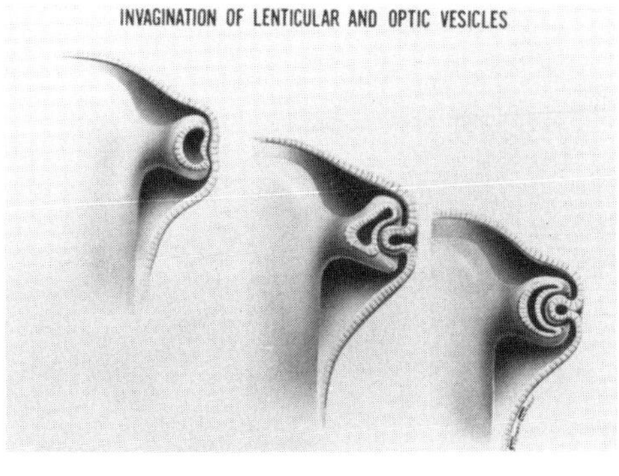

FIG 2–6.
On the left is the beginning of invagination of optic and lenticular vesicles. In center and right is shown the formation of the optic cup and lens. The optic stalk constricts as it emerges from the neural tube.

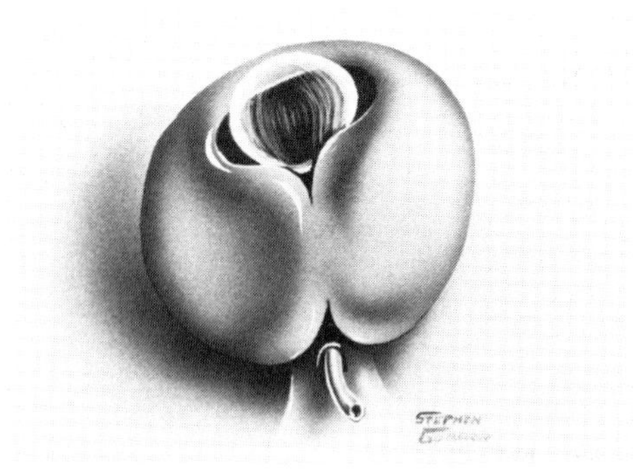

FIG 2–7.
Closure of the embryonic fissure in the inferior nasal portion of the globe traps the hyaloid artery *(below)* in the region of the developing optic disc. Failure of closure of the embryonic fissure can result in a coloboma from the pupillary rim of the iris to the optic nerve.

inner and outer retinal layers meet end to end and fuse. The closure of the fissure begins in the midportion, or the equatorial region of the globe, and proceeds both anteriorly and posteriorly until the entire fissure is closed. The cells at the margin of the fissure are plastic and multipotent at the time of closure and hence are able to form a perfect seal without evidence of the previous cleft as further growth and differentiation of the globe take place.

If there is an ectropion of the cells destined to form the neurosensory retina such that the inner cells push aside the outer cells (those destined to form pigment epithelium), then an imperfect closure results (Fig 2–8). The tissues are thin and disorganized and form a coloboma down the line of the embryonic fissure in the inferior nasal aspect of the globe. A coloboma may be complete but is usually incomplete and has skipped areas where normal tissues alternate with the dysgenetic segments of closure. In certain instances, a cystic coloboma forms when the primary cavity of the optic vesicle is not obliterated with closure of the embryonic fissure.

At this stage the developing eyes are located approximately 180 degrees from each other and are surrounded by undifferentiated mesenchymal cells (Fig 2–9). As the midfacial, cranial, and lateral facial tissues develop, the position of the eyes gradually changes such that the eyes rotate medially and converge toward the midline. The adult configuration of the globes is that of an angle of 68 degrees between the optic axes and is found in the infant shortly after birth. With the development of the optic cup and closure of the embryonic fissure, the basic outlines of the eye are established. From this point we will look at the development of the different ocular structures in greater detail after a brief introduction to the neural crest cells.

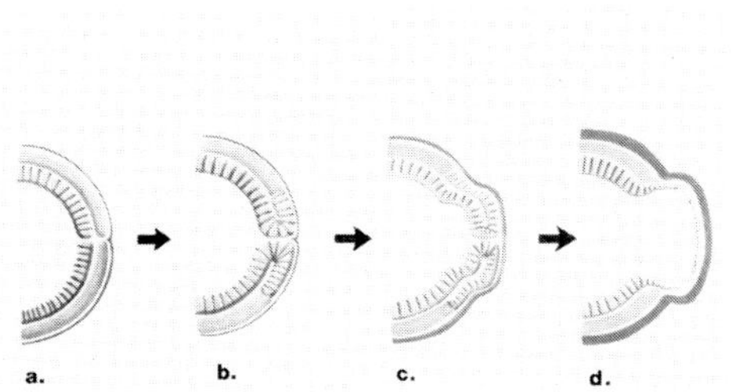

FIG 2–8.
Closure of the embryonic fissure. The end-to-end closure of the neurosensory retina and the retinal pigment epithelium produces normal retina and pigment epithelium (**a**). The neurosensory retina has pushed into the outer layer normally occupied by the retinal pigment epithelium (**b**). This ectropion of predestined neurosensory retinal cells displaces the retinal pigment epithelium laterally (**c**). A coloboma results, and the underlying choroid and sclera develop as thin, dysgenetic layers (**d**).

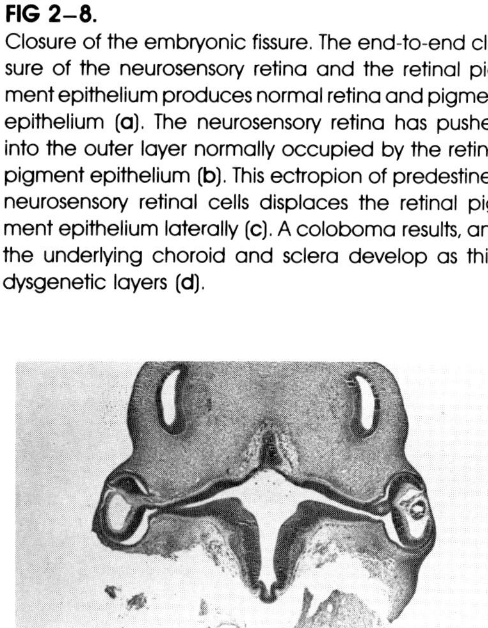

FIG 2–9.
Cross section of the head reigon in a human embryo in the second month of gestation. Undifferentiated cells around the eyes and the neural tube are almost entirely neural crest cells. These cells will develop into the upper facial and ocular mesenchyme (see Table 2–1).

THE NEURAL CREST CELLS

In the past 20 years, one of the most important contributions to our understanding of the development of the eye and the adnexal tissues has been the delineation of the origin of the mesenchymal tissues. Formerly most of the mesenchymal tissues were thought to arise from mesoderm. In 1966, Johnston, using tritiated chick embryos, showed that much of the mesenchyme of the face derived from cranial neural crest cells (CNCC) (see Fig 2–9).[7] When using tritiated thymidine grafts, the cell marker quickly became diluted and could only be followed through a few replications. Later, Le Douarin[8,9] and Le Lievre and Le Dovarin[10] transplanted tissues from Japanese quail embryos, which have a replicating condensation of nuclear heterochromatin, into chick embryos that have no such marker. The replicating nuclear marker enabled the quail tissues to be followed to maturity. The insights that were gained through the study of chick embryos have been expanded to encompass mammalian species, including mice.[11] The migratory patterns of the neural crest cells have been well described by Johnston and Noden.[7,12]

The CNCCs arise in the neural folds in the region of the presumptive fifth nerve nucleus. The crest cells do not extend to the anterior ends of the neural folds (Fig 2–10). The crest cells arise from ectoderm located beween surface ectoderm and neuroectoderm (see Fig 2–3). The CNCCs migrate in two waves.[13] The first wave starts from the middle portion of the head region near the middle of the mesencephalon prior to cranial flexure. A space or cavity filled with hydrated hyaluronic acid and some collagen forms in front of the migrating cells under the surface ectoderm. The neural crest cells move through this acellular matrix ventrally by following the body contour.[14,15] The crest cells, with flexure of the neural tube, growth of the eye, and enlargement of the branchial arches, are carried into the region around the eye. The cells migrate ventrally into the maxillary process and in smaller numbers into the mandibular process.

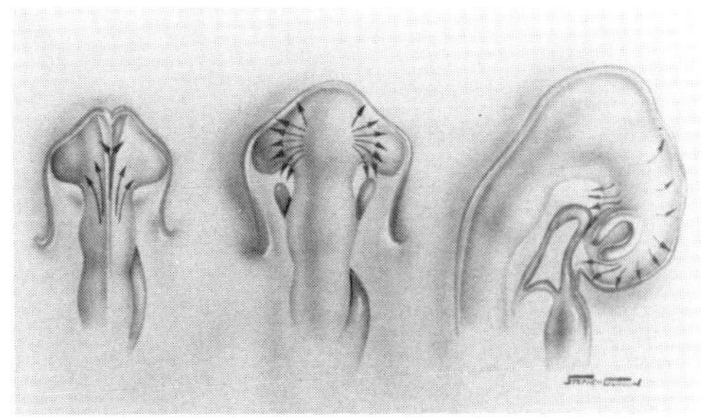

FIG 2–10.
Partially closed neural tube *(left)*. Arrows depict the neural crest cells migrating from the region of the presumptive fifth nerve nucleus rostrally along the midline and beginning to curve around the optic vesicles laterally. The neural tube has totally closed *(middle)*. The neural crest cells have reached the developing optic vesicles. Some cells move rostrally and medially, whereas others surround the eye caudally and more ventrally. The neural tube has flexed, which carries the head region and eye forward *(right)*. Dilations and constrictions in the neural tube begin to occur. The ocular embryonic fissure is open. The arrows depict the movement of the neural crest cells around the eye and medial nasal portion of the face. (From Torczynski E: Ocular development and congenital anomalies, in Lewis RA (ed): *The Basic and Clinical Science Course,* section 1, *Fundamentals and Principles of Ophthalmology.* San Francisco, American Academy of Ophthalmology, 1988–89. Used with permission.)

The remaining cells from the mesencephalic area and cells from the diencephalic neural folds grow dorsally around the optic stalks and then ventrally around each stalk to the embryonic fissure, which at this stage is opposed to the surface ectoderm. With the invagination of the optic vesicle, the crest cells approach the future limbic region of the globe.

The second wave of cells moves anteriorly along the prosencephalon and optic stalk to spread over the front of the head region. The prosencephalic crest cells secondarily move toward the dorsal midline where they will form the skeletal and connective tissues of the face. Some crest cells remain along the neural folds to form the sensory neurons of the trigeminal nucleus. During migration, the crest cells are connected to one another. The collagen fibers in the matrix provide a framework for their movement. Once the crest cells have arrived at their destination, they lose contact with the place of origin except for those that will form sensory neurons of the ganglia. The two waves of crest cells, the frontonasal process and the maxillary process, meet below the eye (Fig 2–11). Failure of appropriate migration or fusion of crest cells results in a cleft lip and palate.[16–18] Failure of midline coalescence of the frontonasal processes results in median cleft face deformity.

The crest cells are precursors of many varied and diverse tissues in the body as well as the head and face. Cells as seemingly unrelated as choroidal melanocytes, orbital fat, and odontoblasts of the teeth, to mention only a few, all arise from neural crest cells.[19–23] Ocular and orbital tissues from neural crest cells are listed in Table 2–1. The neural crest cells supply most of the connective tissue of the eye, orbit, and upper and lower midfacial regions (Fig 2–12). The mesoderm supplies the connective tissues for the remainder of the head.

THE RETINA

The primordium of the retina is identifiable in the neural plate before closure of the

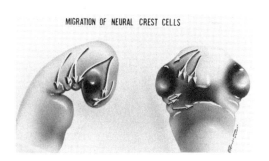

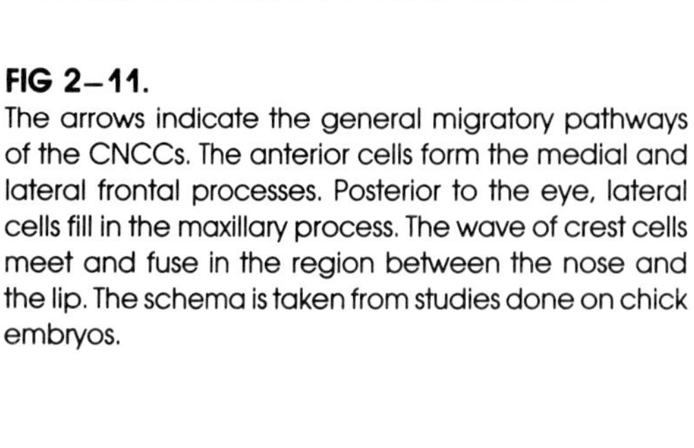

FIG 2–11.
The arrows indicate the general migratory pathways of the CNCCs. The anterior cells form the medial and lateral frontal processes. Posterior to the eye, lateral cells fill in the maxillary process. The wave of crest cells meet and fuse in the region between the nose and the lip. The schema is taken from studies done on chick embryos.

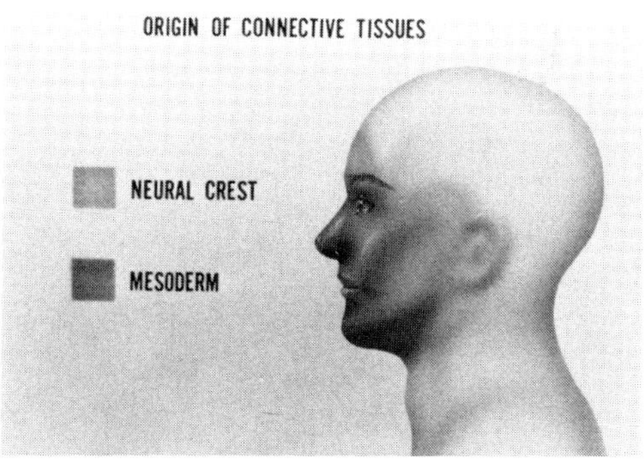

FIG 2–12.
By extrapolating from data obtained for chick and mammalian embryos, it is estimated that the connective tissues of the human head and face derive partially from the neural crest *(darkly shaded areas)* of the facial region while lightly shaded areas of the cranium and posterior cell come from the mesoderm.

tube as a thicker area of columnar cells with mitotic activity. As the optic vesicle balloons outward, the inner side is a ciliated basement membrane. Constriction in the optic stalk serves to separate the optic vesicles from the diencephalic region of the forebrain and the future third ventricle (see Fig 2–9). With invagination, the neuroectoderm destined to become the neurosensory retina is carried inward, and the outer layer of the optic vesicle will become the retinal pigmented epithelium. Cilia project from the future neurosensory retina to the pigment epithelium. Most of the cilia disappear by the seventh week and are replaced over the next few months by the outer segments of the photoreceptors.

From the end of the fifth week, the developing retina is characterized by a rapid proliferation of cells. The single layer of columnar cells present in the optic vesicle with mitotic activity undergoes progressive thickening and develops into the adult thickness by the 20-mm stage (seventh week). With the closure of the embryonic fissure, the retina forms two zones basically, the outer primitive or nuclear zone of neuroepithelium from which cells will migrate into the inner or marginal zone, which at this stage is fibrillar and contains no nuclei (Fig 2–13). The primitive zone contains eight to ten layers of oval nuclei and occupies most of the thickness of the retina at this stage. The

TABLE 2 – 1.
Derivatives of Embryonic Tissues

Ectoderm		
Neuroectoderm	Cranial Neural Crest Cells	Surface Ectoderm
Neurosensory retina	Corneal stroma and endothelium	Epithelium, glands, and cilia of skin of lids and caruncle
Retinal pigment epithelium	Sclera (see mesoderm)	
	Trabecular meshwork	
Pigmented ciliary epithelium	Sheaths and tendons of extraocular muscles	Conjunctival epithelium
		Corneal epithelium
Nonpigmented ciliary epithelium	Connective tissues of iris	Lens
	Ciliary muscle	Lacrimal gland
Pigmented iris epithelium	Choroidal stroma	Lacrimal drainage system
Sphincter and dilator muscles of iris	Melanocytes (all uveal and epithelial)	Vitreous
Optic nerve, axons, and glia	Meningeal sheaths of the optic nerve	
Vitreous	Schwann's cells of ciliary nerves	
	Ciliary ganglion	
	Orbital bones (all midline) and inferior orbital, as well as parts of orbital roof and lateral rim	
	Cartilage	
	Connective and fatty tissues of orbit and lids	
	Muscular layer and connective tissue sheaths of all ocular and orbital vessels	
	Mesoderm	
	Endothelial lining of all orbital and ocular blood vessels including the hyaloid system and tunica vasculosa lentis	
	Portion of sclera temporally	
	Vitreous	
	Muscle fibers of extraocular muscles, levator, and orbicularis	

*From Torczynski E: Ocular development and congenital anomalies, in Lewis RA (ed): *The Basic and Clinical Science Course*, section 1, *Fundamentals and Principles of Ophthalmology*. San Francisco, American Academy of Ophthalmology, 1988–89. Used with permission.

inner marginal layer is shortly invaded by migrating nuclei that arise from the outermost layer of the primitive layer, called the ependymal layer. From the sixth week to the third month, the mitotic activity in the primitive zone is intense, and marked migration of the developing cells quickly results in the formation of an inner and outer neuroblastic layer. These two layers are separated by a narrow fibrillar zone called the transient nerve fiber layer of Chievitz (Fig 2–14). The process of mitosis and migration are most intense in the posterior pole adjacent to the optic papilla and gradually extends anteriorly to the rim of the cup. By the 13-mm stage, the nerve fiber layer of Chievitz is clearly seen in the posterior pole, and by the 65-mm stage, the process of forming the inner and outer neuroblastic layers has extended to the ora serrata (end of the third month).

In the development of the retina, the cells of Müller, which form structure and support for the more specialized neural elements, are identifiable at the 10-mm stage. These cells grow with their long axis at right angles to the surface of the retina and provide scaffolding for the development of the neural cells.

The first cells in the retina to assume identifiable characteristics are the ganglion cells. At about the 17-mm stage, the ganglion cells migrate from the inner neuroblastic layer into the residual marginal zone. The cells are at first small and gradually enlarge and develop more cytoplasm. As they migrate toward the surface of the retina, they send out processes that run toward the optic stalk as the beginning of the nerve fiber layer. The ganglion cell layer is the first layer of the retina to be completely established (130-mm stage, fifth month).[24] Between the fifth and sixth months, cells migrating into the inner neuroblastic layer begin to differentiate into the bipolar and horizontal cells so that, at the 180-mm stage, the inner plexiform and inner nuclear layers are fairly well differentiated. With the development of the three definitive nuclear layers of the retina, the transient nerve fiber layer of Chievitz is slowly obliterated, as are the two separate neuroblastic layers.

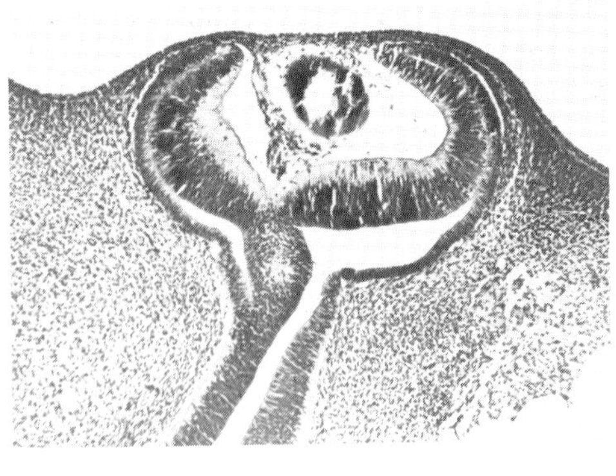

FIG 2–13.
Developing eye at 2 months. Shown are the thin epithelium and endothelium of the cornea anteriorly. The lenticular vesicle has pinched off from the cornea and is surrounded by blood vessels anteriorly and posteriorly from the hyaloid system. The retina shows the marginal and primitive layers, with a few cells having migrated inwardly to begin development of the inner neuroblastic layer. The continuity of the outer layer of the optic cup, the retinal pigment epithelium, with the cells of the optic stalk is evident. No differentiation in the surrounding mesenchyme has yet taken place.

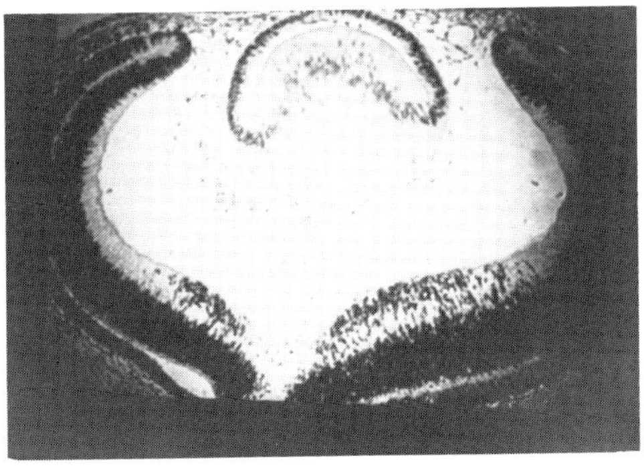

FIG 2–14.
Six-week stage. Primary lens fibers fill in the chamber of the lens vesicle. In the retina posteriorly, migration of nuclei is beginning; the nerve fiber layer of Chievitz is noted.

Although the final differentiation of the cell bodies of the rods and cones is a late occurrence in the development of the retina, there are nuclei and cell bodies in the outer neuroblastic layer that can be identified at a very early stage as the cell bodies of the rods and cones. The first major evidence of this layer occurs at the 48-mm stage when kidney-shaped nuclei are identified beneath the outer limiting membrane.[25]

The development of the macula is accelerated in the first 3 months but then lags behind the rest of the retina until after the eighth month. The macula is not fully developed until 16 weeks after birth. At the sixth month of gestation, the macula is thicker than the surrounding retina and is heaped up and elevated. The thinning of the macula becomes evident in the seventh and eighth months, with a gradual movement of the ganglion cells away from the fovea, until at birth they are reduced to a single layer. The cones in the macula are at first small and ill developed, but gradually the layer becomes thicker and pushes inward. By the fourth month after birth, the ganglion cell nuclei and bipolar cells are essentially absent from the macular area, whereas the number of cone nuclei has increased and the cones have increased in length so that the macular thickness is mainly from cone cells.

THE RETINAL PIGMENT EPITHELIUM

The retinal pigment epithelium is formed by the outer layer of the optic cup. Originally the cells of the outer cup have a pseudostratified appearance, but with growth and development of the globe, they form a monolayer. The pigment epithelium is the first tissue in the eye to form melanin granules and does so by the sixth week of gestation. Melanization begins in the posterior pole and proceeds anteriorly. Mitotic activity is present in the first few weeks of development and then slows after the eighth week when the cells assume a more mature cuboidal state. Bruch's membrane, the outer layer of the basement membrane, is developed between the 14- and 18-mm stage. Pigmentation is widespread by the end of the sixth week, but total pigmentation is not present until the end of the third month when the entire cell becomes filled with pigment granules.[26, 27] The pigment epithelium has an inductive effect on the surrounding tissues. Underlying choroid and sclera do not develop appropriately in the absence of the retinal pigment epithelium (Fig 2–15).

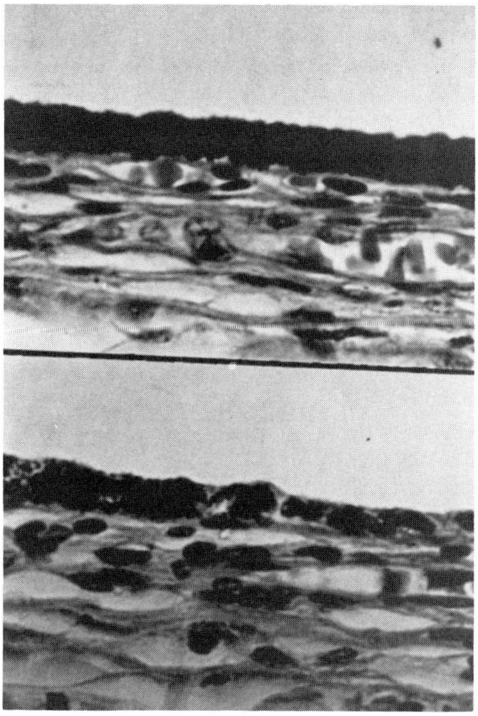

FIG 2–15.
Pigment epithelium is heavily melanized, and the underlying choroid shows well-developed choriocapillaris and choroidal vessels *(top)*. Where pigment epithelium is less well melanized, the development of the underlying choroid is dysgenetic *(bottom)*.

HYALOID VASCULAR SYSTEM

Although originally complicated and extensive, many intraocular vessels are transitory and disappear by birth. The hyaloid artery is a major branch of the primitive dorsal ophthalmic artery, which enters the globe posteriorly through the embryonic fissure and grows forward to the posterior pole of the lens by the end of the fifth week. It is incorporated in the globe by the closure of the embryonic fissure. The hyaloid system develops to form the primary vitreous (Fig 2–16). Anteriorly, twigs of the hyaloid meet the vascular system of the lens, the tunica vasculosa lentis; these twigs come from the annular vessels of the anterior rim of the optic cup and surround the lens vesicle (Fig 2–17). The two together complete the tunica vasculosa lentis. A second set of vessels is sent out from the hyaloid system to the annular vessel (Fig 2–

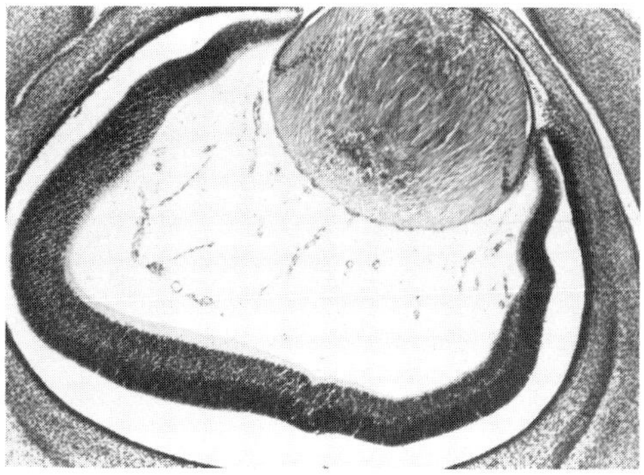

FIG 2–16.
Three-month stage. A nuclear bow of secondary lens fibers is seen at the equator of the developing lens. The cornea has become thickened with the inward migration of the neural crest cells in the stroma. The vitreous is filled with vessels from the hyaloid system as the primary vitreous. Little secondary vitreous has yet developed.

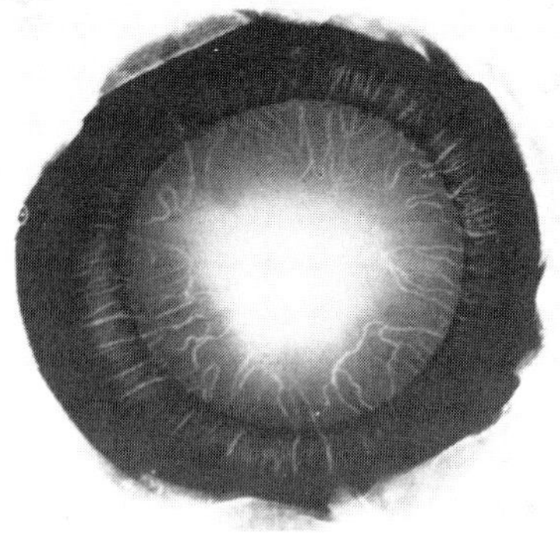

FIG 2–17.
Human eye at 6 months' gestation with the cornea removed. Capillary plexuses of the tunica vasculosa lentis and pupillary membrane are seen. The tunica vasculosa lentis is beginning to disappear centrally. (From Torczynski E: Ocular development and congenital anomalies, in Lewis RA (ed): *The Basic and Clinical Science Course,* section 1, *Fundamentals and Principles of Ophthalmology.* San Francisco, American Academy of Ophthalmologists, 1988–89. Used with permission.)

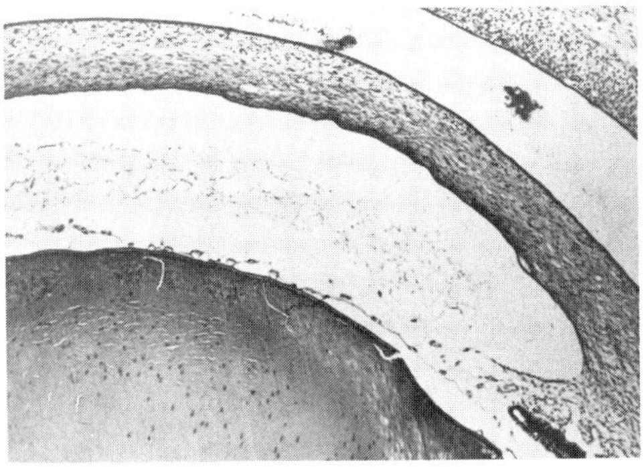

FIG 2–18.
Third month. The anterior segment with the cornea is well populated and thickened with keratocytes and collagen. In the chamber angle a few mesenchymal cells have migrated beyond the anterior tip of the optic cup. A small space in the anterior cup is the marginal sinus of von Szily. The thin vascularized membrane anterior to the lens is the tunica vasculosa lentis (hematoxylin-eosin [HE]).

18). The vascular loops run in the mesodermal layer between the cornea and the lens as the pupillary membrane. The hyaloid vessel attains its greatest development at the 60-mm stage (12th week) when it joins with the tunica vasculosa lentis and fills up the entire posterior portion of the globe. At the 60-mm stage, the anterior portions of the hyaloid vessels begin to atrophy. The hyaloid system is completely obliterated before birth (Fig 2–19).

Vascularization of the retina begins about the fourth month from solid clusters of cells of the hyaloid artery at the disc, the primordium of the superior and inferior branches of the central retinal artery. Buds or strands grow into the nerve fiber layer. Venous channels develop along with the arteries. The rate of growth of the vessels is 0.1 mm/day from the fourth to the seventh month. Temporal vascularization follows nasal vascularization. Irregular nets form first in the nerve fiber layer and gradually grow into the outer layers of the retina. Capillaries reach the ora serrata by the eighth month of gestation. It is not totally clear whether the macula develops by the retardation of capillaries in the central section, which results in an avascular zone, or whether the macula is originally vascularized and by obliteration of existing vessels becomes avascular.[28–30]

THE LENS

As the optic vesicle approaches the unbroken surface of cuboidal epithelium, a thickening of the overlying epithelium takes place. A thin space of fibrillar material separates the basement membrane of the optic vesicle from that of the surface ectoderm. The cells in the surface ectoderm elongate and thicken, thereby producing a plate called the lens placode. The events from placode for-

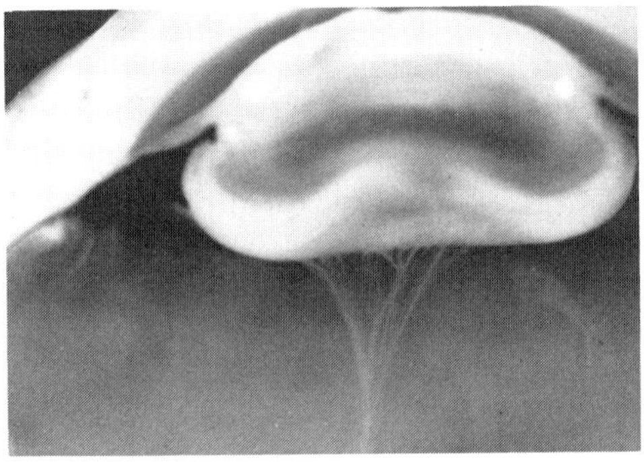

FIG 2–19.
Human eye near term with fine remnants of the hyaloid artery posterior to the lens. Vessels no longer carry blood.

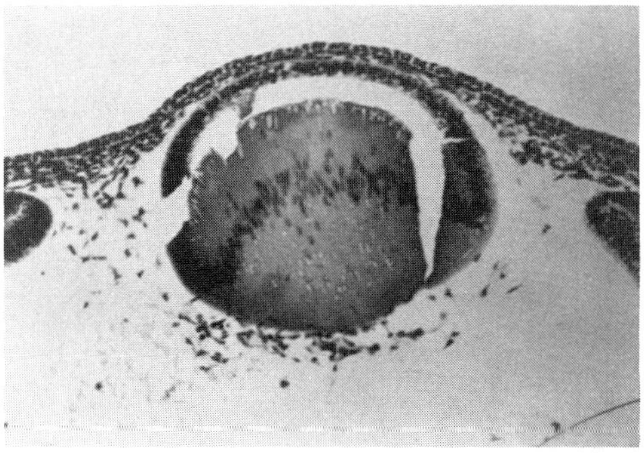

FIG 2–20.
The cornea is present as two cell layers of epithelium. Neural crest cells begin migration over the rim of the optic cup and posterior stroma. Primary lens fibers fill in the lenticular vesicle.

mation on the 26th day to invagination of the lenticular vesicle occur very quickly. With contraction of the apical cytoplasm and terminal bar system of the epithelial cells, invagination of the lens placode begins.[31] Sequentially, the lens pit, the lens cup, and the vesicle are formed. Simultaneously with invagination of the optic vesicle, invagination of the lenticular vesicle occurs. Separation of the lens vesicle from the surface ectoderm occurs at the end of the fifth week. The basal lamina is thickened by increasing layers of material laid on the surface of the lens capsule. A zone of necrosis develops around the pore of the lens vesicle, which isolates the vesicle from the surface ectoderm. The remaining cells then contract and close the pore so that the lens vesicle is separated from the surface ectoderm. The capsule fills in the pore area of the lens.

The cells in the posterior portion of the lens elongate and fill in the lumen of the vesicle (Fig 2–20). These are the primary lens fibers. As the cells elongate, ultrastructural changes occur including a decrease in the size of the cellular nuclei and the number of organelles. The fibrillar protein concentrations begin to increase in the lens fibers. Further enlargement of the lens occurs by the accretion of the secondary lens fibers. The anterior epithelium migrates to the equatorial region; lens nuclei and fibers move internally at the equator and result in the lens bow, a region of nuclei adjacent to the equator from which new lens fibers, the secondary lens fibers, are added to the lens. The epithelial nuclei do not extend posteriorly in the developing lens. The tips of the fibers become elongated and attach to each other along lines called the sutures. The primary sutures marking the fetal nucleus form an upright Y anteriorly and an inverted Y posteriorly. Secondary sutures are complex branching sutures. The first layer of secondary lens fibers is in place by the seventh week. Initially, the anteroposterior diameter of the lens is greater than the equatorial one. After the eighth week, the equatorial diameter becomes greater, and the lens assumes the more adult configuration. At birth, the diameter of the lens is approximately 6 mm. The primary lens fibers form the embryonic nucleus of the lens, which remains as the most central portion of the lens throughout life. The lens continues to grow throughout life by the addition of secondary lens fibers. With the closure of the anterior lens capsule, the lens is isolated from the surrounding structures.[32,33]

The fetal lens is nourished by a prominent system of vessels, the tunica vasculosa lentis, which is totally obliterated before birth. The vascular system posterior to the lens joins with the hyaloid system at the 9-mm stage, and later vessels from the annular vessel at the rim of the optic cup join with lenticular vessels anteriorly at the 25-mm stage. The long posterior ciliary vessels, the early choroidal vessels, and the palisade of vessels that forms the pupillary membrane in the mesoderm anterior to the lens all contribute to the intricate system of vessels that nourishes the anterior segment, lens, and vitreous from the second to the seventh month when this temporary system of fetal vessels is obliterated.

THE CORNEA

The cornea develops from two tissues, the surface ectoderm and the neural crest cells. The surface ectoderm provides the epithelium of the cornea after the lens placode has been pinched off from its central portion. The neural crest cells provide the mesenchymal components, the bulk of the cornea. Shortly after lens separation, the epithelium develops two layers and then three. During the sixth week the crest cells move in from the area near the lens equator and separate the basement membranes of the surface epithelium and the lens capsule, which have been fused (see Fig 2–20). Pseudopodial-like processes from the cells extend between these layers, and shortly thereupon, a double layer of corneal endothelium is formed that migrates across the entire central cornea (12-mm stage). Hyaluronic acid and collagen fibers fill the acellular zone between the epithelium and the endothelium, whereupon neural crest cells move in quickly through the acellular zone. First the crest cells populate the posterior portion of the cornea just anterior to the endothelial layer, and later, the anterior stromal area is filled with crest cells with their long axes parallel to the surface of the cornea. At 8 weeks, the more posterior layers of the corneal stroma are in contact with similar cells of the sclera (Fig 2–21). By the second month, the cornea has approximately 15 layers of stromal cells interspersed with sulfated mucopolysaccharides and collagen lamellae, most prominently in the posterior layer. By the third month, the endothelial layer has stretched into a single layer of cells, and irregular deposits of basement membrane material have appeared, the first indications of Descemet's membrane. The cornea grows in thickness, both by the addition of new cells and by the laying down of collagen fibrils in orderly lamellae. Growth occurs in diameter by extension of the length of the collagen lamellae.[34–39]

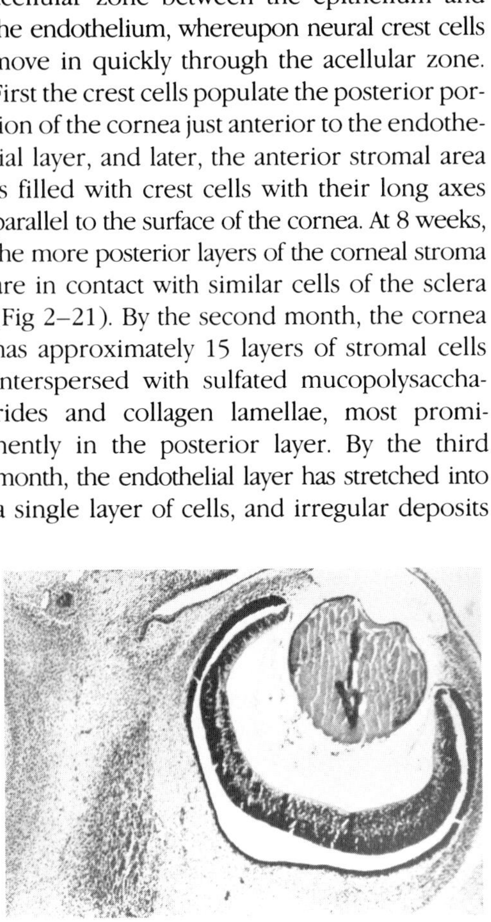

FIG 2–21.
Three-month stage. The sclera condenses adjacent to the anterior rim of the optic cup. The cornea remains thin, and iridic development has barely begun. Posteriorly in central left area dark cells indicate fibers of the extraocular muscle growing in from the paraxial mesoderm (HE).

Bowman's membrane appears in the fourth and fifth months as an acellular layer of randomly distributed collagen produced by the anterior fibroblasts of the stroma. The patches of Descemet's membrane posteriorly gradually become confluent and thicken as more basement membrane material is synthesized by the endothelium.

Hyaluronic acid is the principal ground substance of the fetal cornea. Hyaluronidase appears in the stroma in the fifth and sixth months and removes the hyaluronic acid. With the removal of the hyaluronic acid, the hydration of the cornea subsides, and the cornea thins to a more adult configuration. The production of keratan sulfate, the adult mucopolysaccharide of the cornea, is then noted; it is deposited first posteriorly and then anteriorly.

The nerve fibers first enter the developing cornea at the third month, continue to grow through the stroma, and reach the epithelium by the 20th or 21st week. From then until birth, the nerves increase and branch, thereby forming a diffuse network throughout the stroma and subepithelial tissues. As the lids open, the cornea is highly innervated.

Initially, the cornea and sclera have the same radius of curvature. After the third month, however, as the anterior chamber develops, the corneal curvature becomes greater than that of the sclera. Both the cornea and sclera are initially transparent. The cornea retains the uniform arrangement of parallel bundles and lamellae of its fibers and the thick ground substance of mucopolysaccharide, but the collagen of the sclera becomes progressively less organized, and the ground substance changes. Hence, the cornea maintains the transparent state, whereas the sclera becomes opaque. At birth both the cornea and sclera are highly cellular. With growth of the eye, few cells are added to the fibrous covering, and the addition of collagen and mucopolysaccharide ground substance dilutes the number present.

THE SCLERA

The sclera is one of the later tissues of the eye to develop. It is first noted in the anterior portion of the globe just posterior to the developing cornea. Here the undifferentiated layer of neural crest cells begins to consolidate and condense as the anterior layers of the sclera external to the rim of the optic vesicle. Cells and fibers begin to differentiate posterior to the limbus where the rectus muscles will be inserted. The consolidation and organization of cells proceeds toward the equator by the end of the second month. For the next several months, little activity is noted in the sclera until the late fifth and early sixth months when differentiation of the mesenchymal cells in the posterior pole takes place. From this time on, the sclera becomes thicker by the addition of new cells and fibers peripherally.

THE LIMBUS AND CHAMBER ANGLE

During the second month, the stromal cells of the sclera become more polymorphic and less regularly oriented, and the corneal curvature changes as a rudimentary space destined to become the anterior chamber is noted in the second month. Shortly thereafter, the canal of Schlemm develops from the venous channels within the limbal region of the cornea. The canal of Schlemm arises in the deepest part of the chamber angle and, with growth, gradually shifts more anteriorly. In the fifth month, the sclera adjacent to the chamber angle condenses into the scleral spur, which is both a continuation of and an anchor for the meridional fibers of the ciliary muscle. In the eighth month, the scleral venous channels are connected to the canal of Schlemm to provide an outflow path for aqueous fluid.

The angle of the anterior chamber develops late, during the sixth month, well after the canal of Schlemm has become visible. The angle deepens in the loose, still undifferentiated mesenchymal tissue between the canal of Schlemm and the root of the iris. The mesenchymal tissue from neural crest differentiates into the widely spaced anastomosing strands that form the trabecular meshwork. Through atrophy of cells lying between the trabecular meshwork and the developing stroma of the iris, the chamber angle gradually rounds out starting in the sixth month and continuing to birth. The process of the formation of Schlemm's canal, the chamber angle, and the trabecular meshwork is exceedingly complex, and there is considerable alteration in the topographical relationships between these structures from the fifth month to the time of birth. The final architecture of the limbus and angle are altered by the growth and disappearance of the pupillary membrane, the addition of the stromal tissues of the iris, and the thickening and growth of the ciliary muscle. The classic view that the chamber angle was formed mainly by atrophy or cell death of the mesodermal tissues in the region of the chamber angle has been challenged by Allen et al[40] who suggest that the process is one of separation of dissimilar tissues along a cleavage plane that is stimulated by unequal growth of the neighboring tissues. The angle is probably formed by aspects of both processes, that is, cell death and cleavage along the plane.

THE UVEAL TRACT

The uveal tract consists of the iris, ciliary body, and choroid. The uveal tract is the primary vascular coat of the eye and carries 90% or more of the blood to the mature eye.

Ciliary Body and Iris

The anterior chamber develops before the anterior growth of the rim of the optic cup completes the ciliary body and the iris. In the third month, the anterior rim of the optic cup grows forward rapidly. The leading edge of the cup moves anteriorly and inward, first over the equator and then more centrally along the peripheral edge of the lens. More posteriorly, the epithelial layers destined to become the ciliary epithelium ripple and bulge, thus initiating the formation of the ridges and folds of the ciliary processes. Shortly thereafter, the neural crest cells migrate into the folds to form the ciliary muscles, stroma, and melanocytes. At the 18-mm stage as the growing edge of the optic cup extends over the lens, a third wave of mesenchyme from the anterior portion of the neural crest grows inward to form the iris stroma. The posterior boundary of the anterior chamber is thus definitely established. The ridges and folds of the ciliary body become highly vascularized from vessels from the annular vessel. Seventy to 75 ciliary processes develop in each eye. The condensations of the neural crest cells present in the third month have a longitudinal configuration and become the longitudinal muscle. By the fifth month a triangular portion of muscle emerges as the earliest indication of the meridional muscle. Full development of the meridional and oblique muscles is not complete by birth but continues for a variable period of time after birth. Melanocytes, the pigmented cells, migrate from the neural crest into the ciliary body in a manner similar to that occurring in the choroid.[41–43]

As the optic vesicle grows forward, there is a small opening in the leading tip that is called the marginal sinus. The marginal sinus is the residual of the cavity of the optic vesicle. The sinus is evident at the second month, reaches its maximum size at 5 months, and is gradually obliterated late in the seventh and eighth months. The portion of anterior layer of the optic vesicle that is continuous with the pigmented epithelium of the retina and ciliary body becomes differentiated in the iris into the sphincter and dilator pupillae muscles. In the fifth month (65-mm stage), the sphincter muscle arises from cells just slightly posterior to the marginal sinus. By the sixth month, stromal cells, fibers, and capillaries grow into and divide the sphincter muscle into bundles and by the eighth month separate it from the epithelium. The dilator muscle evolves from the epithelial layer in the sixth month, but it is not fully formed or functional until after birth. The dilator muscle is not separated from the epithelium by mesenchyme and vessels but remains associated with its parent epithelium throughout life (Fig 2–22).

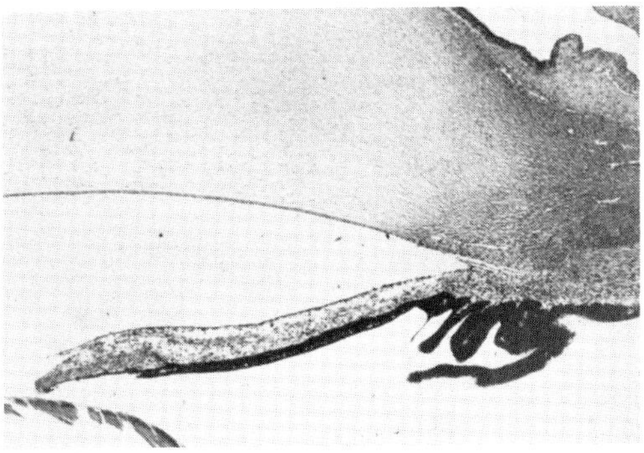

FIG 2–22.
Chamber angle near term. The anterior rim of the optic vesicle has differentiated into the iridic epithelium; differentiation into the sphincter muscle can also be noted at the far left of the iris and dilator muscle. The chamber angle shows a thin slit of Schlemm's canal and attachment of the ciliary muscle to the scleral spur (HE).

The Choroid

By the fourth week, an irregular and somewhat evanescent layer of vascular spaces forms around the developing optic vesicle. These are twigs from the developing internal carotid artery and from the primitive ophthalmic arteries. The pigmented epithelium of the retina induces the underlying tissues to develop as choroid and sclera. If the pigment epithelium does not develop normally, the two outer coats of the eye remain poorly formed and dysgenetic (see Fig 2–15).

Blood spaces forming around the optic vesicle drain into the supraorbital and infraorbital venous plexuses. The vessels develop into an embryonic type of choriocapillaris by the

13-mm stage during the second month. The anterior portion develops a palisaded connection between the vessels of the choroid and those of the ciliary body. During the second month, the long posterior ciliary arteries become established and pass beneath the choroid to the base of the ciliary body. In the fourth month, the larger vessels, mainly veins and tributaries to the vortex veins, begin to form anterior to the equator and proceed to the posterior portion of the globe as Haller's layer. During the fifth month the arteries become interposed between the layer of larger veins and the layer of maturing choriocapillaris. With growth and development, many intra-arterial and intravenous anastomoses take place. By the end of the fourth month, the anterior ciliary and long posterior ciliary arteries have formed the major arterial circle of the iris. The short posterior ciliary arteries invade the macular area and later the remainder of the choroid and send out a few branches to form the circle of Zinn around the optic nerve. In the third trimester, recurrent branches from the greater arterial circle grow posteriorly into the ciliary body and choroid. Anterior to the equator, there are essentially two layers of vessels, the choriocapillaris and a layer of medium-sized vessels (some arteries but mostly veins).[44]

The stroma of the choroid is produced from the neural crest cells, which contribute the melanocytes and the fibroblasts that create a fine matrix of collagen. Melanization of the melanocytes begins posteriorly near the disc in the 24th week, proceeds anteriorly, and is relatively complete by the 27th week. The ultramicroscopic structure of the capillaries of the chroriocapillaris includes diaphragm-covered fenestrae. The open junctions in the endothelial cells of the capillaries develop early in embryonic life. The pericytes along the outer wall of the endothelium develop from the crest cells. Elastic fibers develop from the mesenchymal cells in all areas of the choroid, and with collagen fibers, they form arcades and strata that are parallel to the layers of the vessels.

THE VITREOUS

The vitreous develops in three fairly distinct stages: the primary or vascularized vitreous develops from the hyaloid system in the fourth week to the 13-mm stage (fifth and sixth weeks), the secondary or nonvascularized vitreous from the 13- to 70-mm stage, and the tertiary vitreous or zonule in the fourth month. The primary vitreous develops from the retina and the lenticular epithelium as well as from the hyaloid system, which invades and fills the space between the optic cup and the lenticular vesicle. The primary vitreous is fibrillar in appearance, with the fibers arranged parallel to the surface of the retina and enmeshing the capillaries of the hyaloid system. Fibers form a fanlike configuration at the anterior end of the cup with perpendicular radiations from the retina to the lens. The secondary, or definitive, vitreous is formed principally from the 6th to the 12th week as a cone of nonvascularized fibers and ground substance around the primary vitreous. The secondary vitreous consists of very fine fibers parallel to the retina with fine attachments to the internal limiting membrane and a circular attachment at the periphery of the lens, the hyaloidal capsular ligament.

With growth, the hyaloid fades, and the primary vitreous becomes a progressively smaller triangular zone extending from the posterior portion of the lens to the optic disc. A thin layer of demarcation between the primary and secondary vitreous is evident on many histological preparations although a definite intravitreal membrane is not found. The primary vitreous is attached around the optic disc and persists in adult life as the canal of Cloquet. Occasionally, remnants of the hyaloid vascular system may be seen in a fully mature eye. By the end of the 12th week, two thirds of the optic cup is filled with secondary vitreous.

The anterior and most peripheral fibrils become thicker and form the tertiary vitreous, the zonule, or the marginal bundle of Drualt. Zonular fibers extend from the internal limiting membrane of the ciliary body to the lens capsule by the 170-mm stage (third to the sixth month). On the lens, the fibrils terminate as fine lamellae on the capsule. As the eye grows, the fibrils become progressively longer and stronger, and from these fibers, the zonule is developed.[45] The embryonic progenitors of the vitreous include the surface ectoderm (lens), neuroectoderm (retina), and the neural crest cells, a few of which enter at the closure of the embryonic fissure and mesoderm, which contributes much of the hyaloid system.

THE VASCULAR SYSTEM

The vascular system of the eye and the orbit by the beginning of the fourth week is derived from the primitive internal carotid system. A large branch of the internal carotid, the primitive dorsal ophthalmic artery, supplies almost the entire eye and orbital tissues during the early stages, with only a small contribution from adjacent vessels. From the dorsal ophthalmic artery, the long posterior temporal and nasal ciliary arteries and the hyaloid artery eventually arise. The stapedial artery, a branch of the carotid, supplies the orbit initially, but it eventually anastomoses with the distal branches of the dorsal ophthalmic artery. The venous system develops from the supraorbital and infraorbital plexuses that surround the developing neural tube. From the plexuses the cavernous sinus and other major sinuses of the cerebral system develop. By the 14-mm stage, the primitive maxillary vein and supraorbital vein have developed. The superior ophthalmic vein derives from the superior orbital vein and remains as the permanent drainage system of the orbit.

All the blood vessels of the eye and orbit originate from the paraxial mesoderm that supplies all of the endothelial cells. The muscles of the arteries, the pericytes, and the supporting connective tissues of the vascular system are derived from the neural crest cells. Initially the blood vessels are endothelial tubes without supporting connective tissues. During the seventh week connective tissue and muscular cells invest the tubes and help to differentiate the vessels as an artery or vein.

THE OPTIC NERVE

The optic vesicle is originally connected to the forebrain by a short tube called the optic stalk. The tubular structure is opened to both the cavity of the optic vesicle and the cavity of the forebrain and is lined by a single layer of undifferentiated neuroectodermal cells continuous with those of the outer cup, the retinal pigment epithelium. With invagination of the optic vesicle, invagination of the long axis of the stalk occurs. The stalk near the vesicle develops an invaginated segment that is crescent shaped, while the segment that is closer to the brain is circular. The invaginated distal portion of the nerve originally encircles the hyaloid artery. After closure of the fissure, the nerve gradually fills with glial tissues and axons that have grown from the retina toward the brain. The first retinal cells that turn into the optic stalk are sequestered in the central portion of the nerve around the hyaloid artery as glial cells. The vessel and glia form a cone-shaped zone known as Bergmeister's papilla. As the hyaloid artery and covering glial cells disappear, the papilla atrophies, which produces the physiological optic cup of the disc.

The first axons of the ganglion cells enter the optic nerve at the sixth week. Many of the first axons that enter the invaginated layer of cells become vacuolated and disappear (Fig 2–23). By the 20-mm stage, the nerve is filled with axons. Some of the peripheral cells become transformed into astrocytic cells, and from these, the supporting glial framework and peripheral glial mantle of the optic nerve are derived. By the 45-mm stage, the glial cells assume an orderly arrangement and lie in longitudinal rows between the bundles of axons. Late in the second month, glial cells grow perpendicular to the direction of the nerve fibers and develop the glial portion of the lamina cribrosa, which at this stage is composed entirely of astrocytes. By the fourth month, both astrocytes and oligodendrocytes form the glial

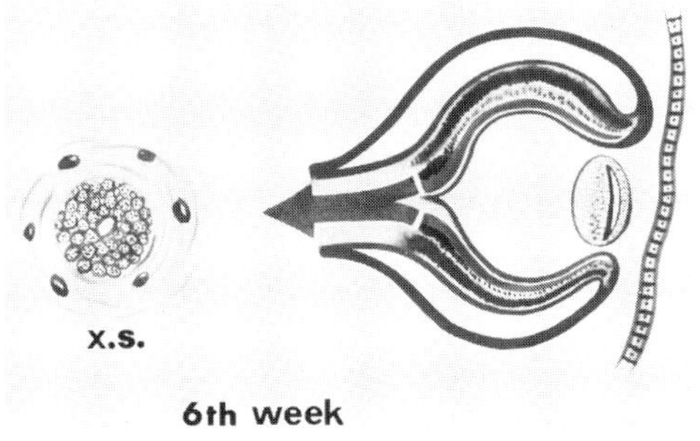

FIG 2–23.
Development of the optic nerve. Axons from the ganglion cells grow in the anterior layers of the retina through the optic nerve and toward the central nervous system. Axons stimulate surrounding neural ectodermal cells of the optic stalk to form glia within the nerve. The mesenchyme from the neural crest condenses as meningeal sheaths. The vascular twigs from the dorsal ophthalmic artery form the blood supply.

framework of the nerve. As the lumen of the stalk is obliterated by invagination distally and the growth of the axons toward the brain, the cavities of the optic vesicle and the third ventricle are no longer in direct communication (25-mm stage). The optic recess on the floor of the third ventricle marks the area of the original connection between the two. The distal portion of the optic nerve becomes vascularized from the hyaloid artery. Closer to the brain, blood vessels invade the periphery of the nerve through the septal system and take with them mesenchymal elements from the neural crest tissues.

The three meningeal sheaths of the optic nerve develop from neural crest cells. As early as the 10-mm stage and definitely by the 17-mm stage, elements of the pial sheath can be identified. At the 50-mm stage, the pia is well developed. During the fifth month, the dura segregates from the surrounding tissue, and in the sixth and seventh months, the arachnoid differentiates between the pia and the dura. By the ninth month, the overall structure of the nerve is well advanced. The collagenous elements of the lamina cribrosa that are first noted in the fifth month are easily identified by the end of the seventh month. Additional collagenous fibers from the sclera, choroid, and dura are evident at the end of the eighth month. An increase in the girth and length of the nerve takes place into the sixth month after birth. After that, some increase in girth and length takes place until puberty.

The myelination of the optic nerve begins in the region of the geniculate bodies about the fifth month and reaches the globe in the eighth month. Myelination occurs by the development of fine lipid droplets that aggregate around the nerve sheaths. The lipid vacuoles develop from the oligodendrocytes.

The optic chiasm forms initially from totally crossed fibers that are present before the 11th week. Between the 11th and 13th weeks, uncrossed fibers find their way into the optic chiasm, and from that point on, the adult configuration is present. About the ninth week, fibers have reached the dorsal nucleus of the lateral geniculate body to develop central connections.

LIDS, CONJUNCTIVA, AND LACRIMAL APPARATUS

The lateral ectoderm of the embryonic disc remains on the surface after closure of the neural folds and provides the basic material for the epithelia of the skin of the lids and the conjunctiva, both the palpebral and the bulbar, the epithelium of the cornea, cilia, glands, and lacrimal gland as well as the nasolacrimal apparatus. While still in the stage of the optic vesicle, there is a thin layer of surface ectoderm covering the vesicles. By the second month, activity in the mesenchymal tissues surrounding the vesicle results in the development of a full circular fold of tissue that gradually encircles the eye (Fig 2–24). Within this mesenchymal fold and covered by surface ectoderm, the structures of the lid arise. The mesenchyme for the upper lid arises from the frontal nasal process of crest cells. Both medial and lateral parts of the lower lid come from the maxillary process. The upper and lower portions of the lid fold elongate horizontally and cover the eye. In the third month, the lids fuse and form an epithelial seal. The process of fusion begins medially and tem-

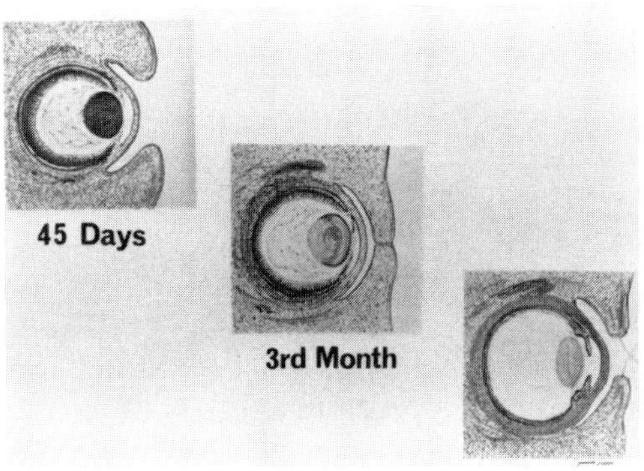

FIG 2–24.
Lid formation. Lid folds are evident by the 45th day. Folds grow over the cornea and meet and fuse by the third month. The folds are filled with vessels and mesenchyme derived from the median nasal process of the neural crest cells. Glands and cilia develop from the epidermis and the orbicularis oculi, from the mesoderm. Starting in the sixth month, cornification and the development of cilia and sebum result in the separation of the lids; this is completed by the end of the seventh month.

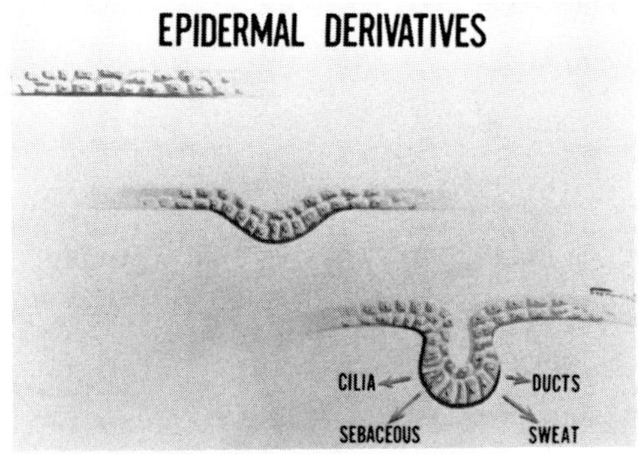

FIG 2–25.
Glands, cilia, and ducts develop from invaginations of the surface ectoderm, with subsequent differentiation into adnexal structures. The lacrimal glands and drainage system also develop by thickenings of the epidermis.

porally and proceeds centrally. It is complete by the 35-mm stage. From this time on, the meibomian glands and cilia develop by epithelial building and ingrowths (Fig 2–25). The orbicularis muscle arises from the mesoderm. The tarsus and connective tissues arise from the neural crest cells. The line of fusion is complete until the sixth or seventh month when a separation begins. Keratinization of the epithelium and formation of meibomian secretions initiate and continue the process of lid separation. Opening of the fissure begins medially and extends temporally. The action of the developing levator palpebrae may also play a part in the separation of the lids.

The caruncle develops as a bud of surface ectoderm from the lower lid after lid fusion has occurred at the end of the third month. The fine lanugo cilia and sebaceous glands develop in the caruncle from the surface epithelium during the fourth and fifth months, but the adenomatous tissue does not develop until after birth.

The orbicularis muscle is part of the facial musculature that develops from the mesoderm of the second visceral arch and has the same origin as the platysma muscle. Muscle cells migrate into the region at the 12-mm stage and, by the 16-mm stage, have surrounded the eye. The muscle appears well formed in the lids by the 11-mm stage, before the cilia and the glands.

DEVELOPMENT OF THE LACRIMAL GLAND

The lacrimal gland is formed by epithelial budding from the basal epithelial layer of the conjunctiva and is first noted at the 25-mm stage. The budding begins in the temporal portion of the upper fornix and results in solid branching outgrowths. As more branches appear, a lumen develops by the breakdown of the central cells in the solid branches. In the second trimester, the tendon of the levator palpebrae superioris divides the gland into two parts. The gland continues to grow and only achieves full development at 3 to 4 years.

THE LACRIMAL PASSAGES

The lacrimal apparatus begins as a solid rod of ectodermal cells that is originally trapped between the maxillary and the lateral nasal processes. The ectodermal fold extends downward into the surrounding mesenchyme and forms a sulcus called the nasal optic fissure. This solid core becomes detached and lies between the future medial canthus and the nasal cavity (sixth week). Simultaneously, a solid core of epithelial cells develops from the primitive nasal cavity and begins to grow toward the superior cord. The superior end of the uppermost rod of cells forms two bud-like growths that develop into the canaliculi, and more distally a thickening occurs that will become the lacrimal sac. Canalization begins by disintegration of the central cells in the solid cores during the third month and proceeds peripherally. Canalization is unequal, and so isolated cavities appear both in the superior and nasal rods of cells. Union between the two epithelial rods occurs about the sixth month, thereby establishing the oculonasal passage. This may be delayed until after birth. The puncta at the lid margin develop at the time the lids are separating, about the seventh month. The lower end of the duct may remain closed by a fusion of mucosal linings of the nasal fossa and the lower end of the duct, a condition that is often present at birth.

EXTRAOCULAR MUSCLES AND ORBIT

The extraocular muscles arise from masses of the paraxial mesoderm posterior to the developing globe (5-mm stage). On each side of the neural tube, the muscle fibers begin to grow anteriorly from three condensations of mesoderm (Fig 2–26). The cranial nerves grow into the muscular primordium between the 7- and 12-mm stages, with the oculomotor nerve the earliest to invest the muscle. The muscles lie parallel to the optic stalk and continue to grow forward. By the end of the second month the muscles have begun to develop their insertions into the sclera. Fibrils and striations can be seen in some of the more anterior muscular fibers. The rectus muscles form before the obliques. The trochlea for the superior oblique muscle appears in the frontal bone at about the 21-mm stage. The levator palpebrae is the last of the striated muscles to appear and is developed at the 60-mm stage but still continues to grow and override the rectus for several weeks. The entire muscle cone slowly develops in length throughout gestation, the muscle bundles becoming progressively longer and narrower and the tendons reaching an adult configuration about the eighth month.[46, 47]

The bones of the orbit, the fat, fascia, Tenon's capsule, and nerve sheaths arise from cranial neural crest cells that have migrated into the upper facial area.[3, 4]

Table 2–1 lists the origin of various ocular tissues from their embryonic progenitors. Table 2–2 is a summary of the time sequence of ocular development.

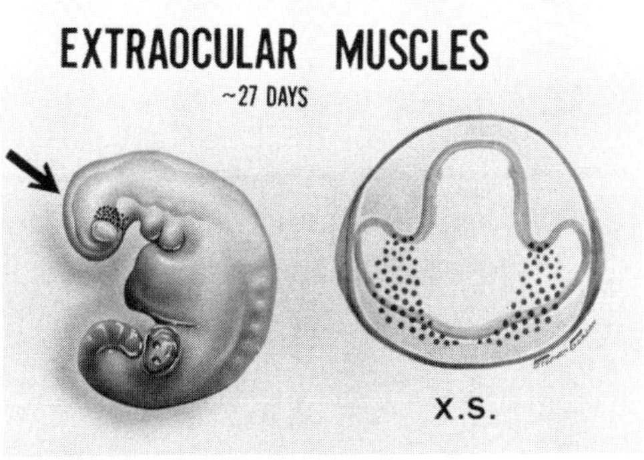

FIG 2–26.
The primordia of the extraocular muscles can be identified behind the developing optic vesicles by the 27th day. The extraocular muscles move forward around the globe over the next several months. The figure on the right shows the approximate distribution of the fibers of the extraocular muscles at the level indicated by the arrow.

TABLE 2–2.
Chronological Development of the Eye*

22 days	Optic primordia appears in neural folds (1.5–3 mm)
25 days	Optic vesicle evaginates. Neural crest cells migrate to surround vesicle
28 days	Vesicle induces lens placode
2nd mo	Invagination of optic and lens vesicles
	Hyaloid artery fills embryonic fissure
	Closure of embryonic fissure begins
	Pigment granules appear in retinal pigment epithelium
	Primordia of lateral rectus and superior oblique grow anteriorly
	Lid folds appear
	Retinal differentiation begins with nuclear and marginal zones
	Migration of retinal cells begins

(Continued.)

TABLE 2–2 (cont.).

	Neural crest cells of corneal endothelium migrate centrally. Corneal stroma follows
	Cavity of lens vesicle is obliterated
	Secondary vitreous surrounds hyaloid system
	Choroidal vasculature develops
	Axons from ganglion cells migrate to optic nerve
	Glial lamina cribrosa forms
	Bruch's membrane appears
3rd mo	Precursors of rods and cones differentiate
	Anterior rim of optic vesicle grows forward, and ciliary body starts to develop
	Sclera condenses
	Vortex veins pierce sclera
	Lid folds meet and fuse
4th mo	Retinal vessels grow into nerve fiber layer near optic disc.
	Folds of ciliary processes appear
	Descemet's membrane forms
	Canal of Schlemm appears
	Hyaloid system starts to regress
	Glands and cilia develop in lids
5th mo	Photoreceptors develop inner segments
	Choroidal vessels form layers
	Iris stroma is vascularized
	Lids begin to separate
6th mo	Ganglion cells thicken in macula
	Recurrent arterial branches join the choroidal vessels
	Dilator muscle of iris forms
7th mo	Outer segments of photoreceptors differentiate
	Central fovea starts to thin
	Fibrous lamina cribrosa forms
	Choroidal melanocytes produce pigment
	Circular muscle forms in ciliary body
8th mo	Iris sphincter develops
	Chamber angle completes formation
	Hyaloid system disappears
9th mo	Retinal vessels reach the periphery
	Myelination of fibers of optic nerve is complete to lamina cribrosa
	Pupillary membrane disappears

*From Torczynski E: Ocular development and congenital anomalies, in Lewis RA (ed): *The Basic and Clinical Science Course*, section 1, *Fundamentals and Principles of Ophthalmology*. San Francisco, American Academy of Ophthalmology, 1988–89. Used with permission.

REFERENCES

1. Duke-Elder S, Cook C: Normal and abnormal development, in Duke-Elder S: *System in Ophthalmology*, vol 3. St Louis, CV Mosby Co, 1963.
2. Ozanics V, Jakobiec FA: Prenatal development of the eye and its adnexa, in Jakobiec FA (ed): *Ocular Anatomy, Embryology and Teratology*, in Duane T, Jaeger E (eds): *Biomedical Foundations of Ophthalmology*, vol 1. Philadelphia, JB Lippincott Co, 1982.
3. Noden DM: Periocular mesenchyme: Neural crest and mesodermal interactions, in Jakobiec FA (ed): *Ocular Anatomy, Embryology and Teratology*, in Duane T, Jaeger E (eds): *Biomedical Foundations of Ophthalmology*, vol 1. Philadelphia, JB Lippincott Co, 1982.
4. Schook P: Cell action and cell interaction during ocular morphogenesis, in Jakobiec FA (ed): *Ocular Anatomy, Embryology and Teratology*, in Duane T, Jaeger E (eds): *Biomedical Foundations of Ophthalmology*, vol 1. Philadelphia, JB Lippincott Co, 1982.
5. Mann I: *Development of the Human Eye*. New York, Grune & Stratton, 1964.
6. O'Rahilly R: The early development of the eye in staged human embryos. *Contrib Embryol Carnegie Inst* 1966; 38:1–42.
7. Johnston MC: A radioautographic study of the migration and fate of cranial neural crest cells in the chick embryo. *Anat Rec* 1966; 156:143–156.
8. Le Douarin NM: Characteristiques ultrastructurales du noyau intephasique chez la caille et chez le poulet et utilisation de cellules de caille comme 'marquers biologiques' en embryologie experimentale. *Ann Embryol Morphol* 1971; 4:125–135.
9. Le Douarin N: A biological cell labelling technique and its use in experimental embryology. *Dev Biol* 1973; 30:217–222.
10. Le Lievre C, Le Douarin N: Mesenchymal derivatives of the neural crest. Analysis of chimaeric quail and chick embryos. *J Embryol Exp Morphol* 1975; 34:125–154.
11. Morriss GM, Thorogood P: An approach to cranial neural crest cell migration and differentiation in mammalian embryos, in Johnson MH: *Development in Mammals*, vol 3. Amsterdam, Elsevier North Holland, 1978.

12. Noden DM: Cytodifferentiation in heterotropically transplanted neural crest cells (abstract). *J Gen Physiol* 1976; 68:13.
13. Noden DM: An analysis of migratory behavior of the avian cephalic neural crest cells. *Dev Biol* 1975; 42:106–130.
14. Noden DM: The migration and cytodifferentiation of cranial neural crest cells, in Pratt RM: *Current Research Trends in Prenatal Craniofacial Development*. New York, Elsevier North Holland, 1980.
15. Erickson CA, Tosney KW, Weston JA: Analysis of migratory behavior of neural crest and fibroblastic cells in embryonic tissues. *Dev Biol* 1980; 77:142–156.
16. Johnston MC, Bhakdinaronk A, Reid Y: An expanded role of the neural crest in oral and pharyngeal development, in Bosma JF (ed): *The Fourth Symposium on Oral Sensation and Perception*. Bethesda, Md. US Department of Health, Education and Welfare Publication No 73-546, National Institute of Health, 1973, pp 37–52.
17. Johnston MC, Listgarten MA: Observations of the migration, interaction and early differentiations of orofacial tissues, in Slavkin HC, Bavetta LA (eds): *Developmental Aspects of Oral Biology*. New York, Academic Press, 1972, pp 53–80.
18. Noden DM: The migratory behavior of neural crest cells, in Bosma JF: *The Fourth Symposium on Oral Sensation and Perception*. Bethesda, Md. US Department of Health, Education and Welfare Publication No 73-546, National Institutes of Health, 1973.
19. Weston JA: The migration and differentiation of neural crest cells, in Abercrombie M, Brachet J, King T (eds): *Advances in Morphogenesis*. New York, Academic Press, 1970, pp 41–114.
20. Johnston MC, Noden DM, Hazelton RD, et al: Origin of avian ocular and periocular tissues. *Exp Eye Res* 1979; 29:27–43.
21. Bartelmez GW: The formation of neural crest from the primary optic vesicle in man. *Contrib Embryol Carnegie Inst* 1954; 35:55–71.
22. O'Rahilly R: The prenatal development of the human eye. *Exp Eye Res* 1975; 21:93–112.
23. Noden DM: The control of avian cephalic neural crest cytodifferentiation. I. Skeletal and connective tissues. II. Neural Tissues. *Dev Biol* 1978; 67:269–329.
24. Spira AW, Hollenberg MJ: Human retinal development: Ultrastructure of the inner retinal layers. *Dev Biol* 1973; 31:1–21.
25. Hollenberg MJ, Spira AW: Human retinal development: Ultrastructure of the outer retina. *Am J Anat* 1973; 137:357–386.
26. Streeten BW: Development of the human retinal pigment epithelium and the posterior segment. *Arch Ophthalmol* 1969; 81:383–394.
27. Mund M, Rodriguez M, Fine B: Light and electron microscopic observation on the pigmented layers of the developing human eye. *Am J Ophthalmol* 1982; 73:167–182.
28. Engerman RL: Development of macular circulation. *Invest Ophthalmol* 1976; 15:835–843.
29. Henkind P, Bellhorn RW, Murphy ME, et al: Development of macular vessels in monkey and cat. *Br J Ophthalmol* 1975; 59:703–709.
30. Wise GN, Dollery CT, Henking P: *The Retinal Circulation*. New York, Harper & Row, 1971, pp 1–18.
31. Wrenn JT, Wessels NK: An ultrastructural study of lens invagination in the mouse. *J Exp Zool* 1969; 171:359–367.
32. Coulombre JL, Coubombre AJ: Lens development: IV. Size, shape and orientation. *Invest Ophthalmol* 1969; 8:251–257.
33. Smelser GK: Embryology and morphology of the lens. *Invest Ophthalmol* 1965; 4:389–410.
34. Hay E, Revel J: Fine structure of the developing avian cornea, in Wolsky, Chem P: *Monographs in Developmental Biology*. Basel, S Karger, 1969.
35. Bard J, Hay E: The behavior of fibroblasts from the developing avian cornea. *J Cell Biol* 1975; 67:400–418.
36. Bard J, Hay E, Meller S: Formation of the endothelium of the avian cornea, study of cell movement in vivo. *Dev Biol* 1975; 42:334–361.
37. Wulle K-G: Electron microscopy of the fetal development of the corneal endothelium and Descemet's membrane of the human eye. *Invest Ophthalmol* 1972; 11:897–904.
38. Ozanics V, Rayborn M, Sagun D: Observations on the morphology of the developing primate cornea: Epithelium, its innervation and anterior stroma. *J Morphol* 1977; 153:263–298.
39. Hay E: Development of the vertebrate cornea. *Int Rev Cytol* 1980; 63:263–322.
40. Allen A, Burian HM, Braley AE: A new con-

cept of the development of the anterior chamber angle. *Arch Ophthalmol* 1955; 53:783.
41. Burian HM, Braley AE, Allen L: A new concept of the development of the angle of the anterior chamber of the human eye. *Arch Ophthalmol* 1956; 55:439–442.
42. Tamura T, Smelser GK: Development of the sphincter and dilator muscles of the iris. *Arch Ophthalmol* 1973; 89:332–339.
43. Hansson HA, Jerndal T: Scanning electron microscopic studies on the development of the iridocorneal angle in human eyes. *Invest Ophthalmol* 1971; 10:252–265.
44. Heinmann K: The development of the choroid in man. *Ophthalmology* 1972; 3:257–273.
45. Balaz EA: Fine structure of developing vitreous. *Int Ophthalmol Clin* 1975; 15:53–63.
46. Gilbert PW: The origin and development of the human extrinsic ocular muscles. *Contrib Embryol Carnegie Inst* 1957; 36:59–78.
47. Sevel D: A reappraisal of the origin of human extraocular muscles. *Ophthalmology* 1981; 88:1330–1338.

3 Physical and Refractive Characteristics of the Eye at Birth and During Infancy

Sherwin J. Isenberg, M.D.

THE ORBIT

Introduction

Ophthalmologists and pediatricians should be concerned about development of the orbit for two reasons. The first is the cosmetic effect of a malformed orbit on the appearance of the child. The second and more important reason is the effect of a malformed orbit on the state of the eye and brain. An orbit that is too shallow can cause eversion of the eyelids, proptosis, and exposure of the conjunctiva and cornea as well as exotropia (see Chapter 24). Maldevelopment of the orbit can affect the optic canal, which may decrease vision through effects on the optic nerve (see Chapters 12 and 21). Over 30 congenital malformation syndromes that involve the orbit and/or produce microphthalmos have been described.[1]

Reciprocally, the state and size of the eye can affect the development and growth of the orbit. There are data in the literature relating the perinatal removal or absence of the eye to impaired orbital growth. Infants requiring enucleation for conditions such as retinoblastoma, trauma to the globe, severe glaucoma, or congenital structural defects including microphthalmos and anophthalmia may require early prosthesis placement, often within the first few weeks of life. In the rapidly developing infantile eye, a replacement of prosthesis may be needed as often as every 2 weeks,[2] especially if expansion of the orbit is desired. Socket development has been reported to be stimulated by the presence of a globe,[2] and the early loss of a globe, produced experimentally in sheep, has been shown to result in a 35% decrease in mature orbital size.[3] Thus, using correctly sized conformers in the developing neonate may ensure adequate conjunctival growth.[3]

Orbital Growth

Between 6 months of gestational age and 18 months following birth, the bony orbit undergoes rapid changes in size and shape.[4]

TABLE 3–1.
Mean, Standard Deviation, and Range of Newborn Parameters and Ocular Measurements in 55 Neonates

Measurement	Mean + SD	Range
Weight	1732 ± 447 gm	820–2,990
Gestational age	34.7 ± 3.0 wk	28.5–44.5
Conjunctival fornix diameter		
Horizontal	17.9 ± 1.3 mm	15.5–21
Vertical	15.0 ± 1.1 mm	12.5–17
Orbital margin diameter		
Horizontal	18.3 ± 1.2 mm	16–21
Vertical	15.5 ± 1.7 mm	11–20
Palpebral fissure width	14.8 ± 1.7 mm	12–18.5

Whitnall described the orbital margin to be circular at birth and to remain so until puberty.[5] Then as the face grows, the vertical diameter of the orbit increases dramatically. Compared with the adult orbit, the orbit at birth has a large flat roof, an increased contribution of the greater wing of the sphenoid bone to the lateral wall, and an anteriorly facing lacrimal sac caused by an accentuated lacrimal crest. The transverse orbital axis of the neonate is more horizontal than is the downward sloping axis of the adult.

However, the palpebral fissures, as opposed to the rapid growth of the orbit, slowly increase in size from early in gestation to term. Sivan and colleagues[6] as well as Mehes[7] found the palpebral fissure length to increase 5 mm in the last 10 to 14 weeks of gestation. Similarly, Jones and associates found a 4-mm increase in the last 8 weeks of gestation.[8] Hymes found a similar infantile growth but also documented a continuous, although slower increase until puberty.[9] Palpebral fissure length appears to be greater in black than in Hispanic infants.[10]

With regard to the development of the conjunctival fornixes, there is nearly no information in the literature. However, it has been stated that "the folds of the fornices (in man) are not obvious until the last month of gestation."[11]

Isenberg et al. prospectively measured the conjunctival fornix and orbital margin dimensions of 55 term and premature neonates within a week of birth.[12] The means, standard deviations, and ranges for gestational age, body weight, horizontal and vertical diameters of the orbital margin, horizontal and vertical diameters of the conjunctival fornix, and palpebral fissure width for the group of infants are shown in Table 3–1.

The relationship between conjunctival fornix dimensions, body weight, and gestational age for each infant are indicated in Figures 3–1 and 3–2. Statistically significant correlation coefficients were calculated for both conjunctival fornix horizontal and vertical diameters in relation to weight, as indicated with P values in Figure 3–1. Horizontal and vertical diameters of the conjunctival fornixes were similarly significantly correlated with gestational age (see Fig 3–2).

Figure 3–3 illustrates the relationship between orbital margin and weight. Statistically significant correlation coefficients were found for the infants' body weight in relation to either orbital margin horizontal or vertical diameter (P values are given). Figure 3–4 similarly depicts the statistically significant correlation between each of these parameters and gestational age. The relation between palpebral fissure width, body weight, and gestational age is given in Figures 3–5 and 3–6; correlation coefficients were statistically significant for these parameters. Statistically significant linear regression equations ($P < .05$) allowing prediction of conjunctival fornix, orbital margin, and palpebral fissure dimensions from weight or gestational age were calculated (Table 3–2).

A comparison of individual ocular parameters with each other revealed statistically sig-

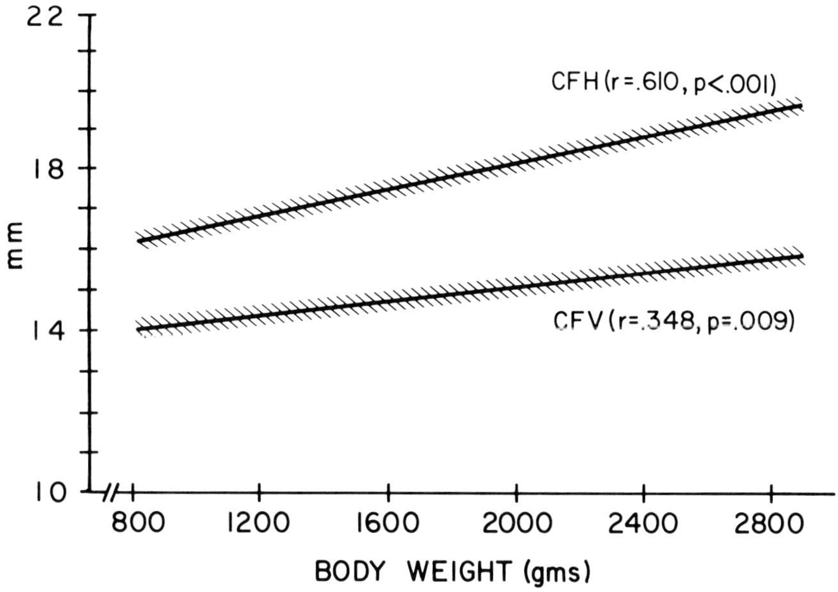

FIG 3–1.
Linear regression relationship (see Table 3–2) and standard error of the estimate between conjunctival fornix horizontal (CFH) and vertical (CFV) diameters and body weight. Correlation coefficients with *P* values are indicated. (From Isenberg SJ, McCarty JAW, Rich R: Growth of the conjunctival fornices and orbital margin in term and preterm infants. *Ophthalmology* 1987; 94:1276. Used with permission.)

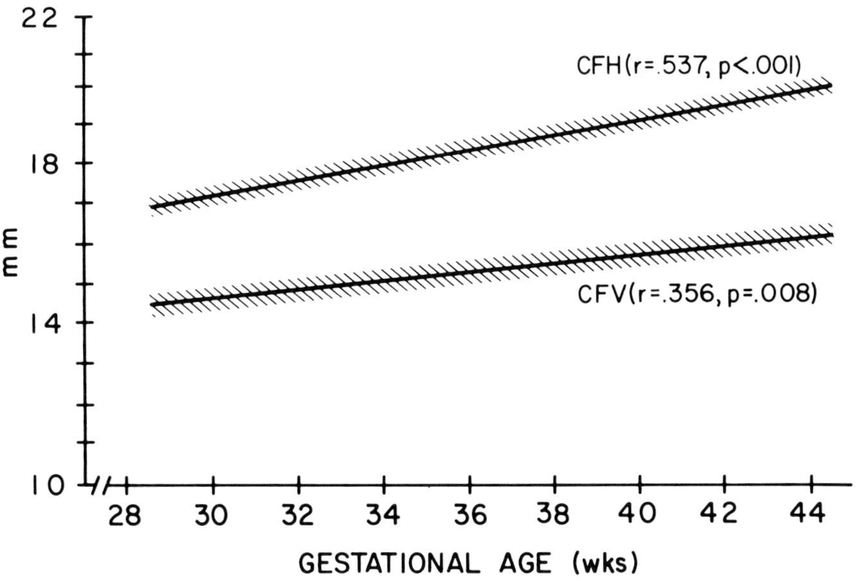

FIG 3–2.
Linear regression relationship (see Table 3–2) and standard error of the estimate between conjunctival fornix horizontal (CFH) and vertical (CFV) diameters and gestational age. Correlation coefficients with *P* values are indicated. (From Isenberg SJ, McCarty JAW, Rich R: Growth of the conjunctival fornices and orbital margin in term and preterm infants. *Ophthalmology* 1987; 94:1276. Used with permission.)

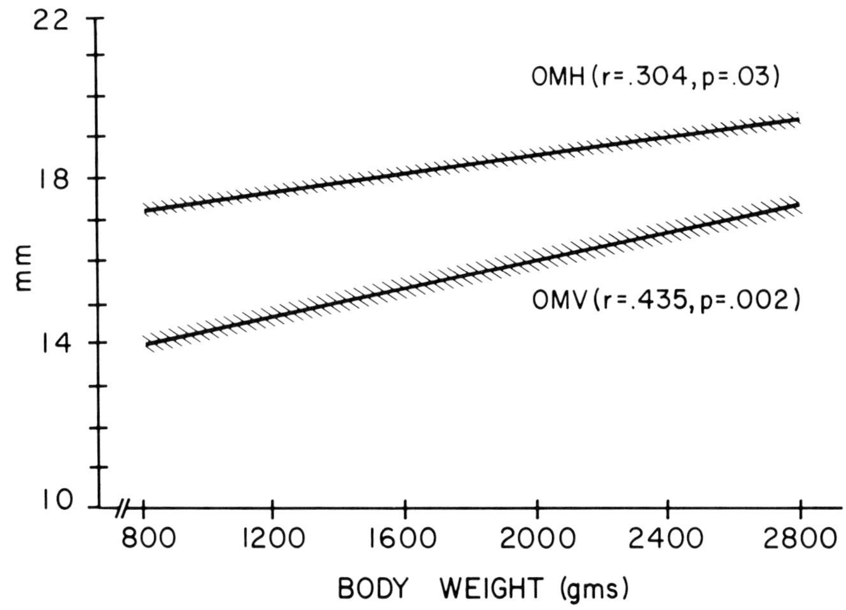

FIG 3–3.
Linear regression relationship (see Table 3–2) and standard error of the estimate between orbital margin horizontal (OMH) and vertical (OMV) diameters and body weight. Correlation coefficients with *P* values are indicated. (From Isenberg SJ, McCarty JAW, Rich R: Growth of the conjunctival fornices and orbital margin in term and preterm infants. *Ophthalmology* 1987; 94:1276. Used with permission.)

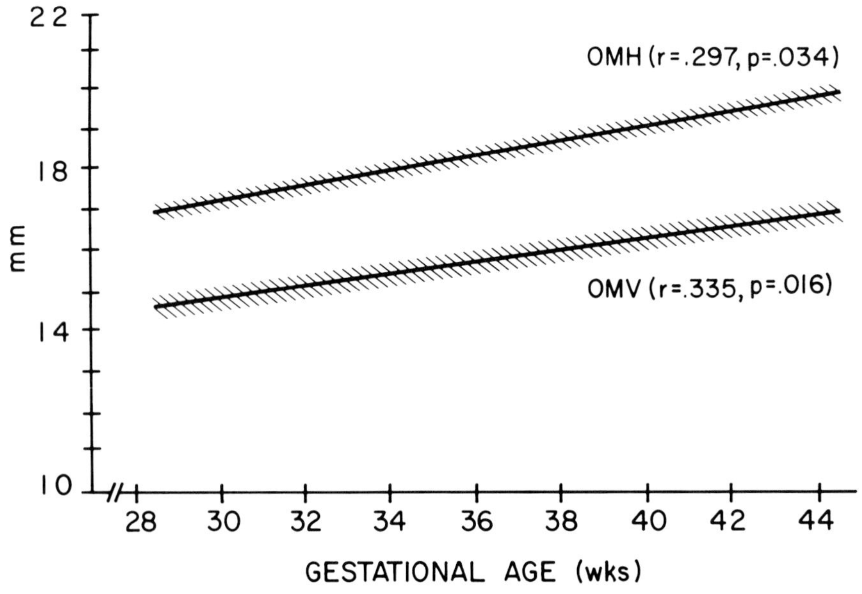

FIG 3–4.
Linear regression relationship (see Table 3–2) and standard error of the estimate between orbital margin horizontal (OMH) and vertical (OMV) diameters and gestational age. Correlation coefficients with *P* values are indicated. (From Isenberg SJ, McCarty JAW, Rich R: Growth of the conjunctival fornices and orbital margin in term and preterm infants. *Ophthalmology* 1987; 94:1276. Used with permission.)

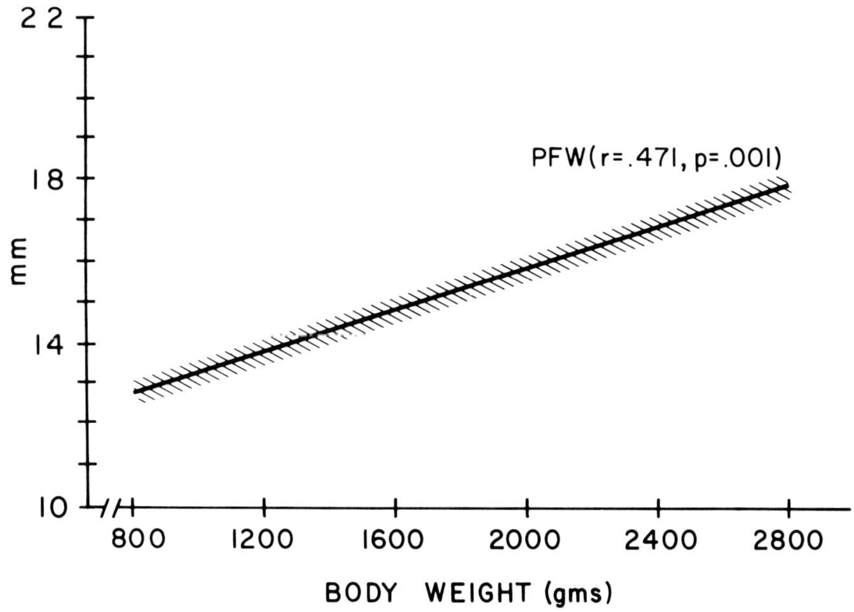

FIG 3–5.
Linear regression relationship (see Table 3–2) and standard error of the estimate between palpebral fissure width (PFW) and body weight. Correlation coefficients with *P* values are indicated. (From Isenberg SJ, McCarty JAW, Rich R: Growth of the conjunctival fornices and orbital margin in term and preterm infants. *Ophthalmology* 1987; 94:1276. Used with permission.)

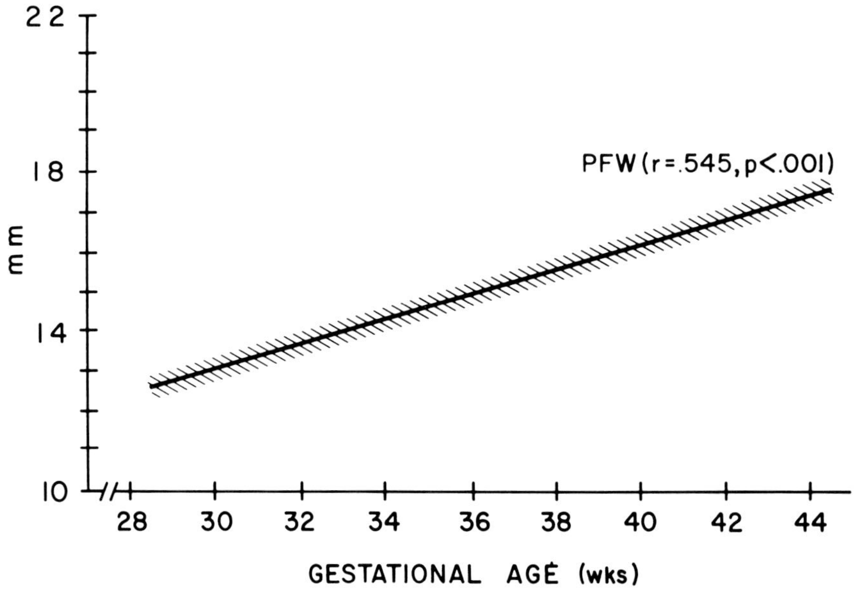

FIG 3–6.
Linear regression relationship (see Table 3–2) and standard error of the estimate between palpebral fissure width (PFW) and gestational age. Correlation coefficients with *P* values are indicated. (From Isenberg SJ, McCarty JAW, Rich R: Growth of the conjunctival fornices and orbital margin in term and preterm infants. *Ophthalmology* 1987; 94:1276. Used with permission.)

TABLE 3–2.
Linear Regression Equations for Neonatal Conjunctival Fornix, Orbital Margin, and Palpebral Fissure Dimensions in Relation to Weight and Gestational Age

Gestational Age (wk)	Weight (gm)
Conjunctival fornix (mm)	
Horizontal = 0.188 (GA) + 11.4*	= 0.0017 (WT) + 14.9*
Vertical = 0.113 (GA) + 11.1†	= 0.0001 (WT) + 13.4†
Orbital Margin (mm)	
Horizontal OMH = 0.182 (GA) + 11.8†	= 0.0012 (WT) + 16.1†
Vertical OMV = 0.148 (GA) + 10.4‡	= 0.0016 (WT) + 12.7*
Palpebral fissure width (mm) = 0.312 (GA) + 3.73*	= 0.0020 (WT) + 11.1*

GA = gestational age; WT = weight.
*$P < .01$.
†$P < .05$.
‡$P = .057$.

nificant correlation coefficients for the conjunctival fornix in relation to orbital margin and palpebral fissure only in the horizontal plane ($r = .500$, $P = .0004$; and $r = .561$, $P = .0001$, respectively). A comparison of the orbital margin horizontal diameter to palpebral fissure width revealed a statistically significant correlation coefficient ($r = .471$, $P = .001$). Significant correlation coefficients were found between orbital margin horizontal and vertical diameters ($r = .3149$, $P = .02$) and between conjunctival fornix horizontal and vertical diameters ($r = .331$, $P = .013$).

The overall proportions of the conjunctival fornix in the premature and term neonate (horizontal diameter:vertical diameter ratio, 18/15 mm = 1.2) vary greatly from those established previously for the adult (25/29 mm = 0.9).[6] Conjunctival fornix dimensions correlate closely and in a linear fashion with the weight and gestational age of the infant. The growth of the conjunctival fornix also parallels the growth of the palpebral fissure width but only partially correlates with orbital margin dimensions. There appears to be a different growth pattern in the palpebral fissure and conjunctival fornixes from that of the orbit. Similar findings were reported by Hymes who concluded that the palpebral fissure followed slow, general body growth in contrast to the rapid postnatal changes observed in the eye.[9]

The axis of the newborn orbit is oriented more laterally than that in the adult. The orbital axis is angulated 115 degrees from the center of the skull in neonates and 45 degrees in adults. In a Belgian population, the distance between the eyes was found to be about 21 mm at birth and, in preterm infants, follow the regression curve 0.47 times weeks of gestational age plus 3.3.[13] This equation should be considered prior to diagnosing certain craniofacial syndromes with hypertelorism or hypotelorism.

DIMENSIONS AND GROWTH OF THE EYE AND ITS STRUCTURES

The Eye: Physical Development

Of all human organs, the eye is one of the most fully developed at birth. While many changes will occur with maturity, the absolute dimensions of the eye are closer to adult size than are nearly any other organ of the body.

In the prenatal period, the eye grows fastest between the 8th and 14th week. Overall, growth of the eye parallels growth of the embryo until the 30th week, after which it slows down. The sagittal diameter increases from 12 mm at 6 months' gestational age to 17 mm at 8 months' gestational age (Fig 3–7). Postnatally, the eye grows fastest in the first year of life (about 3.8 mm in sagittal diameter) and then at a progressively slower rate until puberty (Table 3–3). Swan and Wilkins found that half the expected total increase over one's entire lifetime in ocular diameter, volume, and surface area occurs by 6 months of age.[14]

TABLE 3–3.
Physical Ocular Characteristics in Preterm and Term Infants Pooled From the Literature*

Age	Sagittal Length (mm)	Corneal Diameter (mm)	Refractive Error (D)
Gestational (wk)			
34	15.1	8.2	−0.8
36	16.1	9.2	0.3
Term	17.3	9.9	0.5
Postnatal (mo)			
6	18.2		0.9
12	20.6	11.1	0.9

*Data from Adams RJ, Maurer D, Davis M: Newborns' discrimination of chromatic from achromatic stimuli. *J Exp Child Psychol* 1986; 41:267. Banks MS: The development of visual accommodation during early infancy. *Child Dev* 1980; 51:646. Cook RC, Glassock RE: Refractive and ocular findings in the newborn. *Am J Ophthalmol* 1951; 34:1407. Gwiazda J, Scheiman M, Mohindra I, et al: Astigmatism in children: Changes in axis and amount from birth to six years. *Invest Ophthalmol Vis Sci* 1984; 25:88. Harayama K, Amemiya T, Nishimura H: Development of the eyeball during fetal life. *J Pediatr Ophthalmol Strabismus* 1981; 18:37. Jeanty P, Dramaix-Wilmet M, Van Gansbeke D, et al: Fetal ocular biometry. *Radiology* 1982; 143:513. Larsen JS: The sagittal growth of the eye. IV. Ultrasonic measurement of the axial length of the eye from birth to puberty. *Acta Ophthalmol* 1971; 49:873. Swan KC, Wilkins JH: Extraocular muscle surgery in early infancy—Anatomical factors. *J Pediatr Ophthalmol Strabismus* 1984; 21:44. Thorn F, Held R, Fang LL: Orthogonal astigmatic axes in Chinese and Caucasian infants. *Invest Ophthalmol Vis Sci* 1987; 28:191. Weale RA: Ocular anatomy and refraction. *Doc Ophthalmol* 1983; 55:361. Used with permission.

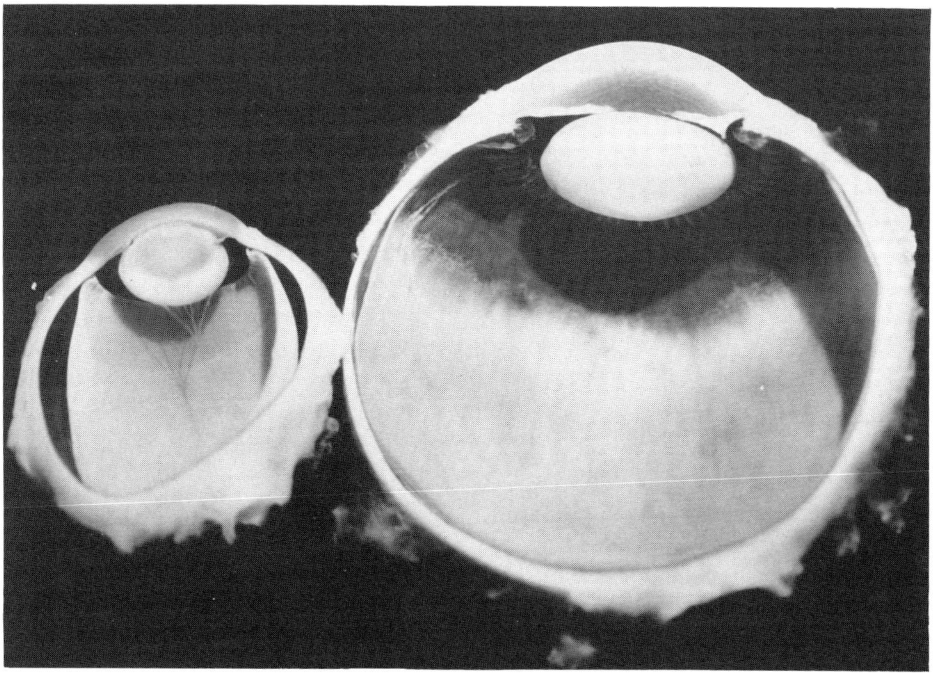

FIG 3–7.
Relative size of sectioned eyes of a normal premature infant compared with an adult. (Courtesy of Dr. Robert Foos.)

Early studies of the sagittal diameter of the eye gave variable results due to the inclusion of preterm infants with term infants. In 23 term infants, Sorsby and Sheridan found the sagittal diameter to be 17.9 mm.[15] Most studies give a figure of about 18.0 mm for this parameter. At birth, the transverse diameter of the globe is slightly greater than the sagittal (mean, 18.3 mm) and the vertical diameter slightly less (17.3 mm). Males average about 0.2 mm more in each diameter. In premature infants, the sagittal and transverse diameters are nearly identical, while the vertical diameters are uniformly shorter. However, Harayama and colleagues reported in a Japanese study that the sagittal diameter was shorter than the transverse or vertical diameters during fetal life.[16] They also showed that the vertical meridian circumference was shorter than the transverse or meridian circumferences during fetal life. When studied by ultrasonography the sagittal diameter appears shorter than that measured directly in the pathology laboratory. Using ultrasonography, both Larsen[17] and Blomdahl[18] found the mean sagittal ocular diameter of term newborns to be about 16.6 mm (range, 15.3 to 17.6).

The weight of the newborn eye varies from 2.3 to 3.4 gm, and the volume is between 2.20 and 3.25 cc.[19] The scleral surface area is about 828 sq mm.

The Anterior Segment

The corneal diameter in infants is an important clinical parameter. Diagnoses such as infantile glaucoma or microphthalmos often depend on or are influenced by measurements of corneal diameter. In 15 term infants, Blomdahl found the corneal diameter to range from 9.0 to 10.5 mm with a mean of 9.8 mm.[18] At birth, the vertical corneal diameter exceeds the horizontal (10.5 vs. 9.9 mm) according to Sorsby and Sheridan.[15] Newborn females have a corneal diameter 0.3 mm greater than do males. The definition of macrocornea and microcornea should be 2 SD away from the mean, which would be approximately greater than 11.0 and less than 9.0 mm in term infants (others feel the parameters should be 12.5 and 10.0, respectively). The gestational age of the infant must be taken into consideration before declaring the corneal diameter as being abnormally small. In preterm neonates, Sorsby and Sheridan found the corneal diameter to range from 7.5 to 9.2 mm without directly relating the diameter to gestational age. Musarella and Morin examined 37 infants with a mean postconceptual age of 34 $\pm$ 2 weeks and found the corneal diameters to average about 8.2 $\pm$ 0.5 mm.[20] They found corneal diameter to correlate best with weight and approximate regression relationship to be corneal diameter $= 0.0014 \times$ weight $+ 6.3$ where the corneal diameter is expressed in millimeters and weight in grams.

The corneal curvature is much steeper in infants than in adults. Donzis and colleagues found the corneal curvature to be about 60 Diopters in a 28-week gestational age infant.[21] At term, the mean curvature was about 51 D. By following a population of premature infants, they found a reduction of about 8 D in corneal curvature in the last 3 months of gestation. Thus, using donor corneas from infants for keratoplasty may cause a significant myopic shift due to the steep curvature, especially in the more premature neonate.[22]

The sclera in neonates has four times the pliability of adult sclera.[23] Therefore, the infant eye has a greater tendency to collapse during intraocular surgery than does the adult eye. The thickness of the sclera in infants is only 0.45 mm, while in adults it is 1.09 mm. Based on scleral stretching experiments, infantile sclera was found to be about half as strong as adult sclera.

The extraocular muscles are much closer to the back of the eye at birth than at any time later in life.[14] Because most of the growth of the sclera is in the posterior portion of the eye, the distance of the extraocular muscles from the posterior pole of the eye increases much more with growth than does the distance from the anterior pole. At birth, the lateral rectus muscle insertion lies just about over the equator, while the insertion of the medial rectus muscle lies only 1 or 2 mm in front of the equator. The width of the rectus muscle insertions is between 6.8 and 7.6 mm at birth.

The depth of the anterior chamber in term newborns averages 2.6 mm and ranges from 2.4 to 2.9 mm as shown by ultrasound.[17] Due to postmortem movement of the lens, in vivo ultrasonographic studies of anterior chamber depth are more reliable.

The iris has a different appearance in preterm than in older infants. The crypts appear less developed in preterm neonates and develop a more detailed architecture of crypts and hillocks with maturation. The color of the uveal tract appears paler in newborns than in older children. At birth, the iris in many white infants appears gray or blue, largely due to the pigment of the iris pigment epithelium, while other infants have a darker, even brown, iris from partial development of stromal mesodermal pigment. With time, the iris darkens as the stromal mesodermal cells mature and progressively develop more pigment. The iris blood vessels may contribute to the observed color of the iris. Due to immaturity of the dilator muscle of the pupil in the newborn, pupils dilate less than might otherwise be expected.

At birth, the lens volume is 90 cu mm, and the weight is 65 mg. The lens thickness in newborns varies from 3.4 to 4.0 mm, and the equatorial diameter is between 6.0 and 6.5 mm. Lens thickness does not correlate linearly with body weight.[15] The curvature of the lens is nearly spherical at birth, with a radius of curvature of 5 mm for the anterior surface and 4 mm for the posterior surface. The curvature increases until 2 years of age. The volume and weight of the lens nearly double by 1 year of age. The greater spherical power in the newborn eye, when compared with the adult eye, contributes to the greater refractive power needed in the shorter eye of neonates, as will be discussed later. While the lens as a whole continues to grow throughout life, it becomes less spherical. The lens diameter decreases 0.3 mm in the first 18 months of life and another 0.2 mm between 2 and 5 years of age.

The lenticulovitreal adhesions (Weiger's hyaloid-capsular ligament) are very strong in infants. Attempts to weaken these with enzymes as α-chymotrypsin have been unsuccessful.[20] Thus, intracapsular cataract surgery in infants can easily cause vitreous loss and is generally contraindicated.

The intraocular pressure in newborns is important since the clinician must occasionally measure it to rule out glaucoma. With various methods, the intraocular pressure in normal neonates has been reported as low as 8 and as high as 28 mm Hg. There are a number of variables that can affect these data, including whether the measurements are taken under anesthesia and, if not, whether the infant is crying, squeezing his eyelids, or straining at the time of measurement. A recent study found the mean intraocular pressure in unanesthetized noncrying premature infants to be 18 $\pm$ 2 mm Hg.[20]

Posterior Segment

At birth, the vitreous cavity measures 16.0 mm in sagittal diameter. By ultrasonography, the vitreous diameter has been shown to be decreased in certain developmental anomalies as fetal alcohol syndrome and holoprosencephaly.[24] Remnants of the hyaloid vascular system can still be found in the eyes of premature infants. Jones found posterior remnants in the eyes of 95% of premature newborns but in only 3% of term babies.[25] All the remnants resolved with time. Renz and Vygantas examined the vitreous cavity of 226 infants.[26] They reported all the premature neonates with a gestational age less than 34 weeks (or 4 lb) to exhibit the complete hydaloid vessel reaching from the optic nerve head to the posterior capsule of the lens. At about 34 weeks, the center of the vessel appeared to resolve, which left a Bergmeister's papilla attached to the optic nerve head and a strand attached to the posterior lens capsule. The frequency of the remnants diminished until they were not observed at all after 41 weeks' gestational age (or greater than 9 lb). After resolution of the hyaloid vasculature, Cloquet's canal, consisting of the multilayered fenestrated sheaths of the vessel, persists in the eye. This canal follows the original course of the hyaloid vasculature and runs from the optic nerve to the posterior lens capsule. In infants, the vitreous is a gel with no liquid vitreous present. With time, the sodium hyaluronate content of the vitreous increases as the collagen fibers, which do not increase in number, become less concentrated.

Of all ocular structures at the time of birth, the retina is the least developed functionally. The retinal vessels first appear in the fourth month of gestational age from spindle cells at Bergmeister's papilla. These mesenchymal vessels advance peripherally toward the ora serrata. By the eighth month of gestation, the vessels have extended almost to the nasal ora serrata but have reached the equator on only the temporal side. Even in term infants, the retinal vessels on the temporal side have often not fully reached the ora serrata but do so within a few weeks. Microscopic maturity of the blood vessels does not necessarily correlate with the extent of vascularization of the anterior retina.[27]

Other than the retinal vessels and the general mild pallor of the retina (as well as the optic nerve) at birth, the retina appears similar to the adult retina. However, there are many differences on a histological level. At birth, the retinal capillaries have a relative endothelial hyperdensity. During the first year of life, the capillary basement membranes thicken, and the intramural pericytes develop. The macula is the last retinal area to reach maturity. Even after birth, the macular cones elongate and undergo other histological changes. In addition, the ganglion and bipolar cells continue to migrate peripherally. The examiner can appreciate some of the macular changes in preterm infants through the ophthalmoscope.[28] Further details of macular development are presented later in this chapter. It is possible that the histologically immature newborn macula accounts for the poor fixation of infants in the first 3 months of life. However, the general inattentive nature of the newborn also contributes to their poor fixation.

VISUAL DEVELOPMENT (OTHER THAN ACUITY)

The development of vision as a whole is covered in Chapter 4. However, there are new data indicating the development of some parameters of vision other than acuity.

The visual field in infants can be used to indicate the development of the peripheral retina as well as the visual cortex. Mohn and Van Hof-van Duin found the visual field in newborns to extend 28 degrees to either side horizontally, 11 degrees superiorly, and 16 degrees inferiorly.[29] The visual field expanded slowly immediately after birth but increased rapidly after 2 months of age. By 1 year of age, the upper visual field had reached adult size, while the horizontal and lower fields were still smaller than those in the adult. They attributed these changes to maturation of cortical and subcortical pathways.

Newborn infants can accommodate very shortly following birth. In a series of studies, Banks reported that accommodation was present as early as 1 month of age, which enables the newborns to intermittently fixate on near targets as determined by retinoscopy.[30] Because the depth of focus of newborns is greater than that of adults for a number of reasons including a smaller pupil and poorer central visual acuity, their accommodation does not have to be as exact.

Color vision develops earlier than previously thought. Adams and colleagues tested 240 infants within the first week of life for discrimination between checkerboards by preferential forced looking techniques.[31] They showed discrimination between gray and green, yellow, and red stimuli. However, they did not show discrimination between gray and blue stimuli. Contrast and illumination were controlled during these investigations. Thus, newborns have a limited ability to discriminate chromatic from achromatic stimuli.

DEVELOPMENT OF REFRACTION

When considering the development of refraction, one must examine the contribution of each refractive surface. Then, the net effect of these components on overall refraction can be evaluated. The steep nature of the newborn cornea and subsequent flattening was discussed before, as was the high refractive power of the lens at birth. In the first 3 months of life, the lens power decreases approximately 4 D for term infants and 7.5 D for preterm infants.[32] The sagittal (or axial) length of the eye increases dramatically in the first 2 years of life and less thereafter. Larsen reported the axial length to increase from about 16.5 mm at birth to about 20.8 mm at 2 years of age.[17] In the next 11 years of development, he found the axial length to increase only another 2 mm.

Refractive Error

Most early studies of refraction in neonates were not done with the use of cycloplegic eyedrops and are subject to the criticism that the powerful accommodation present in infants introduced error. By administering atropine to infants, Cook and Glassock studied the refractive error of 1,000 newborn infants.[33] They found simple hyperopia in 43.9%, simple myopia in 16.7%, hyperopic astigmatism in 29.1% and myopic astigmatism in 6.4% of the infants. Goldschmidt performed retinoscopy on 356 term newborns less than 10 days old who had received atropine eyedrops.[34] He found the mean refractive error to be 0.62 D of hyperopia (± 2.24 with a 0.1 SEM). Myopia was found in 24.2% of his study population.

Gordon and Donzis reported that ten term newborns had a mean axial length of 16.8 mm, corneal curvature of 51.2 D, and lens power of 34.4 D which yielded a mean refractive error of 0.4 D of hyperopia.[35] They confirmed the rapid elongation of the globe and corneal flattening in infants as previously reported. In addition, they calculated that lens power rapidly decreased from 43.5 D in premature neonates to about 24 D by 2 years of age. The mean net refractive error remained between 0.3 and 1 D of hyperopia until 10 years of age.

Astigmatism

Astigmatism in neonates is more frequent and bears a different axis than that later in life. Utilizing a near-retinoscopy procedure without cycloplegia, Gwiazda and colleagues examined 521 children under 1 year of age.[36] This method can be questioned because a number of assumptions were made in regard to the accommodative status of the subjects. Nonetheless, they found about half the children to have an astigmatism of 1 D or greater. The axis was as likely to be against the rule as with the rule. They longitudinally followed 29 children with significant astigmatic errors from 6 months to 6 years of age. The amount of astigmatism significantly decreased over that period. Of 16 children with against-the-rule astigmatism, only one had greater than 1 D remaining at 6 years of age. Of 8 with with-the-rule astigmatism, the astigmatism decreased or vanished in all cases.

Fulton and coworkers, utilizing retinoscopy following instillation of 1% cyclopentolate, examined 75 infants under 1 year of age.[37] They reported 19% to have an astigmatism of greater than 1 D. Between 7 and 12 months of age, the astigmatism rate increased to about 25%. Of their astigmatic infants, 82% had an against-the-rule axis, and 18% had a with-the-rule axis. Only 5.7% of their subjects had an astigmatism exceeding 2 D. The use of cycloplegic agents may have made their data more accurate than previous noncycloplegic studies. The prevalence of against-the-rule astigmatism may only be true for white infants. Thorn and colleagues compared a group of white infants with Chinese infants.[38] They confirmed the high incidence of against-the-rule astigmatism in whites but found the majority of Chinese infants to have a with-the-rule astigmatism. They felt that the difference could not be attributed to the difference in eyelid shape. In adults, the axis of astigmatism appears to be similar in the two groups.

Most studies have shown a decrease in the against-the-rule astigmatism so commonly found in infants with increasing age, especially after the age of 4. Without proof, this decrease is usually attributed to the effect of the pressure of the upper eyelid against the superior aspect of the cornea. This would induce a tendency toward with-the-rule astigmatism. Indirect support of this hypothesis comes from Robb who showed that hemangiomas of the eyelids can exert pressure on the cornea and cause an astigmatism with the positive axis pointing in the direction of the hemangioma.[39] Bogan and associates have demonstrated that astigmatism may also be caused by dacryoceles and dermoid tumors as well as hemangiomas.[40]

Refraction in Premature Infants

Premature neonates have a different refractive status than do term infants. Shapiro and associates performed cycloplegic refractions on 236 children with a birth weight of 2,000 gm or less.[41] In 22 eyes under 1 year of age, the mean refractive error was 1.5 D of hyperopia ($\pm$0.8). The mean birth weight of 1,707 gm (range, 1,300 to 1,960) indicates that this population was not very premature. This may explain the lack of a significant difference from a population of term infants.

On the other hand, Dobson and colleagues reported the cycloplegic refractions of 146 infants at a mean postconception age of 34.2 weeks $\pm$ 2.9.[42] These infants had normal retinal examination results. The mean refractive error was 0.55 D of myopia ($\pm$2.8). The mean amount of astigmatic correction was about 1.6 D. Full-term infants were not found to be myopic ($P < .001$). Infants who were born more prematurely tended to have more myopia and greater astigmatism than infants who were born less prematurely. Of the 101 infants with greater than 1 D of astigmatism, 83% had against-the-rule, 10% had with-the-rule, and 7% had oblique axes. Nissenkorn and coworkers examined 155 premature infants weighing between 600 and 2,000 gm.[43] They reported that the 113 infants without retinopathy of prematurity had an average of 1.50 D of myopia. Prematurity appears to be a more important cause of myopia than does low birth weight since it has been shown that full-term infants with intrauterine growth retardation have refractive errors and visual acuities resembling those of normal birth weight infants.[44]

Myopia in Infants

It must also be recognized that there are special circumstances, besides prematurity, that can cause myopia in neonates. Hoyt and colleagues reported eight children who developed unilateral axial myopia associated with neonatal eyelid closure.[45] The eyelid closure resulted from various causes such as congenital third cranial nerve palsy, blepharoptosis from hemangioma or neuroma of the eyelid, and periorbital edema from obstetric trauma. The myopia ranged from 4.25 to 7.00 D and resulted primarily from an increase in the sagittal diameter of the posterior ocular segment as shown by ultrasonography.

Retinopathy of prematurity has been shown to be associated with myopia. In 42 premature infants with retinopathy of prematurity, Nissenkorn and colleagues reported an average of 4 D of myopia, with half of the children demonstrating between 0.25 and 15.5 D of myopia.[43] The greater the birth weight of the infants with retinopathy of prematurity, the smaller the amount of myopia. The cause of the myopia appears to be multifactorial. Some cases seem to result from increased axial length, while others arise from increased lenticular power or a combination of both these factors.[46] Increased corneal curvature may also contribute to the myopia.

MARKERS OF GESTATIONAL AGE

Although almost all aspects of the neonatal eye change with maturation, only two have been carefully correlated to gestational age in living neonates. This relationship has been exact enough for these parameters to be considered indicative of a neonate's postconceptual age by virtue of their degree of maturation.

TABLE 3–4.
Assessing Gestational Age by Dissolution of the Anterior Vascular Capsule of the Lens*

Grade	Age, wk	Finding
4	27–28	Lens surface entirely covered by vessels
3	29–30	Central vessels begin to atrophy Peripheral vessels thin
2	31–32	Central lens area more visible Peripheral vessels thin more
1	33–34	Only a few vessels remain at lens periphery

*From Hittner HM, Hirsch NJ, Rudolph AJ: Assessment of gestational age by examination of the anterior vascular capsule of the lens. *J Pediatr* 1977; 91:455. Used with permission.

Tunica Vasculosa Lentis

At the 17-mm stage of embryogenesis, small buds from the annular vessel form vascular loops carrying mesodermal tissue onto the anterior surface of the lens even before development of the anterior chamber. By the 22-mm stage, the lamina iridopupillaris is a richly vascularized layer of mesodermal cells closely opposed to the anterior surface of the lens. The peripheral part thickens to form the embryonic iris. The central portion is much thinner, composed almost entirely of blood vessels. It is this plexus of blood vessels that constitutes the tunica vasculosa lentis (also known as the anterior vascular capsule of the lens). With time, this plexus further thins, only to eventually disappear.

In 1977, Hittner and colleagues reported that the degree of dissolution of the tunica vasculosa lentis could be closely correlated to gestational age.[47] They examined the anterior vascular capsule of the lens on the first day of life with a direct ophthalmoscope after pupillary dilation with tropicamide, 0.5%, and phenylephrine, 2.5%. Their grading system can be found in Table 3–4 and Figure 3–8.

Subsequently, these investigators found

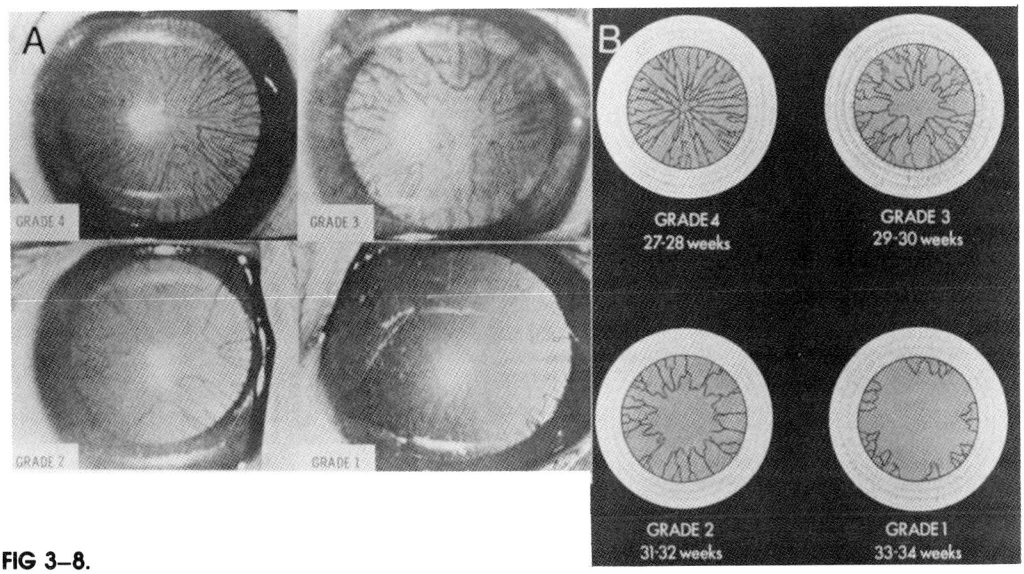

FIG 3–8.
Grading system for assessment of gestational age by examination of the anterior vascular capsule of the lens. (From Hittner HM, Hirsch NJ, Rudolph AJ: Assessment of gestational age by examination of the anterior vascular capsule of the lens. *J Pediatr* 1977; 91:455. Used with permission.)

that this method of gestational age assessment was valid for 33 newborns who were small for gestational age.[48] They also studied six newborns with congenital infections of toxoplasmosis, rubella, cytomegalovirus, and herpes simplex virus.[49] These infants, who had various ocular anomalies including microphthalmos, demonstrated persistence, hypertrophy, or asymmetry of the anterior vascular capsule of the lens. Thus, this method of gestational age determination may be invalid in the presence of systemic infection or other ocular anomalies.

Development of the Macula

In 1986, Isenberg described the ophthalmoscopic appearance of the macula in 129 premature infants.[50] He was able to correlate the observed developmental changes to gestational age. The classification for the 92 infants without retinopathy of prematurity appears in Table 3–5. The stages of development are depicted in Figures 3–9 through 3–12. For these normal infants, there was an overlap in gestational age at stages 1 and 2, but the 37 infants with retinopathy of prematurity demonstrated a delay of 3.2 weeks between stages 1 and 2. It was suggested that the appearance of the annular reflex of the macula (stages 1 and then 2) is largely dependent on migration of the ganglion cells from the macular area to the retinal periphery. The retinal changes of retinopathy of prematurity, including formation of a line or ridge in the anterior retina, may impose a barrier to ganglion cell migration. This would delay the appearance of the annular ring of the macula. An alternative explanation for this hypothesis can be found in the subsequent histological report of Johnson and Ahdab-Barmada.[51] They observed karyorrhexis (nuclear fragmentation and dispersion) in the ganglion cells of the central retina of premature neonates who had received supplemental oxygen. They found these changes more frequently in infants with lower birth weight and younger gestational age. This hyperoxemic cytological injury may explain part or all of the aforementioned delay in ganglion cell migration to the retinal periphery.

One should not expect normal visual acuity in neonates despite the fact that their maculae resembles adult maculae by 42 weeks after conception. As indicated in Chapters 4 and 5, the visual acuity at birth is approximately 20/400. Even at 42 weeks after conception, the cone inner and outer segments are short and thick, and many rods can still be found in the foveal region.[52] Electrophysiological tests also indicate an immaturity of the newborn visual system. The electroretinogram at birth has a normal configuration but a low amplitude.[53] Visually evoked potentials have been reported to be totally absent at birth in some infants, only to become normal at a later date.[54] Thus, while the maculae of term neonates may appear mature, histological changes are still underway that will bring their visual systems to functional maturity.

TABLE 3–5.
Development of the Macula in Normal Preterm Infants*

Stage	Gestation (wk)	Observations in Macular Area
0	31.5 ± 1.5	No pigmentation
1	34.8 ± 1.0	Dark red pigmentation appears
2	34.7 ± 2.4	Annular reflex is partially evident
3	36.3 ± 2.2	Complete annular reflex is present
4	37.6 ± 3.3	Foveolar pit seen with difficulty
5	41.7 ± 4.0	Foveolar light reflex is present

*From Isenberg SJ: Macular development in the premature infant. *Am J Ophthalmol* 1986; 101:74. Used with permission.

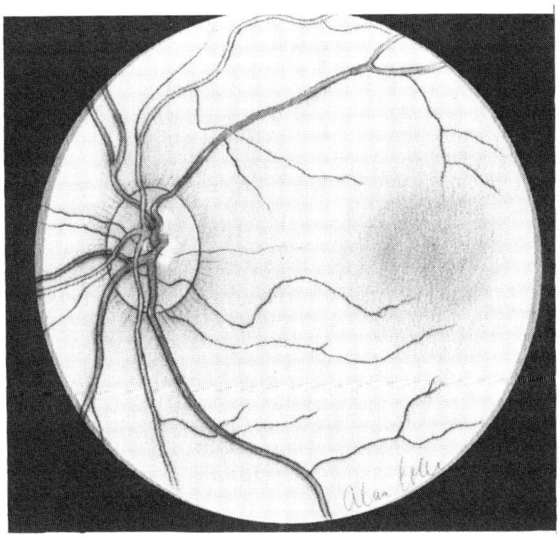

FIG 3–9.
Macular development, stage 1 (see Table 3–5). (From Isenberg SJ: Macular development in the premature infant. *Am J Ophthalmol* 1986; 101:74. Used with permission.)

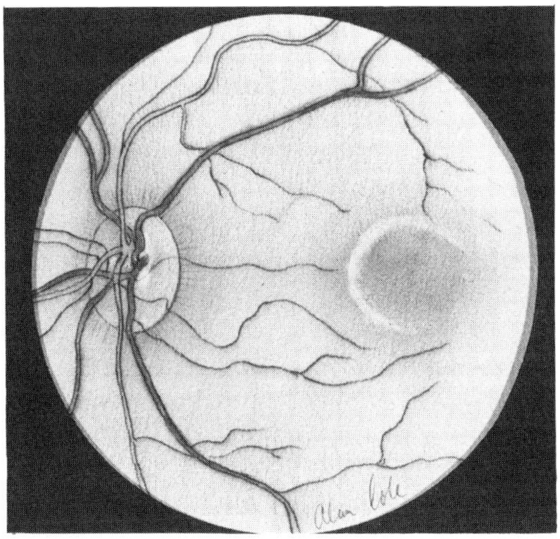

FIG 3–10.
Macular development, stage 2. (From Isenberg SJ: Macular development in the premature infant. *Am J Ophthalmol* 1986; 101:74. Used with permission.)

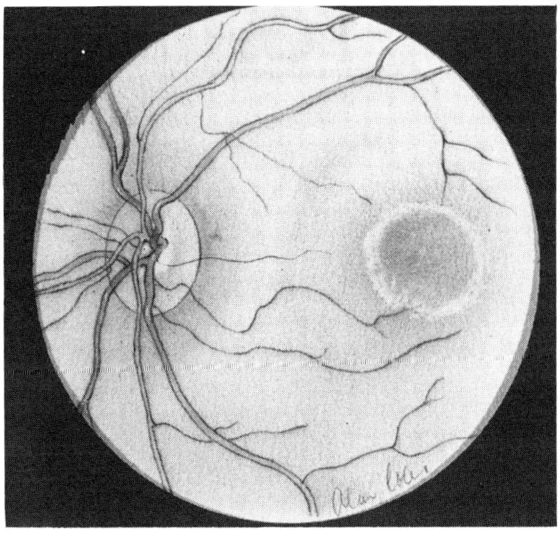

FIG 3–11.
Macular development, stage 3. (From Isenberg SJ: Macular development in the premature infant. *Am J Ophthalmol* 1986; 101:74. Used with permission.)

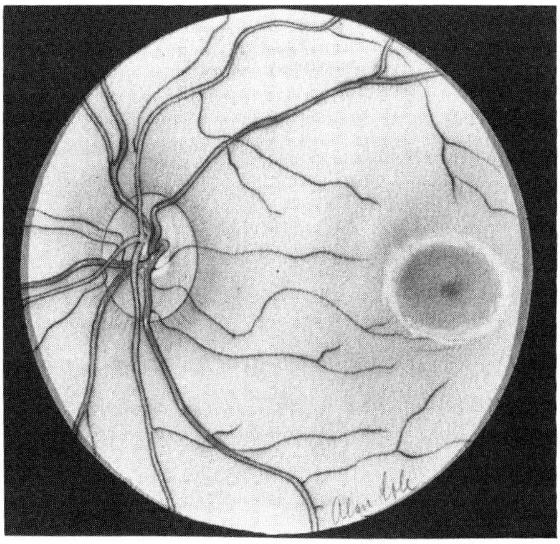

FIG 3–12.
Macular development, stage 4. (From Isenberg SJ: Macular development in the premature infant. *Am J Ophthalmol* 1986; 101:74. Used with permission.)

REFERENCES

1. Smith DW, Jones KL: *Recognizable Patterns of Human Malformation: Genetic, Embryologic and Clinical Aspects*. Philadelphia, WB Saunders Co, 1982, pp 620–622.
2. Smith B, Guberina C: Congenital ocular anomalies, in Kwitko ML (ed): *Surgery of the Infant Eye*. New York, Appleton-Century-Crofts, 1979, pp 53-65.
3. Apt L, Isenberg S: Changes in orbital dimensions following enucleation. *Arch Ophthalmol* 1973; 90:393.
4. Mann IC: *The Development of the Human Eye*. London, Cambridge University Press, 1928, p 41.
5. Whitnall SE: *Anatomy of the Human Orbit*, ed 2. Oxford, Oxon, 1932, pp 98–103.
6. Sivan Y, Merlob P, Reisner SH: Eye measurements in preterm and term newborn infants. *J Craniofac Genet Dev Biol* 1982; 2:239.
7. Mehes K: Palpebral fissure length in newborn infants. *Acta Pediatr Acad Sci Hung* 1980; 21:55.
8. Jones KL, Hanson JW, Smith DW: Palpebral fissure size in newborn infants. *J Pediatr* 1978; 92:787.
9. Hymes C: The postnatal growth of the cornea and palpebral fissure, and the projection of the eyeball in early life. *J Comp Neurol* 1928; 48:415.
10 Iosub S, Fuchs M, Bingol N, et al: Palpebral fissure length in black and Hispanic children: Correlation with head circumference. *Pediatrics* 1985; 75:318.
11. Duke-Elder S: *System of Ophthalmology*, vol 3, pt 1. St Louis, CV Mosby Co, 1963, pp 211–271, 291–313.
12. Isenberg SJ, McCarty JAW, Rich R: Growth of the conjunctival fornices and orbital margin in term and premature infants. *Ophthalmology* 1987; 94:1276–1278.
13. Jeanty P, Dramaix-Wilmet M, Van Gansbeke D, et al: Fetal ocular biometry. *Radiology* 1982; 143:513.
14. Swan KC, Wilkins JH: Extraocular muscle surgery in early infancy—Anatomical factors. *J Pediatr Ophthalmol Strabismus* 1984; 21:44.
15. Sorsby A, Sheridan M: The eye at birth: Measurement of the principal diameters in forty-eight cadavers. *J Anat* 1960; 94:192.
16. Harayama K, Amemiya T, Nishimura H: Development of the eyeball during fetal life. *J Pediatr Ophthalmol Strabismus* 1981; 18:37.
17. Larsen JS: The sagittal growth of the eye. IV. Ultrasonic measurement of the axial length of the eye from birth to puberty. *Acta Ophthalmol* 1971; 49:873.
18. Blomdahl S: Ultrasonic measurements of the eye in the newborn infant. *Acta Ophthalmol* 1979; 57:1048.
19. Goes F: Ocular biometry in childhood. *Bull Soc Belge Ophtalmol* 1982; 202:159.
20. Musarella MA, Morin JD: Anterior segment and intraocular pressure measurements of the unanesthetized premature infant. *Metab Pediatr Syst Ophthalmol* 1982; 8:53.
21. Donzis PB, Insler MS, Gordon RA: Corneal curvature in premature infants. *Am J Ophthalmol* 1985; 99:213.
22. Koenig S, Graul E, Kaufman HE: Ocular refraction after penetrating keratoplasty with infant donor corneas. *Am J Ophthalmol* 1982; 94:534.
23. Girard LJ, Neely W, Sampson WG: The use of alpha chymotrypsin in infants and children. *Am J Ophthalmol* 1962; 54:95.
24. Birnholz JC: Ultrasonic fetal ophthalmology. *Early Hum Dev* 1985; 12:19.
25. Jones HE: Hyaloid remnants in the eyes of premature babies. *Br J Ophthalmol* 1963; 47:39.
26. Renz BE, Vygantas CM: Hyaloid vascular remnants in human neonates. *Ann Ophthalmol* 1977; 9:179.
27. Foos RY, Kopelow SM: Development of the retinal vasculature in paranatal infants. *Surv Ophthalmol* 1973; 18:117.
28. Isenberg SJ: Macular development in the premature infant. *Am J Ophthalmol* 1986; 101:74.
29. Mohn G, Van Hof-van Duin JV: Development of the binocular and monocular visual fields of human infants during the first year of life. *Clin Vis Sci* 1986; 1:51.
30. Banks MS: The development of visual accommodation during early infancy. *Child Dev* 1980; 51:646.
31. Adams RJ, Maurer D, Davis M: Newborns' discrimination of chromatic from achromatic stimuli. *J Exp Child Physchol* 1986; 41:267.
32. Grignolo A, Rivara A: Observations biometriques sur l'oeil des enfants nes terme et des prematures au cours de la premier annee. *Ann Oculist* 1968; 201:817.
33. Cook RC, Glassock RE: Refractive and ocular findings in the newborn. *Am J Ophthalmol* 1951; 34:1407.
34. Goldschmidt E: Refraction in the newborn. *Acta Ophthalmol* 1969; 47:570.

35. Gordon RA, Donzis PB: Refractive development of the human eye. *Arch Ophthalmol* 1985; 103:785.
36. Gwiazda J, Scheiman M, Mohindra I, et al: Astigmatism in children: Changes in axis and amount from birth to six years. *Invest Ophthalmol Vis Sci* 1984; 25:88.
37. Fulton AB, Dobson V, Salem D, et al: Cycloplegic refractions in infants and young children. *Am J Ophthalmol* 1980; 90:239.
38. Thorn F, Held R, Fang LL: Orthogonal astigmatic axes in Chinese and Caucasian infants. *Invest Ophthalmol Vis Sci* 1987; 28:191.
39. Robb RM: Refractive errors associated with hemangiomas of the eyelids and orbit in infancy. *Am J Ophthalmol* 1977; 83:52.
40. Bogan S, Simon JW, Krohel GB, et al: Astigmatism associated with adnexal masses in infancy. *Arch Opthalmol* 1987; 105:1368.
41. Shapiro A, Yanko L, Nawratzki I, et al: Refractive power of premature children at infancy and early childhood. *Am J Ophthalmol* 1980; 90:234.
42. Dobson V, Fulton AB, Manning K, et al: Cycloplegic refractions of premature infants. *Am J Ophthalmol* 1981; 91:490.
43. Nissenkorn I, Yassur Y, Mashkowski D, et al: Myopia in premature infants with and without retinopathy of prematurity. *Br J Ophthalmol* 1983; 67:170.
44. Rutstein RP, Wesson MD, Gotlieb S, et al: Clinical comparison of the visual parameters in infants with intrauterine growth retardation vs. infants with normal birth weight. *Am J Optom Physiol Opt* 1986; 63:697.
45. Hoyt CS, Stone RD, Fromer C, et al: Monocular axial myopia associated with neonatal eyelid closure in human infants. *Am J Ophthalmol* 1981; 91:197.
46. Gordon RA, Donzis PB: Myopia associated with retinopathy of prematurity. *Ophthalmology* 1986; 93:1593.
47. Hittner HM, Hirsch NJ, Rudolph AJ: Assessment of gestational age by examination of the anterior vascular capsule of the lens. *J Pediatr* 1977; 91:455.
48. Hittner HM, Gorman WA, Rudolph AJ: Examination of the anterior vascular capsule of the lens: II. Assessment of gestational age in infants small for gestational age. *J Pediatr Ophthalmol Strabismus* 1981; 18:52.
49. Hittner HM, Speer ME, Rudolph AJ: Examination of the anterior vascular capsule of the lens: III. Abnormalities in infants with congenital infection. *J Pediatr Ophthalmol Strabismus* 1981; 18:55.
50. Isenberg SJ: Macular development in the premature infant. *Am J Ophthalmol* 1986; 101:74.
51. Johnson BL, Ahdab-Barmada M: Hyperoxemic retinal neuronal necrosis in the premature neonate. *Am J Ophthalmol* 1986; 102:423.
52. Abramov I, Gordon J, Hendricksen A, et al: The retina of the newborn human infant. *Science* 1982; 217:265.
53. Horsten GPM, Winkelman JE: Electrical activity of the retina in relation to histological differentiation in infants born prematurely and at full-term. *Vision Res* 1962; 2:269.
54. Hoyt CS, Jastrzebski G, Marg E: Delayed visual maturation in infancy. *Br J Ophthalmol* 1983; 67:127.
55. Weale RA: Ocular anatomy and refraction. *Doc Ophthalmol* 1983; 55:361.

4 Visual Acuity Assessment of the Preverbal Patient

David S. Friendly, M.D.

Visual assessment of an infant, like the evaluation of other biologic functions, requires a history, physical examination, and appropriate laboratory studies. The history can be divided into medical and ophthalmologic portions. The ocular examination centers on evaluation of both fixation and following. New laboratory methods including optokinetic nystagmus (OKN), preferential viewing (PV), and pattern-evoked visual potentials (PEVP) have recently been introduced and may improve the accuracy of diagnosis. This article presents updated approach to visual assessment of the preverbal child.

HISTORY AND PHYSICAL EXAMINATION

If serious medical disorders are present, the medical history requires the development of a family pedigree. The mother should be questioned about viral infections, use of legal and illegal drugs, and exposure to ionizing radiation during pregnancy. Complications during pregnancy or at the time of delivery that might affect the fetus should likewise be recorded; included are conditions such as toxemia, maternal bleeding, premature rupture of membranes, and premature birth. Severe health problems involving the neonate may also be relevant. Of particular interest are events that might cause central nervous system damage and signs of such damage such as fetal distress, seizures, respiratory arrest, and low Apgar scores.

Growth and development should be evaluated. The possibility of delayed growth, mental retardation, and physical retardation should be explored.

Established medical or neurological abnormalities should be made known. Questions should be asked concerning hospitalizations, medications, and surgery. The patient's general medical records may contain pertinent information. It is therefore useful to obtain the names of all nonophthalmologic physicians previously consulted, laboratory studies ordered, and the results obtained.

The eye history should be elicited in some detail. If there is a family history of ocular disorders, particularly those commencing early in life, a family tree should be constructed, with affected individuals appropriately noted. It may be helpful to obtain the eye office records of other family members.

Parental observations of the child's eyes and visual behavior may suggest which diagnostic procedures should be emphasized. Any suspected eye abnormalities should be noted. A history of visual deprivation as suggested by cataracts or other opacities of the media, severe ptosis, or prolonged patching is ex-

TABLE 4–1.
Normal Human Visual Development

Function	Age
Visual fixation present	Birth
Fixation well developed	6–9 wk
Visual following	3 mo
Accommodation	4 mo
Stereopsis	4 mo

tremely relevant. Information on past ocular treatment including patching, glasses, and extended use of eye drops is essential. If the child has already been seen by an eye specialist, examination and laboratory findings, diagnoses, treatments, and recommendations from these consultations should be obtained.

Thorough medical and eye examinations are essential. Particular attention should be directed to light-induced pupillary reflexes; a swinging light test for a Marcus Gunn pupillary defect should be done. The examiner should be aware that lid closure to bright light (such as that of the indirect ophthalmoscope) and intact pupillary light reflexes do not necessarily indicate cortical visual function. Because the pathways that subserve pupillary light reflexes are subcortical, their presence is compatible with cortical blindness.

Tests for ocular alignment (Hirschberg, Krimsky, and cover tests) and range of ocular movements (induced, if necessary, by turning the child's head rapidly) are essential. Abnormal eye movements in one or both eyes (such as nystagmus) should be noted. Thorough study of the ocular anatomy is also important; this may require hand-held slit-lamp biomicroscopy of the anterior segment. Cycloplegic retinoscopy and careful indirect ophthalmoscopy, with particular attention to the macula and optic disc, are essential. Ocular examination of the child's parents and siblings may also provide useful information.

It may be worthwhile to refer the patient to other specialists, particularly if other defects are suspected or known. Dysmorphologists, geneticists, neurologists, neonatologists, and pediatricians can all be helpful in this regard.

Laboratory tests, including electroretinography, and computed tomography (CT) scans of the orbits and brain as well as the laboratory tests mentioned in detail in the following sections may be informative.

CLINICAL ASSESSMENT OF CENTRAL VISION

The development of central vision is outlined in Table 4–1. Newborns have ocular fixation, but their pursuit movements consist of course, jerky, hypometric saccades. Pursuit movements do not become smooth until about 3 months of age. It should be emphasized, however, that there are wide variations in the rate of visual development; Table 4–1 provides only mean values. Some infants have significant delays in fixation and following; these visually late bloomers frequently have other medical problems as well, including premature birth and delayed generalized motor development.[1] The lack of other ophthalmologic findings, particularly the absence of nystagmus, helps to distinguish patients in this group from those with organic pathology. Disorders of eye movement such as those found in patients with ocular motor apraxia can be confused with blindness in young individuals. Conspicuous head thrusts suggest this uncommon neuro-ophthalmologic condition.[2]

Assessment of vision in the preverbal child centers on evaluation of the fixation and following ability of each eye under both monocular and binocular conditions. In infants, these reflexes are studied at close range; in toddlers, they are studied at a distance as well as at close range. For infants, a human face and hand-held lights are suitable fixation targets. For young preverbal children, moving, lighted toys, movies, wiggle pictures, or other targets that require accurate accommodation are appropriate.

To evaluate fixation and following, one eye is covered. The examiner's thumb is probably the least threatening and best tolerated means of occluding the infant's eye. A flashlight beam is directed to the patient's face, and the examiner attempts to obtain fixation with the nonoccluded eye by tapping the light, flashing it, or moving it slightly. If accomodative-type targets are used, they may be touched by the toddler or moved about to heighten interest and attention.

Patient cooperation may be difficult to obtain, particularly, if the infant is hungry, frightened, or tired. A pacifier or fluid-filled bottle that permits the child to suck or swallow during the examination may be helpful. The possibility that the child will associate the visit with previous unpleasant office experiences may be reduced by avoiding white coats and other nonessential medical paraphernalia and paying attention to office decor. A homelike environment, which is generally less threatening to the young patient, may promote better cooperation. If the child is extremely somnolent, it may be advisable to postpone the examination. The examiner should ascertain the time of day the child is most alert (frequently early morning) and schedule the appointment as close as possible to that time.

The position of the corneal light reflex in reference to the center of the cornea is noted. If it is centrally located, the letter C is recorded, and fixation is assumed to be foveal. Next, the target (or if necessary, the child's head) is slowly moved, and the patient's ability to follow the object is observed. If the eye maintains alignment with both the stationary and moving object, fixation and following are said to be steady, and the letter S is recorded. Note that S implies both good fixation and following ability. Also note that fixation and following are both studied under monocular testing conditions.

The occluder is then removed. The examiner seeks to determine whether, under binocular conditions, the previously fixating eye continues to fixate or whether the previously occluded eye takes up fixation. This maintenance (M) or failure of maintenance of fixation can be evaluated only in the presence of strabismus, either natural or optically induced with a vertical prism. If both foveas are aligned with the target at the moment the occluder is withdrawn, foveal fixation preference cannot be appreciated because in this test foveal fixation preference is revealed by eye movement.

Binocular fixation preference can be quantitated by assessing the ability of each eye to maintain fixation on the basis of time, through one or more blinks, or despite movement of the object. Attempts to correlate fixation behavior with Snellen acuities have been only partially successful.[3] The greatest discrepancy between the two measures occurs in patients with small-angle esotropia, who may show very strong fixation preferences despite equal or nearly equal Snellen acuities.[4]

The binocular fixation preference can be examined in straight-eyed patients by means of a ten-prism, diopter prism held vertically before one or the other eye. Unfortunately, many patients with amblyopia will alternate fixation with this test.[5]

Conventional fixation preference techniques, although sensitive, generally lack sufficient specificity. Diagnoses based on such techniques will lead to some unnecessary treatment. This is not of major concern, however, because such treatment is unlikely to harm the patient if follow-up is obtained at frequent intervals to guard against occlusion-induced amblyopia. Inadequate treatment is the much more common error.

Avoidance movements, manifested by the patient's repeated attempts to maneuver around an occluder applied to one eye and an absence of such movements when the occluder is applied to the other, are at times quite helpful in establishing the presence of a significant difference in visual acuity between the two eyes. In the author's experience, it is often difficult to reproduce such avoidance movements consistently in infants, even in those with profound amblyopia. Nontheless, such behavior when present can be very helpful in diagnosis.

The Visuscope projects a target on the patient's retina. With this modified ophthalmoscope, one may directly observe both the retinal area selected for fixation and the fixation target through a dilated pupil. This per-

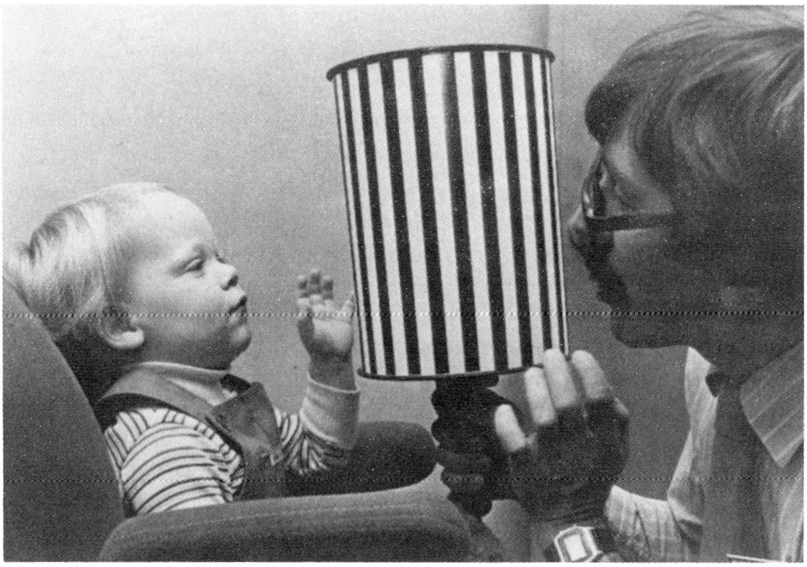

FIG 4–1.
OKN eye movements are elicited by rotating a striped drum before a subject's eyes. (From Nelson LB: *Pediatric Ophthalmology.* Philadelphia, WB Saunders Co, 1984, p 22. Used with permission.)

mits documentation of eccentric fixation. Micronystagmus is readily apparent by visuscopy because of the retinal magnification obtained. This technique is occasionally suitable for toddlers, but not for infants because of the degree of cooperation required.

The use of fixation, following, and avoidance movements to diagnose unilateral central visual loss in infants is still more an art than a science. The experienced pediatric ophthalmologist uses the patient's medical history, caretaker observations, and previous ophthalmologic findings as well as office observations in making a tentative diagnosis. A unilateral visual loss is far easier to detect than bilateral loss because of the ease of comparing visual behavior between the two eyes. Bilateral symmetrical visual loss, unless profound, is much more difficult to determine by conventional clinical methods.

Obviously, clinical measures of visual acuity in the preverbal child are quite imperfect. Specialized laboratory methods are now being introduced. These include OKN; PV, with and without operant conditioning; and PEVP. Each of these relatively new techniques has certain advantages and disadvantages. All require visual attention and accurate accommodation. In sleepy infants, this can be a significant problem.

LABORATORY METHODS—OPTOKINETIC NYSTAGMUS, PREFERENTIAL VIEWING, AND PATTERN-EVOKED VISUAL POTENTIAL

Optokinetic Nystagmus

OKN is the familiar type of nystagmus that occurs when a subject fixates on a moving target such as stripes on a rotating drum. Following-type eye movements and quick restorative eye movements occur. The slow following eye movements are at the same velocity as the target, while the fast restorative eye movements are independent of the speed of movement of the target. The combination of slow movements in one direction and fast movements in the opposite direction constitute a jerk-type nystagmus known as OKN (Fig 4–1).

A motor response is required for OKN; what is measured is a combination of sensory and motor functions. This probably explains why acuity scores obtained with both this method and PV, which also requires a motor

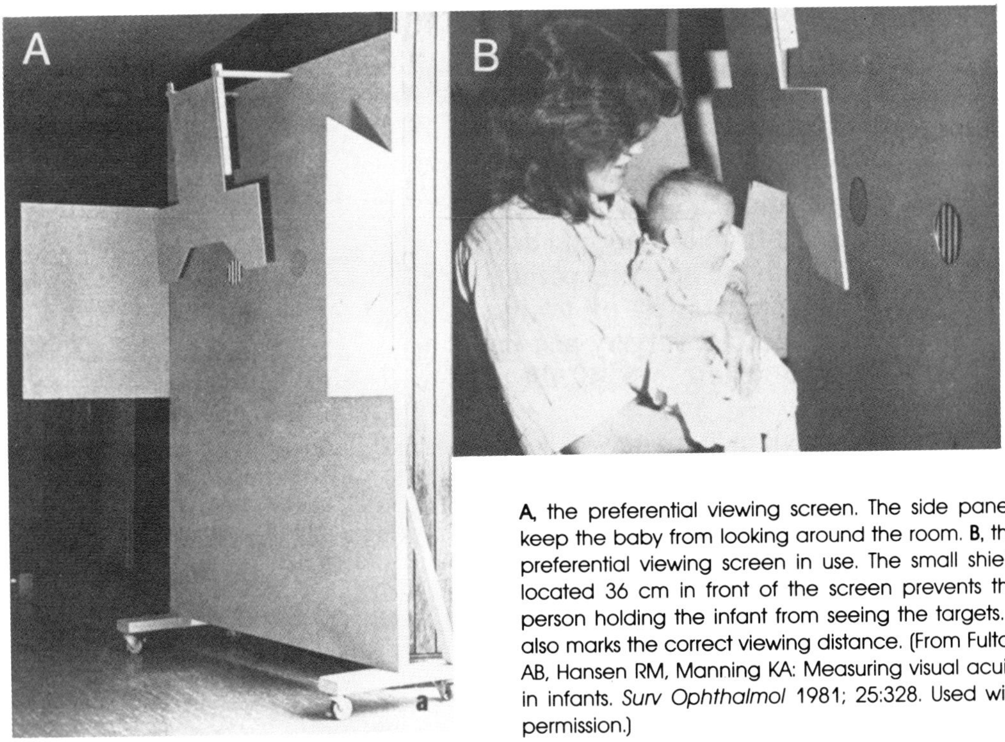

A, the preferential viewing screen. The side panels keep the baby from looking around the room. **B**, the preferential viewing screen in use. The small shield located 36 cm in front of the screen prevents the person holding the infant from seeing the targets. It also marks the correct viewing distance. (From Fulton AB, Hansen RM, Manning KA: Measuring visual acuity in infants. *Surv Ophthalmol* 1981; 25:328. Used with permission.)

response, are lower than those obtained with PEVP. Early cortical PEVP responses mature more rapidly, perhaps because they are purely sensory and represent earlier stages of visual neural processing.

Optokinetic responses may be difficult to detect by simple observation. Eye movement sensing devices can be used for this purpose; however, infants and young children do not tolerate them well, and they are expensive. Test parameters such as speed of movement of the target, eye-target distance, and target characteristics are not standardized. Moreover, some investigators have shown a poor correlation between the dynamic visual acuities obtained with OKN methods and Snellen acuities.[6,7] Normal infants under 3 months of age have asymmetrical OKN responses.[8] OKN may be driven monocularly if the motion of the patterned field is from a temporal to a nasal direction (i.e., toward the nose), but not if the direction is reversed. This may be a reflection of the adaptive mechanism seen in some primitive adult mammals that allows suppression of visual stimuli associated with forward motion.

For these reasons, OKN testing is not widely used for the assessment of visual acuity at the present time. When an infant or young child responds to OKN testing, some vision must be present; however, lack of response in such a patient has uncertain significance.

Preferential Viewing

PV has received more publicity than either OKN or PEVP. There are many variations of the test; however, all are based on the tendency of subjects to fixate on a patterned stimulus in preference to a target of similar size and space-averaged luminance. Grating patterns and homogeneous test objects are randomly assigned to right or left viewing ports and are shown to infants at a known distance. An observer who does not know which side the test pattern is on judges on which object the infant fixates by making note of head and eye movements (Fig 4–2). The width of stripes that compose the grating may be reduced until there is no preference to fixate on the patterned stimulus. At this point, both objects presumably appear the same to the infant. In practice, a 75% correct response level is usually used as the end point of the psychometric function. This point is numerically halfway between the two extreme possible end points of the function—100% correct and 50% correct. (The latter would be the expected performance if the infant could not resolve the stripes).

The results of PV testing are usually expressed in terms of spatial frequency or cycles per degree. A one-octave difference in spatial frequency corresponds to a halving or doubling of the spatial frequency. Thus, there are one-octave differences between 30 and 60 and between 60 and 120 cycles per degree. By definition, the 20/20 Snellen E symbol subtends overall 5 minutes of arc. Each component letter stroke width subtends one minute, or 1/60 degree of arc at 20 ft. A complete cycle or wave would correspond to two stroke widths, or 2/60 (1/30) degree of arc. In other words, 20/20 Snellen corresponds in a strictly geometric sense to 30 cycles per degree.

Conventional two-alternative, forced-choice PV is possible only up to about 6 months of age. Patients become too inattentive after that age unless behavioral reinforcement is provided. By offering rewards for correct responses in the form of moving toys[9] or food such as Cheerios,[10] the breakfast cereal, the testable range can be extended to the age of 3 years.

Conventional laboratory forced-choice testing involves more than 100 separate stimulus presentations. Such testing takes an hour or more and requires the use of three adults. Because such rigorous laboratory methods are impractical in terms of testing time and personnel, clinical modifications of the test have been made. One approach is to use diagnostic gratings.[11] In this stratagem, an exact acuity value is not determined; instead, the infant's vision is located between predetermined values. This method is much faster than conventional testing; it requires only 5 to 10 minutes per eye and is useful for screening purposes. Another approach is to use a staircase paradigm, In such testing procedures, the visual acuity threshold is straddled by predetermined step increases or decreases in target size, depending on the correctness of the infant's response. The acuity levels produced by such methods are, however, misleading if only a small number of trials are used. The most recent variation of the PV technique is the use of "acuity cards."[12] In this method, cards with gratings on one side and a gray luminance matched target on the other are shown to infants at a known distance. The examiner observes the child's responses through a peephole in the center of the card. Progressively finer gratings are shown until the 50% correct level is reached. Binocular acuity may be measured in 3 to 5 minutes with this test. Monocular acuity testing is usually more difficult than binocular, presumably because of the irritation and distraction produced by the occluder. The examiner is not masked to the grating, and all the infant's behavior is used in determining whether the pattern is seen. Because customary safeguards to prevent bias are not used, this test lacks methodological vigor. Some have claimed that this less strict testing technique provides information similar to that obtained in more rigorous PV testing[12]; however, sufficient clinical experience from different centers has not been accumulated to verify this hypothesis.

In a recent study,[13] reasonably close agreement between acuity card estimates was found by two highly experienced, masked examiners. Validity comparisons with conventional PV testing was also good. Whether less experienced examiners can perform as well has yet to be established.

One of the most significant problems with the PV approach is that for each presentation there is a 50-50 chance of correctly guessing which side the patterned stimulus is on. Consequently, many iterations are required to obtain small confidence intervals. In fact, after 20 trials of optimally sized gratings presented in a staircase fashion, there is at least a $1\frac{1}{2}$ octave error in the acuity estimate. Thus, if a 20-trial staircase procedure yields a nominal acuity estimate of 20/140, the procedure has really shown only that the child's visual acuity is between 20/50 and 20/400.[12]

With a 20-trial staircase procedure, a difference of at least $1\frac{1}{2}$ octaves between the two eyes must be demonstrated before the test can be considered reliable at an α level of .05, and this assumes optimum selection of grating target spatial frequencies.[14] The lack of sensitivity of PV with small sample sizes substantially limits its utility; in fact, PV tests performed with small sample sizes may provide little additional useful information to that obtained by standard clinical methods.

Another serious difficulty with this procedure is that gratings (the most frequently used targets) provide falsely high acuities in many patients with amblyopia. The reasons for this phenomenon are somewhat speculative; nonetheless, the observation has been made so frequently[15–17] that there can be little doubt as to its validity. In this regard, the common practice of equating spatial frequencies of grating targets used in PV testing and Snellen acuities should be questioned.

Modifications of the forced-choice PV test are convenient for office use. A version of the acuity cards is presently commercially available.

Pattern-Evoked Visual Potentials

The PEVP is recorded by means of occipitally placed scalp electrodes. The normally large amplitude background electroencephalographic (EEG) activity can be separated from the small-amplitude cortical waves generated by a visual stimulus only through the use of computer averaging. Over many iterations, background EEG waves will tend to sum to zero at specific time intervals after the visual stimulus if the latter occur at random in relationship to the EEG waves. If the stimulus (which often consists of rapidly alternating black and white checkerboard squares or stripes) is shown 50 to 100 times, the characteristic complex wave form of the PEVP may be discriminated by computer averaging. The technique reduces the background noise by the square root of N, where N is the number of iterations.

Accurate accommodation on the target is essential; fixation should be monitored continuously. Electrodes must be accurately applied to the scalp in order to receive the time-locked, computer-average signal. This can be difficult in young patients. PEVP also requires expensive equipment and specially trained technicians. Older techniques such as presenting reversing squares of a single size (for example, 15-minute squares) are associated with both false-negative and false-positive results.[18] Steady-state PEVP, a newer method, holds considerable promise.[19] In this technique, the visual stimuli are presented in very rapid succession rather than once or twice per second.

When a pattern is rapidly alternated, the detailed waveform of the transient PEVP is no longer discernible; instead, the tracing resembles a sine wave at the frequency of the pattern reversal. By presenting a continuously changing pattern size and analyzing response characteristics by fast Fourier transform methods, it is possible to obtain the stimulus size-response amplitude function. Visual acuity may be estimated in as little as 10 seconds by this sweep technique,[19] in contrast to transient PEVP methods that require recording over a 30- to 60-second interval for each spatial frequency (stimulus size) tested.

Insufficient pediatric clinical experience has yet been obtained to determine the reliability, validity, and cost-benefit ratio of PEVP testing for acuity measurement.

Comparisons of OKN, PV, and PEVP acuity data from normal subjects according to age are shown graphically in Figure 4–3.

CONCLUSION

As the reader can readily appreciate, a wholly satisfactory method of accurately assessing visual acuity in the preverbal child has yet to be developed; however, rapid progress is being made in this important field. Based on the advances made in the past 10 to 15 years, there is ample cause for optimism.

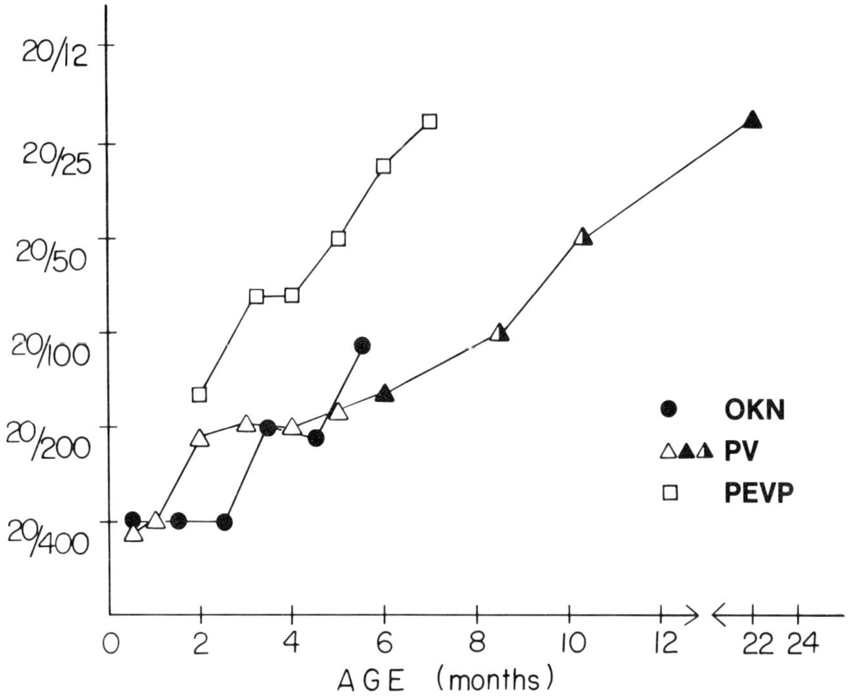

FIG 4–3.
Visual acuity is shown as a function of age according to three techniques: OKN, PV, and PEVP. All methods show improvement in visual acuity with age. (From Fulton AB, Hansen RN, Manning KA: Measuring visual acuity in infants. *Surv Ophthalmol* 1981; 25:326. Used with permission.)

REFERENCES

1. Hoyt CS, Jastrzebski G, Marg E: Delayed visual maturation in infancy. *Br J Ophthalmol* 1983; 67:127.
2. Cogan DG: Congenital ocular motor apraxia. *Can J Ophthalmol* 1966; 1:253.
3. Wilcox LM, Sokol S: Changes in the binocular fixation patterns and the visually evoked potential in the treatment of esotropia with amblyopia. *Ophthalmology* 1980; 87:1273.
4. Zipf RF: Binocular fixation pattern. *Arch Ophthalmol* 1976; 94:401.
5. Wright KW, Edelman PM, Walonker F, et al: Reliability of fixation preference testing in diagnosing amblyopia. *Arch Ophthalmol* 1986; 104:549.
6. Khan SG, Chen KFC, Frenkel M: Subjective and objective visual acuity testing techniques. *Arch Ophthalmol* 1976; 94:2086.
7. Atkinson J, Braddick O, Pimm-Smith E, et al: Does the Catford drum give an accurate assessment of acuity? *Br J Ophthalmol* 1981; 65:652.
8. Atkinson J: Development of optokinetic nystagmus in the human infant and monkey infant: An analogue to development in kittens, in Freeman RD (ed): *Developmental Neurobiology of Vision*. New York, Plenum Publishing Corp, 1979.
9. Mayer DL, Dobson V: Assessment of vision in young children: A new operant approach yields estimates of acuity. *Invest Ophthalmol Vis Sci* 1980; 19:566.
10. Birch EE, Naegele J, Bauer JA, et al: Visual acuity of toddlers tested by operant and preferential looking techniques. *Invest Ophthalmol Vis Sci* (suppl.) 1980; 20(suppl):210.
11. Dobson V, Salem D, Mayer DL, et al: Visual acuity screening of children 6 months to 3 years of age. *Invest Ophthalmol Vis Sci* 1985; 26:1057.
12. McDonald MA, Dobson V, Sebris SL, et al: The acuity card procedure: A rapid test of infant acuity. *Invest Ophthalmol Vis Sci* 1985; 26:1158.
13. Preston KL, McDonald M, Sebris SL, et al: Validation of the acuity card procedure for assessment of infants with ocular disorders. *Ophthalmology* 1987; 94:644.
14. Teller DY: Measurement of visual acuity in

human and monkey infants: the interface between laboratory and clinic. *Behav Brain Res* 1983; 10:15.

15. Mayer DL, Fulton AB, Rodier D: Grating and recognition acuities of pediatric patients. *Ophthalmology* 1984; 91:947.
16. Gstalder RJ, Green DG: Laser interferometric acuity in amblyopia. *J. Pediatr Ophthalmol Strabismus* 1971; 8:251.
17. Harris SJ, Hansen RM, Fulton AB: Assessment of acuity of amblyopic subjects using face, grating, and recognition stimuli. *Invest Ophthalmol Vis Sci* 1986; 27:1184.
18. Friendly DS, Weiss IP, Barnet AB, et al: Pattern-reversal visual-evoked potentials in the diagnosis of amblyopia in children. *Am J Ophthalmol* 1986; 102:329.
19. Norcia AM, Tyler CW: Spatial frequency sweep VEP: Visual acuity during the first year of life. *Vision Res* 1985; 25:1399.

5 Examination Methods

Sherwin J. Isenberg, M.D.

When examining the adult eye, we assume that we will have full cooperation from the patient, and we usually receive it. When examining the eyes of children and even older infants, we use many unusual fixation devices and are pleasantly satisfied when the children cooperate a good part of the time. However, when examining the eyes of newborns, we should not expect any cooperation. Instead, because of the precarious stability of neonates, ophthalmologists and pediatricians should concentrate on obtaining the needed information with concern for the safety of the neonate. As will be explained, the information one tries to obtain from the examination of an infant's eye is not quite the same as that desired from the eyes of older children or adults.

HISTORY

When the physician is called to examine a newborn in the nursery, a parent is usually not available to provide a history. Fortunately, the baby's chart will usually have the desired information. From the chart, one can learn details of the pregnancy, including the use of medications, fevers, skin rashes, infections (venereal or otherwise), and social history such as drug or alcohol abuse. All newborn charts will contain extensive documentation of the delivery. Concerning the eye, we are most interested in the newborn's gestational age, birth weight, Apgar scores, evidence of anoxic episodes such as seizure activity, resuscitative efforts, duration and level of supplemental oxygen, birth trauma, and any congenital anomalies (especially those of the head and neck). In addition, for infants hospitalized 1 or 2 days beyond birth, the chart will document any subsequent illnesses and medications. While it may still be important to interview the mother to answer other questions such as a family history of ocular disease, we must be sensitive to the state of mind and body of the newly delivered mother.

For the infant presenting in the office, the parent can be a better source of information. In addition to the aforementioned desired historical information, one should also ask about visual and nonvisual milestones. The nonvisual milestones will indicate the overall progress of the child. If the child is delayed in all his other milestones, the visual milestones will usually be delayed. The three most important visual milestones to inquire about are (1) turning toward light (phototropism is present even in flowers!), which is present shortly after birth; (2) following the mother's face, which is also apparent shortly after birth; and (3) following (or "tracking") objects by about 2 to 3 months of life.

VISUAL ACUITY TESTING

Ophthalmologists are taught on the first day of residency that the most important and therefore the first information to be obtained in the ocular examination is visual acuity. In newborns, however, the assessment of vision can be quite difficult. These problems arise from the tendency of neonates to fall asleep at the most inopportune times. To improve

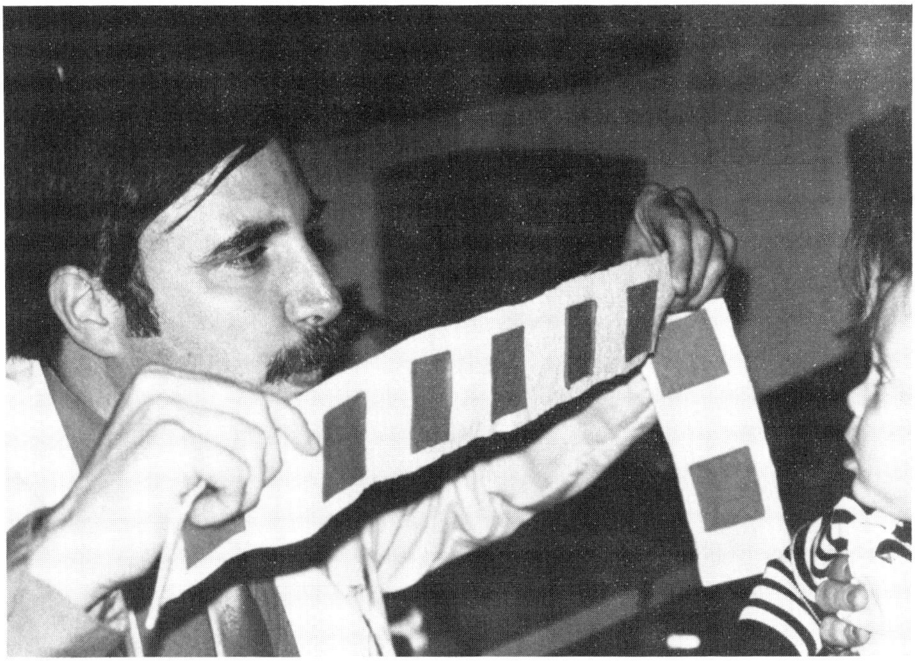

FIG 5–1.
Optokinetic nystagmus in a newborn can be induced with colored squares on a white background.

the chances of even the most minimal amount of cooperation, one should try to examine the newborn just before his feeding. Even while the baby is crying, you can assess his response to visual stimuli.

To which stimuli will a neonate respond beyond 32 weeks of gestational age? Newborns will generally not respond to accommodative targets, i.e., targets with form. However, they will transiently follow faces, especially that of the mother.[1] This may be used as evidence of vision. A light should not be used as a target since one needs only bare light perception to briefly follow a light. In the best of circumstances, one may observe the newborn turn to a diffuse light source such as a window in a dimly lit room in daytime.[2] Neonates will often demonstrate aversive behavior to very bright lights such as the indirect ophthalmoscope. The aversive behavior may be manifested by turning the head away from the light, blinking, or rotating the eyes away from the direct light. An absence of these signs should not be interpreted as a sign of blindness since the newborn may only be inattentive. The presence of these signs does not preclude absent or poor vision in one eye.

The newborn's visual acuity can be assessed by several methods. These methods include preferential forced looking and electrophysiological tests. Because these tests are not generally available to clinicians, they will not be discussed here but are presented in detail in Chapters 4 and 29. Optokinetic nystagmus (OKN), however, is of practical value in the nursery or the office and can be elicited from neonates even shortly after birth. In newborns, the central retina is quite immature.[3] Laboratory studies have established the visual acuity in the first 2 months of life to be no better than 20/400.[4] However, the peripheral portion of the retina can be stimulated by these OKN mechanisms, even in newborns.[5]

OKN can be induced by the use of either a rotating drum or cloth flag (Fig 5–1). Because the examiner often works in tight quarters, whether in the nursery huddled over an incubator, or in the office with the mother holding the infant, a cloth flag is easier to use. To maximize the newborn's fleeting attention, the flag should be held very close to the infant's eye with the other eye patched. It is preferable for the flag to contain rather wide (about 1 in.) black or colored strips on a white field to maximize contrast.

One must be cautious in interpreting responses to OKN. The neonate must be somewhat attentive to perceive the stimulus. The examiner must present the stimulus in vertical and horizontal orientations and not declare the response as positive unless the baby responds with both vertical and horizontal nystagmus appropriately. The examiner should not be fooled by considering the random movements of neonates as a nystagmus response.[6] While visual acuity values have been assigned to neonates on the basis of the size of the stripes to which the newborn responds,[5] the clinician should generally look for any definitely positive response as evidence that the child has vision. The absence of responses should not be considered conclusive evidence that babies are blind since they may be inattentive or actually sleeping. Producing nystagmus requires involvement of the oculomotor system, which may be defective or simply immature. Finally, neonates have been found to initially demonstrate poor vision in addition to absent electrophysiological responses only to later develop normal vision.[7]

Nystagmus can also provide information in another way. The vestibulo-ocular reflex can be stimulated by opposing the face of the newborn to that of the examiner and rotating around the infant. If the infant properly fixates on the face, nystagmus will be inhibited. In addition, after cessation of rotation, a sighted infant will generally stop nystagmus before the third beat or within 5 seconds, while a blind infant will allow nystagmus to endure longer.[8]

At 2 to 4 months of age, infants will begin following targets that are the size of conventional finger puppets (Fig 5–2). Enhancing these targets with a light placed within the puppet will engender more interest by the baby. With one of the infant's eyes occluded, the examiner should evaluate whether the infant fixates on the target centrally and steadily and then follows the target as it moved horizontally and vertically. Fulfillment of these

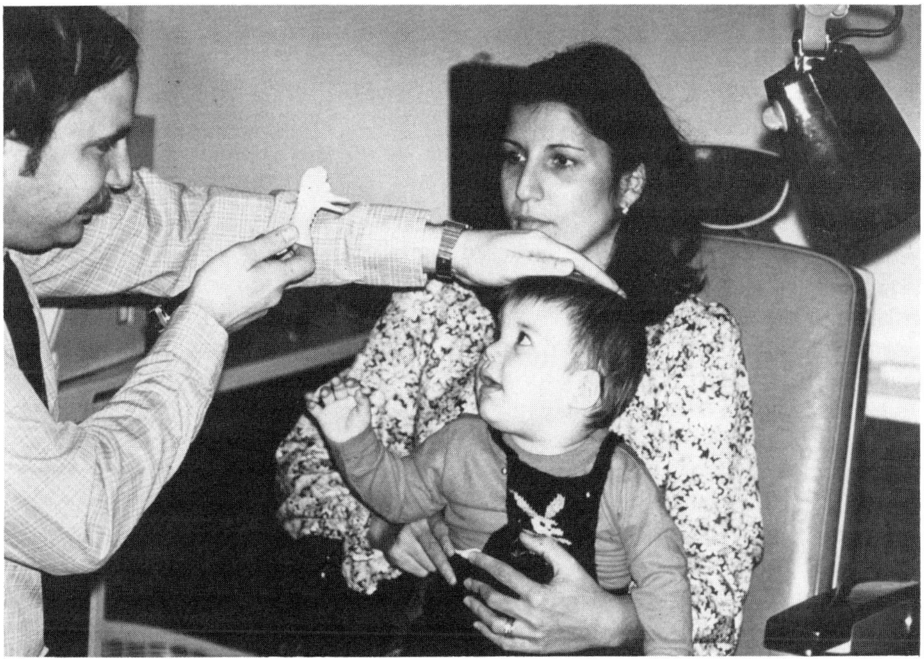

FIG 5–2.
Infant visually tracking a near target of interest.

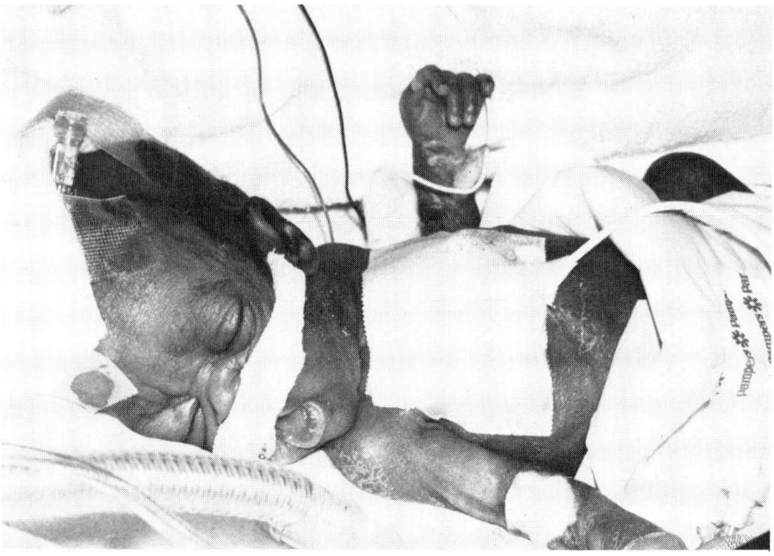

FIG 5–3.
An intubated newborn surrounded by monitors and other equipment is difficult to examine properly.

criteria by each eye usually signifies normal vision of each in the absence of strabismus. With strabismus, the examiner should also compare the ability of each eye to hold fixation relative to the other. If the infant spontaneously alternates fixation between the eyes or holds indefinitely with either eye, amblyopia is probably absent. However, if the baby consistently switches to one eye, one must consider the diagnosis of amblyopia in the nonpreferred eye. As amblyopia is treated, the duration that fixation is held by the nonpreferred eye can be used as an indication of the effectiveness of therapy. Any eye considered amblyopic should be carefully examined to rule out organic disease.

When congenital esotropia is present, the examiner may find that the infant will fixate on objects to his left with his right eye and on objects to his right with his left eye. One should not be overly impressed with this cross-fixation since amblyopia may still be present. The fixation pattern with the target held directly in front of the baby must still be carefully evaluated.

An uncooperative infant should not discourage the examiner from assessing the visual acuity. A mildly hungry infant will often cooperate better than a very hungry infant, who will be irritable, or a recently fed infant, who will probably be sleeping. Should doubts remain about the child's visual acuity after the examination, one should not hesitate to reexamine the patient after a partial feeding or on another day.

GENERAL TECHNIQUES

Nursery

Performing an ophthalmic examination in the nursery is a challenge for the ophthalmologist. To many ophthalmologists, the nursery environment may be as strange as a visit to a distant planet. During daytime hours, there is constant action and movement by nurses, physicians, phlebotomists, radiology technicians, and microbiological technicians. The incubators are surrounded by many different types of monitors, respirators, and infusion machines (Fig 5–3). The noise of the machinery and the frequent beeping, chirping, and ringing of the various alarms can make the ophthalmologist uncomfortable. The infant may have tubes and lines seeming to enter or exit every conceivable port in his body. Nurseries are illuminated at high intensities, which makes the darker working environment of ophthalmologists very difficult to achieve. While darkening the room for an ophthalmic examination may be beneficial for the infant to be examined, the darkness will often interfere with the care of a nearby neonate.

To minimize these difficulties, the ophthalmologist should familiarize himself with the routine in his nursery. Often, the late afternoon is a time of less noise and action than the morning. Movable screens can be used to block nearby lights and noises. Some incubators are constructed to permit manipulation of the infant and his eyes with less repositioning of the infant than are others. Infants requiring frequent ocular examinations can be positioned in a darker part of the nursery or in an area that has individual light controls. Finally, it is advisable never to examine the infant in the presence of his family in the nursery. Parents may easily misinterpret comments or actions or become concerned at the alarms that occasionally ring during the examination. In addition, parents will nearly always be disturbed by the sight of the ophthalmologist performing scleral depression.

Despite these problems, the nursery can be a fascinating place in which to appreciate the role of systemic physiological changes and their effect on the eye, and vice versa. Only in the nursery can an ophthalmologist examine an eye that should still be in utero and experience "in vivo embryology."

The Office

Examining neonates and infants in the office strains the ophthalmologist's ability to innovate and entertain. The short attention span of these babies forces the examiner to be quick, energetic, noisy, childish, and yet thorough. One needs to obtain as much information in as short a period of time as possible while maintaining the child's interest. To accomplish this, it is convenient to divide the ophthalmic examination into two groups of techniques—those that require cooperation from the child and those that do not. Certainly, under the age of 2 months (following 39 weeks of true or partially artificial gestation), we should not expect any cooperation from the child. In older infants, tasks that demand some cooperation include visual acuity determinations, ocular motility testing, and the anterior segment examination. For these tasks, the examiner should be armed with a variety of toys, especially larger toys that are noisy and colorful to better maintain the child's attention. However, silent toys are preferable when determining the fixation pattern to be sure that the baby is following the target visually and not following a noise with his eyes. Infants tire of any target after about 1 minute; therefore it is helpful to have a sizable collection. If it is desirable for the examiner to have both hands free for the examination, he may use toys held in his mouth such as kazoos or airplanes that make noise and spin propellers upon blowing.

For tasks that do not require the infant's cooperation such as retinoscopy, ophthalmoscopy, portable biomicroscopy, and pupil examination, one can still use the aforementioned toys to maintain the child's goodwill and increase the speed of examination. The ophthalmologist should not hesitate to make animal sounds or other noises to keep the baby interested. If the child is too irritable to cooperate, the ophthalmologist's ultimate weapon is have the child fed. With baby under the influence of the bottle or breast, one can usually easily perform the aforementioned tasks and even the removal of superficial corneal foreign bodies! If these measures fail, restraining the child by having the mother sit the child upright in her lap, placing his legs between hers, and maintaining the child's elbows over his ears with his arms extended facilitate exposing and examining the eye.

EXAMINATION OF OCULAR MOTILITY

In the first few weeks of life, the position of the eyes varies greatly.[6] Thus, one should not be overly concerned about the eye position prior to 1 month of age unless an abnormal eye position is constant or nearly constant. To test the eye position in primary (or straight ahead) near gaze, use noisy toys either on or immediately adjacent to a light. The examiner should then note an abnormal displacement of the light reflex away from the center of the cornea in term of Hirschberg values (15 degrees at the pupillary margin, 25 degrees midway between the pupillary margin and the corneoscleral junction, and 45 degrees at the junction). This Hirschberg determination is an approximation and should be seriously considered only if the infant does not permit a more objective test. For better precision, the prism-light reflex test may then be used in which a prism is used to move the abnormal light reflex to the normal visual axis. However, when the prism-reflex test can be performed, the infant will almost always cooperate with the cover test, which is more objective. In this test, the examiner gently places his palm on the child's head and covers one eye and then the other with his thumb. Normally, neither eye should move. If the uncovered eye moves to pick up fixation, strabismus is present. Prisms can then be used to neutralize the shift and quantitate the strabismus.

After 6 months of age, infants will generally begin to fixate on distant targets, thereby permitting the use of noisy mechanical toys located 20 ft away from the patient. While fixating on the distant target, the examiner can perform the cover test as just described. Finally, a noisy near target can be moved into various positions to evaluate ocular versions.

EXAMINATION OF THE PUPILS

Examination of the pupils is very important in infants. While most other ophthalmic tests in infants either demand some cooperation or can be misinterpreted if the child is inattentive, pupils never lie. In a darkened room, the pupils should respond to light regardless of the infant's state of mind.

Pupillary responses should not be expected in very premature newborns. Robinson found that pupils began to constrict to the light of a penlight only after 29 weeks gestational age.[2] Pupillary reactions to light first appear between 30 and 31 weeks of gestational age. Those neonates who display a direct response also demonstrate a consensual response.

If the pupillary examination seems difficult because of their smaller size in newborns, magnification can be obtained with a magnifying lens (even the 20-D lens used for indirect ophthalmoscopy) or a portable slit lamp. First the pupil should be evaluated for roundness, size equal to the other pupil in room light, amount of constriction to light, and consensual response. Because neonates have poor near fixation, constriction to accommodation is usually not tested, and interpretation of the swinging flashlight test becomes quite difficult. If the pupil responds poorly to the light of a penlight, one should use a brighter light source such as an indirect ophthalmoscope.

If the pupillary responses are abnormal, one should carefully evaluate the ocular media, size and appearance of the optic nerve, and the retina. If doubts remain, electrophysiological tests such as the electroretinogram and visually evoked potential may be ordered.

EXAMINATION OF THE ANTERIOR SEGMENT

For infants, the anterior segment may be examined in three different ways. One may use a simple penlight, which is often adequate but gives no magnification. Since the infantile eye is small and the palpebral fissure narrow, magnification can be helpful. A second method is to wear loupes to improve magnification while using a penlight. By replacing the penlight with a slit-projecting light, one can simulate a slit lamp and focus by moving the light closer to or farther from the eye (Fig 5–4). The best way to examine the anterior segment is with a portable slit lamp (Fig 5–5). This instrument not only magnifies but also permits biomicroscopy (examining a "cross section" of the cornea, anterior chamber, lens, and anterior vitreous humor by observing the slit beam image of the structure from a different angle with the oculars).

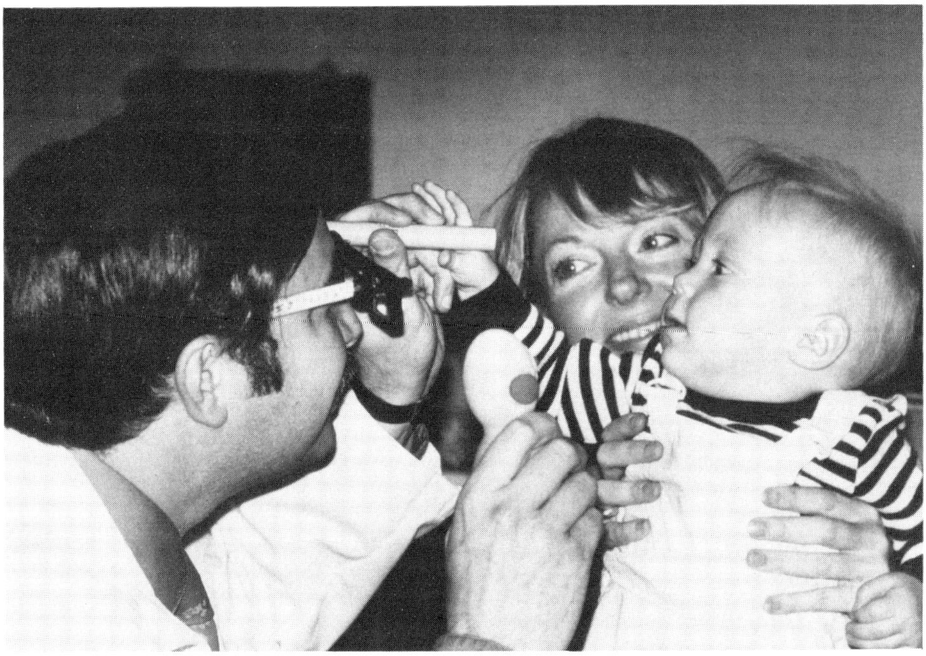

FIG 5–4.
Performing biomicroscopy by the use of loupes with a projected slit beam.

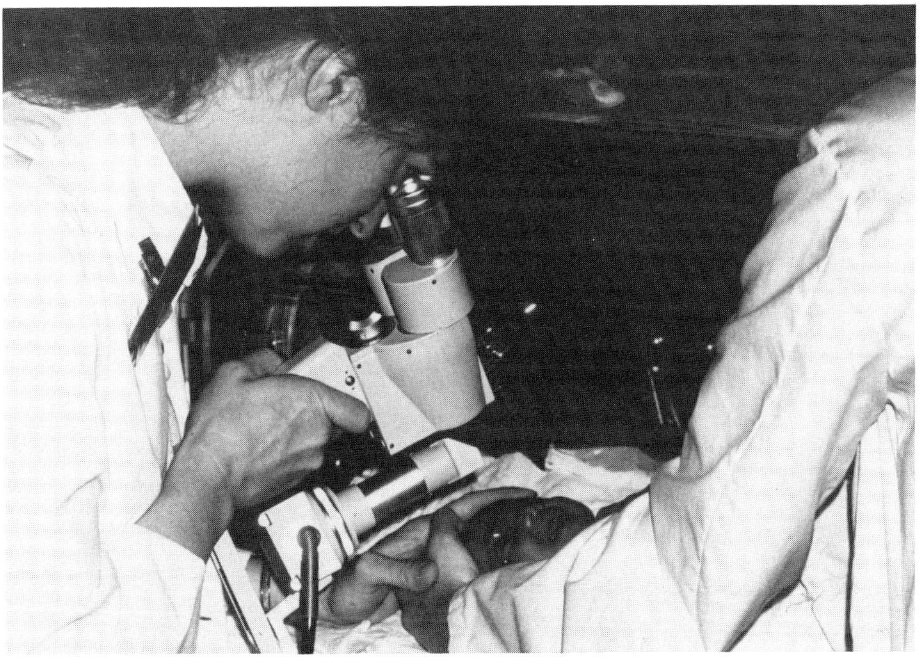

FIG 5–5.
Using a portable slit lamp yields the best biomicroscopy.

One should approach this examination in a systematic way. First, the eyelids and eyelid margins should be examined for any irregularities in shape, discharge on the lashes or margins, or other abnormality. Then the lower eyelids can be gently everted to expose the lower bulbar and palpebral conjunctival. One should compare the color and consistency of each conjunctiva by looking specifically for follicles, papillae, discharge, or edematous changes. The cornea can be examined for clarity by noting any irregularities or opacities. If there is any doubt about the latter, fluorescein dye should be applied to the ocular surface and a cobalt blue light used to uncover or emphasize any superficial changes. The anterior chamber is observed for depth and the presence of cells or flare. The iris is examined for any irregularities of shape or vessels. The lens and vitreous humor are then carefully tested for opacities or other abnormalities.

If the infant has a cloudy or possibly enlarged cornea, it is important to measure the intraocular pressure. In most infants, general anesthesia is not justified for the main purpose of determining the intraocular pressure. Most small infants are somewhat sedated by the simple act of feeding. Thus, the examiner should have the infant feed at the bottle or breast or possibly place a clean finger in the infant's mouth, apply a topical anesthetic (possibly with a drop of fluorescein dye) to the cornea, and then measure the intraocular pressure in the most inobtrusive method possible (Fig 5–6). I have found the portable applanation tonometer to be both reliable and effective for this task. Second choices would be a pneumotonometer, "pencil"-type tonometer, or the Schiotz tonometer. If doubts remain regarding a possibly elevated intraocular pressure, examination under anesthesia (EUA) may be warranted.

EXAMINATION OF THE POSTERIOR SEGMENT

The most frequent reason the ophthalmologist is called to the nursery is to examine the retina to rule out retinopathy of prematurity. The first consideration prior to examination is the choice of eyedrops to dilate the pupils. The ideal eyedrop would be completely safe and still maximally dilate the pupils for a period just sufficient for the examination. To accomplish this, one should use a sympathomimetic agent to stimulate dilation and a parasympatholytic (or cycloplegic) agent

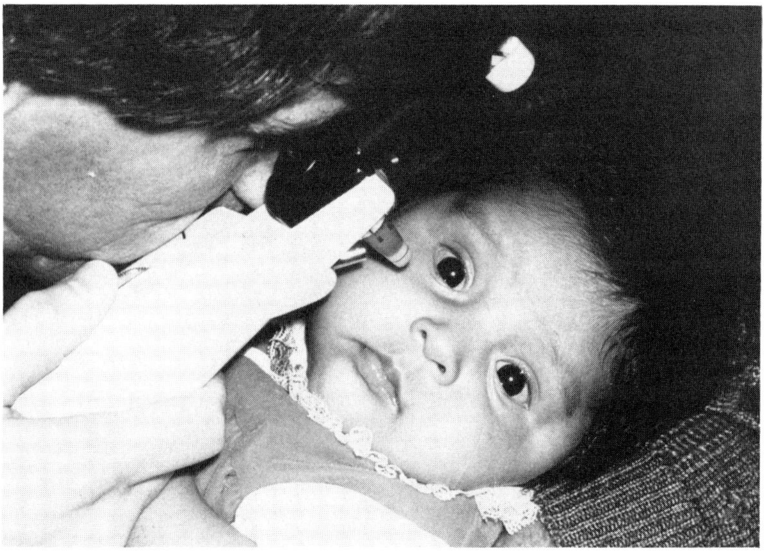

FIG 5–6.
Performing tonometry with a portable hand-held applanator.

to inhibit constriction. For the purposes of this examination, the parasympatholytic agent is used to provide mydriasis and not cycloplegia. Newborns who develop retinopathy of prematurity tend to have a low birth weight and often have bronchopulmonary problems. Thus, an eyedrop that may be safe for older children or even full-term newborns may be dangerous for low-weight neonates because of their smaller mass and immature physiological mechanisms.

For low-weight neonates, the sympathomimetic agent of choice is phenylephrine 1%. It has been demonstrated that when added to a parasympatholytic agent, phenylephrine 2.5%, causes a 20% increase in mean blood pressure while 1% phenylephrine has no effect on blood pressure.[9] Three of the 12 babies receiving 2.5% phenylephrine actually had an increase in mean blood pressure of more than 50%. With 1% phenylephrine, the net mydriasis was less than with the 2.5% strength (2.7 vs. 3.5mm) but still adequate for examination.

The parasympatholytic agent of choice in low-weight neonates is cyclopentolate in a concentration of 0.25% or less. This drug has long been used for pupillary dilation because of its appropriate duration of action. Only recently has it been appreciated that the commonly used 0.5% strength significantly decreases gastric acid secretion and volume while placebo and the 0.25% concentration have no significant effect on these gastric parameters.[10]

A commercially available eyedrop, Cyclomydril (Alcon Laboratories, Inc), contains phenylephrine, 1%, and cyclopentolate, 0.2%. At this time, this combination eyedrop appears to be the agent of choice to dilate the pupils of low-weight neonates. For babies weighing more than 3,000 gm, more concentrated solutions (phenylephrine, 2.5%, and cyclopentolate, 0.5%) may be used, especially for infants with dark irides.

It is difficult to attempt to examine the fundus of newborns without assistance. Although these babies cannot yet turn over, they can squirm, turn their heads, and otherwise avoid the light of the ophthalmoscope. An assistant can be very helpful by stabilizing the infant's body and head, and, if necessary, placing a clean finger in the infant's mouth to calm him. At the same time the assistant can mind the newborn's general health by either watching the monitoring equipment or the infant's physical signs. The babies most likely to develop retinopathy of prematurity are, unfortunately, those most likely to be physiologically unstable. These infants tend to be premature and small and often have bronchopulmonary problems. They can also respond to ocular manipulation with the oculocardiac reflex in as much as 31% of cases.[11] This reflex, usually generated by applying traction to an extraocular muscle, travels from the trigeminal nerve to the vagus nerve and results in a bradycardia or other dysrhythmia.[12] Thus, it is preferable that the assistant be knowledgeable in the diagnosis of cardiopulmonary distress and techniques of resuscitation in neonates.

The aforementioned physiological instability of the neonate provides one of the two principal reasons for completing the retinal examination in as efficient a manner as possible. The second is the strong tendency of neonates to develop conjunctival chemosis during the course of the examination, which is exacerbated by crying. The increasing chemosis can make the conjunctiva overlap the cornea, thereby making visualization of the retina quite difficult. In addition, the chemosis can rotate the eyelid speculum and cause expulsion. To increase efficiency, the examiner should have all the needed equipment ready in a kit. The suggested contents of this kit are listed in Table 5–1.

TABLE 5–1.
Necessary Items for Posterior Segment Examination

1. A strong, compassionate assistant
2. Eyelid speculum for infants (Sauer or Cook)
3. A bottle of balanced salt solution or its equivalent and a topical anesthetic
4. Indirect ophthalmoscope
5. Indirect lenses—28 (or 30) and 20 D
6. Scleral depressor
7. Alcohol swabs to clean the speculum and depressor
8. A flexible examiner
9. Plenty of patience

Once the infant is stabilized, a drop of a topical anesthetic should be applied to both eyes to make the use of the speculum and scleral depressor more comfortable. After the special eyelid speculum for infants is inserted, the examiner should begin his examination with the indirect ophthalmoscope and lens. A 28- (or 30)-D lens may be preferable for the initial examination since one can see a larger expanse of retina in a single view, which makes the examination quicker. If an abnormality is observed, the examiner may then elect to use a 20-D lens for greater magnification. He should first examine the posterior pole while realizing that neonates normally have a more pallid optic nerve and retina then one sees in adults regardless of race. The macular may not yet fully resemble the adult macula.[3] Then attention should be paid to the retina in the equatorial region, which can be appreciated by having the examiner bend or stoop over as the head is tilted away. If the area of furthest vascularization is visualized at this point, there is no need to depress the sclera in that clock hour. Usually, one needs to use scleral depression to observe the most advanced edge of retinal vascularization due to its anterior location (Fig 5–7). It is at this "edge" that retinopathy of prematurity may develop. While retinopathy is more common in the temporal periphery, it may also occur in other areas. Thus, scleral depression should be started on the temporal side but then completed around the anterior retina. This will require a degree of cooperation from the assistant as he consistently tilts the head away as the examiner moves around the infant's head.

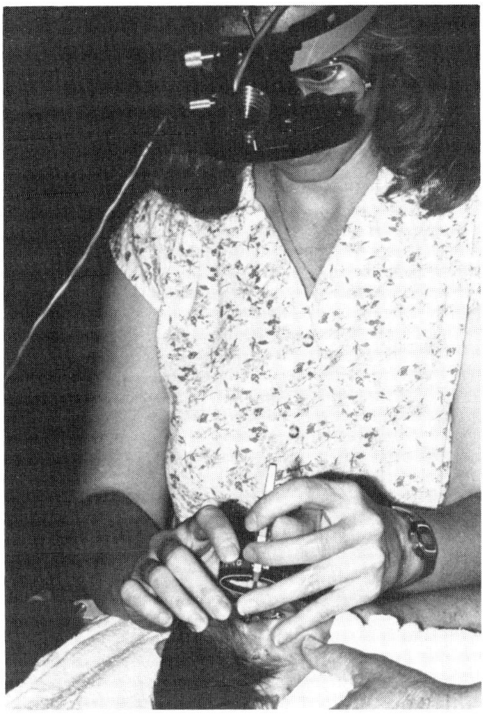

FIG 5–7.
Scleral depression is essential in most examinations for retinopathy of prematurity.

There are a number of precautions that the examiner should observe (Table 5–2). The first consideration is which babies should be examined. It is often fruitless for the ophthalmologist to examine a baby who is so surrounded by tubes and catheters that the infant may not be moved. This is especially true for intubated neonates. At our current state of knowledge regarding treatment, active therapy would not be applied to such neonates. Thus, the ophthalmologist should suggest postponing the retinal examination until the infant is more stable. The cornea will tend to dry due to exposure and the heat of the indirect ophthalmoscope. The examiner should be prepared to intermittently apply a drop of a lubricant such as balanced salt solution to the cornea. The examiner must be very careful to avoid continuous scleral depression for more than about 1 minute. Each time the depressor is applied to the sclera, the central retinal artery is immediately occluded, probably because of the elastic quality of the infantile sclera elevating the intraocular pressure. It is not difficult to imagine ischemic damage to the retina if the sclera is depressed for a significant time. Scleral depression that is too vigorous may result in retinal hemorrhage (especially over an area of retinopathy) or increased chemosis of the conjunctiva.

More specific suggestions for examination and follow-up of the baby with retinopathy of prematurity can be found in Chapter 26.

TABLE 5–2.
Possible Pitfalls of the Posterior Segment Examination

1. Systemic effects of mydriatic agents
   a. Sympathomimetic agents such as phenylephrine can cause hypertension
   b. Parasympatholytic agents such as cyclopentolate can inhibit gastric acid volume and concentration
2. Tubes and catheters everywhere! Wait until the baby is more stable.
3. Ocular complications
   a. Retinal hemorrhages (especially in retinopathy of prematurity)
   b. Central artery occlusion (especially during scleral depression)
   c. Conjunctival hemorrhage and chemosis
   d. Oculocardiac reflex (potentially lethal)

EVALUATION UNDER ANESTHESIA

With advancing technology, EUAs are becoming less frequent. If the corneal diameter or the intraocular pressure needs to be measured, this can be accomplished quite readily when the infant is nursing or otherwise feeding. Even the peripheral retinal can be evaluated with proper restraint of the child. Contact lenses trial with high hyperopic lenses can be fitted in the office. However, when operating on the second eye in cases of bilateral infantile cataracts, contact lens measurement can be facilitated by applying contact lenses to the first operated eye and evaluating the base curve and refractive error. The surgeon may then order contact lenses for each eye on the basis of these measurements unless a disparity exists such as an unequal corneal diameter.[13]

When is it appropriate to perform an EUA? The obvious answer is anytime important information is needed to preserve sight that can be obtained in no other way. If glaucoma may be present and the intraocular pressure cannot be measured when the child is awake, an EUA is indicated. If a very detailed retinal examination is necessary such as evaluation of the uninvolved eye in a child who has had the other eye enucleated for a retinoblastoma, EUA may be indicated. If one needs to remove corneal sutures after infantile keratoplasty, an EUA would provide the greatest safety for the child.

The form of anesthesia should conform to the duration and type of examination and should be comfortable for the anesthesiologist to perform. In recent years, we have found anesthetic gas delivered through intranasal catheters to provide excellent anesthesia and generally not interfere with the procedure.[14] We have often used this technique for nasolacrimal duct probing and had the anesthesiologist temporarily remove one catheter for aspiration of marker fluid from the nose or nasopharynx with no problems. Using nasal catheters avoids the morbidity of laryngeal intubation and extubation while freeing the anesthesiologist from holding a mask on the child's face (and often obstructing the ophthalmologist). The use of ketamine is often unsatisfactory for the ophthalmologist because the eyes can move under it's influence and the extraocular muscles can tighten, which elevates the intraocular pressure.

It is wise to have a routine technique in mind when approaching an EUA. The nature of any particular case can dictate departures from this routine. Prior to anesthesia, the ophthalmologist must decide whether to dilate the pupil. Under anesthesia, the pupil becomes constricted, and accommodation is stimulated.[15] Therefore, to properly evaluate the retina outside the posterior pole or to perform a meaningful retinoscopy (to assess the refraction), dilation with cycloplegic and sympathomimetic agents is necessary. If it is possible that gonioscopy may be necessary or that mydriasis in this patient may affect intraocular pressure, dilation should be delayed until after gonioscopy and/or tonometry.

The following sequence is a good general order to follow. First, a portable slit lamp is routinely used to examine the eyelids, conjunctiva, cornea, iris, and lens. Then, the corneal diameters are carefully measured with a caliper or ruler. These determinations should be performed without exerting any pressure upon the eye. The intraocular pressure is then measured. It is a good idea to use at least two different instruments to measure intraocular pressure to permit confirmation and comparison. One may use a portable applanation tonometer, Schiotz tonometer, pneumotonometer, pencil-type tonometer, or other similar instrument. Gonioscopy may then be performed. Subsequently, retinoscopy and ophthalmoscopy may then be carried out. If ultrasound is needed, it should be done after tonometry since the weight of the ultrasound probe or water bath may affect the intraocular pressure.

CONCLUSION

The examination of the newborn and infantile eye is a different experience than the examination of adults. Not only are the techniques themselves disparate, but the very approaches to those techniques are also dissimilar. Despite these differences, one should remember that the information obtained by the ophthalmologist from a baby's examination is potentially among the most important he may ever gather since it will ensure or provide vision for a lifetime.

REFERENCES

1. Goren CC, Sarty M, Wand-Wu PYK: Visual following and pattern discrimination of face-like stimuli by newborn infants. *Pediatrics* 1975; 56:544.
2. Robinson RJ: Assessment of gestational age by neurological examination. *Arch Dis Child* 1966; 41:437.
3. Isenberg SJ: Macular development in the premature infant. *Am J Ophthalmol* 1986; 101:74.
4. Fulton AB, Hansen RM, Manning KA: Measuring visual acuity in infants. *Surv Ophthalmol* 1981; 25:325.
5. Dayton GO, Jones MH, Aiu P, et al: Developmental study of coordinated eye movements in the human infant. I. Visual acuity in the newborn human: A study based on induced optokinetic nystagmus recorded by electro-oculography. *Arch Ophthalmol* 1964; 71:865.
6. Hoyt CS, Mousel DK, Weber AA: Transient supranuclear disturbances of gaze in healthy neonates. *Am J Ophthalmol* 1980; 89:708.
7. Mellor DH, Fielder ER: Dissociated visual development. Electrodiagnostic studies in infants who are "slow to see." *Dev Med Child Neurol* 1980; 22:327.
8. Hoyt CS, Nickel BL, Billson FA: Ophthalmological examination of the infant. Developmental aspects. *Surv Ophthalmol* 1982; 26:177.
9. Isenberg SJ, Everett S: Cardiovascular effects of mydriatics in low-birth-weight infants. *J Pediatr* 1984; 105:111.
10. Isenberg SJ, Abrams C, Hyman PE: Effects of cyclopentolate eyedrops on gastric secretory function in pre-term infants. *Ophthalmology* 1985; 92:698.
11. Clark WN, Hodges E, Noel LP, et al: The oculocardiac reflex in premature infants. *Am J Ophthalmol* 1985; 99:649.
12. Apt L, Isenberg SJ, Gaffney WJ: The oculocardiac reflex in strabismus surgery. *Am J Ophthalmol* 1973; 76:533.
13. Feldman S, Isenberg SJ: Is a third anesthesia necessary following bilateral cataract surgery in children? *Ann Ophthalmol* 1987; 19:228.
14. Durazo M: Intranasal catheters for evaluation under anesthesia. Presented at the Western Anesthesia Residents Conference, 1983.
15. Saunders RA, Andrews CJ: Refractive changes in children under general anesthesia. *J Pediatr Ophthalmol Strabismus* 1981; 18:38.

6 Transient Phenomena of the Newborn Eye

Andrew Q. McCormick, B.S., M.D., C.M.

The development of intensive care units for newborn infants over the past 25 years has been accompanied not only by impressive technical advances for the care of babies but also by an increasingly diverse array of physicians and other health care professionals who have an interest in these small patients and who can contribute to the infants' better clinical care. More and more ophthalmologists and residents in training are finding their way into these units, predominantly for the detection of retinopathy of prematurity and its possible therapy. In addition, they are called upon to examine infants who have chromosomal disorders, possible congenital infections, and a wide variety of other illnesses and developmental abnormalities. To the inexperienced observer, the eye of the newly born infant can present a number of unusual features that are not seen in the ophthalmic examination of older children or adults. In no other aspect of the newborn examination are changes so prominent as those that can be seen in the eye. If we include the very premature infant, the changes to be viewed over the first few weeks following birth are dramatic ones indeed.

It is the purpose of this chapter to outline these changes and emphasize that the phenomena to be described are either all normal or else are seen so commonly, with no adverse sequellae, that they must be considered "normal" in our present state of knowledge.

EYELID FUSION

The eyelids develop by superior and inferior folds of epithelium with a mesodermal core that elongate and grow to fusion in the horizontal midline in front of the globe at the 40-mm stage.[1] As seen in Figure 6–1, the fusion is an epithelial one only, and separation of the lids is achieved as keratinization proceeds through the center of this epithelial bridge. Separation of the lids can always be accomplished by a little downward pressure on the lower lid and some upward pressure on the upper one. The gentle release of these anatomic adhesions by such pressure never distresses the infant and can be done with equanimity.

Duke-Elder suggested that the eyelids become unfused between 7 and 9 months of postconceptual age.[2] No indication was given as to how these time limits were established. At the practical clinical level, I consider that the lids are always fused until 27 weeks' gestation and are never fused after 28 weeks' gestation. There are likely exceptions to this generalization, but it has been a helpful clinical guide.

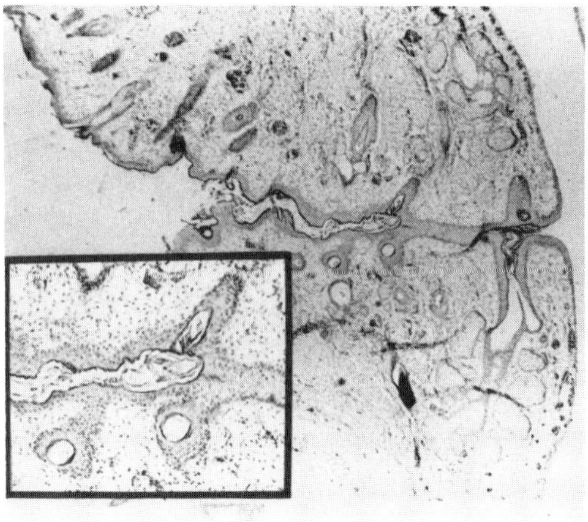

FIG 6–1.
The fused lids of a 24-week stillborn infant. The inset under greater magnification shows the progress of keratinization along the epithelial bridge.

CORNEAL INTRANSPARENCY

Congenital developmental abnormalities of the anterior segment of the eye are not common but are often associated with variable corneal clouding, or opacification. The trained observer will be able to examine such cases and carry out the necessary investigations to establish the proper diagnosis and initiate appropriate treatment. What will surprise the inexperienced observer is the frequency of slight to moderate corneal intransparency in otherwise normal eyes. This cloudiness is of a uniform nature, affects the whole corneal area, and is symmetrical in the two eyes. The corneal epithelial surface is smooth and does not resemble the roughened surface of a cornea that is edematous.

Slightly cloudy corneas are very occasionally seen in healthy newborn infants, and normal clarity is achieved in a day or two. They are more commonly seen in infants who are small for their gestational age, and differences in corneal clarity may even be seen between twin or triplets, particularly if there are large discrepancies in their birth weights—the more opaque corneas seen in the smaller babies (Fig 6–2).

Corneal cloudiness is universally seen in very small premature infants, and its degree is porportional to the degree of prematurity. The cornea of a 26-week-gestation fetus is virtually always sufficiently intransparent as to prevent an evaluation of the iris structure. Along with the pupillary membrane and the hyaloid vascular system, it absolutely prevents a view of fine fundus detail.

The clearing of the intransparency associated with prematurity may well take at least 4 to 6 weeks in the very preterm baby. It is unlikely to interfere with the examination of the interior of the globes after 32 or 34 postconceptual weeks have been completed.

TRANSIENT "CATARACTS"

Transient vacuolar lens changes were first reported in 1968 in 7 of 17 premature infants examined,[3] and in 1973, similar changes were reported to occur in 3.7% of infants with a birth weight of less than 2,500 gm.[4] The vacuoles first appeared at the three apices of the inverted-Y suture, which at 27 to 28 weeks lies immediately beneath the posterior lens capsule, and in some cases spread to involve the whole sutural area (Fig 6–3). They tended to disappear in a reverse fashion, the apical areas

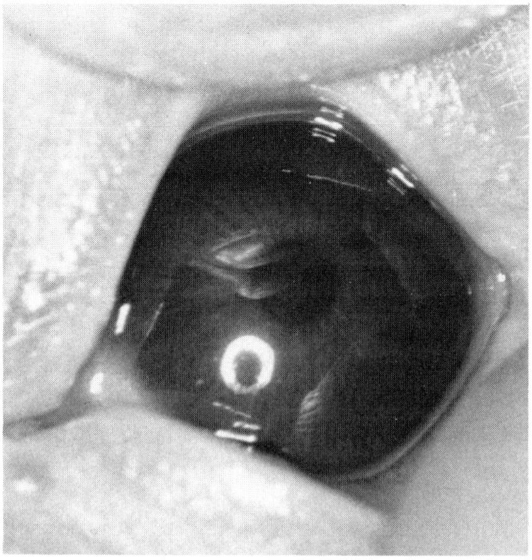

FIG 6–2.
This hazy cornea was seen in a second twin who weighed 450 gm less than his brother. They were born at 36 weeks and were otherwise normal.

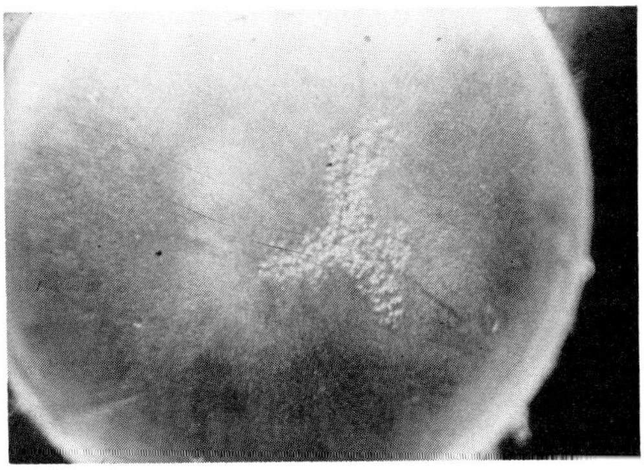

FIG 6–3.
This lens was removed from the eye of a 27-week-gestation baby who died at 2 weeks of age. The vacuoles can be seen lying in relation to the posterior inverted-Y suture, which at this stage of development lies just under the posterior lens capsule.

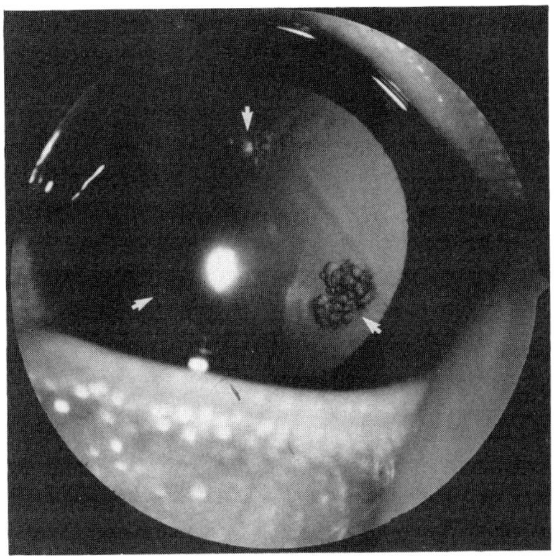

FIG 6–4.
Clusters of vacuoles are seen in the 12, 4, and 8 o'clock meridians as indicated by arrows.

clearing last. Once the changes had appeared, they tended to remain for several days to several weeks. In Figure 6–4, the presence of three clusters of vacuoles lie in the 12, 4, and 8 o'clock meridians.

No etiology for these unusual lens changes has ever been established. Curiously, a baby exhibiting these lens changes was virtually always present in our nursery during the late 1960s and through the 1970s, whereas only three or four cases have been seen in the past 5 years. This may be because very tiny premature infants are not examined as early in their life now as they were previously, but the suspicion remains strong that these vacuolar changes are occurring less frequently.

TRANSITORY INTRAOCULAR BLOOD VESSELS

The pupillary membrane is a network of blood vessels continuous with iris blood vessels whose function probably is the nourishment of the anterior portion of the developing fetal lens. At its greatest extent, it covers the pupillary aperture (Fig 6–5). As development progresses there is a "retraction" of blood vessels away from the central region until there are just a few remnants around the pupil border. It has been suggested that the extent of this structure[5] is an accurate guide to the infant's gestational age, and in many cases it is. Figure 6–6 shows the pupillary membrane in one of a set of twins, the other having no remnant of this structure whatever. The pupillary membrane is best seen with the magnification provided by a direct ophthalmoscope focused at the pupil plane with the pupil well dilated.

The hyaloid vascular system cannot be completely viewed in the infant eye, but its

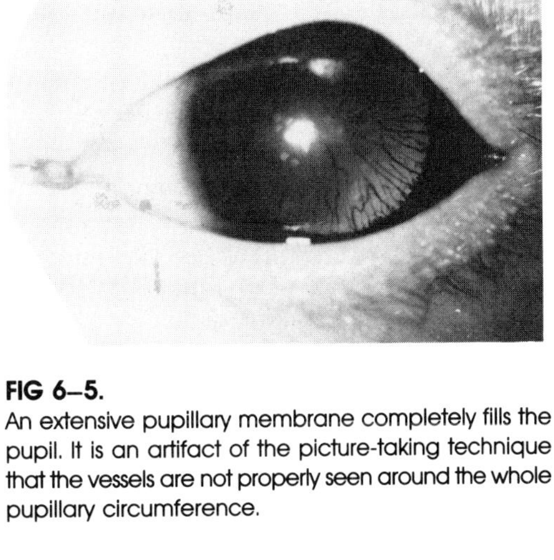

FIG 6–5.
An extensive pupillary membrane completely fills the pupil. It is an artifact of the picture-taking technique that the vessels are not properly seen around the whole pupillary circumference.

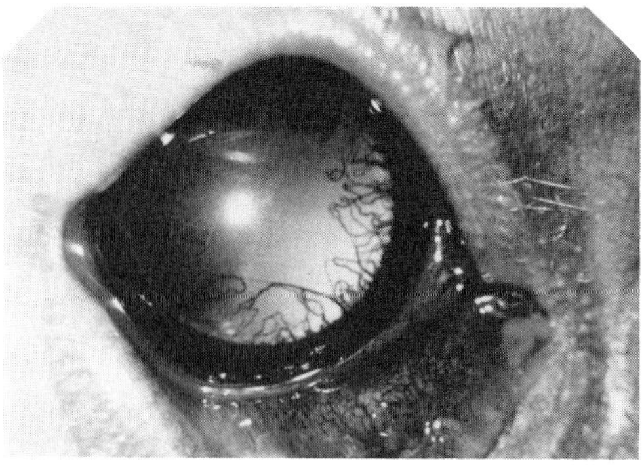

FIG 6–6.
This pupillary membrane has retracted to the point that the interior of the globe could now be assessed.

presence can be verified with two techniques. The anterior vitreous portion of the hyaloid artery can be seen as an indistinct gray stalk behind the pupillary membrane as this structure is being viewed. If the examiner's head is moved from side to side while looking through the ophthalmoscope, the anterior portion of the hyaloid artery can be seen in parallax. When the fundus is examined, the vessel can be seen to extend from the optic nerve head into the vitreous, again by parallax as the examiner's head and the condensing lens are moved slightly from side to side (Fig 6–7). The embryology literature is inconsistent about when this hyaloid vascular system disappears,[6] and the clinical literature never seems to discuss it. There is doubtless some variation in the exact time of its disappearance, but my clinical impression is that it is always visible until 32 weeks' gestational age.

THE DEFINITIVE OCULAR BLOOD VESSELS

The redness of the conjunctivae in the newborn has traditionally been attributed to the irritant effects of silver nitrate given prophylactically at birth. But now with the use of nonirritant antibiotic ointment, the conjunctival blood vessels are still seen to be more prominent immediately after birth than they are several hours or a day later (Fig 6–8). The cause of the prominent blood vessels clearly lies elsewhere.

In addition to the changes seen in the conjunctival blood vessels during the first hours or days of life, similar changes can also be seen in the iris and retinal blood vessels following birth.

The iris shows an elaborate network of blood vessels on its surface and a prominent circumferential vessel at the junction of the inner third of the iris with its outer two thirds,

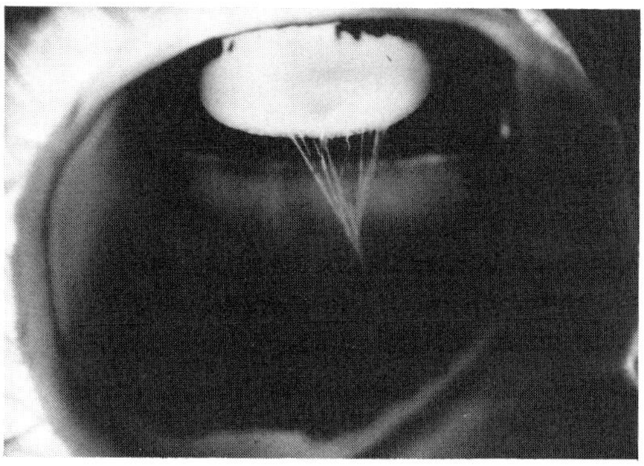

FIG 6–7.
The hyaloid artery as it branches behind the lens. This autopsy specimen was obtained from a 27-week-gestation infant who died shortly after birth.

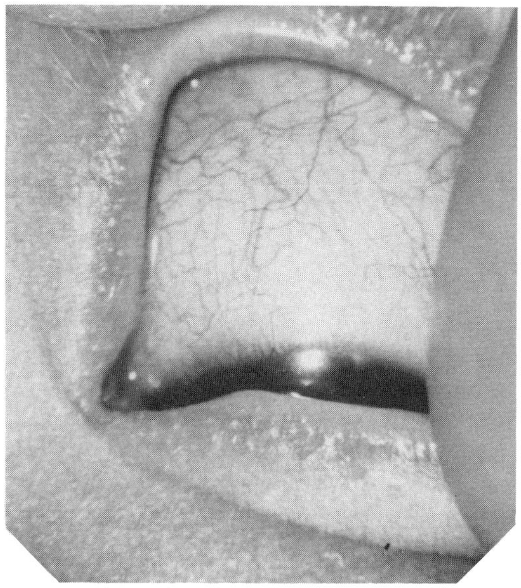

FIG 6–8.
Prominent conjunctival blood vessels are shown in a term infant shortly after birth. No medication has yet been given for eye prophylaxis.

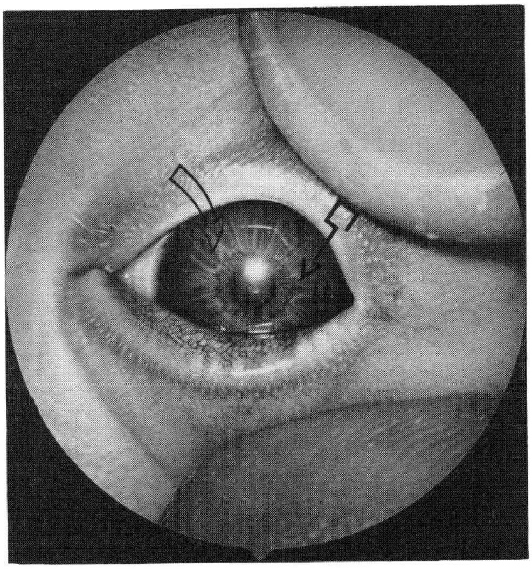

FIG 6–9.
The iris 5 minutes after birth. The open arrow indicates a circumferential iris blood vessel near the pupil border. The closed arrow indicates radial blood vessels.

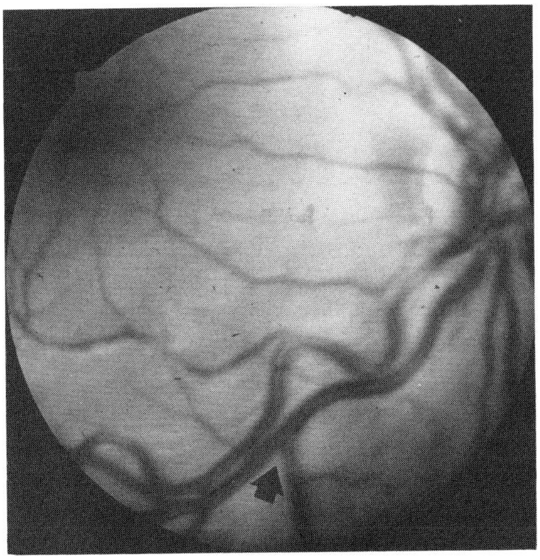

FIG 6–10.
The retina 6 hours following birth. The baby was a term, East Indian infant with a birth weight of 2,400 gm.

with radial vessels extending peripherally to the root of the iris and centrally to the pupil border (Fig 6–9). These vessels may be completely hidden by the heavy anterior pigment layer in the dark brown irides of heavily pigmented races but are readily observed in paler irides of most white babies.

Veins and arteries in this network cannot be distinguished from each other, but rhythmic changes can be readily seen if looked for with good focal illumination and magnification. At one moment the vascular complex is engorged, while 15 to 30 seconds later the vessels are much less easily seen, only to become more prominent again after another short time lapse. The trend is for them to become less prominent until they are no longer visible, which may occur within a few hours or a few days.

Although retinal blood vessels cannot be evaluated as soon after birth as iris vessels because of the need to dilate the pupils, they nevertheless all show caliber and pattern changes as time elapses. Retinal arteries are always of wider caliber immediately after birth than later, and they always become straighter in their courses. The proof of this statement lies in photographic documentation as illustrated in Figures 6–10 and 6–11.

It is unlikely that the eye is the only organ in which blood vessels decrease in caliber as the baby adapts to its extrauterine existence.

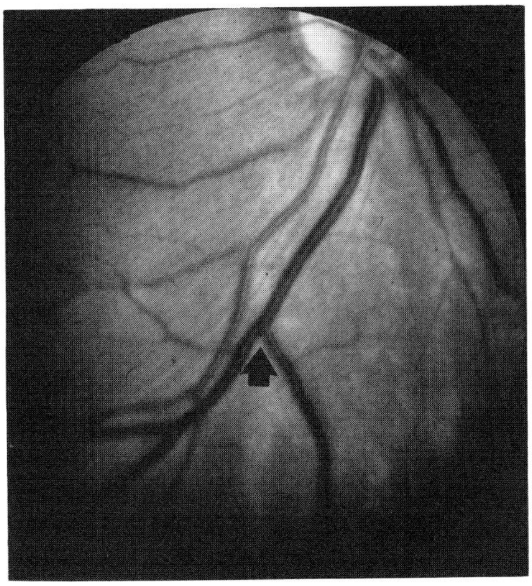

FIG 6–11.
This is the same retina shown in Figure 6–10, 48 hours later. Vascular changes are obvious. The arrows indicate similar anatomic points.

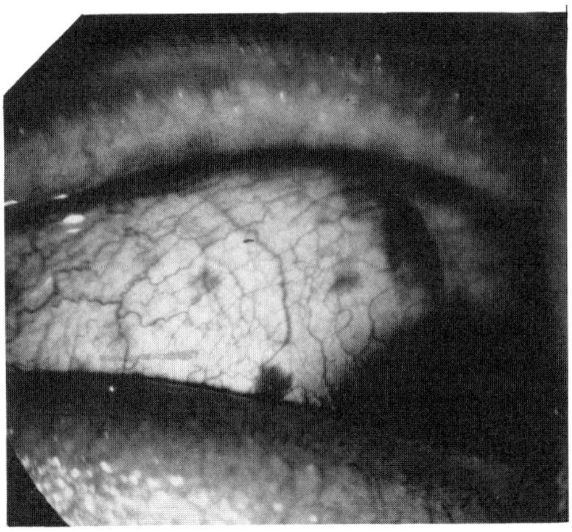

FIG 6–12.
In addition to the prominent conjunctival blood vessels, there are a number of scattered conjunctival hemorrhages. The baby was a normal, term infant.

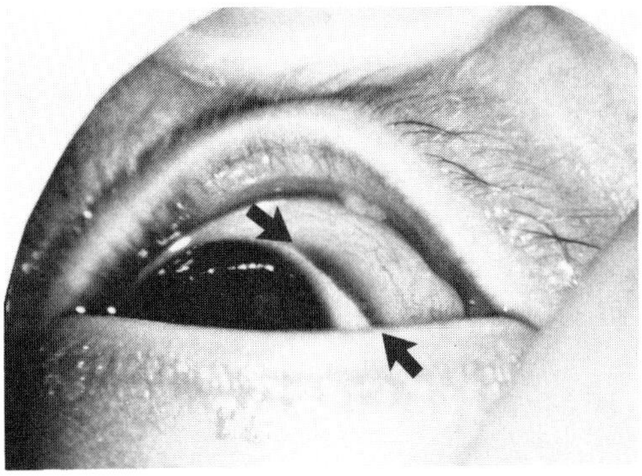

FIG 6–13.
The dark line *(arrows)* is a "limbal trough" hemorrhage The baby was a normal, term infant.

NEWBORN HEMORRHAGES

The infant palpebral aperture is small in relation to globe size, and very little conjunctiva is seen even in the awake baby. Because of this, conjunctival hemorrhages are often not noticed by anyone, including the mother, in spite of their frequent occurrence. These hemorrhages may be small or large, isolated or widespread (Fig 6–12), and they are often prominent in the limbal trough (Fig 6–13) where their absorption may be quite delayed.

Retinal hemorrhages have been reported in 2.5% to 50% of all births[7] while two large personal studies confirmed them in 25% of normal, term infants and found them unilaterally in half. These hemorrhages vary widely in extent and are often both intraretinal and preretinal in location. Like conjunctival hemorrhages, retinal hemorrhages are absorbed without a trace, and they tend to do so quickly. Figures 6–14 and 6–15 are retinal photographs of the same infant. Figure 6–14 was taken on the day of the baby's birth, and Figure 6–15 was taken 6 days later. Large preretinal hemorrhages may not be resorbed as quickly.

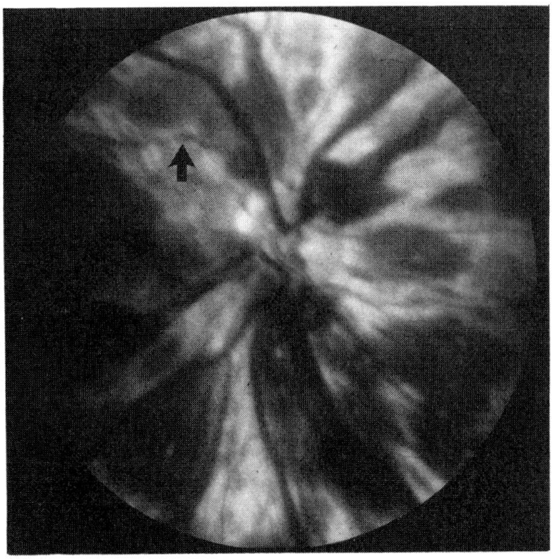

FIG 6–14.
Retinal hemorrhages 4 hours after a normal delivery. Many of the retinal hemorrhages have pale centers.

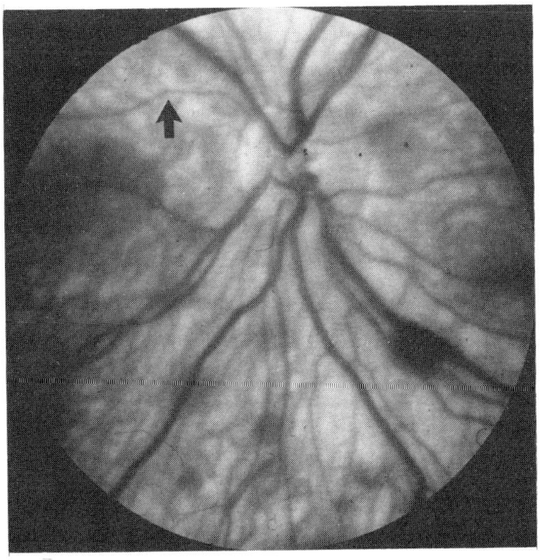

FIG 6–15.
This retinal photograph was taken 6 days after that in Figure 6–14. The *arrows* indicate similar anatomic locations.

REFERENCES

1. Andersen H, Ehlers N, Matthiessen ME: Histochemistry and development of the human eyelids. *Acta Ophthalmol* 1980; 43:624–648.
2. Duke-Elder S: *System of Ophthalmology*, vol III, pt 1. *Normal and Abnormal Development*. London, Henry Kimpton, 1963.
3. McCormick AQ: Transient cataracts in premature newborn infants—A new clinical entity. *Can J Ophthalmol* 1968; 3:202–205.
4. Alden ER, Kalina RE, Hodson WA: Transient cataracts in low birth weight infants. *J Pediatr* 1973; 82:314–318.
5. Hittner HM, Hirsch NJ, Rudolph AJ: Assessment of gestational age by examination of the anterior vascular capsule of the lens. *J Pediatr* 1977; 91:455–458.
6. Jakobiec FA: *Ocular Anatomy, Embryology and Teratology*. Philadelphia, Harper & Row Publishers, Inc, 1982.
7. Duke-Elder S: *System of Ophthalmology*, vol X. *Diseases of the Retina*. London, Henry Kimpton, 1967.

7 Workup of Common Differential Diagnostic Problems

Sherwin J. Isenberg, M.D.

This chapter is not meant to completely cover any of the entities mentioned in it. For details about the presentation and treatment of any specific disorders, the reader should refer directly to the chapter that deals with that entity.

Instead, this chapter is intended to aid the reader when confronting a patient who presents with one of these signs. It will guide him in the proper mental algorithm by suggesting those physical signs and aspects of the history that are helpful in seeking the diagnosis as well as appropriate tests to investigate or confirm the correct diagnosis.

LEUKOKORIA

The term *leukokoria* is a Greek phrase meaning "white pupil." As in adults or older children, upon simple observation an infant usually displays a black pupil, or upon shining a bright light into the pupil, an orange or red reflex emerges. However, when the examiner notices any other color in or behind the pupillary space, with or without a light, the patient is considered to have leukokoria (Fig 7–1).

Since leukokoria can refer to any mass at or behind the pupillary space, the first part of the differential diagnosis is to determine the anatomic location of the lesion. If the lesion is immediately in the pupillary space, a cataract is usually present (Fig 7–2). This can be easily confirmed with the use of a slit lamp. One should remember that the presence of a cataract does rule out the possibility of pathology located behind the cataract that can cause or contribute to the cataract. Indeed, some entities such as advanced retinopathy of prematurity or persistent hyperplastic primary vitreous can initially present as a simple cataract, with the true diagnosis discovered only after further testing.

To the ophthalmologist, the presence of leukokoria in an infant is an urgent situation for two reasons. First, the potentially lethal retinoblastoma often presents as leukokoria. A delay in the diagnosis of retinoblastoma can allow metastases to arise, which greatly increases the mortality of this tumor. The second reason for urgent diagnosis and treatment is the specter of amblyopia. If leukokoria is present unilaterally, deprivation amblyopia will almost always arise in the unaffected eye. This type of amblyopia is particularly destructive to vision unless it is treated promptly. In fact, unless a congenital unilateral leukokoria affecting the visual axis is reversed in the first 3 to 4 months of life, the amblyopia will leave

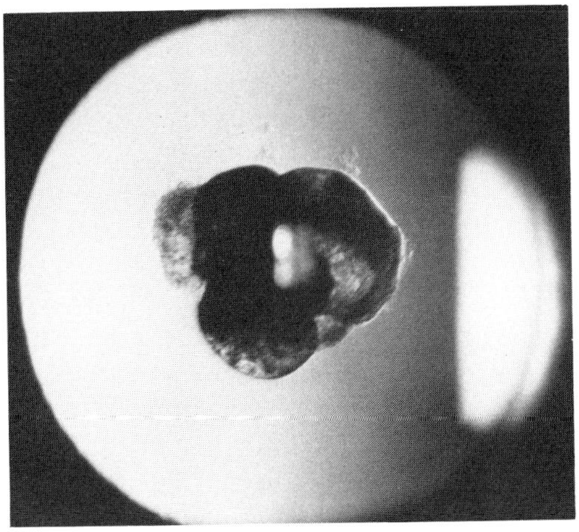

FIG 7–1.
Leukokoria caused by a posterior subcapsular cataract and made evident by retroillumination.

permanent visual deficits even if it is totally reversed later.[1]

History

A detailed history from the parents can be helpful in the differential diagnosis of leukokoria. Questions about the pregnancy should include duration since retinopathy of prematurity can present as leukokoria if the retina detaches. If the mother was ill while pregnant, one should inquire about the nature of the illness since such disorders as rubella, toxoplasmosis, and cytomegalovirus infections can cause leukokoria. In addition, medications or drugs taken during pregnancy can lead to leukokoria.

Information about the birth can be useful. The physician should not hestitate to acquire the medical records of the child's delivery if they may be helpful. If the birth weight is low, again retinopathy of prematurity should be considered. A traumatic birth, suspected from the size of the neonate or difficulties encountered by the obstetrician, could account for such diverse entities as cataract, opacities of the cornea, vitreous hemorrhages, or retinal detachment, which may all present as leukokoria (see Chapter 24). During the neonatal period, prolonged oxygen administration (even in the absence of significant prematurity based on birth weight) can lead to retinopathy of prematurity. A history of anomalies outside the orbits can indicate a systemic disorder that may explain the leukokoria. Deafness can suggest rubella or Norrie's disease. A seizure disorder would be consistent with toxoplasmosis or tuberous sclerosis. Unusual skin lesions can be found in incontinentia pigmenti or tuberous sclerosis. The diagnosis of mental retardation should be made carefully in the presence of bilateral leukokoria since poor vision alone can delay development in otherwise normal children (see Chapter 29). A social history can reveal possible sociopathic behavior by the parents that may have lead to child battering. Unusual eating habits or the presence of pets can imply *Toxocara* infection (although not usually in the first year of life). If the child is male, the diagnoses of Coat's disease, Norrie's disease, and juvenile retinoschisis are more likely than in females. Incontinentia pigmenti is found exclusively in females. Although not diagnostic, if the leukokoria is bilateral, retinopathy of prematurity, Norrie's disease, retinal dysplasia, and familial exudative chorioretinopathy are more likely. If unilateral, the diagnoses of persistent hyperplastic primary vitreous, Coat's disease, intraocular foreign body, and toxocariasis are more likely.

Either before or after examination of the child, examination of the parents can be very helpful. A parent can demonstrate a regressed retinoblastoma, an unappreciated congenital

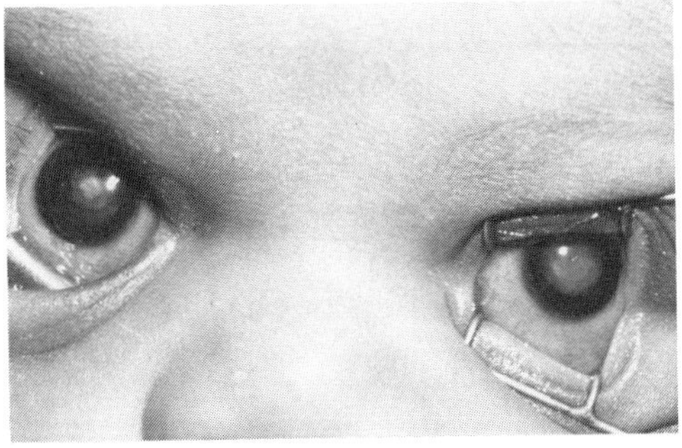

FIG 7–2.
Bilateral congenital cataracts present behind the pupil.

cataract, or the findings of familial exudative chorioretinopathy. Any of these findings would simplify and accelerate treatment of the child.

Physical Examination

The size of the eyes can be a very helpful sign. In the office, the ophthalmologist should measure the corneal diameter as an indication of ocular size. If the corneal diameter is at least 0.5 mm less than normal (see Chapter 3 for the normal values), the eyes are probably small. If in doubt, ocular ultrasonography can accurately determine the axial length. If the eyes are small and leukokoria is present, the most likely diagnoses are persistent hyperplastic primary vitreous (especially when bilateral), coloboma associated with microphthalmos, or cataract associated with microphthalmos (as rubella).

Persistent hyperplastic primary vitreous is essentially an arrest of ocular development that leaves, among other findings, some of the primary vitreous along with a retrolental membrane exerting traction on the ciliary processes. Either the membrane itself or a secondary cataract can cause the leukokoria. While microphthalmos is frequent in persistent hyperplastic primary vitreous, it is not always present. Rubenstein reported 14 cases of posterior hyperplastic primary vitreous in which normal-sized eyes contained glial deposits in the retina and optic nerve, preretinal membranes usually affecting the macula, distortion and tortuosity of the blood vessels, and pigmentary disturbances.[2]

Colobomas are not uncommon in microphthalmic eyes. If a coloboma of the retina and choroid is large enough, the white color of the sclera will replace the normal red or orange retinal reflex. The diagnosis of coloboma can be inferred from related ocular defects, especially notching or an absence of the inferior portion of the iris usually affecting the pupil. Fortunately, the diagnosis of retinal or choroidal coloboma can easily be made with ophthalmoscopy. Similarly, retinal dysplasia can also occur in microphthalmic eyes, especially in the presence of trisomy 13. Again, a good ophthalmoscopic examination should determine that diagnosis. In addition, certain types of congenital cataracts can occur in microphthalmic eyes, including those caused by maternal rubella.

If the cornea is opaque, the examiner might mistakenly refer to it as leukokoria. However, a simple penlight examination should indicate that the opacity is in the cornea and not within the eye. The differential diagnosis of an opacified cornea is discussed in the section on the cloudy cornea.

An iris coloboma, which causes the pupil to simulate a "keyhole," will support the diagnosis of retinal coloboma. If there are signs of inflammation on the iris, cornea, or within the anterior chamber (such as flare or white blood cells), inflammatory explanations for the leukokoria should be sought. Among the inflammatory causes of leukokoria are such congenital infections as rubella, toxoplasmosis, cytomegalovirus, and herpes as well as such acquired infections as toxocariasis (rare in infants) and endophthalmitis possibly following trauma.

The presence of a cataract should not end the workup for the cause of leukokoria. While the cataract may be the only pathology in the eye, there may also be a mass or detached retina behind the cataract that contributes to the lenticular opacity. Ocular ultrasound and computerized tomography will demonstrate most abnormal findings behind the lens that are large enough to cause a cataract. As described in Chapter 20, the morphology of the lens opacity in terms of its location, shape, and density can help determine the etiology of the cataract. It should be noted that retinoblastoma very rarely presents with a cataract.

The vitreous chamber is often the location of the leukokoria. Ophthalmoscopy can usually distinguish among the many entities that can cause opacities in the vitreous chamber. For example, if a persistent hyaloid vessel is observed, the diagnosis of persistent hyperplastic primary vitreous should be entertained. Many small vitreous opacities may represent the vitreous seeding of a retinoblastoma or the inflammatory cells of active

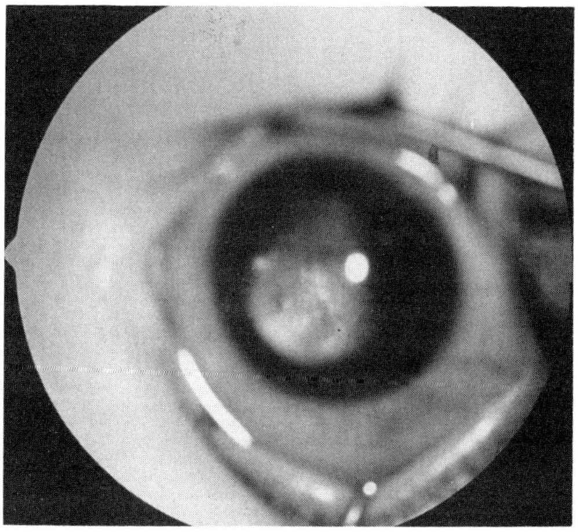

FIG 7–3.
A retinoblastoma extending to the vitreous chamber.

toxocariasis or toxoplasmosis. Certainly, any mass in the vitreous chamber that is contiguous with the retina must be considered a retinoblastoma until proved otherwise (Fig 7–3). However, other disorders can present with a retrolental mass involving the retina, including Norrie's disease (Fig 7–4) and toxocariasis.

A careful retinal examination is mandatory in the workup of leukokoria. Due to the lack of cooperation of the infants and the gravity of the disorder, an evaluation under anesthesia is usually warranted in these cases. At the time of anesthesia, the ophthalmologist can unhurriedly obtain additional valuable information including the intraocular pressure, electroretinogram (ERG), electro-oculogram (EOG), visually evoked potential (VEP), an ultrasound of the lesion with a determination of the axial length of the eye, corneal diameters, retinoscopy, and any invasive tests as indicated.

Noninvasive Tests

The advent of ocular ultrasound greatly simplified the workup of leukokoria. Behind a cataract, ultrasound might reveal the funnel-shaped retinal detachment of retinopathy of prematurity or the anterior membrane and hyaloid artery of persistent hyperplastic primary vitreous. A retinoblastoma may demonstrate the characteristics of intralesional calcifications, high attenuation, and a nonhomogeneous consistency. In Coat's disease, the vitreous is sometimes opaque, with a solid mass that is generally mobile behind the detached retina. Determination of the axial length

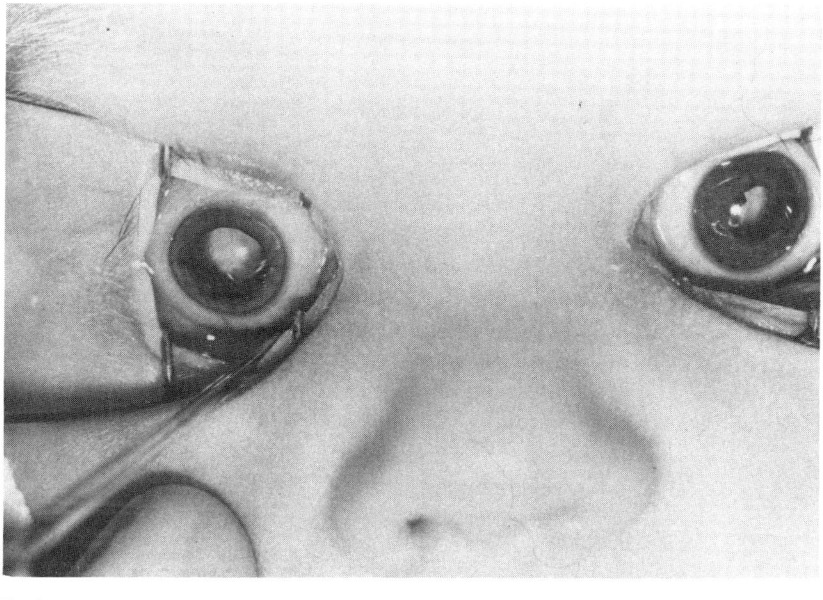

FIG 7–4.
This infant with retrolental opacities was found to have Norrie's disease, as did his maternal uncle.

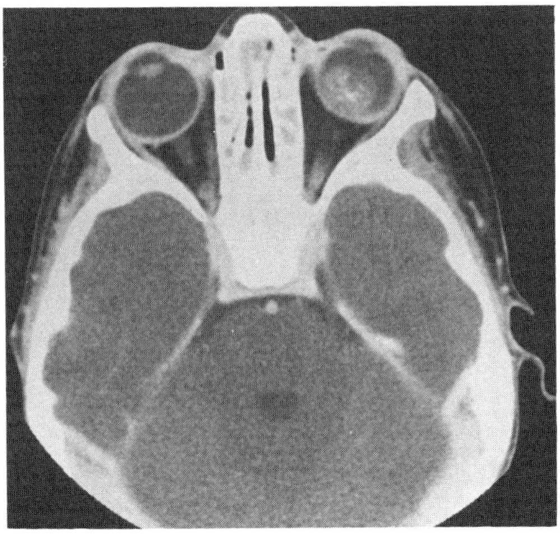

FIG 7–5.
Computed tomography of a child with retinoblastoma. Note the calcifications evident as hyperdensities within the mass. (Courtesy of Dr. Steven Cobb.)

can be very helpful in determining the presence of microphthalmos since this is found commonly with persistent hyperplastic primary vitreous or rubella but almost never in retinoblastoma or Coat's disease.

Computerized tomography has also been valuable in the workup of leukokoria (Figs 7–5 and 7–6).[3] The presence of calcifications within an intraocular tumor makes retinoblastoma the most likely diagnosis; however, some retinoblastomas will not have radiologically (or ultrasonographically) evident calcifications. Other ocular disorders may contain calcifications such as medulloepitheliomas, phthisis bulbi, teratomas, optic disc drusen, and hamartomas. Computerized tomography of persistent hyperplastic primary vitreous has demonstrated microphthalmos. subhyaloid blood, and intravitreal opacities. Unfortunately, the computerized tomography of Coat's disease and toxocariasis may resemble a noncalcified retinoblastoma with a homogeneous intravitreal and/or subretinal density.

Magnetic resonance imaging is now proving to be helpful in securing a diagnosis in leukokoria according to Haik and associates.[4] Retinoblastoma has been found, especially on T2-weighted images, to demonstrate calcifications as well as exudates and subretinal hemorrhages. In Coat's disease, the T2-weighted images are also informative by accentuating the subretinal exudates. In *Toxocara* infection, these authors found marked enhancement and thickening of the sclera that gave the impression of microphthalmos. Longstanding vitreous hemorrhages were evident on magnetic resonance imaging, while acute hemorrhages were not.

If one is convinced that the lesion is actually a retinoblastoma, other noninvasive tests become mandatory. These tests are selected to seek metastases. Usually, the pediatric oncologist will order such tests as a bone scan, liver scan, complete blood count, and urinalysis. A blood test for the enzyme-linked immunoabsorbent assay (ELISA) for toxocariasis can be helpful in questionable cases.

Invasive Tests

Although not always necessary, invasive tests occasionally prove to be important. From the ocular standpoint, the invasive tests pri-

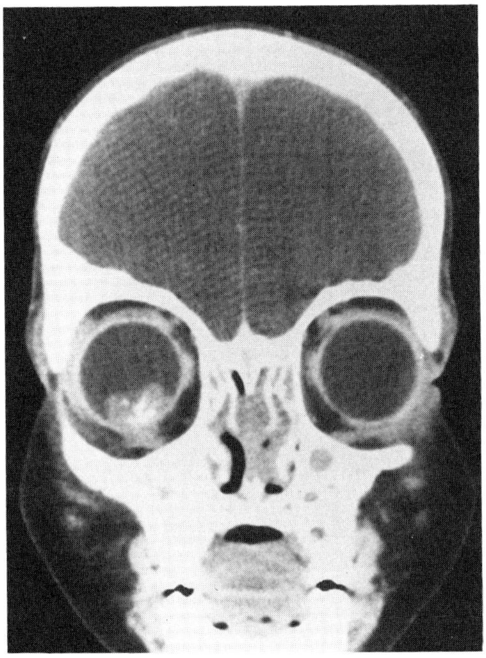

FIG 7–6.
Coronal view of the same child as in Figure 7–5. (Courtesy of Dr. Steven Cobb.)

marily consist of tapping the anterior chamber to withdraw aqueous humor for analysis. Due to the fear of spreading a possible tumor by performing anterior-chamber paracentesis, this procedure should only be considered if a reasonable doubt remains after completing all of the noninvasive tests. Generally, the aqueous humor is analyzed for two factors, cells and enzyme levels.

By direct cytological examination, a pathologist can identify the cells withdrawn from the anterior chamber. The finding of eosinophilic leukocytes implies inflammation and is very suggestive of toxocariasis. Of course, neoplastic cells suggest the presence of retinoblastoma.

The aqueous humor can also be analyzed for its enzymes. Lactic dehydrogenase (LDH) has been found to be in increased concentration in the presence of a retinoblastoma.[5] The LDH test response is considered positive if the level of LDH in the aqueous humor exceeds that in the serum[6] or if the aqueous humor concentration exceeds known normal aqueous humor values. The LDH test has a false-negative rate of about 7% and a false-positive rate of about 1%. Unfortunately, most of the false-positive cases are of the difficult-to-differentiate Coat's disease.

To complete the workup for metastatic disease if retinoblastoma is seriously suspected, the pediatric oncologist will usually desire a lumbar puncture and bone marrow analysis. These two tests are typically performed when the child is undergoing evaluation under anesthesia for his ocular disease.

POOR VISION AND NYSTAGMUS

The pediatrician and ophthalmologist is occasionally confronted by parents who believe that their infant does not appear to have normal visual function. While the new parent may simply not be familiar with the poor vision all newborns initially display (see Chapters 3, 4, and 5), we must treat this complaint seriously if the parent has had previous children, especially if nystagmus is present.

Nystagmus resulting from or accompanying poor vision is usually of the "pendular" type. Nystagmus alone does not always indicate poor vision. Oculomotor nystagmus affects eye movements; however, the eye is otherwise normal. If the nystagmus is of the "jerk" variety, the child may, later in life, adopt mechanisms to minimize the nystagmus. These mechanisms, which include convergence and anomalous head position, can improve visual acuity to the 20/20 level in some patients.

History

The physician must first assess whether the child has a generalized delay in development or a systemic syndrome, with poor vision being only one manifestation. Inquiring about the usual infantile milestones can be very revealing. With a pure visual handicap, the nonvisual milestones should be achieved only slightly later than normal. The assistance of a pediatrician experienced in infant development can be very valuable. A history of any cause of brain damage should be sought. This event could occur during the pregnancy or delivery or following birth. A nonocular cause of poor vision should be suspected if there is a history of low birth weight, neonatal asphyxia as caused by the umbilical cord, seizure disorder, meningitis, hydrocephalus, or poor Apgar scores. Blindness due to ocular pathology should be suspected if one elicits a history of little or no skin or ocular pigmentation, photosensitivity, or poor pupillary responses. Endocrine abnormalities would be consistent with optic nerve hypoplasia.[7] A history of any family members with decreased vision can be very helpful. If the child appears quite fair, the family should be asked about any other relatives who may be as fair as the infant.

Physical Examination

First, the examiner should ascertain whether the vision is indeed below normal. Chapter 5 details the clinical findings of visual acuity determinations at different ages. All of those suggested tests, including optokinetic nystagmus, should be performed. In the presence of nystagmus, the examiner must be even more vigilant than normal for signs of visual perception. Often, moving a static or optokinetic nystagmus target in a different direction than the nystagmus, i.e., vertically when the child has horizontal nystagmus, will make the responses more evident. In the office, the ophthalmologist should then conduct a full ocular examination to rule out any apparent causes of blindness that present with an opacity of the ocular media such as cataract or a retinal mass (see Chapter 5). If there is no apparent cause, the ophthalmologist must be mindful of the retinal and optic nerve disorders that can cause blindness.

The pupils can be helpful in the workup. If the pupillary response to light is slow or nonexistent, the pathology probably lies in the eyes or optic nerves. With normal pupillary responses, the pathology probably lies in the subgeniculate visual pathway. As current experience shows, one should be sure that the infant is awake before assessing pupillary responses. Physicians should not mistake the constricted pupil of a sleeping infant as indicative of poor ocular function.

The retinal examination is critical in this evaluation. One should first look at the integrity of the entire retina to rule out retinal folds, detachment, or dysplasia. Then one should pay attention to the overall color and vascular development. Normally, the retina and optic nerve of a newborn will have more pallor than later in life. An albinotic-looking retina will of course be found in albinism (Fig 7–7) but also may be present in achromatopsia or other panretinal degenerations including Leber's amaurosis. Leber's amaurosis is usually characterized in infancy by a normal-appearing retina; however, some variants can display abnormal pigmentary patterns. The development of the macular should then be considered and compared with normal values for the infant's age.[8] Retinal hemorrhages are suggestive of trauma, possibly from battering. An absence of retinal tissue can result from a coloboma that is a developmental defect. If the coloboma involves the macula, vision will be decreased.

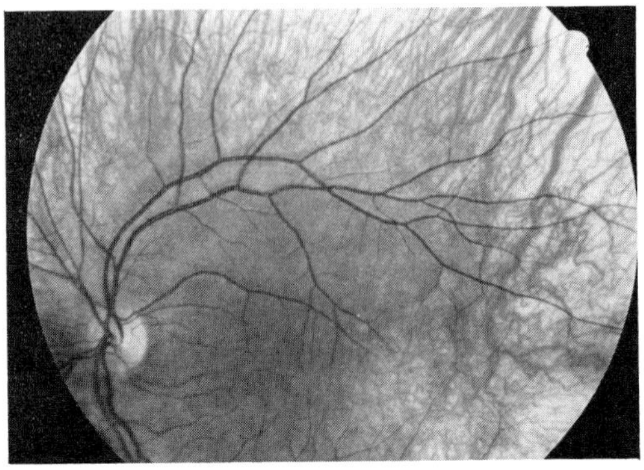

FIG 7–7.
The fundus of a black child with albinism. Note the prominence of the choroidal vasculature.

Unless the optic nerve is profoundly pale, one should hesitate to diagnose infantile optic atrophy because of the normal, somewhat pale color in infants. The size and vascular pattern of the arterioles of the optic nerve should be carefully evaluated. The size can be judged by comparison with the other eye or the eyes of similarly aged infants. However, the latter practice should consider the refractive error of the eye since refractive error can alter the apparent size of intraocular structures. More helpful is the appearance of one or two rings around a hypoplastic optic nerve (see Chapter 21). In addition, the retinal vessels appear to emerge from the center of hypoplastic discs rather than the more nasal location observed in normal discs. A decrease in the number or caliber of the small arterioles of the optic nerve can indicate optic atrophy. An enlarged optic nerve may result from a coloboma and can profoundly affect vision (Fig 7–8).

The refractive error determined after cycloplegia can be suggestive of the diagnosis. If the eyes are found to be significantly hyperopic (greater than 6.00 D), Leber's congenital amaurosis should be considered.[9] Achromatopsia can present with high hyperopia or myopia. A high astigmatic error would support the diagnosis of ocular albinism.

Unfortunately, the pattern of nystagmus is not usually helpful in determining the diagnosis. However, the presence of nystagmus may confirm the impression of poor vision, particularly if it has a pendular or "wandering" pattern. Simon and colleagues found that many patients diagnosed as having nystagmus and poor vision without a specific etiology actually had a form of albinism.[10] They based their diagnosis on the signs of detectable iris transillumination, choroidal depigmentation, and a history of abnormal tanning. It is imperative in cases of acquired nystagmus in infancy to obtain appropriate radiological studies. Lavery and coworkers reported nystagmus that generally presented before 10 months of age to be the presenting sign of life-threatening chiasmal or parachiasmal gliomas in ten infants.[11]

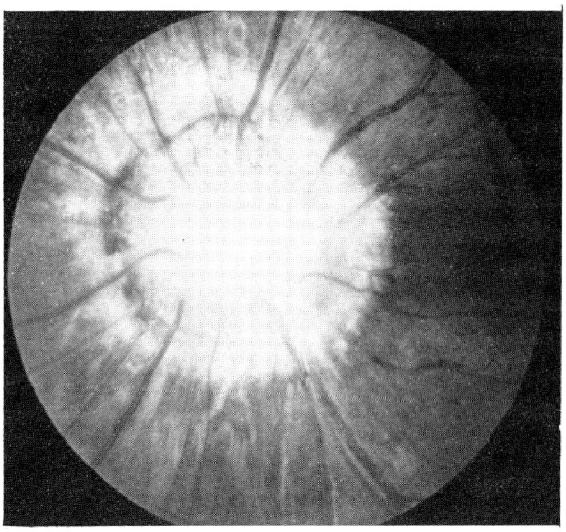

FIG 7–8.
A coloboma of the optic nerve head.

Tests

To simplify interpretation of the various tests one can order, it is convenient to divide the possible etiologies in these cases into three groups. The first is when the pathology is primarily in the eye such as in Leber's amaurosis or albinism. In this group, the electrophysiological tests will be the most useful. The second group are disorders of the optic nerves. For this group, VEP and computerized tomography are beneficial. The last group consists of those patients with pathology either of the brain as a whole or of the subgeniculate visual pathways. Magnetic resonance imaging, computerized tomography, VEP, and sometimes an electroencephalogram will aid this diagnosis.

Electrophysiological tests of the eye are always indicated in these children if the diagnosis is not obtained from the examination. This is due to the fact that retinal degenerations can have a retinal appearance that can vary from normal to gross pigmentary abnormalities. Since each laboratory has different standards, it is difficult to give absolute numbers for abnormalities. The most helpful test in understanding whether a panretinal problem is present is the ERG that tests separately both the cone and rod systems. In Leber's amaurosis, both the light-adapted, cone-mediated and dark-adapted, rod-mediated ERGs will be either nonrecordable or have a markedly abnormal response. In achromatopsia, the light-adapted cone or flicker ERG will be minimal or nonrecordable, while the rod ERG will be normal. In albinism, both responses will be normal to supernormal. If a minimal response is discovered on any of the tests, it is generally worthwhile to repeat them for confirmation in 3 to 6 months. The EOG is not very helpful in the diagnosis of infantile blindness.

VEPs can be very useful. The ERG should be performed first since a grossly abnormal retina will produce abnormalities in the VEP by itself even if the rest of the visual pathways are normal. If the ERG is normal, then an abnormal VEP indicates a problem in the optic nerves or cerebral cortex. Indeed, optic nerve hypoplasia can yield a grossly abnormal VEP. Because infants generally display waves of low amplitude compared with adults, the laboratory must have normal standards established for babies. Otherwise repetitive testing may be necessary prior to establishing a diagnosis.

Computerized tomography or magnetic resonance imaging can be useful in the investigation of the visual pathways including the optic nerves. An experienced radiologist may be able to diagnose optic nerve hypoplasia from the size of the optic nerves apparent on these tests. Hypodensities in the visual cortex may result from previous ischemic events, which can explain visual deficits (Fig 7–9). These tests can also disclose such central nervous system diagnoses as septooptic dysplasia, porencephalic cysts, Aicardi syndrome, and many of the phakomatoses. Lambert and associates have demonstrated that computer tomography and magnetic resonance imaging are particularly useful in infants who sustained hypoxic insults.[12] They reported that normal scans were consistent with a better visual prognosis, while asphyxia in premature infants was associated with a poor visual prognosis.

The Final Diagnosis

The physician should be cautious about giving definitive diagnostic and prognostic statements to the family until some time has passed since blindness was first suspected. The electrophysiological tests noted earlier can demonstrate improvement with time in some disorders. The child's visual performance may improve significantly with maturation even in the presence of a visual handicap. Finally, a specific group of infants with decreased vision is now being more frequently recognized. These infants are thought by both their parents and physicians to be blind or nearly blind, only to eventually develop normal or nearly normal vision.[13] In these infants, the electrophysiological test results are initially grossly abnormal but become normal with time. Another group of infants who appeared to be clinically blind in infancy and later develop near-normal vision were finally diagnosed as having congenital stationary night blindness.[14] However, the improvement in both these groups of infants should be appreciated by 6 to 12 months of age.

The diagnosis of blindness is not only crucial to the future of the infant but can be shattering to the child's parents and siblings. These important considerations are discussed in Chapter 29.

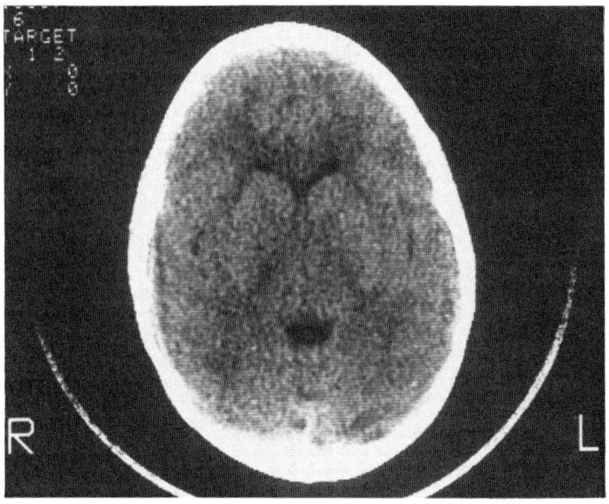

FIG 7–9.
Computerized tomography demonstrating occipital hypodensities in a child with 20/200 visual acuity.

THE CLOUDY CORNEA

Opacities of the cornea are usually noted very soon after birth. Not only will the eyes lack the red reflex sought by pediatricians, but the parents will appreciate a lack of corneal luster. An eye born with a significant corneal opacity will almost always develop amblyopia either from deprivation of formed vision reaching the retina or from refractive errors caused by corneal changes. Because the former type of amblyopia can only be reversed within the first few months of life, early recognition and treatment of this disorder is crucial.

Many corneal opacities will clear with time. To understand which disorders persist to the point where corneal transplantation is necessary, one needs to review published studies. In one series dealing only with congenitally opaque corneas, 60% of the cases were due to Peter's anomaly and 26% to sclerocornea with microphthalmos (Fig 7–10).[15] In a later series, the analysis of congenital corneal opacities was 60% Peter's anomaly, 13% residual corneal edema from glaucoma, 11% posterior polymorphous dystrophy, 9% multiple anomalies, and 7% sclerocornea.[16] It should be appreciated that these series reflect the feeling of the surgeons that the eyes were operable and that satisfactory vision might result from the procedure. The final visual acuity ranged from 20/40 to no light perception, with most patients attaining a vision of 20/100 to counting fingers.

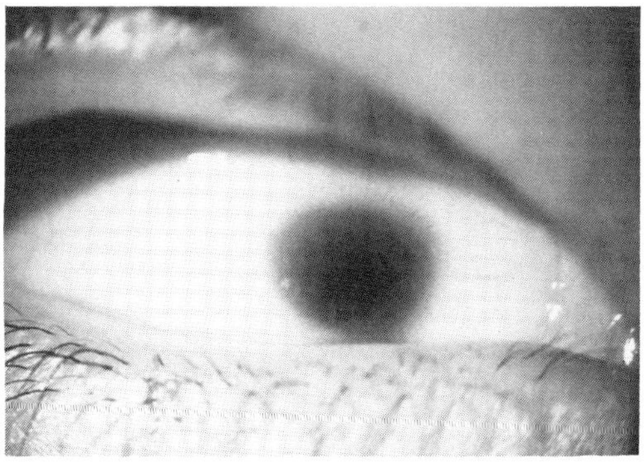

FIG 7–10.
Microphthalmos with sclerocornea. Note the absence of the normal limbal sulcus.

History

The parents should be asked about any illnesses during pregnancy since intrauterine keratitis can result from such infections as herpes, rubella, and syphilis. Drugs taken during pregnancy should be evaluated. A delivery by forceps of a particularly large infant would be suggestive of birth trauma. Since birth, a history of any infections, particularly if systemic or periocular, as well as structural abnormalities (as the umbilical hernia associated with Rieger's syndrome or the cutaneous manifestations of Sturge-Weber syndrome) may be helpful. The presence of photophobia and tearing support the diagnosis of glaucoma. A family history of congenital glaucoma, large eyes, poor vision from birth, or metabolic disease would aid in attaining a diagnosis.

Physical Examination

Other than inspection of the cornea, the most important test of the opacified infantile cornea is the intraocular pressure. If the pressure is elevated, the logical progression would be the differential diagnosis of primary vs. all the various secondary glaucomas (see Chapter 19). If possible, one would like to associate an elevated intraocular pressure with an increased corneal diameter and optic nerve cup to confirm the diagnosis of glaucoma. If the intraocular pressure is normal, either the glaucoma has "burned out," or the etiology lies elsewhere.

The eyelids should be examined for any evidence of infection or any unusual structures suggestive of the phakomatoses. The conjunctiva should be examined for any evidence of hemorrhage since birth trauma severe enough to cause corneal clouding usually engenders subconjunctival hemorrhages (Fig 7–11). The conjunctiva should also be carefully evaluated for such signs of inflammation as hyperemia and vascular pannus of the cornea. These findings would support either the diagnosis of a secondary glaucoma, possibly from a pupillary block, or one of the inflammatory etiologies. The latter possibility would generate a workup of intrauterine or postnatal infectious agents, trauma, etc.

The corneal examination can often indicate the diagnosis. First, the corneal diameters should be measured. An opacified cornea with an enlarged diameter strongly suggests glaucoma, although other diagnoses should be considered. An opacified cornea with a diameter smaller than normal can be found in rubella, trisomy 13, sclerocornea, and glaucoma in the presence of microphthalmos. If striae, which result from ruptures in Descemet's membrane, can be seen, their orientation can be revealing. Horizontally oriented corneal striae suggest glaucoma. However, vertically or obliquely oriented corneal striae

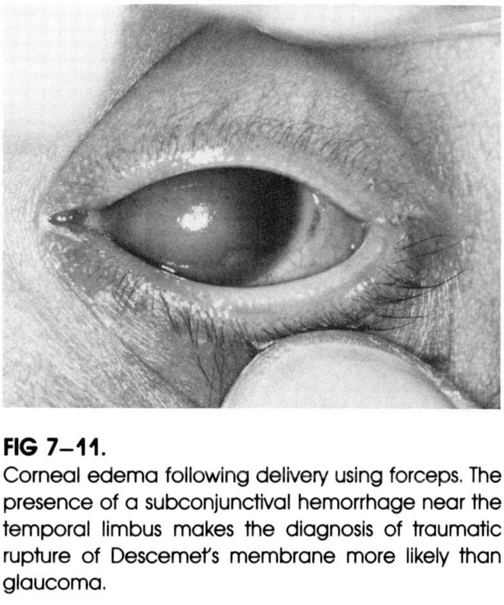

FIG 7–11.
Corneal edema following delivery using forceps. The presence of a subconjunctival hemorrhage near the temporal limbus makes the diagnosis of traumatic rupture of Descemet's membrane more likely than glaucoma.

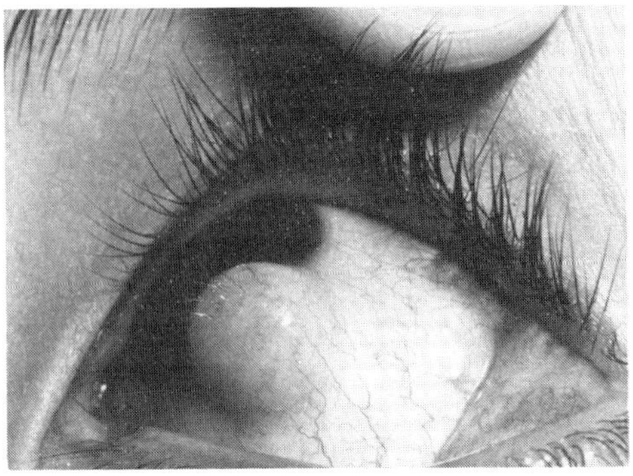

FIG 7–12.
A large limbal dermoid bearing hair follicles.

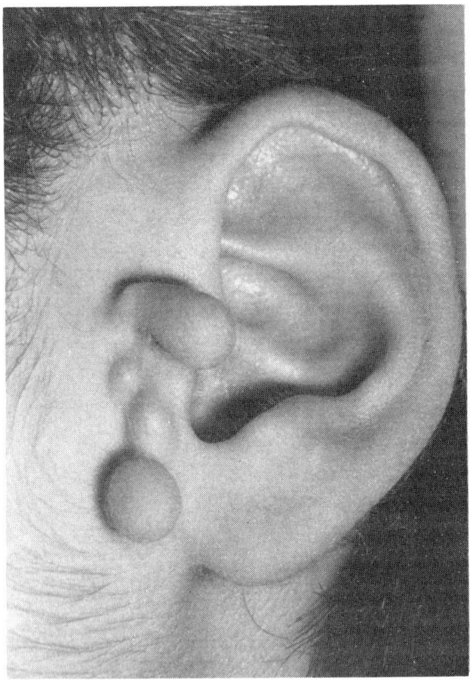

FIG 7–13.
The preauricular skin appendages commonly found in Goldenhar syndrome.

are consistent with birth trauma. A gray or yellowish mass overlying the cornea and containing hair follicles and glands is probably a dermoid tumor (Fig 7–12). Some dermoids are so large as to occlude the visual axis directly or by the lipid infiltrate around the tumor base. These tumors may be isolated or be part of Goldenhar syndrome (Fig 7–13). The sensation of the cornea should be tested since hypesthesia can result from neurotrophic keratopathy (Fig 7–14). This disorder, which may cause corneal ulcers with secondary infection, is sometimes treatable with tarsorrhaphy and other modalities. If the opacification is total, either the intraocular pressure is quite elevated, or another abnormality is present that may be structural (as sclerocornea or congenital endothelial dystrophy)[17] or metabolic (as mucolipidosis IV).[18] However, the extent of the opacity usually expresses the severity of the disorder and is not, by itself, diagnostic. The limbus should be carefully inspected. If one finds the limbus to lack a true sulcus, the diagnosis of sclerocornea or other structural abnormality is likely.

If the corneal opacity permits, the anterior chamber should be inspected. Any evidence of inflammation, especially flare and white blood cells, in the anterior chamber would favor the diagnoses of intraocular infection, uveitis, or trauma. The depth of the anterior chamber may be shallow in the secondary glaucomas with an opaque cornea on the basis of a force in the vitreous or posterior chambers that makes the anterior chamber shallow. The causes of this phenomenon are quite diverse and range from a dislocated lens to the detached retina of retinopathy of prematurity.

The iris, if visualized, may be useful in attaining a diagnosis. Adhesions between the

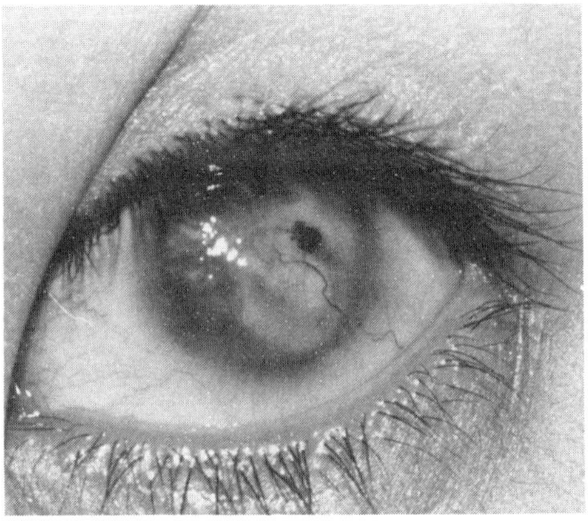

FIG 7–14.
Neurotrophic keratopathy caused recurrent corneal ulcers with subsequent scarring and vascularization in this infant.

iris and cornea often suggest a mesodermal dysgenesis syndrome (see Chapter 19). Indeed, Peter's anomaly can cause corneal clouding without causing glaucoma. Inflammatory iris changes such as nodules are rarely seen in infancy.

If the lens is cataractous, rubella, Lowe's syndrome, and birth trauma should be considered. An anterior polar or subcapsular lenticular opacity suggests Peter's anomaly. A dislocated lens in an infant would suggest birth or postnatal trauma as well as all the other recognized causes.

Examination of the vitreous and retina can be helpful, especially when considering rubella (pigmentary retinal changes) or a leukokoria disorder (see the section "Leukokoria") causing a secondary glaucoma. However, usually, the corneal opacity precludes a clear view of the posterior segment of the eye. Thus, one must often rely on diagnostic tests, especially ultrasonography, in making the diagnosis.

Tests

Ultrasonography is not only helpful in finding pathology in the posterior of the eye but can also indicate its size and shape. The cornea may be so opacified that the anterior chamber or iris is not visible. By using a "standoff" water bath, the ultrasound probe is moved away from the cornea but is still acoustically coupled to the eye. This permits visualization of the cornea, anterior chamber, iris, and lens, which are not visualized in the usual B scan. Occasionally the diagnosis of Peter's anomaly in the presence of a completely opacified cornea can be made with ultrasonography. As mentioned earlier, the size of the eye can imply a diagnosis. While ocular size is suggested by the corneal diameter, it is best to document it with an A scan axial length determination when possible.

OPHTHALMIA NEONATORUM

Conjunctivitis occurring within the first month of life is defined as ophthalmia neonatorum. When confronted with this entity, the ophthalmologist or pediatrician must consider a variety of possible causes since, like any infection or inflammation, the therapy depends on the diagnosis.

History

Since infants appear to acquire their conjunctival bacteria at birth from the mother during passage down the birth canal, it would be advantageous to inquire whether the mother had any recent disease of a venereal or genital sort.[19] Even if the mother admits to a previously treated venereal disease, it should be assumed that the infant has acquired that infection because the infection may not have been properly treated or the mother may have been reinfected. The father should also be asked the same questions.

The onset of infection is an important indicator of the diagnosis. If the symptoms began within 48 hours of birth, one should strongly consider that the child is not really infected but has a toxic reaction to the silver nitrate solution. This was more frequent when the silver nitrate solution was kept in a large bottle in the delivery room. Occasionally, the bottle would not be adequately mixed, thus causing the solution at the bottom to be more concentrated. This more concentrated solution would cause the toxic reaction. However, even the 1% concentration administered from a small ampule can engender a toxic reaction. An onset between 2 and 5 days following birth would be consistent with gonococcal infection. Herpes simplex, type 2, can present from 2 to 30 days of age. From 4 days to 1 week after birth, a variety of bacteria, with *Staphylococcus aureus* the most prominent, may cause a clinically evident conjunctivitis. Chlamydial conjunctivitis can present 1 to 4 weeks following birth, with the second week being the most frequent. These figures for the inception of the disease should be considered only estimates. With the exception of silver nitrate conjunctivitis, the onset of all of these conditions may vary from these times.

If the infant has a history of a severe sys-

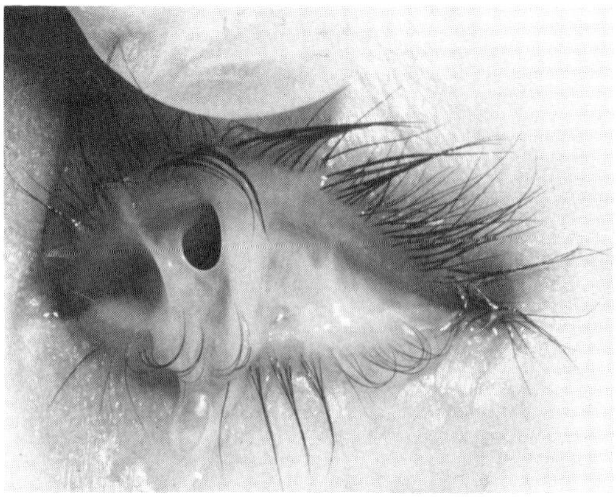

FIG 7–15.
Purulence of the severe degree found in this infant should always suggest the possibility of gonococcal conjunctivitis.

temic illness, herpes should be ruled out since herpes simplex can present in a disseminated form including in the eye. This disseminated form can affect the central nervous system, lungs, liver, and adrenal glands. The actual clinical findings are nonspecific. The mortality is said to be 80%.

Physical Examination

If the eyelids demonstrate intense edema, gonococcal infection should be strongly suspected. Do not separate the eyelids for inspection without wearing glasses or a form of goggles! Gonococcal conjunctivitis has been noted to pass from infant to the examiner by squirting into the examiner's eye. Mild eyelid edema can be found in almost any case of neonatal conjunctivitis.

Most patients with neonatal conjunctivitis will present with red injected eyes, conjunctival edema, and a secretion varying from a scant watery discharge to copious purulence. With conjunctivitis, neonates generally do not demonstrate follicles or papillae as do adults. However, follicles can appear in chlamydial infections. In newborns, one depends heavily on laboratory tests for a diagnosis. However, there are some minor physical findings of the conjunctiva that are helpful. If the purulent discharge is very copious in the presence of a beefy red conjunctiva, gonococcus should be suspected (Fig 7–15). Pseudomembranes can be found with chlamydial and streptococcal infections. If keratitis develops relatively early in the disease and there has not been a significant purulent exudate, herpes must be ruled out.

Tests

The laboratory evaluation of this disorder requires numerous types of cultures and cytological analyses to achieve a diagnosis. The eyelids should be everted with a lid speculum or a paper clip bent in the shape of the letter *C*. First, a moistened, cotton-tipped applicator should be placed deeply into the conjunctival fornix to avoid contact with the speculum or clip. Specimens should be inoculated on blood agar, chocolate, and Thayer-Martin agar plates and cultured appropriately. Second, conjunctival epithelial cells should be obtained with a spatula and not with applicator sticks. After the cells have been spread on a microscope slide, Giemsa and Gram stains should be applied. On Gram stain, one should look for the gram-negative intracellular diplococci indicative of gonococci (Fig 7–16) or the gram-positive response and morphology of such organisms as staphylococci or streptococci. On the Giemsa-stained slides, one should look for the paranuclear cytoplasmic inclusion bodies found in chlamydial infections (Fig 7–17) as well as the intranuclear inclusion bodies and

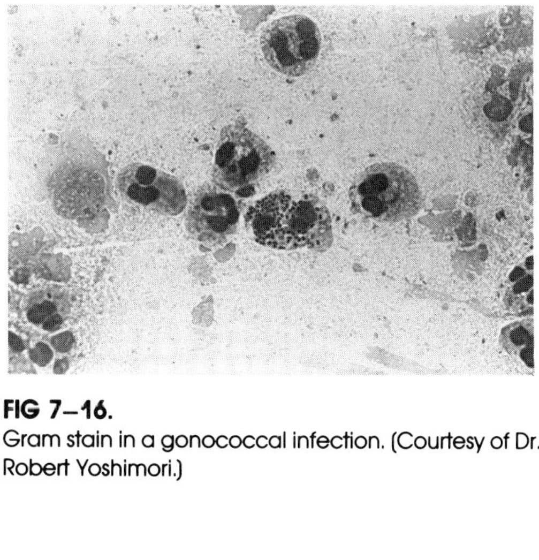

FIG 7–16.
Gram stain in a gonococcal infection. (Courtesy of Dr. Robert Yoshimori.)

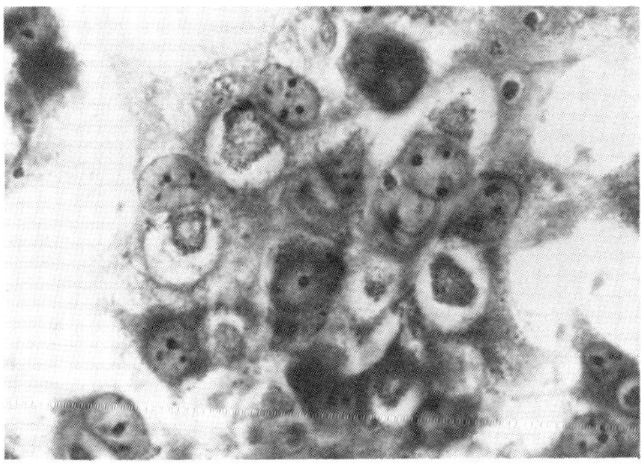

FIG 7–17.
Modified Giemsa stain of a chlamydial infection. (Courtesy of Dr. Robert Yoshimori.)

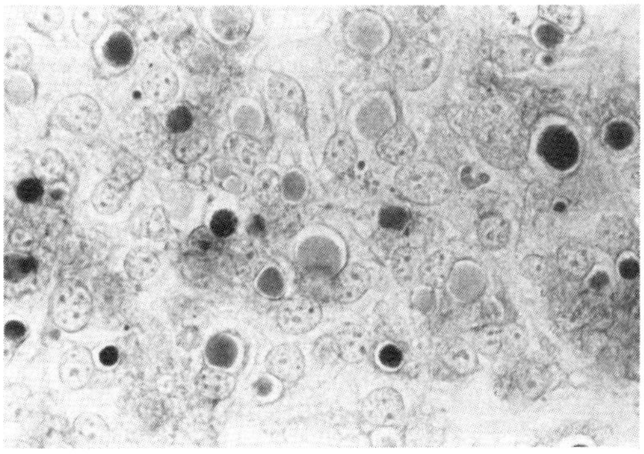

FIG 7–18.
Iodine test response is positive in this chlamydial culture. (Courtesy of Dr. Robert Yoshimori.)

multinucleated giant cells indicative of herpetic infection. One can also utilize an iodine stain to enhance the chlamydial organisms (Fig 7–18). Third, the direct slide immunofluorescent monclonal antibody test for chlamydia should be obtained since this is proving to be sensitive and specific (Fig 7–19).

A faster technique has been recently described for diagnosing neonatal chlamydial conjunctivitis.[20] Impression cytology permits the acquisition of conjunctival epithelial cells by applying precut cellulose acetate filter paper to the conjunctiva. The specimen is then fixed in 95% alcohol and stained with hematoxylin-eosin. Maskin and colleagues were then able to identify basophilic cytoplasmic inclusions characteristic of chlamydial infections.

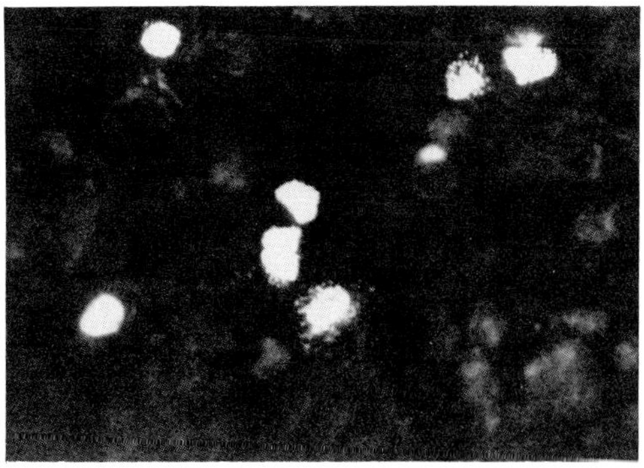

FIG 7–19.
Positive immunofluorescent test response for chlamydial culture using a monoclonal antibody. (Courtesy of Dr. Robert Yoshimori.)

REFERENCES

1. Beller R, Hoyt CS, Marg E, et al: Good visual function after neonatal surgery for congenital monocular cataracts. *Am J Ophthalmol* 1981; 91:559.
2. Rubenstein K: Posterior hyperplastic primary vitreous. *Br J Ophthalmol* 1980; 64:105.
3. Katz NNK, Margo CE, Dorwart RH: Computerized tomography with histopathological correlation in children with leukokoria. *J Pediatr Ophthalmol Strabismus* 1984; 21:50.
4. Haik BG, Saint Louis L, Smith ME, et al: Magnetic resonance imaging in the evaluation of leukocoria. *Ophthalmology* 1985; 92:1143.
5. Kabak J, Romano PE: Aqueous humor lactic dehydrogenase isoenzymes in retinoblastoma. *Br J Ophthalmol* 1975; 59:268.
6. Swartz M, Herbst RW, Goldberg MF: Aqueous humor lactic acid dehydrogenase in retinoblastoma. *Am J Ophthalmol* 1974; 78:612.
7. Skarf B, Hoyt CS: Optic nerve hypoplasia in children. *Arch Ophthalmol* 1984; 102:62.
8. Isenberg SJ: Macular development in the premature infant. *Am J Ophthalmol* 1986; 101:74.
9. Wagner RS, Caputo AR, Nelson LB, et al: High hyperopia in Leber's congenital amaurosis. *Arch Ophthalmol* 1985; 103:1507.
10. Simon JM, Kandel GL, Krohel GB, et al: Albinotic characteristics in congenital nystagmus. *Am J Ophthalmol* 1984; 97:320.
11. Lavery MA, O'Neill JF, Chu FC, et al: Acquired nystagmus in early childhood: A presenting sign of intracranial tumor. *Ophthalmology* 1984; 91:425.
12. Lambert SR, Hoyt CS, Jan JE, et al: Visual re-

covery from hypoxic cortical blindness during childhood. *Arch Ophthalmol* 1987; 105:1371.
13. Mellor DH, Fielder ER: Dissociated visual development. Electrodiagnostic studies in infants who are "slow to see." *Dev Med Child Neurol* 1980; 22:327.
14. Weleber RG, Tongue AC: Congenital stationary night blindness presenting as Leber's congenital amaurosis. *Arch Ophthalmol* 1987; 105:360.
15. Schanzlin DJ, Goldberg DB, Brown SI: Transplantation of congenitally opaque corneas. *Ophthalmology* 1980; 87:1253.
16. Stulting RD, Sumers KD, Cavanagh HD, et al: Penetrating keratoplasty in children. *Ophthalmology* 1984; 91:1222.
17. Kenyon KR, Maumenee AE: The histological and ultrastructural pathology of congenital hereditary corneal dystrophy: A case report. *Invest Ophthalmol* 1968; 7:475.
18. Merin S, Nemet P, Livni N, et al: The cornea in mucolipidosis IV. *J Pediatr Ophthalmol* 1976; 13:289.
19. Isenberg SJ, Apt L, Yoshimori R, et al: Bacterial flora of the conjunctiva at birth. *J Pediatr Ophthalmol Strabismus* 1986; 23:284.
20. Maskin SL, Heitman KF, Yee RW: Use of impression cytology in neonatal chlamydial conjunctivitis. *Arch Ophthalmol* 1987; 105:1626.

8 Pharmacology

Leonard Apt, M.D.

GENERAL CONSIDERATIONS

In prescribing a safe yet effective drug dosage for premature infants, newborns, and young infants the physician must understand that certain physiological factors are unique in these changing, developing patients. Drug metabolism may be impaired because of enzyme (principally hepatic) immaturity; drug excretion is diminished because of renal immaturity; gastrointestinal absorption of drugs modified by variations in gastric pH, delayed gastric emptying time, and intestinal motility; intramuscular absorption of drugs is altered by differences in relative blood flow to various muscle groups; and distribution of drugs to their sites of action is determined by differences in the size of the body fluid compartments, muscle mass and fat store, tissue blood flow, and protein binding.

Bioavailability of drugs in newborns is not always in one direction. For example, oral penicillin preparations usually are absorbed well because of relative achlorhydria during the first few weeks of life, whereas the oral absorption of phenobarbital is decidedly reduced; the metabolism of chloramphenicol is impaired because of deficient hepatic glucuronidation ("gray-baby syndrome"), yet other metabolic pathways such as demethylation permit satisfactory biotransformation of mepivacaine.

Though many drugs are given to newborns in reduced dosages because of the immaturity of physiological functions, some drugs must be given in relatively large amounts to achieve a given serum concentration. Explanations for this requirement include the following: (1) since total-body, extracellular fluid, and blood volumes of newborns are larger on a weight basis than those of older children and adults, the initial larger volume for distribution of a given drug necessitates a higher dose; and (2) the metabolic rate is higher in the young patient.

Pediatric patients, especially the younger ones, are not miniature adults. Their physiological functions differ and are ever changing as they develop and grow. Dosage schedules based solely on proportions of an adult dose by weight or age often are not satisfactory. Schedules based on surface area are more reliable. Usually the popular published schedules for drug dosage on a weight basis have been derived from clinical and laboratory monitoring by expert physicians. The figures are a good starting point. However, drug schedules for newborns and young infants need to be individualized. Complex medicolegal issues of experimentation in young patients have hindered progress in these studies. Thus Food and Drug Administration (FDA) clearance for use of many beneficial drugs in infants has not been given.

Topical eye drug therapy in pediatric patients is on an even less sound basis than are dosing guides for oral and parenteral drug therapy. Topical medication is primarily for action on the anterior structures of the eye. A good portion of the dose, however, leaves the eye and may be absorbed systemically. The eyelid and cul-de-sac retain only one fifth of an instilled eyedrop (0.05 ml is average eyedrop size). Systemic absorption may occur through the conjunctival epithelium; through the mucous membrane lining of the nasolacrimal duct, nose, and oropharynx; through the digestive system if drainage is swallowed; or through the skin from the overflow. Since most topical eye drug preparations are available only in one concentration, the pediatric patient receives the adult dose. Adult dosing with potent ocular drugs can then lead to serious systemic toxicity because the dose relative to blood volume, body weight, and surface area is much greater for infants and children. Also, neonates and young infants are particularly susceptible to overdosage because of the immaturity of their metabolic and excretory systems.

The factor of the relationship of the dose to body weight and surface area is particularly important. If drops only are considered, an approximation can be made of the total dose delivered to the eyes following a routine instillation. The dose per drop is listed in Table 8–1 for certain topical eye drugs used in the pediatric age group for examination and therapeutic purposes. The usual systemic pediatric therapeutic dose and the lethal dose, if it is known, also are included.

A relative overdosage of all of the drugs listed in Table 8–1 may occur in the pediatric patient, particularly if repeated doses are given. Up to 80% of an eyedrop dose may be absorbed into the systemic circulation. If systemic absorption is only 50% of the instilled medication, however, the systemic dose can be dangerously large. For example, one drop of 10% phenylephrine (100 mg/mL) instilled into each eye delivers 10.0 mg of drug. Assuming that only 50% of the administered drug (5 mg) is absorbed, a 5-kg infant receives ten times the usual subcutaneous (SC) or intramuscular (IM) therapeutic dose (0.5 mg) or five times the usual intravenous (IV) therapeutic dose (0.1 mg). Similar comparisons can be made for other drugs in Table 8–1.

Measures to reduce excessive absorption and toxicity of topical eye medication in pediatric patients include proper immobilization of the infant and of the eyelids to avoid instilling more than the prescribed dose, digital pressure on the punctum to avoid the entrance of eyedrops into the nasolacrimal system, decreasing the drop size by modifying the present eyedroppers, dissolving the drug in an oily solution or an ointment base to decrease the passage of drug into the nasolacrimal duct, and combining two or more drugs into one solution so multiple instillation with each drug is avoided.

SELECTED EYE DRUGS USED IN INFANTS

A summary of selected drugs used in the examination and treatment of eye problems in newborns and young infants follows. For more details on the respective drugs, standard pharmacology and ocular pharmacology texts should be consulted.

MYDRIATICS AND CYCLOPLEGICS

Mydriatics and cycloplegics both dilate the pupils. Cycloplegics also cause paralysis of accommodation. The more potent agents such as atropine and scopolamine should not be used if only mydriasis is needed. Both types of drugs often are used together to maximize mydriasis.

Mydriatics (Sympathomimetics)

Phenylephrine Hydrochloride (Neo-Synephrine)

Preparations.—Solution, 2.5% and 10% (avoid in infants).

Dosage.—1 drop, repeated in 30 minutes if needed.

Onset and Duration of Action.—Effect is within 30 minutes. Maximum response occurs in about 60 minutes. The pupil returns to normal in 2 to 3 hours.

Comment.—Phenylephrine is of little

TABLE 8–1.
Administered Dose of Commonly Used Topical Ophthalmic Drug*

Drug and Concentration	Amount Drug (mg) in 1 Drop (20 Drops/mL)	Amount Drug (mg) (1 Drop Each Eye)	Pediatric Systemic Therapeutic Dose†
Phenylephrine, 10% (Neo-Synephrine)	5.0	10	0.1 mg/kg SC, IM; or 0.02 mg/kg IV‡ 5-kg infant = 0.5 mg SC, IM; or 0.1 mg IV 20-kg child = 2.0 mg SC, po; or 0.4 mg IV Minimum lethal dose, 10 mg SC or 1.5 mg IV (young adult)
Epinephrine HCl, 2.0%	1.0	2.0	0.01 mL 1:1,000/kg SC (maximum, 0.5 mg q4h) 5-kg infant = 0.05 mg 20-kg child = 0.2 mg Minimum lethal dose = 4 mg§
Atropine sulfate, 1.0%	0.5	1.0	0.01 mg/kg po or SC q4–6h (maximum, 0.4 mg total) 5-kg infant = 0.05 mg 20-kg child = 0.2 mg Minimum lethal dose = 10 mg (infant), 10–20 mg (child)‖
Scopolamine, 0.25% (Isopto Hyoscine)	0.125	0.25	0.03 mg/kg IM, IV, or SC 5-kg infant = 0.15 mg 20-kg child = 0.6 mg Minimum lethal dose = 10 mg‖
Cyclopentolate, 2.0% (Cyclogyl)	1.0	2.0	Too toxic for systemic use Estimated lethal dose = 10–100 mg/kg‖
Ecthotiophate iodide, 0.25% (Phospholine Iodide)	0.125	0.25	Too toxic for systemic use Systemic lethal dose not known Estimated lethal dose intraocularly = 10 mg‖
Prednisolone acetate, 1.0%	0.5	1.0	Physiological replacement dose (po)¶ Infant = 2–4 mg/day Child = 4–10 mg/day
Dexamethasone, 0.1%	0.05	0.1	Infant = 0.4–0.8 mg/day Child = 0.8–2.0 mg/day Pharmacological dose is up to four times replacement dose

*From Apt L, Gaffney WL: Toxic effects of topical eye medication in infants and children, in Duane TD, Jaeger EA (eds): *Biomedical Foundations of Ophthalmology.* Hagerstown, Md, Harper & Row, Inc, 1982, p 2. Used with permission.
†Data from Shirkey HC: Table of drugs. In Vaughan VC III, McKay RJ (eds): *Nelson Textbook of Pediatrics,* 10th ed. p 1713. Philadelphia, WB Saunders Co, 1975, p 1713.
‡Data from Keys A, Violente A: The cardiocirculatory effects in man of Neo-Synephrine. *J Clin Invest* 1942; 21:1.
§Data from Freedman BJ: Accidental adrenaline overdosage and its treatment with piperoxan. *Lancet* 1955: 2:575.
‖Data from Dreisbach RH: *Handbook of Poisoning: Prevention, Diagnosis and Treatment,* 10th ed. pp 343, 350. Los Altos, Calif, Lange Medical Publications, 1980, pp 343, 350.
¶Data from Gardner LI: *Endocrine and Genetic Diseases of Childhood and Adolescence,* 2nd ed. Philadelphia, WB Saunders Co, 1975, p 531.

value when used alone for ophthalmoscopy because of its limited dilating effect. The drug usually is used with a less potent cycloplegic drug such as tropicamide or cyclopentolate (see the section on cycloplegics). Avoid the use of concentrations higher than 2.5% to avert a rise in blood pressure and heart rate.

Hydroxyamphetamine Hydrobromide (Paredrine)

Preparations.—Solution, 1%.

Dosage.—1 drop, repeated in 30 minutes if needed.

Onset and Duration of Action.—Similar to phenylephrine.

Comment.—The drug is used to produce mydriasis for ophthalmoscopy but is a weaker mydriatic than phenylephrine in infants and children. Hydroxyamphetamine has been reported to produce greater than normal mydriasis in patients with Down syndrome. No side effects have been reported, but the drug has not been used widely in infants.

Cycloplegics (Parasympatholytics)

Atropine Sulfate

Preparations.—Solution, 0.5%, 1%, 2%, and 3%; ointment, 0.5% and 1%; 0.25% atropine in oil (not available commercially—see the comment later in this section).

Dosage.—For refraction, 1 drop or 1 drop size of ointment is less likely to be absorbed systemically than the solution and thus should decrease the toxicity risk. For anterior uveitis and postoperative mydriasis/cycloplegia, 0.5% solution or ointment 1 to 2 times daily.

Onset and Duration of Action.—Onset of action is within 30 to 40 minutes, and maximal cycloplegia is reached in about 32 hours. The duration of the cycloplegic effect is 1 to 2 weeks.

Comment.—I prefer the use of 0.25% atropine in sesame oil for infants. The drug is specially prepared at the UCLA Medical Center pharmacy. I found in a group of young children that this preparation was comparable in action to a 1% aqueous solution (unpublished data), which is probably explained by the longer contact time of the medication in the eye. Furthermore, less toxicity has been encountered, presumably because of the lower concentration of available drug and the lessened chance of systemic absorption since the base is an oil rather than water. Acute systemic reactions from atropine usually are dose-related. Idiosyncratic responses, however, may occur. Lightly pigmented, Down syndrome, and brain-damaged infants seem especially susceptible to the toxic effects of atropine. Parents need to be advised of the early signs of toxicity so that the administration of medication is not continued. In the event of systemic atropine toxicity, prompt treatment with physostigmine salicylate (Antilirium) reverses both the central and peripheral toxicity. The dosage of physostigmine salicylate for infants is 0.02 to 0.03 mg/kg IV, IM, or SC; the dose is repeated in 30 minutes if no effect is obtained and then given every 1 to 2 hours as needed. Contact dermatitis and allergic conjunctivitis are uncommon in infants.

Scopolamine Hydrobromide (Isopto Hyoscine)

Preparation.—Solution, 0.25%.

Dosage.—For refraction (author's preference): 1 drop in each eye the night before and 1 hour before examination. For anterior uveitis and postoperative mydriasis/cycloplegia: 1 drop once or twice daily.

Onset and Duration of Action.—Maximum cycloplegia occurs within 1 hour. Recovery of some accommodation in infants begins within 24 hours (author's observation). Cycloplegia lasts 3 to 5 days in normal eyes.

Comment.—Scopolamine is similar to atropine in its action and toxicity manifestations. It has been used as a substitute when atropine allergy occurs. Systemic toxicity is treated with physostigmine salicylate (see the dosage recommended in the comment on atropine).

Homatropine Hydrobromide (Isopto Homatropine)

Preparations.—Solution, 2% and 5%.

Dosage.—For refraction: 1 drop of 2% solution in each eye, repeated in 15 minutes. For anterior uveitis: 1 drop of 2% solution twice daily.

Onset and Duration of Action.—Onset of cycloplegia is in 10 to 30 minutes, with maximum cycloplegia reached in 30 minutes to 2 hours. Cycloplegia lasts 36 to 48 hours.

Comment.—Homatropine is a weaker cycloplegic and mydriatic agent than either atropine or scopolamine. The drug is not often used at present because its cycloplegic action is less complete than that of atropine and lasts longer than that of cyclopentolate, which is at least as effective. Systemic toxic reactions from homatropine drops are similar to those from atropine and scopolamine. Physostigmine salicylate reverses the systemic anticholinergic effects of homatropine (see the dosage recommended in the comment on atropine).

Cyclopentolate Hydrochloride (Cyclogyl)

Preparations.—Solution, 0.5%, 1%, and 2% (avoid in infants).

Dosage.—For refraction and ophthalmoscopy; 1 drop of 0.5% solution in newborns and 0.5% or 1% solution in older or darkly pigmented infants in each eye, repeated in 10 mintues.

Onset and Duration of Action.—Onset of mydriasis and cycloplegia is 15 minutes, with maximum cycloplegia reached in 30 to 75 minutes. Maximum cycloplegia lasts for an additional hour. Recovery of accommodation is complete in 6 to 24 hours.

Comment.—Cyclopentolate is identical to atropine in its pharmacological action, but the intensity and duration of its anticholinergic action is considerably shorter. Since the period of maximal cycloplegia in young infants is brief, refraction must be performed within about 1 hour after instillation of the drug. Otherwise, refraction during the recovery phase may result in an erroneous measurement.

Systemic toxicity induced by cyclopentolate eyedrops is similar to that produced by atropine except that visual and tactile hallucinations are a more striking feature. Abdominal distention, paralytic ileus, and necrotizing enterocolitis have been reported in newborns, but this author has seen the same complications after the use of atropine eyedrops. As with atropine, systemic toxicity is seen more often in patients with brain damage, Down syndrome, and light pigmentation. Physostigmine salicylate reverses the central and peripheral toxicity of cyclopentolate (see the dosage recommended in the comment on atropine).

Toxic reactions are more likely to occur with the 2% concentration, even in older children and adults. The use of this concentration should be avoided in newborns and young infants.

Ophthalmoscopic examination of premature infants and neonates often requires maximum mydriasis that is sustained during binocular indirect ophthalmoscopy. The combination of 1 drop of cyclopentolate, 0.5%, and 1 drop of phenylephrine, 2.5%, instilled either separately 5 minutes apart or together in a single-instillation solution produces excellent and sustained mydriasis, especially if the drops are preceded by a drop of local anesthetic. A local anesthetic such as proparacaine enhances the mydriatic effect of the drugs by increasing transcorneal absorption and decreasing the dilution effect of tearing by preventing the stinging sensation of the dilating drugs. Cyclomydril is a commercially available combination of cyclopentolate, 0.2%, and phenylephrine, 1%, that is safe in premature infants and newborns and produces wide mydriasis.

Tropicamide (Mydriacyl)

Preparations.—Solution, 0.5% and 1%.

Dosage.—For mydriasis: 1 drop of 0.5% solution in each eye and repeat in 5 minutes.

Onset and Duration of Action.—Maximal mydriasis occurs within 30 minutes and lasts for about 30 minutes, with recovery over the following 2 to 4 hours. Cycloplegia is insignificant in infants.

Comment.—Tropicamide should be considered exclusively a mydriatic in infants. Cycloplegia even with the 1% concentration is minimal and transient. Tropicamide is an effective mydriatic in infants with darkly pigmented irides as well as those with blue irides.

Tropicamide, 0.5% or 1% eyedrops, combined with phenylephrine, 2.5% eyedrops, given either separately 5 minutes apart or combined in one drop, produces wide pupillary dilation for indirect ophthalmoscopy in premature infants and neonates. A drop of local anesthetic such as proparacaine preceding the combination of mydriatic eyedrops enhances the mydriatic effect of the drugs. Tropicamide also has been used in combination with cyclopentolate and phenylephrine in one solution to obtain wide mydriasis for indirect ophthalmoscopy in premature babies and newborns. The single-instillation solution contains cyclopentolate, 0.5%, tropicamide, 0.5%, and phenylephrine, 2.5%. The solution is prepared by combining 3.75 mL of cyclopentolate, 2%, with 7.5 mL of tropicamide, 1%, and 3.75 mL of phenylephrine, 10%. Tropicamide rarely causes either local or systemic adverse reactions.

ANTIBIOTIC THERAPY

Intelligent antibiotic treatment of infections in and around the eyes of newborns and premature infants requires knowledge of the types of microorganisms likely to be causative at this time of life, the means to identify the etiologic agent, selection of the appropriate anti-infective drug, and familiarity with the dosage schedule of the drug that ensures a suitable and safe blood level.

The various ocular infections that may be encountered in newborns such as conjunctivitis, keratitis, corneal ulcer, dacryocystitis, preseptal and orbital cellulitis, and endophthalmitis will not be dealt with here. Details on these diseases, including information on the likely causative bacteria and the recommended antibiotics for treatment, can be found in Chapter 25, in regular pediatric and ophthalmic textbooks, and in published papers.

Commercial topical ophthalmic antibiotic solutions and ointments usually are made only in one concentration. Thus no special dosage discussion is needed. The amount of antibiotic absorbed systemically from these drugs usually is negligible and rarely creates a problem. Local allergic reactions (especially with neomycin) and eye irritation seen in adults are uncommon in young infants. Antibiotics that are commonly used systemically should not be used topically, if possible, because sensitization of the patient will preclude future use of the drug.

Nontoxic dosages of antibiotics for subconjunctival and intravitreal injections have been established in adults. These routes of administration usually are reserved for serious intraocular infections. Dosage schedules are found in standard ocular pharmacology and therapeutics texts and in ophthalmic publications. The dosage of drugs in these injections seems safe for infants when used briefly. However, little experience with therapy by these routes of administration in infants has been made known. Subconjunctival and intravitreal antibiotic therapy usually is used only over a short period and generally in conjunction with the systemic administration of antibiotics.

Dosage guidelines for antibiotics given systemically to premature and newborn infants are presented. Comments on possible adverse reactions to the drugs listed are given when known.

Systemic Antibiotic Dosages

Amikacin (Amikin)

Dosage.—7.5 mg/kg IV or IM every 12 hours for newborns less than 1 week old, every 8 hours for those older than 1 week. IV dose is given over 30 minutes. Premature infants may need higher doses, up to 20 mg/kg/day. Blood level monitoring is recommended (10 to 25 μg/mL is desirable).

Toxicity.—Renal and eighth nerve toxicity; fever, rash.

Ampicillin (Numerous Tradename Products)

Dosage.—25 to 50 mg/kg IV or IM every 12 hours for newborns less than 1 week old, every 8 hours for those older than 1 week.

Toxicity.—See penicillin G.

Carbenicillin Disodium (Geopen, Pyopen)

Dosage.—100 mg/kg IV every 12 hours to newborns less than 1 week old; after 1 week old the same dose is given every 8 hours to infants 2,000 gm or less, and every 6 hours to those over 2,000 gm.

Toxicity.—See penicillin G. Bleeding diathesis secondary to platelet dysfunction also is reported but is rarely seen in newborns. Hypokalemia may also occur.

Cefotaxime (Claforan)

Dosage.—50 mg/kg IV (given over 3 to 5 minutes) or IM every 12 hours for infants up to 1 week old; every 8 hours for infants older than 1 week.

Toxicity.—Bleeding diathesis is possible because of impairment of vitamin K synthesis and alteration of prothrombin time. Vitamin K therapy is recommended during use of drug. Rash, fungal overgrowth, and neutropenia are uncommon.

Ceftazidime (Fortaz)

Dosage.—50 mg/kg IV or IM every 12 hours for infants less than 1 week; same dose every 8 hours for infants older than 1 week.

Toxicity.—See cefotaxime.

Ceftriaxone (Rocephin)

Dosage.—50 mg/kg IV every 12 hours for newborns and infants.

Toxicity.—See cefotaxime with regard to bleeding potential and other side effects. Ceftriaxone can displace bilirubin from serum albumin, so avoid use in hyperbilirubinemic neonates, especially prematures. The prothrombin time may be altered because of possible impairment of vitamin K synthesis and thus cause a bleeding problem. Vitamin K therapy is recommended during the use of ceftriaxone.

Chloramphenicol (Chloromycetin)

Dosage.—12.5 mg/kg IV (over 30 minutes) every 12 hours for infants up to 1 week of age; after 1 week of age low–birth weight infants receive 12.5 mg/kg IV (over 30 minutes) every 12 hours, and normal–birth weight infants receive 25 mg/kg IV (over 30 minutes) every 12 hours.

Toxicity.—Gray-baby syndrome (cardiovascular collapse), cardiac toxicity, and bone marrow suppression usually are avoided by blood level monitoring (therapeutic level, 10 to 25 μg/mL).

Clindamycin (Cleocin)

Dosage.—5 mg/kg IV or IM every 8 hours for low–birth weight infants less than 1 month old and for full-term infants less than 1 week old; 5 mg/kg IV or IM every 6 hours for normal–birth weight infants over 1 week of age.

Toxicity.—Rash, thrombophlebitis, and pseudomembranous colitis are uncommon in neonates.

Erythromycin (Numerous Tradename Products)

Dosage.—Oral (estolate), 10 mg/kg, every 12 hours for infants less than 1 week old; every

8 hours if older than 1 week. Intravenous (lactobionate), 10 mg/kg, every 8 hours for infants less than 1 week old; 7.5 to 12.5 mg/kg every 6 hours for infants older than 1 week.

Toxicity.—Pain at injection site, drug fever, gastrointestinal symptoms. Intrahepatic cholestatic jaundice from the estolate form is rare in pediatric patients when the drug is used for a short period.

Gentamicin (Garamycin)

Dosage.—2.5 mg/kg IV (over 30 minutes) or IM once daily for premature infants less than 1 week old, with the same dose every 12 hours for normal–birth weight infants less than 1 week old; 2.5 mg/kg IV (over 30 minutes) or IM every 8 hours for infants over 1 week old.

Toxicity.—Impaired hearing and vestibular function. Minimize or avoid toxicity by monitoring blood level (optimum serum level, 4 to 8 μg/mL).

Kanamycin (Kantrex)

Dosage.—7.5 mg/kg IV (over 20 minutes) or IM every 12 hours for infants less than 1 week old; after 1 week of age, 7.5 to 10 mg/kg IV (over 20 minutes) or IM every 12 hours for low–birth weight infants and every 8 hours for normal–birth weight infants.

Toxicity.—Deafness (cumulative with other ototoxic drugs), renal damage (usually transient unless there is previous renal impairment). Deter toxicity by monitoring blood level (15 to 25 μg/mL is desirable) and limit use of the drug to 10 days.

Methicillin (Staphcillin), Nafcillin (Unipen), Oxacillin (Prostaphlin)

Dosage.—25 to 50 mg/kg IV (over 10 minutes) or IM every 12 hours for infants less than 1 week old; same dosage every 6 to 8 hours for infants older than 1 week.

Toxicity.—See penicillin G. IV route is preferred because IM injection may cause a sterile abscess.

Mezlocillin (Mezlin)

Dosage.—75 mg/kg IV (over 30 minutes) or IM every 12 hours for infants less than 1 week old; same dose every 8 hours for infants older than 1 week.

Toxicity.—See carbenicillin.

Penicillin G (Numerous Tradename Products)

Dosage.—25,000 to 50,000 units/kg IV or IM every 12 hours for infants less than 1 week old; same dose every 6 to 8 hours for infants older than 1 week.

Toxicity.—Hypersensitivity reactions, diarrhea and candidiasis due to bowel flora change, hemolytic anemia, and neurotoxicity. All are uncommon in young infants with the dosage given.

Ticarcillin (Ticar)

Dosage.—75 mg/kg IV or IM every 12 hours for low–birth weight infants less than 1 week old; same dose every 8 hours for normal–birth weight infants less than 1 week old; same dose every 6 to 8 hours for infants older than 1 week.

Toxicity.—See carbenicillin.

Tobramycin (Nebcin)

Dosage.—See gentamicin.

Toxicity.—See gentamicin.

Vancomycin (Vancocin)

Dosage.—15 mg/kg IV (given over 1 hour) every 12 hours for infants less than 1 week old; same dose every 8 hours for infants older than 1 week.

Toxicity.—Deafness, drug rash and fever, thrombophlebitis at injection site. Renal damage is rare except when used in combination with aminoglycosides.

GLAUCOMA DRUGS

The most common cause of glaucoma in the neonatal and early infancy period is a developmental abnormality of the angle of the anterior chamber that prevents normal outflow of aqueous humor. Treatment therefore is primarily surgical (see Chapter 19). Medical therapy with topical antiglaucoma drugs such as timolol maleate, pilocarpine, and epinephrine products or a systemic agent such as acetazolamide (Diamox) are rarely of long-term value and are generally ineffective.

The topical drugs sometimes are used to help control residual elevation of intraocular pressure between surgical procedures. Acetazolamide is used in infants only for a short period (for example, preoperatively) because of its potential to produce metabolic acidosis and electrolyte imbalance. Acetazolamide is available in tablets of 125 mg and 250 mg; a vial containing a sterile powder of 500 mg is made by Lederle Laboratories for parenteral use (reconstitute with at least 5 mL of sterile water for injection). The oral dosage of acetazolamide for infants and children is 10 to 20 mg/kg/day in three or four divided doses; the IV dosage is 5 to 10 mg/kg every 6 hours. In neonates, start with the lower dosages at 12-hour intervals.

The hyperosmotic agent mannitol is occasionally used immediately preoperatively to lower the ocular tension. In pediatric patients the drug is given IV over a 30- to 40-minute period as a 10% solution. The total dose is 1 to 1.5 gm/kg body weight. The maximal ocular hypotensive effect is reached in 1 hour, and the effect may last up to 6 hours. If used during surgery when the patient is receiving a general anesthetic, catheterization is advisable.

This chapter attempts to give a short review of pediatric pharmacology information that relates to a select group of drugs used for eye disorders in premature, newborn, and young infants. A special plea is made to ophthalmologists who may need to use systemic therapy in this age group, namely, that they first consult with a pediatrician or neonatologist with regard to the choice and dosage of drugs and their possible side effects.

BIBLIOGRAPHY

1. Apt L, Gaffney WL: Toxic effects of topical eye medication in infants and children, in Duane TD, Jaeger EA (eds): *Biomedical Foundations of Ophthalmology*. Hagerstown, Md, Harper & Row, 1982, pp 1–13.
2. Apt L, Henrick A: Pupillary dilation with single eyedrop mydriatic combinations. *Am J Ophthalmol* 1980; 89:553–559.
3. Caputo AR, Schnitzer RE, Lindquist TD, et al: Dilation in neonates: A protocol. *Pediatrics* 1982; 69:77–79.
4. Ellis PP: *Ocular Therapeutics and Pharmacology*, 7th ed. St Louis, CV Mosby Co, 1985.
5. Havener WH: *Ocular Pharmacology*, 5th ed. St Louis, CV Mosby Co, 1983.
6. Isenberg S, Everett S: Cardiovascular effects of mydriatics in low birth weight infants. J Pediatr 1984; 105:111–112.
7. MacLeod SM, Radde IC: *Textbook of Pediatric Clinical Pharmacology*. Littleton, Mass, PSG Publishing Co, 1985.
8. Marx CM: Medications used in the newborn, in Cloherty JP, Stark AR (eds): *Manual of Neonatal Care*, 2nd ed. Boston, Little, Brown, & Co, 1985, pp 507–512.
9. Roberts FJ: *Drug Therapy in Infants*. Philadelphia, WB Saunders Co, 1984.

9 Amblyopia

Thomas D. France, M.D.

Amblyopia can be defined as a reduction of visual acuity in the absence of apparent organic cause that, in appropriate cases, is correctible by therapeutic measures.[1] The lay term *lazy eye* is often used to describe amblyopia on the conception that the visual loss is due to lack of use of the eye by the child, also called *amblyopia ex anopsia* or *amblyopia of disuse*. (Note that in this connotation, lazy eye does *not* indicate a deviation of the eye, only visual loss.) While the loss of vision may be related to the inability of the child to use the eye due to cataract, ptosis, etc (see the discussion of deprivation amblyopia, later), the cause of visual loss is much more commonly related to an active suppression of the vision of one eye to prevent diplopia or aniseikonia (unequal image size).

Amblyopia is the most common cause of visual loss in children before the age of 6 years, with a prevalence of 1% to 2% in this age group.[2] It is readily treatable if detected before the age of 4 years with decreasing success of correction between the age of 4 and 8 or 9 years.[3] After the age of 9 it is unusual to see a full restoration of vision (see the section on treatment at the end of this chapter).

CLASSIFICATION

Amblyopia can be classified on the basis of the associated etiology[4] (see Table 9–1).

Strabismic amblyopia and anisometropic amblyopia are the most common types and account for the majority of cases. In such patients the amblyopia is always unilateral. Ametropic amblyopia is less commonly seen and is always bilateral. These three types have been called "functional" amblyopias. They respond well to treatment and do not appear to be related to any changes in the anatomy or pathophysiology of the visual system, at least in the early stages of onset.[5]

Deprivation amblyopia can be either unilateral or bilateral and, with the so-called congenital amblyopias, is considered to be "organic" in nature. It responds poorly to treatment and is thought to be due to changes in the basic structures of the visual system.

Occlusion amblyopia is iatrogenic, being secondary to prolonged occlusion of the preferred eye during treatment of amblyopia in the fellow eye. The reversal of visual loss is almost never permanent and would, therefore, be considered functional.

The cause of amblyopia is not clearly understood. Recent laboratory and clinical investigations have given us better insights into the etiology of this common disorder but do not explain all the phenomena associated with amblyopia, nor have they, as yet, given us newer, more successful modes of therapy.

Visual development in the newborn has been discussed in Chapter 4. Any deficit in the visual image can lead to changes in both the anatomic and physiological strata of the immature visual system. That visual maturity does not occur until the age of 8 or 9 years is in keeping with the aforementioned clinical experience. Unfortunately, there is good evidence that irreversible changes occur during the first months of life if the two visual images are not equal. Even before birth, the development of the visual centers is dependent upon the presence of binocular competition.[6] If one eye is malformed or, in the case of the animal model, one eye is removed prenatally, there are permanent changes in the cellular organ-

TABLE 9–1.
Classification of Amblyopia[4]

1. Strabismic amblyopia
2. Anisometropic amblyopia
3. Ametropic amblyopia
4. Deprivation amblyopia
5. Congenital amblyopia
6. Occlusion amblyopia

ization and synaptic connectivity of the visual centers. In these animal models, the lateral geniculate nucleus develops only two cellular layers and one interlaminar fiber band instead of the normal six layers and five bands, aberrant synaptic connections form between the intact eye and the geniculate neurons that have lost their normal input, and ocular dominance columns fail to develop in the visual cortex. That such significant changes can occur in the visual system even before birth and the onset of visual stimulation indicates the importance of binocular input to the development of the visual system. Of apparently equal importance is that these visual impulses must be nearly equal in their quality if the visual system is to develop normally postnatally. von Noorden and Crawford have shown that it is not a decrease in the amount of light in the lid-sutured animal model (and, therefore, in the infant with congenital cataract) that is critical to visual development but that the visual image must be clearly focused on the retina as well if deprivation amblyopia is to be avoided.[7]

Animal models have shown that misalignment of the visual axes, induced anisometropia, and lid closure will all lead to abnormal development of the normal visual system. This may include loss of binocular input at the cortical level,[8–10] loss of visual cortical cells tuned to a specific orientation,[11, 12] and a marked decrease in visual acuity in one or both eyes.[13, 14] These models along with the use of laboratory techniques to define parameters of human amblyopia have helped explain some of the specific aspects of this condition.

Strabismic Amblyopia

Strabismic amblyopia is most commonly associated with a convergent strabismus (or esotropia) that is acquired after birth. Recent work by Helveston[15] has shown that babies do not have a persisting esotropia present in the first few days after birth. This indicates that such deviations are not due to a mechanical or developmental defect present at birth. They must, therefore, be due to neurogenic influences of either a sensory or motor component that develops in the first few months of life since, by definition, infantile, or congenital, esotropia must be present by 6 months of age.[16] Amblyopia is not a common constituent of infantile esotropia. It is thought that this is due to the lack of development of binocular function in these children with the resultant absence of visual confusion and diplopia normally leading to amblyopia.[17] Cases of acquired esotropia developing after binocular vision has been established are more commonly associated with amblyopia,[18, 19] perhaps confirming the need for active suppression in order to develop amblyopia.

Intermittent divergent strabismus (exotropia) and/or vertical strabismus, if not paralytic, are less commonly associated with amblyopia. Acute-onset paralytic strabismus, most usually a fourth or sixth nerve palsy due either to trauma or infection, is well known to lead to amblyopia in this young age group unless a compensatory head position permits fusion.

Strabismic conditions caused by anatomic or neurological abnormalities in development such as Brown's syndrome[20] or Duane's syndrome[21] where there is an inability of the child to move the eyes into a certain field of gaze due to a structural or innervational anomaly are not associated with the development of amblyopia if a compensatory head posture that allows binocularity can be found.

The most widely held view is that strabismic amblyopia develops as a result of diplopia and image confusion caused by the misalignment of the visual axes.[22] Since dissimilar images are falling on corresponding retinal areas (areas of the retina that have similar visual direction such as the foveae), these two dissimilar images will appear to be in the same place in space and lead to visual confusion. In the case of dissimilar images falling on the fovea of each eye, the physiological phenomenon of retinal rivalry will prevent superimposition and subsequent central confusion.[23] In addition to the case of dissimilar images, similar images will now fall on noncorresponding retinal elements. They will, therefore, appear to lie in two different directions in visual space, thus leading to diplopia both centrally and in the visual periphery. In addition, peripheral confusion may also occur due to the increased size of the retinal receptor fields in the peripheral retina.

Ikeda and Wright[24] have suggested that the most significant factor in the development of strabismic amblyopia is the lack of image resolution due to the fact that the mechanism for clearing the image on the retina, accommodation, is dependent on the fixing eye. Since the deviating eye will not have the same images on the fovea as does the fixing eye, the foveal image will be out of focus and thereby lead to a lack of stimulation of those cells that are tuned to only sharply focused images (the sustained cells, or "X" cells).[25] Subsequent investigations by Hess and colleagues have shown that patients with strabismic amblyopia have a deficient contrast sensitivity function for stationary targets at both high and low spatial frequencies while retaining normal sensitivity to targets that are allowed to move.[26,27] Thus patients with strabismic amblyopia have reduced central vision by using the physiological method of retinal rivalry and by a more "central" mechanism, as yet unknown, that inhibits the sustained (X-cell) system while allowing the transient (Y-cell) system to remain intact.

Anisometropic Amblyopia

A significant difference in the refractive error between the two eyes can lead to amblyopia and is a very common cause of this condition in children. Early in the course there is often no strabismus present. With persistently poor vision, it is not unusual to see a deviation develop secondarily. Due to the lack of obvious ocular malalignment, the poor vision is often not suspected until the child reaches school age and vision is tested during a routine school examination.

The amount of difference in refractive error necessary to produce anisometropic amblyopia varies according to the type of refractive error. Children with farsightedness (hypermetropia) in each eye (the norm for most infants) may need as little as 1.5 to 2.0 D of difference between the two eyes to develop a significant amblyopia in the more hypermetropic eye. In this case the child has apparently favored the eye that required less effort to focus to a clear image and ignored the second eye even if it would normally have been expected to be the dominant eye. (Eye dominance is usually associated with hand and foot dominance, so it may be predictable if hand dominance is known.) If amblyopia is present in the *less* hypermetropic eye, one should suspect an organic cause of visual loss.

A difference of a least 6 D between the two eyes is likely to be associated with anisometropic amblyopia if both eyes are myopic or if one is slightly hypermetropic and the other is myopic. Clinical studies have shown that children will tend to use the less myopic, more hypermetropic (within the usual norms of hypermetropia) eye for distance fixation and the more myopic eye for near fixation if the amount of myopia in the second eye is less than 6 D. If the myopia exceeds this amount, the child apparently finds it easier to accommodate for near work with the normal eye rather than holding the object closer for clear viewing with the myopic eye. Significant degrees of myopic anisometropia may be associated with anatomic changes in the retina including abnormal myelination of the nerve fiber layer, axial length change with myopic conus development around the optic nerve, and changes in the macula that may lead to an organic loss of vision. Myelinated nerve fibers associated with high degrees of myopia (greater than 13 D) have been shown to have a poor prognosis for visual rehabilitation when using the usual antiamblyopia therapy.[28]

Significant anisometropia involving astigmatic refractive errors usually require that the anisometropia be at least 2 to 3 D of difference. Oblique astigmatic errors in one eye may lead to amblyopia if the other eye has vertical or horizontal astigmatism.

The high frequency of myopic anisometropic amblyopia in patients with prematurity and low birth weight should make one suspicious of this entity in all such children, even in the absence of other signs of retinopathy of prematurity.

The etiology of the amblyopia in anisometropia has long been thought to be similar to that seen in strabismus. Many of these patients have strabismus at the time of first examination[29] to confirm this concept. Ikeda and Wright have again suggested that the abnormality is caused by a blurred retinal image in the ametropic eye that is caused by unbalanced accommodation due to the hypermetropic or myopic anisometropia or an uncorrected unilateral astigmatism.

Animal models of anisometropic amblyopia have shown changes in the visual system similar to those seen in strabismic animal models.[30] In particular, there is a loss of binocularly driven cells in the visual cortex of cats with anisometropia, with those cells driven by the defocused (amblyopic) eye tending to have lower contrast sensitivity than the normal eye. Clinical work has shown that there is the expected loss of function of the sustained (X-cell) system with persistence of the transient (Y-cell) system in patients with anisometropia and amblyopia.[31,32]

Surprisingly, however, there is a significant difference in the contrast sensitivity between strabismic and anisometropic amblyopia when these patients are tested under different levels of illumination.

It has been known for a number of years that if a neutral density filter is placed before first the normal and then the amblyopic eye it will cause a reduction in the vision of the normal eye that is greater than that seen in the amblyopic eye if the cause of the amblyopia is strabismic.[33] Hess et al. found that there was a similar lack of degrading of contrast sensitivity in strabismic amblyopic eyes as compared with the normal eye with reduced illumination.[34] However, this was not the case in patients with anisometropic amblyopia who showed an equal loss of vision in each eye with reduced illumination. A similar finding has been shown to be present when neutral-density filters are used in these patients.[35] In spite of the differences in the laboratory findings between these two types of amblyopia, we have not found differences in the level of vision or in therapeutic results in these two groups.

Ametropic Amblyopia

When both eyes have significant refractive errors, vision may not be improved with simple correction by glasses. Such *bilateral* amblyopia is considered to be due to the lack of a clear visual image on the retina due to the ametropic state. This condition is seen in patients with high degrees of refractive error, either spherical or astigmatic. In the later case amblyopia may only occur at one axis, a so-called meridional amblyopia.

The degree of refractive error necessary to create ametropic amblyopia differs depending on the type of ametropia present. A significant degree of hypermetropia may be +6.00 D of error, while in the myopic patient it may not be present until −10.00 or −12.00 D of refractive error is present. In the former, the effort of accommodation required to clear vision may lead to enough convergence to cause a manifested strabismus with secondary diplopia. If the child "chooses" to remain blurred to avoid diplopia, bilateral amblyopia will result. If the patient accommodates and clears vision in the fixing eye but suppresses the vision in the deviating eye to avoid diplopia, then only the deviating eye will develop amblyopia, due to the strabismus and not due to the ametropia.

The myopic child is able to provide a clear image on the retina by holding the object of regard close to the eye. Only if the degree of ametropia is so high as to require the patient to hold the object so close that it exceeds the fusional convergence capability will a blurred image be tolerated. It is for this reason that myopic ametropic amblyopia is much less common than hypermetropic ametropic amblyopia.

Significant astigmatic refractive errors can lead to ametropic amblyopia. In astigmatism one meridian (or axis) is blurred when the complementary axis (at 90 degrees to the first) is in focus. When bilateral, astigmatic errors of 2.50 D or more of cylinder can cause amblyopia.

Cells in the visual system have been shown to be sensitive to orientation as well as to form and movement.[36] In animal models raised in environments with only one contour orientation, only those visual cells sensitive to that orientation persisted.[37] In patients with significant astigmatism, contrast sensitivity function has been shown to be reduced for gratings oriented to the astigmatic (amblyopic) meridian.[38]

Mohindra et al. have shown that infants show ten times the incidence and considerably greater amounts of astigmatism than do children of school age.[39] This degree of astigmatic refractive error becomes less during the first year of life and does not appear to be related to an equally high incidence of meridional amblyopia. So it appears that the development of meridional amblyopia is limited to those patients with persistence of a significant astigmatism after the first year of life and that a high degree of astigmatism during the first year of life does not produce an irreversible amblyopia.

Initial treatment of ametropic amblyopia is to correct the existent refractive error. Either glasses or contact lenses may be used. Careful repeat refractions are often needed to obtain the best final vision. Often, vision cannot be fully recovered to the 20/20 level in spite of early detection and correction.

Deprivation Amblyopia

Deprivation amblyopia, which is much less common than strabismic or anisometropic amblyopia (accounting for approximately 10% of all cases), is the most serious type of amblyopia because although it is preventable, once present, it is not treatable by any known therapy. In addition, it is an amblyopia that is found in infants before the age of 3 months, usually as a consequence of infantile cataract, congenital ptosis, or corneal leukoma. It may be unilateral or bilateral.

Prior to 1963 it was well known that visual results in unilateral congenital cataracts were not as good as in the acquired cataracts of adults,[40] but the cause of this difference was not understood. In 1963 the reports of Wiesel and Hubel[8,9] outlining the effect of unilateral or bilateral lid closure in kittens showed us that significant changes occur with deprivation of the normal visual stimulus during visual development. These changes included both anatomic and physiological abnormalities in the visual system. Later work in kittens and in monkeys showed that it was the loss of form vision during a "critical period" of development that led to these changes.[7,41] This critical period is about 3 months after birth in the animal model. The exact period in which stimulus deprivation can lead to visual loss in humans is not known but is at least 3 months and may be considerably longer.*

Psychophysical testing in humans with deprivation amblyopia has shown that there is a significant loss of function in addition to visual acuity.[42] Contrast sensitivity testing showed a marked reduction in threshold from the normal for *both* spatial and temporal frequency tests. Some patients showed a complete absence of form vision, with only movement perception remaining. Testing at low luminance levels showed a reduced response at all luminance levels. Thus deprivation amblyopia, while significantly different from anisometropic amblyopia, is more similar to that condition than to strabismic amblyopia.

*In an unpublished review, the author found in a series of 18 patients with acquired, unilateral cataracts occurring after the age of 3 years that the best visual acuity attained was 20/40 if the cataract occurred before the age of 8 years. In those patients who developed their cataract after the age of 8, final vision was 20/30 or better. This may suggest that the critical period for visual development in humans may persist well beyond the 3-month period seen in animal models.

Congenital Amblyopia

Patients with reduced vision associated with nystagmus or with systemic or ocular anomalies should probably not be included in our definition of amblyopia. Nystagmus associated with a central nervous system (CNS) abnormality such as hydrocephalus or a porencephalic cyst can lead to poor vision due to the inability of the patient to maintain fixation with the fovea.

In the case of nystagmus associated with ocular anomalies such as achromatopsia or albinism, the cause of the poor vision is less certain. Reduced visual acuity in children with albinism has been thought to be due to a number of possible abnormalities in the visual system, each one of which could account for the poor vision. These include transillumination of the iris with poor collimation of light on the retina; lack of macular development; scatter of light in the posterior pole due to lack of choroidal pigment; pendular nystagmus; and most recently described, abnormal retinogeniculate pathways wherein retinal axons normally destined to remain ipsilateral have been found to cross to the opposite side.[43] With so many possible causes of poor vision, amblyopia would not be the likely *primary* cause of low vision.

The poor vision seen in congenital achromatopsia is most likely due to the lack of cone function in these patients. The presence of significant nystagmus and photophobia also would be expected to lead to low vision. Amblyopia, if present, would have to be secondary to the severe ocular abnormalities.

Treatment of the amblyopia in such cases is not likely to succeed due to the multiple ocular and visual system abnormalities. Conversely, it is important to rule out the possible presence of a treatable amblyopia, especially if one eye appears to have significantly decreased vision as compared with the other. For this reason, a trial of occlusion therapy should be considered to see whether some improvement in vision can be attained.

Occlusion Amblyopia

Prolonged occlusion therapy of the preferred eye can lead to loss of vision in that eye to the point of inducing an amblyopia. In such cases the vision in the previously amblyopic eye is usually improved to normal, but occasional cases have been reported with a loss of vision in the preferred eye *without* improvement of vision in the amblyopic eye.

In general, vision can be easily restored by reversing the occlusion to the other eye. Infrequently, there is a permanent loss of vision due to excessive occlusion. Careful adherence to patching guidelines (see the next section) should prevent such occurrences.

TREATMENT

In spite of the significant advances in our understanding of amblyopia from laboratory and clinical investigations, there has been little change in our basic approach to therapy. The use of an occluder over the preferred eye to force visual function in the amblyopic eye was first described in the 18th century. It remains the treatment of choice 200 years later!

Before beginning occlusion therapy it is important to correct any refractive errors and to ensure that any medial opacities are treated. Strabismus therapy is usually deferred until the amblyopia is corrected.

In the case of anisometropic or ametropic amblyopia, frequently all that may be necessary to restore vision is to determine and correct the refractive error. In infants this may seem to be a significant problem, but we have found that even the younger children can be fit with glasses and will wear them quite happily if their vision is improved. The use of contact lenses is, in our practice, usually confined to children with unilateral aphakia following cataract extraction. The contact lens is fit at the time of cataract surgery and worn constantly following surgery. In some cases of high-myopic anisometropia we have found contact lenses to be of help as well. In general, however, we have used glasses for most of our patients.

Cataract extraction in unilateral or bilateral congenital cases must be carried out as soon as possible after detection. If a unilateral congenital cataract is not corrected before the age of 3 months, the visual results are likely to be poor. Other types of lesions leading to visual deprivation such as hemangiomas of the lid, congential ptosis, or corneal opacities should similarly be corrected as soon as they are determined to be causing a visual problem. In every such case a careful refraction is imperative to allow correction of any significant astigmatism or other refractive error. (In the case of congenital ptosis, early treatment is often indicated if there is a significant abnormal head position leading to poor motor development.)

Once the refractive error is determined and, if necessary, corrected, occlusion therapy can be started. The type of occlusion required is, however, not generally agreed upon. In general, most pediatric ophthalmologists prefer to use a patch that adheres to the face rather than the more easily displaced cloth patch with a headband or the clip-on patch for glasses. A variety of manufactured patches are available, some with black facing to reduce light transmission and some with colorful stickers for the more fashion minded. The critical concern is to provide occlusion of the preferred eye that cannot be easily removed by the child and does not lead to serious skin disruption. Frequent removal of the adherent patches by either the child or the parents will almost always lead to erosion of the epithelium. This is often interpreted by the parents as an "allergic" reaction to the patch. Occasionally a true dermatitis will occur. Hypoallergenic patches are available; however, simply changing to a different manufacturer may be all that is necessary to correct the problem.

The amount of patching that is carried out in terms of hours per day or days per week is also not uniformly agreed upon. In general I prefer to prescribe wearing patches all waking hours of the day and 7 days a week without any respite. The patch is removed only at night when the child goes to sleep. This allows time for the skin to recover but ensures that the child does not lose ground by having the patch off during waking hours.

In order to avoid occlusion amblyopia, careful attention is paid to how long the child wears patches between vision assessments. In the infant age group (less than 1 year of age), the child is initially assessed on a weekly basis. Over the age of 1, the child is seen at intervals of 1 week per year of age to a total of 4 weeks. Thus, if the child is 3 years old, he is seen every 3 weeks to reassess vision. The need to see the child and to encourage continued occlusion requires that the child be seen at least once a month.

Once vision is normalized, it may be possible to reduce the time of occlusion to less than full time. This may be done by reducing the time of full occlusion to half a day, every day, or to a full day every other day. I prefer the former since it is a "regular" method that is easier for the child to understand and for the parent to remember.

Approximately one half of children with amblyopia will require some occlusion therapy to the age of 8 or 9 years in order to maintain normal vision. This may only be 1 day per week of occlusion or the use of a penalizing lens.

Not all infants can be made to wear a patch. Other forms of occlusion include opaque contact lenses, high-minus contact lenses, and cycloplegic agents (atropine). The use of an occluder contact lens has been advocated by Parks[44] for those patients who will not tolerate traditional occlusion. I have not found this method to be particularly useful due to the high rate of lost lenses. In addition, it is a rather expensive way to occlude an eye.

Cycloplegic agents, especially the long-acting atropine, have been advocated as a means of blurring the vision of the preferred eye, particularly at near distances. This seems to work best if the child has a significant hypermetropia in the preferred eye and a mild degree of amblyopia. If such is not the case, I have found that the child will continue to use the (atropinized) preferred eye in spite of the induced cycloplegia.

The use of a combination of atropine for the preferred eye with a miotic (diisopropyl fluorophosphate [DFP]) in the amblyopic eye has been suggested by Knapp and Capobianco.[45] This method has the advantage of improving the resolving power of the amblyopic eye by producing miosis while penalizing the preferred eye. The problem of installing two medications, each with significant side effects, may have kept this from becoming a popular method of therapy.

Penalization of the preferred eye with glasses has been described in school-age children unwilling to continue occlusion in school. Overcorrection of the preferred eye by 3.00 D of plus lens allows clear near visual acuity with that eye for reading, etc., but forces the amblyopic eye to be used for distance viewing. For the most part, cases with visual acuity in the range of 20/70 or better in the amblyopic eye have been found to be successfully treated by this method.[46]

Other methods of treatment of amblyopia including red lens therapy,[47] pleoptics,[48] and stimulation with rotating spatial frequency grids[49] have been described in children with long-standing amblyopia with varying degrees of success. Since most of these are confined to older children, I will not include them in this discussion.

CONCLUSION

Amblyopia is the most common cause of visual loss in children. It is usually related to strabismus or a refractive error (anisometropia or ametropia) but can be the result of early deprivation of visual stimulation in infants. When detected early it is usually treatable by simple occlusion of the preferred eye. Our increasing knowledge of the development of the visual system during the first months of life has given us some insight into the problems associated with visual deprivation in this age group. Further advances in the treatment of amblyopia in infants can be expected with newer techniques of visual assessment that allow a better determination of visual function. Treatment still depends on carefully following the response to therapy by monitoring the frequent changes in vision with changes in patient compliance. Only when we can accurately and consistently determine the vision in infants can we expect to be able to assess the results of differing therapies.

REFERENCES

1. Burian HM: Thoughts on the nature of amblyopia ex anopsia. *Am Orthopt J* 1956; 6:5–12.
2. Flom MC, Neumaier RW: Prevalence of amblyopia. *Public Health Rep* 1966; 81:329–341.
3. Parks MM, Friendly DS: Treatment of eccentric fixation in children under 4 years of age. *Am J Ophthalmol* 1966; 61:395–399.
4. von Noorden GK: Classification of amblyopia. *Am J Ophthalmol* 1967; 63:238–244.
5. Burian HM: Pathophysiologic basis of amblyopia and of its treatment. *Am J Ophthalmol* 1969; 67:1–12.
6. Rakic R: Development of visual centers in the primate brain depends on binocular competition before birth. *Science* 1981; 214:928–931.
7. von Noorden GK, Crawford MLJ: Form deprivation without light deprivation produces the visual deprivation syndrome in *Macaca mulatta. Brain Res* 1977; 129:37–44.
8. Wiesel TN, Hubel DH: Single-cell responses in striate cortex of kittens deprived of vision in one eye. *J Neurophysiol* 1963; 26:1003–1017.
9. Hubel DH, Wiesel TN: Binocular interaction in striate cortex of kittens reared with artificial squint. *J Neurophysiol* 1965; 28:1041–1059.
10. Smith EL, Bennett MJ, Harwerth RS, Crawford MLJ: Binocularity in kittens reared with optically induced squint. *Science* 1979; 204:875–877.
11. Hirsch HVB, Spinelli DN: Visual experience modifies distribution of horizontally and vertically oriented receptive fields in cats. *Science* 1970; 168:869–871.
12. Blakemore C, Cooper GF: Development of the brain depends on the visual environment. *Nature* 1970; 228:477–478.

13. von Noorden GK, Dowling JE: Experimental amblyopia in monkeys. II. Behavioral studies in strabismic amblyopia. *Arch Ophthalmol* 1970; 84:215–220.
14. von Noorden GK: Experimental amblyopia in monkeys. Further behavioral observations and clinical correlations. *Invest Ophthalmol* 1973; 12:721–726.
15. Helveston EM: Origins of congenital esotropia. *Am Orthopt J* 1986; 36:40–48.
16. Costenbader FD: The management of convergent strabismus, in Allen JH (ed): *Strabismus Ophthalmic Symposium*. St Louis, CV Mosby Co, 1950, p 343.
17. Parks MM: *Ocular Motility and Strabismus*. New York, Harper & Row, Publishers, Inc, 1975, pp 67–72.
18. Pollard Z: Accommodative esotropia during the first year of life. *Arch Ophthalmol* 1976; 94:1912–1913.
19. Baker JD, Parks MM: Early onset accommodative esotropia. *Am J Ophthalmol* 1980; 90:11–18.
20. Brown HW: Congenital structural muscle anomalies, in Allen J (ed): *Strabismus Ophthalmic Symposium*. St Louis, CV Mosby Co, 1950, p 205.
21. Duane A: Congenital deficiency of abduction associated with impairment of adduction, retraction movements, contraction of palpebral fissures and oblique movements of the eye. *Arch Ophthalmol* 1905; 34:133–159.
22. von Noorden GK: Factors involved in the production of amblyopia. *Br J Ophthalmol* 1974; 58:158–164.
23. Bishop PO: Binocular vision, in Moses RA (ed): *Adler's Physiology of the Eye: Clinical Application*. St Louis, CV Mosby Co, 1981, p 590.
24. Ikeda H, Wright MJ: A possible neurophysiological basis for amblyopia. *Br Orthopt J* 1975; 32:2–13.
25. Ikeda H, Wright MJ: Is amblyopia due to inappropriate stimulation of the "sustained" pathways during development? *Br J Ophthalmol* 1971; 58:165–175.
26. Hess RF, Howell ER: The threshold contrast sensitivity function in strabismic amblyopia. Evidence for a two type classification. *Vision Res* 1977; 17:1047–1056.
27. Hess RF, Howell ER, Kitchen J: On the relationship between pattern and movement detection in strabismus amblyopia. *Vision Res* 1978; 18:375–379.
28. Hittner HM, Antoszyk JH: Unilateral peripapillary myelinated nerve fibers with myopia and/or amblyopia. *Arch Ophthalmol* 1987; 105:943–948.
29. Phelps WL, Muir J: Anisometropia and strabismus. *Am Orthopt J* 1977; 27:131–133.
30. Eggers HM, Blakemore CB: Physiological basis of anisometropic amblyopia. *Science* 1978; 201:264–267.
31. Levi DM, Harwerth RS: Contrast evoked potentials in strabismic and anisometropic amblyopia. *Invest Ophthalmol Vis Sci* 1978; 17:571–575.
32. Manny RE, Levi DM: Psychophysical investigations of the temporal modulation sensitivity function in amblyopia: Uniform field flicker. *Invest Ophthalmol Vis Sci* 1982; 22:515–524.
33. von Noorden GK, Burian HM: Visual acuity in normal and amblyopic patients under reduced illumination. *Arch Ophthalmol* 1959; 61:53–55.
34. Hess RF, Campbell FW, Zimmern R: Differences in the neural basis of human amblyopias. The effect of mean luminance. *Vision Res* 1980; 20:295–305.
35. France TD: Amblyopia update: Diagnosis and therapy. *Am Orthopt J* 1984; 34:4–12.
36. Blakemore C, Campbell FW: On the existence of neurones in the human visual system selectively sensitive to the orientation and size of retinal images. *J Physiol (Lond)* 1969; 203:237–260.
37. Blakemore C, Cooper GF: Development of the brain depends on the visual environment. *Nature* 1970; 228:477–478.
38. Freeman RD: Contrast sensitivity in meridional amblyopia. *Invest Ophthalmol* 1975; 14:78–81.
39. Mohindra I, Held R, Gwiazda J, Brill S: Astigmatism in infants. *Science* 1978; 202:329–331.
40. Costenbader FD, Albert DG: Conservatism in the management of congenital cataract. *Arch Ophthalmol* 1957; 58:426–430.
41. Hubel DH, Wiesel TN: The period of susceptibility to the physiological effects of unilateral eye closure in kittens. *J Physiol (Lond)* 1970; 206:419–436.
42. Hess RF, France TD, Tulunay-Keesey U: Residual vision in humans who have been monocularly deprived of pattern stimulation in early life. *Exp Brain Res* 1981; 44:295–311.
43. Guillary RW, Okoro AN, Witkop CJ Jr: Abnormal visual pathways in the brain of a human albino. *Brain Res* 1975; 96:373–377.

44. Parks MM: *Ocular Motility and Strabismus.* Hagerstown, Md, Harper & Row, Publishers, Inc, 1975, pp 97–98.
45. Knapp P, Capobianco NM: Use of miotics in esotropia. *Am Orthopt J* 1956; 6:40–46.
46. Frank JW, France TD: Penalization revisited: Refractive penalization in the treatment of amblyopia. *Am Orthopt J* 1982; 32:90–95.
47. Brinker WR, Katz SL: New and practical treatment of eccentric fixation. *Am J Ophthalmol* 1963; 55:1033.
48. Bangerter A: The purpose of pleoptics. *Ophthalmologica* 1969; 158:334.
49. Banks RV, Campbell FW, Hess RF, et al: A new treatment for amblyopia. *Br Orthopt J* 1978; 35:1–12.

10 Teratogenic Agents

Earl A. Palmer, M.D.

Teratogens are agents in the environment of the developing fetus that produce developmental anomalies resulting in birth defects. The word *teratogenic* is defined as "producing monsters" (which is defined as living things lacking or with malformed parts).[1] The term *monster* has fallen into disfavor in the field of human medicine because it connotes a "hideously wrong or evil being." We now apply the more neutral term *birth defect* to these malformations. In view of this etymological background, it is understandable that parents of an infant with such a malformed body part may experience feelings of guilt and may seek an external agent to blame. As physicians, we must be sensitive to these feelings as we communicate with parents of children with birth defects.

It is important to understand the variability of the syndromes associated with teratogens. Often, known exposure to a teratogen has no apparent effect on the fetus, presumably because of fortunate timing (at a point in embryogenesis when the fetus is insensitive to the teratogenic influence), insufficient exposure of the teratogenic agent, or protection offered by the genetic makeup of the mother or fetus. Abnormalities in affected offspring cover a broad spectrum of severity. As Shepard has noted, "The borderline between a minor congenital defect and normal variation is most difficult to define, and this accounts for a large difference in incidence rates."[2] When Koch's postulates for microbiology are translated into the field of teratology, one derives the following characteristics of a "teratogenic agent":

1. The agent must be present during the critical periods of development.
2. The agent should produce congenital defects in an animal model in a controlled and statistically valid experiment.
3. Experimental proof (through organ culture, for example) should indicate that it is the agent itself acting directly on the fetus or placenta that causes the abnormality.

The presence of the first two characteristics alone defines a teratogenic agent. The third is desirable but not essential, except toward a basic understanding that would eventually lead to prevention of malformations.[2]

This chapter will focus on those birth defects in which malformed ocular structures affect visual function or cause the patient's facial appearance to deviate from the usual range of human variation. Ocular birth defects are thus generally taken to include such variations of orbitofacial structure as hypertelorism, epicanthal folds, unusual eyelid fissure slants, and moderate exophthalmos. While any one of these features alone could be viewed as a normal variant, it is their overall pattern that suggests abnormality. This combination of seemingly minor anomalies is of great importance to geneticists and dysmorphologists, who are trained or gifted in a *gestalt* method of diagnosis whereby an unusual constellation of facial features in a patient may suggest a specific syndrome. For many health care professionals, however, syndromes "... depending mainly on craniofacial anomalies can often be hard to identify, particularly for those with poor visual memories."[3]

There seems to be an inherent curiosity in human nature, to know the cause of such undesirable occurrences as birth defects. We who provide care to the families of children with birth defects would like to be able to answer the inevitable question, "What caused it, doctor?", whether that question be expressed or assumed.

An analysis of more than 50,000 children revealed 3 instances of eye abnormalities per 2,000 children.[4] In a pathologic study of 60 fetuses with various external anomalies, ocular malformation was found in about a third of the specimens. Of these, microphthalmos was the most common severe ocular anomaly.[5] Examination of 993 visually impaired and mentally retarded people disclosed that 86 had microphthalmos or coloboma. Of these 86 cases, 16 were attributed to prenatal infection and 6 to chromosomal aberration.[6] A great many ocular birth defects have no known cause; these are described elsewhere in this text.

In the future, it may be possible to list a teratogenic etiology for many presently cryptogenic defects. Many possibilities exist for postzygotic fetal environmental factors to influence ocular development. Regardless of speculation on causal relationships between various environmental factors and birth defects, it is clear that the *timing* of a particular teratogenic influence is critical in determining how the eyes are affected. The eye is believed to be most susceptible to teratogens during the 4th to 8th week of gestation.[7,8]

Epicanthal skin folds represent an especially difficult variant to evaluate. Because epicanthal folds are common in children who appear otherwise normal, the usefulness of listing this variant among craniofacial anomalies may seem dubious. Indeed, whether the presence of epicanthal folds in a particular individual is the result of genetic predispositions or of a teratogenic influence may be impossible to determine.

Strabismus (ocular misalignment) is often listed among birth defects of the eye and is thereby perceived as a structural anomaly; yet it is perhaps more practical to consider strabismus to be a disturbance of function. At times, strabismus represents an indirect effect of structural abnormalities within the orbit or of an ill-defined functional abnormality of the brain that impairs ocular motor coordination or binocular fusional capability. Most children with strabismus are otherwise normal, although the incidence of strabismus is increased in children with cerebral palsy or mental retardation. Thus, except for relatively rare cases with an identifiable physical defect causing the strabismus, strabismus should be considered merely an associated finding rather than a specific birth defect.

TERATOGENIC AGENTS KNOWN OR SUSPECTED TO AFFECT THE HUMAN EYE

Drugs and Medicines

Anticonvulsants

Of the several anticonvulsant agents linked to the production of birth defects, many involve the eye. In 1968, certain ocular defects were suspected to be generated by anticonvulsant therapy for epileptic pregnant women. In particular, it was noted that widely spaced and prominent eyes were characteristic in the unusual facial appearance of these children.[9]

Trimethadione.—Eye defects reported in children whose mothers had taken trimethadione during pregnancy primarily include a V-shaped configuration of the eyebrow line. In addition, epicanthal folds and myopia have been noted.[10,11] Although the isolated coexistence of epicanthal folds and myopia is rather nonspecific, the eyebrow feature is striking in published photographs.

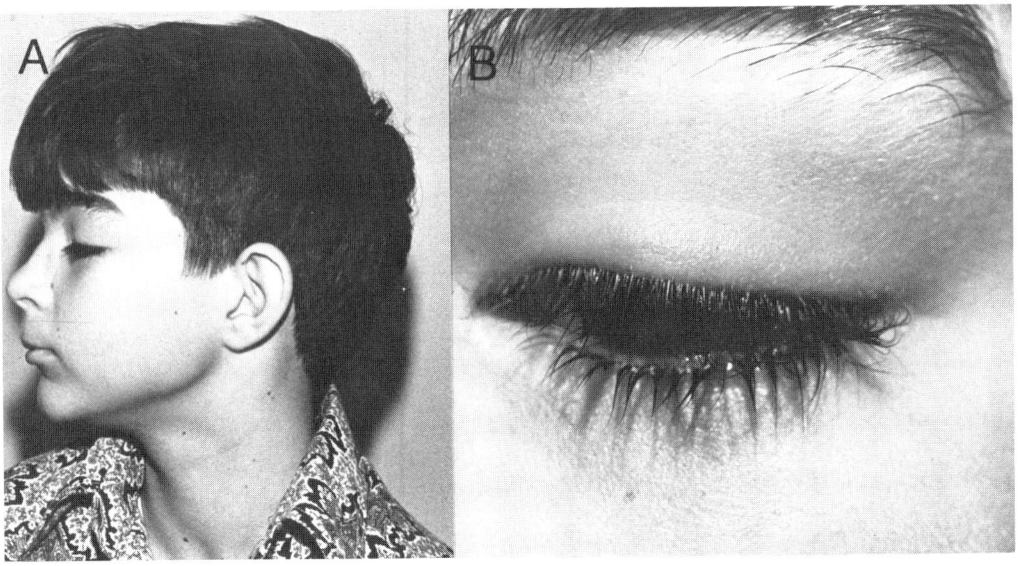

FIG 10–1.
Fetal hydantion syndrome. **A,** ptosis and trichomegaly. **B,** closer view of the trichomegaly. (From Wilson RS, Smead W, Char F: Diphenylhydantoin teratogenicity: Ocular manifestations and related deformities. *J Pediatr Ophthalmol Strabismus* 1978; 15:137–140. Used with permission.)

Phenytoin (Hydantoin).—The most common medication in this class is diphenylhydantoin. The facial appearance and physical findings of patients with the "fetal hydantoin syndrome"[12] are distinct from those with the trimethadione syndrome. Eye defects include hypertelorism, epicanthal folds, blepharoptosis, and strabismus (Fig 10–1). A full listing of reported eye findings, including some that have only rarely been associated, is given in Table 10–1. The eye findings alone would not necessarily suggest a syndrome such as this, and the diagnosis is based upon a constellation of other physical findings, as listed in Table 10–2.

In a study involving over 50,000 pregnancies, 98 mothers were identified as having been exposed to phenytoin during pregnancy. The rate of fetal malformations was 2 to 3 times higher in those cases than in women who had *no history of seizures*. Nevertheless, for each 100 children exposed to diphenylhydantoin in utero no more than 3.5 malformations can be estimated to have been caused by the diphenylhydantoin.[21] On the basis of a prospective study, it has been estimated that some 30% of infants exposed to diphenylhydantoin in utero would have craniofacial and digital anomalies of varying degrees, usually minor.[22] However, the rates of mental or growth retardation and major malformations may have been underestimated in that study because the duration of follow-up of the children may have

TABLE 10–1.
Fetal Hydantoin Syndrome: Eye Findings

Blepharoptosis[12]
Trichomegaly[13]
Hypertelorism[9]
Telecanthus[12]
Epicanthus[13]
Antimongoloid slant of palpebral fissure[13]
Defective lacrimal apparatus[14]
Prominent eyes[9]
Strabismus[10]
Prominent iris vessels[15]
Glaucoma[16]
Microphthalmos[15, 17]
Persistent hyperplasia of primary vitreous[17]
Retinoschisis[13]
Retinal coloboma[18]
Retinal dysplasia[15]
Cystic maculas[13]
Uveal coloboma[15]
Bergmeister's papilla[13]
Optic nerve anomalies[13, 17, 19]

TABLE 10–2.
General Findings in Fetal Hydantoin Syndrome*

This syndrome has been confused with Coffin-Siris syndrome and Noonan's syndrome
Craniofacial
Cleft lip and palate[9]
Mild skull anomalies
Facial asymmetry[17]
Mildly anomalous external ears
Nose short, upturned, with broad, low bridge
Wide mouth with prominent lips
Limbs
Hypoplasia of distal phalanges and nails
Fingerlike thumb
Anomalies of palmar creases and dermatoglyphics
Growth and development; impaired, including intelligence
Cardiac defects[17,19]
Possible transplacental carcinogenesis (neuroblastoma)[20]

*From Hanson JW, Smith DW: The fetal hydantoin syndrome. *J Pediatr* 1975; 87:285–290. Used with permission.

been too short. It has been suggested that studies designed to precisely ascertain these rates should include the exact timing of fetal exposure to diphenylhydantoin, the maternal dosage, and maternal plasma levels of phenytoin. In addition, the age of the child at the time of diagnosis should be standardized, the period of follow-up should extend up to perhaps school age, and genetic factors should be considered more fully.[23]

Hanson and Smith estimated that 7% to 11% of exposed children are affected by the fetal hydantoin syndrome.[12] Schinzel considered that half of the offspring of epileptic mothers who were treated with hydantoin during pregnancy are mentally retarded and advised in 1979 that "hydantoin should be strictly avoided in epileptic women of childbearing age unless safe contraceptive measures are taken. In the event of pregnancy, therapeutic abortion should be considered if hydantoin therapy must be maintained."[24]

It is a vexing dilemma as to how far one should apply general observations to a particular patient,[25,26] yet there are fairly solid reasons to believe in the validity of the fetal hydantoin syndrome.[27] Genetically determined metabolic variations in the detoxification of phenytoin may account for the rather small percentage of women in whom the drug is teratogenic.[28]

Barbiturates.—The facial appearance that characterizes the fetal hydantoin syndrome has also been observed in patients receiving phenobarbital and primidone (a barbiturate precursor).[29] The distal finger anomalies have been attributed to exposure to both hydantoin and barbiturate.[30] One infant with severe bilateral coloboma was born to a mother taking both phenobarbital and phenytoin.[31]

Warfarin

The vitamin K antagonist warfarin, used medically as an anticoagulant in the mother, has been associated with an embryopathy involving multiple congenital anomalies, some of which include the eye. Warfarin embryopathy[32] is characterized by nasal and upper airway defects, skeletal anomalies with stippled epiphyses seen on radiographs (present only during early childhood), persistent truncus arteriosus, developmental delay, and seizures. Central nervous system defects, including optic atrophy, are stated to result from midtrimester exposure.[33] The following are reported eye defects associated with maternal warfarin therapy:

1. Cataract[34]
2. Optic atrophy[33,34]
3. Microphthalmos[35]
4. Hypertelorism[35]
5. Posterior embryotoxon/mesodermal dysgenesis[35]

Warfarin embryopathy is a phenocopy (mimic) of the genetically transmitted syndrome chondrodysplasia punctata.[36] This provides an example of the distinction between a supposed "familial" disorder wherein the mother has been exposed to a teratogen during multiple pregnancies and a "genetic" disorder.[35]

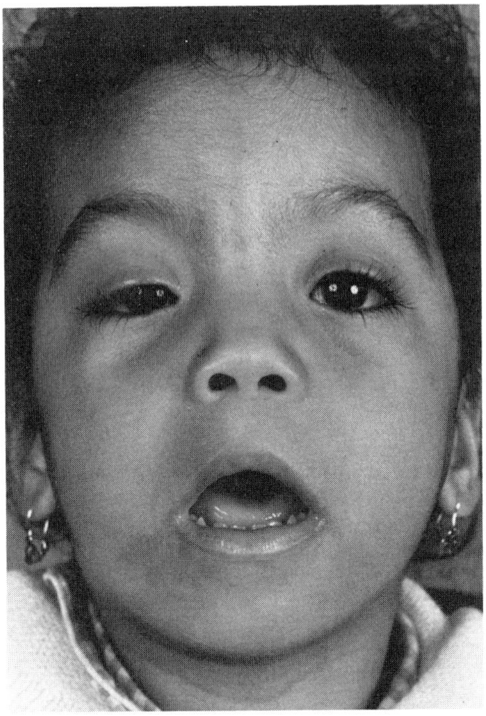

FIG 10–2.
Fetal alcohol syndrome. Frontal view demonstrates the bow-shaped mouth, thin upper lip, and right ptosis. (From Miller M, Israel J, Cuttone J: Fetal alcohol syndrome. *J Pediatr Ophthalmol Strabismus* 1984; 29:8. Used with permission.)

Psychoactive, "Self-Prescribed" Drugs

Alcohol.—Infants born to alcoholic mothers have a high incidence of a particular collection of anomalies now known as the fetal alcohol syndrome. The first major collection of patients with this syndrome was reported by Lemoine and colleagues in 1968.[37]

The minimal criteria for the diagnosis of fetal alcohol syndrome are summarized in Table 10–3.

Cases of fetal alcohol syndrome are usually first recognized by the particular facial appearance of the affected infant or child (Fig 10–2). This facial appearance has been confused with Cornelia de Lange syndrome[39] or Noonan syndrome.[40] The general features of fetal alcohol syndrome include prenatal and postnatal growth retardation, microcephaly, and short palpebral fissures. The craniofacial malformations are attributed to disturbed development of the neural plate and its derivatives. Based upon a mouse model, the critical embryogenic period in humans is the third week of gestation.[41] About 85% of patients have neurodevelopmental deficiencies including subnormal fine motor coordination. About half of the patients have abnormal dermatoglyphics, cardiac malformation, midface hypoplasia, and/or epicanthal folds. The history and the accumulation of data about the fetal alcohol syndrome during the 1960s and 1970s have been documented by Streissguth and colleagues.[42]

Reported eye findings are summarized in Table 10–4.

A third-trimester developmental arrest of cells originating in the neural crest may explain the anterior segment anomalies.[50] Fundus abnormalities have been reported to be

TABLE 10–3.
Minimal Criteria for Diagnosis of Fetal Alcohol Syndrome*†

Low birth weight and growth retardation
Central nervous system dysfunction
At least two of the following:
Microcephaly
Microphthalmos and/or short palpebral fissures
Midface hypoplasia (flat or absent philtrum, thin upper lip, and hypoplastic maxilla)

*From Chermoff GF: introduction: A teratologist's view of the fetal alcohol syndrome, in Gallanter M (ed): *Currents in Alcoholism: Recent Advances in Research and Treatment,* Vol 7. New York, Grune & Stratton, 1980, pp 7–13.
†Note: if alcohol is taken throughout the first trimester, only one of the three main criteria is needed.

TABLE 10–4.
Ocular Findings Associated With Fetal Alcohol Syndrome

1. Short palpebral fissures[39] (a cardinal feature, present in more than 80%)[43, 44]
2. Frequent features (26%–50%)[40]
   a. Epicanthal folds[39, 40]
   b. Blepharoptosis[40, 45]
   c. Strabismus[40, 45]
3. Occasional features (1%–25%)[40]
   a. Hypertelorism[40, 43]
   b. Telecanthus[46]
   c. Microphthalmos[46]
   d. Cataract[42, 46]
   e. Retinal vascular tortuosity[44, 46, 47]
   f. Pigmentary retinal abnormalities[43]
   g. Optic nerve hypoplasia[44, 47, 48]
   h. Myopia[40, 45]
   i. Blepharophimosis[40, 46]
   j. Glaucoma[49]
   k. Peters' anomaly[46, 49]
   l. Axenfeld's anomaly[49]
   m. Microcornea[47]
   n. Trichomegaly[47]

the most frequent eye abnormality, with approximately half of the 30 cases in a recent series showing optic nerve hypoplasia and/or increased tortuosity of retinal vessels.[48]

There is no established minimal amount of alcohol which may be considered absolutely safe for a pregnant woman to imbibe without affecting the fetus. Only a minority of chronically alcoholic women who continue heavy drinking throughout pregnancy produce offspring with the fetal alcohol syndrome. This is consistent with the concept that susceptibility to teratogenesis is multifactorial, resulting from both environmental and genetic components.

Lysergic Acid Diethylamide.—Inconclusive reports of chromosomal breakage due to lysergic acid diethylamide (LSD) were reviewed by Smart and Bateman.[51] Clinical evidence that maternal ingestion of LSD may cause ocular birth defects includes case reports of optic nerve anomalies[52] anophthalmia[53]; and persistent hyperplasia of the primary vitreous with retinal dysplasia, cataract, microphthalmos, and intraocular cartilage.[54] In addition, there is a report of multiple eye anomalies in a child who died at the age of 13 months. The specific anomalies in that case included central nervous malformation, microphthalmos, cataract, retinoschisis, and optic atrophy.[55]

Marijuana (Cannabis).—Transient neurobehavioral alterations have been noted in newborn offspring of mothers who used marijuana. These effects include tremulousness, an increased startle response, and a diminished behavioral response to light stimulation.[56, 57] In addition, five cases of epicanthus and small head size have been reported as possibly resulting from the maternal use of cannabis.[58]

Cocaine.—A fundus abnormality resembling retinopathy of prematurity was observed in one eye of an infant born to a mother who had used cocaine throughout pregnancy. The fellow eye showed persistent hyperplasia of the primary vitreous. There had also been significant maternal alcohol intake in this case.[59] Infants born to mothers who have taken cocaine may exhibit transient engorgement of iris vasculature.[60] Other reported effects on infants have been of a neurobehavioral nature and manifested by depression of interactive behavior and a poor organizational response to environmental stimuli.[61]

Cocaine given to pregnant mice causes eye defects in offspring including anophthalmia and absent lenses.[62]

Anticancer Agents

Both methotrexate and aminopterin, when maternally administered, have been associated with a congenital syndrome that includes shallow orbits and hypertelorism. Three cases were reviewed by Milunsky and colleagues.[76]

Anti-inflammatory Agents

Corticosteroids.—In one case of Aicardi's syndrome, a rare and lethal X-chromosomal anomaly affecting the eyes, the mother had received a 10-day course of adrenocorticotropic hormone (ACTH) during the first trimester. Chhabria reviewed evidence to support the hypothesis of chromosomal damage from the ACTH.[63] Otherwise, there is only a case report of infantile cataracts after the mother received 15 to 60 mg prednisone daily throughout pregnancy.[64] Corticosteroids have been shown to affect ocular development in mice and in the chick retina.[65–68]

Nonsteroidal.—An infant was born with midfacial cleft, cerebral dysgenesis and cyclopia to a mother who took 3.0 to 4.5 gm of aspirin daily during the first trimester and then switched to acetaminophen, 6 to 10 tablets daily, for the remainder of her pregnancy. The patient was also described as a heavy smoker, but no other drugs were taken. There is some peripheral support for the possibility that aspirin could have had a causal relationship[69] despite earlier evidence that aspirin is not teratogenic.[70]

Antimalarials

Chloroquine.—A child was found to have a mottled honeycomb pattern or retinal pigmentary disturbance in the peripheral fundus; the mother, who took chloroquine during pregnancy, had the same eye defect.[71] This case likely represents direct toxicity rather than teratogenicity. Another case in which chloroquine was suspected to have caused ocular birth defects in an infant was reported to the National Registry of Ocular Drug Side Effects in Portland, Ore. In this case chloroquine was taken in early pregnancy, and the infant was born with anophthalmia, microphthalmos, and retinal defects.[72]

Quinine.—After a pregnant woman took at least 60 grains of quinine at $4^1/_2$ months of gestation, her infant was born with multiple anomalies including congenital glaucoma.[73] In another case, after 30 to 40 grains was taken daily for weeks during the last trimester, the infant was born blind, with optic atrophy and attenuated fundus vessels. These same features were noted in a third case wherein 30 grains was taken only 1 day before delivery.[74] Optic nerve hypoplasia may result from maternal ingestion of quinine.[75] The cases of optic nerve atrophy and retinal vascular attenuation could possibly be duplicated by exposure during early infancy and may represent direct toxic effects instead of effects on embryogenesis.

Maternal busulfan treatment during the third trimester has been associated with one case of atypical retinal degeneration in an infant and one case of microphthalmos.[77]

Thalidomide

Paralytic strabismus has been noted in children with birth defects from the maternal administration of thalidomide.[78] Instances of paralytic strabismus, alacrima, gustolacrimal reflex, and blepharoptosis were found among 300 British children with birth defects following the maternal administration of thalidomide. One patient was noted to have fixed pupils.[79] Among 19 cases reported in Germany, 8 patients showed peripheral pigment degeneration in the retina, and some patients had abnormal pigmentation in the anterior chamber angle.[80] One adolescent patient with these changes experienced bilateral retinal detachment.[81]

In Sweden 3 cases of microphthalmos were found among 150 affected children as well as 2 cases of choroidal coloboma.[82] In 1967, Rafuse et al. reviewed ocular findings in these patients.[83]

Isotretinoin (Accutane)

Isotretinoin (13-*cis*-retinoic acid) inhibits sebaceous gland function and is used for the treatment of acne. It is a known teratogen and is not knowingly prescribed to pregnant women. Birth defects reported with in utero exposure to isotretinoin include microtia,[84] dysmorphic nose,[85] and abnormalities of the brain and heart.[84, 86, 87] In one case, the infant had a hepatocellular abnormality.[86]

Ocular findings in affected infants include microphthalmos,[84, 86] neurological damage with minimal reaction of the pupils to a bright light,[85] hypertelorism, and downward-slanted palpebral fissures with facial features reminiscent of Treacher Collins syndrome.[87]

Radiation

A girl was born with microphthalmos, retinal degeneration, and cataract after the mother underwent radiation therapy at 30 to 35 weeks of pregnancy. Other anomalies included microcephaly with mental retardation, stunted growth, and defective teeth.[88] Although eye defects are not specifically emphasized in the literature, ionizing radiation may be involved in the pathogenesis of some cases of trisomy 21 (Down's syndrome).[89] Extensive partial-body exposure to medium-kilovoltage irradiation produces considerable chromosomal damage, some of which persists for up to 20 years and possibly longer. Patients who were treated with irradiation for ankylosing spondylitis had approximately a tenfold increase in risk for dying of leukemia.[99]

Hicks et al. studied the chronology of radiation-induced defects in fetal rats including malformation of the optic nerve and retina. Developmental arrest of the eyes resulted from irradiation on the 9th to 15th day.[91] In a review of this subject, Mole stated that the most common fetal eye sequela of radiation therapy to the mother is microphthalmos (13 of 26 cases). Of 26 cases in which the mother had received radiation therapy, pigmentary degeneration of the retina was seen in 6 infants and cataract in 3.[92]

Infectious Agents

It appears that the ability to produce chromosomal breakage is a property of many viruses.[93, 94]

Rubella Virus

Rubella embryopathy can include multiple congenital anomalies, with ocular defects including cataract and glaucoma,[95–97] microphthalmos,[97] and chorioretinitis.[97] Increased chromosomal breakage is noted in children with congenital rubella. Although genetic damage may be one mechanism by which some of these eye defects are produced, rubella virus may also directly interfere with embryogenesis since it inhibits cell multiplication in vitro.[94]

Epstein-Barr Virus

Epstein-Barr virus (EBV) is the cause of infectious mononucleosis. In 1949, outcomes were reported for five infants born to mothers with infectious mononucleosis during pregnancy. Of these, three were born with congenital defects, one with cataract.[97] A case of cortical blindness has been linked with this same background.[98] Another case resulted in the infant's death at birth. This infant's defects included microphthalmos, hypertelorism, and epicanthal folds.[99]

Finally, another newborn infant with in utero EBV infection was reported with multiple anomalies including cataracts. In this case, however, the mother already had a cataract in one eye.[100]

Cytomegalovirus

Cytomegalovirus has been implicated as one possible cause of optic nerve hypoplasia.[101]

Acquired Immunodeficiency Syndrome

Acquired immunodeficiency syndrome (AIDS) is caused by the human T-cell lymphotropic virus, type III (HTLV-III). It is classified among distinctive RNA viruses sharing some features with retroviruses, which have previously been linked to animal diseases, including leukemia and neurological and immunodeficiency disorders. The HTLV-III kills T lymphocytes of the helper type, which renders the immune system incompetent and leads to diverse fatal infections and tumors.[102]

An AIDS embryopathy recently has been described. This embryopathy is a dysmorphic syndrome that includes a distinct facial appearance (Fig 10–3), with hypertelorism, mild upward or downward obliquity of the eyes, blue scleras, and long palpebral fissures. In this latter feature it differs diametrically from fetal alcohol syndrome which has, as one of its features, *short* palpebral fissures.[103]

As the epidemic of the 1980s expands, more information regarding eye deformities in this fetopathy will undoubtedly become available.

Amniotic Band Syndrome

Amniotic band syndrome is believed to represent the physical effects of intrauterine

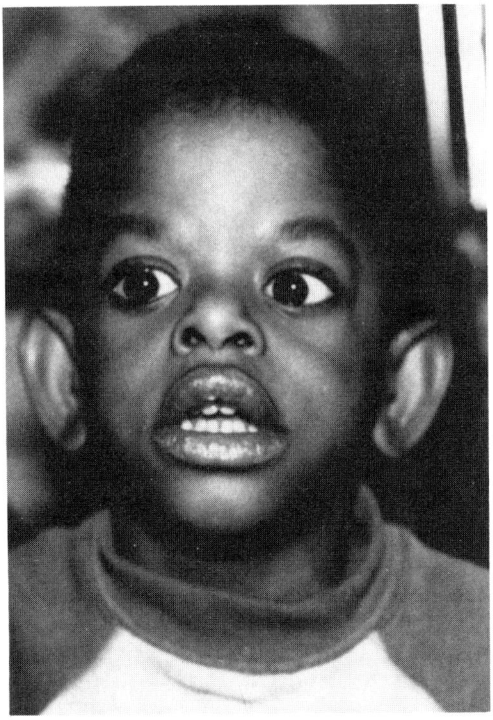

FIG 10–3.
HTLV-III embryopathy patient demonstrates hypertelorism, obliquity of the eyes, blue sclerae, and long palpebral fissure. (From Marion RW, Wiznia AA, Hutcheon G, et al: Human T-cell lymphotropic virus type III (HTLV-III) embryopathy: A new dysmorphic syndrome associated with intrauterine HTLV-III infection. *Am J Dis Child* 1986; 140:638–640. Used by permission.)

impingement on fetal structures by disordered bands of amnion. Three cases of paralytic strabismus have been attributed to this syndrome.[104] In another case one eye was microphthalmic and aphakic and had metaplasia of the cornea. The nose was malformed on the same side.[105] Additional possible ocular defects from this syndrome include eyelid coloboma, corneal opacity, and anophthalmia.[106]

Hyperthermia

Fraser and Skelton reported a possibly significant association of maternal fever during pregnancy with microphthalmos in the newborn.[107] In addition, central nervous system and facial defects have been found associated with maternal hyperthermia at 4 to 14 weeks of gestation.[108]

Agent Orange

The defoliant Agent Orange has been implicated in delayed illness of veterans of the Vietnam War. A case of ocular deformity has been reported in a child of one of the veterans who was exposed to this agent, which was sprayed on foliage by aircraft. The child had a malformed anterior chamber angle with an enlarged globe and retinal dysplasia. The significance of Agent Orange exposure in this case is unclear.[109]

Clomiphene

A case of congenital retinal aplasia has been reported in an infant whose mother received 3 months of clomiphene therapy to achieve pregnancy.[110] Again, this report must be considered only as an alert to the physician to consider this association in future cases and by no means as a proven causal relationship.

TERATOGENIC AGENTS THAT AFFECT EXPERIMENTAL ANIMAL EYES

In addition to the animal effects that previously have been mentioned in the context of possible human teratology, the following agents have been noted to influence animal eye development in a way that would suggest a need for vigilance for possible occasional human manifestations.

1. Radioactively labeled chlorpromazine has been found to concentrate in the retinas of fetal mice and persist 5 months after disappearing from other tissues.[111]
2. L-Asparaginase, an anticancer drug, has caused anophthalmia in rats.[112]
3. Vitamin A deficiency caused anophthalmia in pigs.[113]

Apt and Gaffney have reviewed additional ocular teratogens in animals.[114]

FUTURE PROSPECTS

Several resources are at work to expand our knowledge about teratogenic agents. The federal government operates a National Center for Toxicology Research in Pine Bluff, Ark, which performs basic research in teratology as part of its reproductive and developmental research. In addition, a national registry of birth defects is maintained for approximately 1,700 hospitals by the Centers for Disease Control in Atlanta. Several municipalities and states have registries for birth defects.

Specifically relating to the eye, the National Registry for Drug Induced Ocular Side effects in Portland, Ore, receives requests for information about teratogenic effects on the eye, although a relatively low volume of reports of suspected teratogenic agents is received. A national registry specifically for ocular birth defects and geared to the needs of pediatric ophthalmologists could be useful in identifying possible environmental influences on eye development. These associations could then be investigated by appropriate research. Efforts are under way toward establishing such a registry.

REFERENCES

1. *Webster's New Twentieth Century Dictionary*, ed 2. New York, Simon & Schuster, 1979.
2. Shepard TH: *Catalog of Teratogenic Agents*, ed 3. Baltimore, Johns Hopkins University Press, 1980.
3. Gordon N: Fetal drug syndromes. *Postgrad Med J* 1978; 54:796–798.
4. Heinonen OP, Slone D, Shapiro S: *Birth Defects and Drugs in Pregnancy*. Littleton, Colo, Publishing Sciences Group, 1977.
5. Warburg M: Microphthalmos and colobomata among mentally retarded individuals. *Acta Ophthalmol (Copenh)* 1981; 59:665–673.
6. Amemiya T, Nishimura H: Ocular malformations in human fetuses with external malformations. *J Pediatr Ophthalmol Strabismus* 1977; 14:165–170.
7. Moore KL: *The Developing Human*. Philadelphia, WB Saunders Co, 1973.
8. Sadler TW: *Langman's Medical Embryology*, ed 5. Baltimore, Williams & Wilkins, 1985.
9. Meadow SR: Anticonvulsant drugs and congenital abnormalities. *Lancet* 1968; 11:1296.
10. German J, Kowal A, Ehlers KH: Trimethadione and human teratogenesis. *Teratology* 1970; 3:349–362.
11. Zackai EH, Mellman WJ, Neiderer B, et al: The fetal trimethadione syndrome. *J Pediatr* 1975; 87:280–284.
12. Hanson JW, Smith DW: The fetal hydantoin syndrome. *J Pediatr* 1975; 87:285–290.
13. Wilson RS, Smead W, Char F: Diphenylhydantoin teratogenicity: Ocular manifestations and related deformities. *J Pediatr Ophthalmol Strabismus* 1978; 15:137–140.
14. Wallar PH, Genstler DE, George CC: Multiple systemic and periocular malformations associated with the fetal hydantoin syndrome. *Ann Ophthalmol* 1978; 10:1568–1572.
15. Hampton GR, Krepostman JI: Ocular manifestations of the fetal hydantoin syndrome. *Clin Pediatr (Phila)* 1981; 20:475–478.
16. Tunnessen WW Jr, Lowenstein EH: Glaucoma associated with the fetal hydantoin syndrome. *J Pediatr* 1976; 89:154–155.
17. Bartoshesky LE, Bhan I, Nagpaul K, et al: Severe cardiac and ophthalmologic malformations in an infant exposed to diphenylhydantoin in utero. *Pediatrics* 1982; 69:202–203.
18. Dabee V, Hart AG, Hurley RM: Teratogenic effects of diphenylhydantoin. *Can Med Assoc J* 1975; 112:75–77.
19. Hoyt CS, Billson FS: Maternal anticonvulsants and optic nerve hypoplasia. *Br J Ophthalmol* 1978; 62:3–6.
20. Allen RW, Ogden B, Bentley FL, et al: Fetal hydantoin syndrome, neuroblastoma, and hemorrhagic disease in a neonate. *JAMA* 1980; 244:1464–1465.
21. Monson RR, Rosenberg L, Hartz SC, et al: Diphenylhydantoin and selected congenital malformations. *N Engl J Med* 1973; 289:1049.

22. Kelly TE: Teratogenicity of anticonvulsant drugs. I: Review of the literature. *Am J Med Genet* 1984; 19:413–434.
23. Finnell RH, Chernoff GF: Genetic background: The elusive component in the fetal hydantoin syndrome. *Am J Med Genet* 1984; 19:459–462.
24. Schinzel A: Fetales Hydantoin-syndrom bei Geschwistern. *Schweiz Med Wochenschr* 1979; 109:68–72.
25. Pai GS: Cardiac and ophthalmic malformations and in utero exposure to Dilantin (letter). *Pediatrics* 1982; 70:327–328.
26. Krauss CM, Holmes LB, Van Lang Q, et al: Four siblings with similar malformations after exposure to phenytoin and primidone. *J Pediatr* 1984; 105:750–755.
27. Hanson JW, Buehler BA: Fetal hydantoin syndrome: Current status. *J Pediatr* 1982; 101:816–818.
28. Shepard TH: Detection of human teratogenic agents. *J Pediatr* 1982; 101:810–815.
29. Seip M: Growth retardation, dysmorphic facies and minor malformations following massive exposure to phenobarbitone in utero. *Acta Paediatr Scand* 1976; 65:617–621.
30. Majewski F, Raff W, Fischer P, et al: Zur Teratogenitaet von Antikonvulsiva. *Dtsch Med Wochenschr* 1980; 105:719–723.
31. Laughnan PM, Gold H, Vance JC: Phenytoin teratogenicity in man. *Lancet* 1973; 1:70–72.
32. Kerber IJ, Warr OS III, Richardson C: Pregnancy in a prosthetic mitral valve: Associated with a fetal anomaly attributed to warfarin sodium. *JAMA* 1968; 203:223–225.
33. Stevenson RE, Burton OM, Ferlauto GJ, et al: Hazards of oral anticoagulants during pregnancy. *JAMA* 1980; 243:1549–1551.
34. Becker MH, Genieser NB, Finegold M, et al: Chondrodysplasia punctata. Is maternal warfarin a factor? *Am. J Dis Child* 1975; 129:356–359.
35. Harrod MJE, Sherrod PS: Warfarin embryopathy in siblings. *Obstet Gynecol* 1981; 57:673–676.
36. Spranger JW, Opitz JM, Bidder U: Heterogeneity of chondrodysplasia punctata. *Hum Genet* 1971; 11:190–212.
37. Lemoine P, Harousseau H, Borteyou JP, et al: Les enfants de parents alcooliques: Anomalies observees: Apropos de 127 cas. *Quest Med* 1968; 25:476–482.
38. Chernoff GF: Introduction: A teratologist's view of the fetal alcohol syndrome, in Gallanter M (ed): *Currents in Alcoholism: Recent advances in research and treatment*, vol 7. New York, Grune & Stratton, 1980, pp 7–13.
39. Jones KL, Smith DW: Recognition of the fetal alcohol syndrome in early infancy. *Lancet* 1973; 2:999–1001.
40. Clarren SK, Smith DW: The fetal alcohol syndrome. *N Engl J Med* 1978; 298:1063–1067.
41. Sulik KK, Johnston MC, Webb MA: Fetal alcohol syndrome: Embryogenesis in a mouse model. *Science* 1981; 214:936–938.
42. Streissguth AP, Landesman-Dwyer S, Martin JC, et al: Teratogenic effects of alcohol in humans and laboratory animals. *Science* 1980; 209:353–362.
43. Hanson JW, Jones KL, Smith DW: Fetal alcohol syndrome: Experience with 41 patients. *JAMA* 1976; 235:1458–1460.
44. Rabinowicz M: Ophthalmologic findings in the fetal alcohol syndrome (Abstract of oral presentation, American Academy of Ophthalmology, Nov. 5, 1980). *Opthalmology* 1980; 87(suppl):93. Detailed in *Ophthalmology Times,* March 1981, p 71.
45. Jones KL, Smith DW, Ulleland CN, et al: Pattern of malformation in offspring of chronic alcoholic mothers. *Lancet* 1973; 1:1267–1271.
46. Miller M, Israel J, Cuttone J: Fetal alcohol syndrome. *J Pediatr Ophthalmol Strabismus* 1981; 18:6–15.
47. Stromland K: Ocular abnormalities in the fetal alcohol syndrome. *Acta Ophthalmol [Suppl] (Copenh)* 1985; 171:1–50.
48. Gonzales ER: New ophthalmic findings in fetal alcohol syndrome. *JAMA* 1981; 245:108–110.
49. Miller MT, Epstein RJ, Sugar J, et al: Anterior segment anomalies associated with the fetal alcohol syndrome. *J Pediatr Ophthalmol Strabismus* 1984; 29:8.
50. Shields MB, Buckley E, Klintworth GK, et al: Axenfeld-Rieger syndrome: A spectrum of developmental disorders. *Surv Ophthalmol* 1985; 29:387–409.
51. Smart RG, Bateman K: The chromosomal and teratogenic effects of lysergic acid diethylamide. *Can Med Assoc J* 1968; 99:805–810.
52. Hoyt CS: Optic disc anomalies and maternal ingestion of LSD. *J Pediatr Ophthal-*

mol Strabismus 1979; 16:225–240.
53. Margolis S, Martin L: Anophthalmia in an infant of parents using LSD. *Ann Ophthalmol* 1980; 12:1378–1381.
54. Chan CC, Fishman M, Egbert PR: Multiple ocular anomalies associated with maternal LSD ingestion. *Arch Ophthalmol* 1978; 96:282–284.
55. Bogdanoff B, Rorke LB, Yanoff M, et al: Brain and eye abnormalities; possible sequelae to prenatal use of multiple drugs including LSD. *Am J Dis Child* 1972; 123:145.
56. Fried PA: Marihuana use by pregnant women and effects on offspring: An update. *Neurobehav Toxicol Teratol* 1982; 4:451–454.
57. Fried PA: Marihauna use by pregnant women: Neurobehavioral effects in neonates. *Drug Alcohol Depend* 1980; 6:415–424.
58. Qazi QH, Mariano E, Milman DH, et al: Abnormalities in offspring associated with prenatal marijuana exposure. *Dev Pharmacol Ther* 1985; 8:141–148.
59. Teske MP, Trese MT: Retinopathy of prematurity-like fundus and persistent hyperplastic primary vitreous associated with maternal cocaine use. *Am J Ophthalmol* 1987; 103:719–720.
60. Isenberg SJ, Spierer A, Inkelis SH: Ocular signs of cocaine intoxication in neonates. *Am J Ophthalmol* 1987; 103:211–214.
61. Chasnoff IJ, Burns WJ, Schnoll SH, et al: Cocaine use in pregnancy. *N Engl J Med* 1985; 313:666–669.
62. Mahalik MP, Gautieri RF, Mann DE Jr: Teratogenic potential of cocaine hydrochloride in CF-1 mice. *J Pharm Sci* 1980; 69:703–706.
63. Chhabria S: Aicardi's syndrome: Are corticosteroids teratogens? (letter) *Arch Neurol* 1981; 38:70.
64. Kraus AM: Developmental cataracts. *NY State J Med* 1975; 75:1757–1758.
65. Fraser FC, Fainstat TD: Production of congenital defects in offspring of pregnant mice treated with cortisone. *Pediatrics* 1951; 8:527–533.
66. Rogoyski A, Trzcinska-Dabrowska Z: Corticosteroid-induced cataract and palatoschisis in the mouse fetus. *Am J Ophthalmol* 1969; 68:128.
67. Harris MJ, Juriloff DM: Eyelid development and fusion induced by cortisone treatment in mutant, lidgap-Miller, foetal mice. A scanning electron microscope study. *J Embryol Exp Morphol* 1986; 91:1–18.
68. Gremo F, Marchisio AM, Vernadakis A: Muscarinic receptor subclasses in the chick embryo retina: Influence of corticosterone treatment. *J Neurochem* 1985; 45:345–351.
69. Benawra R, Mangurten HH, Duffell DR: Cyclopia and other anomalies following maternal ingestion of salicyltes. *J Pediatr* 1980; 96:1069–1071.
70. Slone D, Heinonen OP, Kaufman DW, et al: Aspirin and congenital malformations. *Lancet* 1976; 1:1373–1375.
71. Hart CW, Naunton RF: The ototoxicity of chloroquine phosphate. *Arch Otolaryngol* 1964; 80:407–412.
72. *National Registry of Ocular Drug Side-Effects.* Report #2312, ref 423, 5th Annual Report, Portland, Ore, 1980–1981.
73. Reed H, Briggs JN, Martin JK: Congenital glaucoma, deafness, mental deficiencies, and cardiac anomaly following attempted abortion. *J Pediatr* 1955; 46:182.
74. Richardson S: The toxic effect of quinine on the eye. *South Med J* 1936; 29:1156–1164.
75. Hoyt CS, Billson FA: Maternal anticonvulsants and optic nerve hypoplasia. *Br J Ophthalmol* 1978; 62:3–6.
76. Milunsky A, Graef W, Gaynor MF: Methotrexate-induced congenital malformations. *J Pediatr* 1968; 72:790–795.
77. Saraux H, Lefrancois A: Degenerative retinal condition after treatment with busulfan during pregnancy (German). *Klin Monatsbl Augenheilkd* 1977; 170:818–820.
78. d'Avignon M, Barr B: Ear abnormalities and cranial nerve palsies in thalidomide children. *Arch Otolaryngol* 1964; 80:136–140.
79. Newman CGH: Clinical observations on the thalidomide syndrome. *Proc R Soc Med* 1977; 70:225–227.
80. Schuette E, Klaas D, Lizin F: Serial investigations on thalidomide children (German). *Berl Zusammenkunft Dtsch Ophthalmol Ges* 1977; 74:578–580.
81. Klaas D, Schuette E, Lizin F: Atypical retinal detachment in an adolescent victim of thalidomide embryopathy (German). *Berl Zusammenkunft Dtsch Ophthalmol Ges* 1977; 74:575–577.
82. Zetterstroem B: Ocular malformations caused by thalidomide. *Acta Ophthalmol* 1966; 44:39–45.
83. Rafuse EV, Arstikaitis M, Brent HP: Ocular

findings in thalidomide children. *Can J Ophthalmol* 1976; 2:222–225.
84. Rosa FW: Teratogenicity of isotretinoin (letter). *Lancet* 1983; 1:513.
85. Lott IT, Bocian M, Pribram HW, et al: Fetal hydrocephalus and ear anomalies associated with maternal use of isotretinoin. *J Pediatr* 1984; 105:597–600.
86. de la Cruz E, Sun S, Vangvanichyakorn K, et al: Multiple congenital malformations associated with maternal isotretinoin therapy. *Pediatrics* 1984; 74:428–430.
87. Fernhoff PM, Lammer EJ: Craniofacial features of isotretinoin embryopathy. *J Pediatr* 1984; 105:595–597.
88. Gustavson KH, Jagell S, Blomquist HK, et al: Microcephaly, mental retardation and chromosomal aberrations in a girl following radiation therapy during late fetal life. *Acta Radiol [Oncol]* 1981; 20:209–212.
89. Sigler AT, Lilienfeld AM, Cohen BH, et al: parental age in Down's syndrome (mongolism). *J Pediatr* 1965; 67:631.
90. Buckton KE, Jacobs PA, Court Brown WM, et al: Study of chromosome damage persisting after x-ray therapy for ankylosing spondylitis. *Lancet* 1962; 2:676–682.
91. Hicks SP, O'Brien RC, Newcomb EC: Developmental malformations produced by radiation. A timetable of their development. *AJR* 1953; 69:272–293.
92. Mole RH: Consequences of pre-natal radiation exposure for post-natal development. A review. *Int J Radiat Biol* 1982; 42:1–12.
93. Hecht F, Bryant JS, Gruber D, et al: The nonrandomness of chromosomal abnormalities. *N Engl J Med* 1964; 271:1081–1086.
94. Nusbacher J, Hirschhorn K, Cooper LZ: Chromosomal abnormalities in congenital rubella. *N Engl J Med* 1967; 276:1409–1413.
95. Cooper LZ, Green FH, Krugman S, et al: Neonatal thrombocytopenic purpura and other manifestations of rubella contracted in utero. *Am J Dis Child* 1965; 110:416.
96. Sever JL, Nelson KB, Gilkeson MR: Rubella epidemic, 1964: Effect on 6000 pregnancies. *Am J Dis Child* 1965; 110:395–407.
97. Miller HC, Clifford SH, Smith CA, et al: Special report from the committee for the study of congenital malformations to maternal rubella and other infections: Preliminary report. *Pediatrics* 1949; 3:259–270.
98. Visintine AM, Gerber P, Nahmias AJ: Leukocyte transforming agent (Epstein-Barr virus) in newborn infants and older individuals. *J Pediatr* 1976; 89:571–575.
99. Brown ZA, Stenchever MA: Infectious mononucleosis and congenital anomalies. *Am J Obstet Gynecol* 1978; 131:108–109.
100. Goldberg GN, Fulginiti VA, Ray CG, et al: In utero Epstein-Barr virus (infectious mononucleosis) infection. *JAMA* 1981; 246:1579–1581.
101. Hittner HM, Desmond MM, Montgomery JR: Optic nerve manifestations of human cytomegalovirus infection. *Am J Ophthalmol* 1976; 81:661–665.
102. Important AIDS Information. *Bulletin from US Dept of Health and Human Services.* Public Health Service, Food and Drug Administration, Rockville, Md, 1985.
103. Marion RW, Wiznia AA, Hutcheon G, et al: Human T-cell lymphotropic virus type III (HTLV-III) embryopathy. A new dysmorphic syndrome associated with intrauterine HTLV-III infection. *Am J Dis Child* 1986; 140:638–640.
104. Ben Ezra D, Frucht Y, Paez JH, et al: Amniotic band syndrome and strabismus. *J Pediatr Ophthalmol Strabismus* 1982; 19:33–36.
105. Klauss V, Riedel K: bilateral and unilateral mesodermal corneal metaplasia. *Br J Ophthalmol* 1983; 67:320–323.
106. Braude LS, Miller M, Cuttone J: Ocular abnormalities in the amniogenic band syndrome. *Br J Ophthalmol* 1981; 65:299–303.
107. Fraser FC, Skelton J: Possible teratogenicity of maternal fever (letter). *Lancet* 1978; 2:634.
108. Pleet HB, Graham JM, Smith DW: Central nervous system and facial defects associated with maternal hyperthermia at 4 to 14 weeks gestation. *Pediatrics* 1981; 67:785–789.
109. Presland MW, Beauchamp GR, Zakov ZN: Congenital glaucoma and retinal dysplasia. *J Pediatr Ophthalmol Strabismus* 1985; 22:166–170.
110. Laing IA, Steer CR, Dudgeon J, et al: Clomiphene and congenital retinopathy (letter). *Lancet* 1981; 2:1107–1108.
111. Ullberg S, Lindquist NG, Sjostrand SE: Accumulation of chorio-retinotoxic drugs in the foetal eye. *Nature* 1970; 227:1257–1258.
112. Sanfeliu C, Nebot-Cegarra J, Domenech-Mateu JM: Teratogenic effects of L-asparaginase in rat embryos in vitro. *Acta*

Anat (Basel) 1986; 125:152–160.
113. Hale F: Relation of vitamin A to anophthalmos in pigs. *Am J Ophthalmol* 1935; 18:1087.
114. Apt L, Gaffney WL: Congenital eye abnormalities from drugs during pregnancy, in Leopold IH (ed): *Symposium on Ocular Therapy*, vol 7. St Louis, CV Mosby Co, 1974, p 1.

PART II

Congenital Malformations Evident in the First Month of Life

11 Chromosome Abnormalities

Roberta A. Pagon, M.D.
Christine Disteche, Ph.D.

GENERAL CONSIDERATIONS

In 1956 Tijo and Levan first reported the number of human chromosomes to be 46.[1] In 1959 Lejeune published his discovery of trisomy 21, the first known chromosome abnormality in humans. Subsequently, an ever-increasing number of human chromosome abnormalities has been recognized as cytogenetic methodologies have improved and as chromosome analysis of children with congenital anomalies has become routine. This chapter reviews some principles of human cytogenetics and describes those chromosome abnormalities associated with ocular malformation and disease. The reader is referred to other excellent resources for more detailed information on human cytogenetics,[2] chromosomal syndromes,[3–5] and genetic eye disease.[6]

Each chromosome consists of a continuous double strand of DNA that encodes the genes. The DNA is packaged in a higher-order structure called chromatin. In the interphase nucleus between cell divisions, the chromosomes are not identifiable as discrete entities. During cell division, the chromatin condenses, and individual chromosomes are identifiable with a light microscope. When stained by techniques such as G- and R-banding, each metaphase chromosome takes on a characteristic banding pattern identifying it as one of the 22 autosomes (numbered 1 through 22) or one of the 2 sex chromosomes (X or Y). The normal chromosome constitution is 46,XX for a female and 46,XY for a male.

Chromosomes have a short arm, termed *p* for the French *petit* (small), and a long arm termed *q* in lieu of *g* for the French *grand* (large). The centromere is the constricted portion of the chromosome where separation of the chromosome is initiated at cell division. A band is a region of the chromosome that can be distinguished from a neighboring region on the basis of a difference in staining intensity. The bands have been established and identified numerically by convention so as to permit a precise description of any chromosome aberration.[7] A karyotype shows the chromosomes from a single cell arranged in numerical sequence.

Chromosome abnormalities may be numerical or structural and may affect the autosomes or the sex chromosomes. Chromosome abnormalities are to be distinguished from single-gene defects. Chromosome abnormalities involve visible alterations in the chromosomes that result in an imbalance in gene dosage. Single-gene defects (monogenic or mendelian disorders) are caused by submicroscopic alteration of the DNA. Monogenic disorders cannot be detected through chromosome analysis.

The major types of chromosome abnormalities are briefly reviewed.

I. Abnormal number of chromosomes.
   A. Aneuploidy—any deviation in number of chromosomes: missing chromosome (monosomy), three copies of a given chromosome (trisomy), four copies of a given chromosome (tetrasomy), etc.
   B. Polyploidy—there is an extra haploid set of chromosomes: 3n (69) chromosomes is triploidy; 4n (92) chromosomes is tetraploidy.

II. Structural abnormalities of an individual chromosome.
   A. Duplication—part of a chromosome is duplicated thereby causing a partial trisomy.
   B. Deletion—part of a chromosome is missing thus resulting in a partial monosomy. Deletions may be "terminal" (involving loss of the terminal portion of a chromosome) or interstitial (involving loss of a segment within a chromosome arm) or may result in a ring chromosome (loss of material from both the long and short arm, causing the ends to join and form a ring).
   C. Isochromosome—a chromosome composed of two short arms (iso p) or two long arms (iso q).
   E. Inversion—part of a chromosome is inverted with no gain or loss in chromosome material. These can be pericentric (around the centromere) or paracentric (not involving the centromere).

III. Rearrangement between two chromosomes (translocation).
   A. Robertsonian translocation—the joining together of any two acrocentric chromosomes (nos. 13, 14, 15, 21, 22) at the centromeric region.
   B. Balanced translocation—an exchange of chromosome material between any two chromosomes without gain or loss in genetic information.
   C. Unbalanced chromosomal translocation—rearrangement between two chromosomes in which there is gain or loss in chromosome material.

IV. Chromosomal mosaicism.
   A. Mosaicism is the presence of two or more cell lines with different chromosome constitution. Often one cell line is euploid (diploid) and the other aneuploid, although diploid/triploid mosaicism occurs as well as mosaicism for euploid cell lines in which there is a structural abnormality of one chromosome.

Children who have a chromosome imbalance, whether from an abnormal number of chromosomes or from a duplication or deficiency of part of a chromosome, usually have multiple congenital anomalies, growth retardation, and mental retardation. Any organ system can be involved when a chromosome abnormality is present. In general, the type and severity of malformations vary depending on the chromosome abnormality present; however, patients with identical chromosome abnormalities may have different congenital malformations and varying severity of involvement.

There are no chromosome abnormalities that exclusively affect the eye without other organ system involvement. While there are ocular disorders that strongly suggest certain chromosome abnormalities, there are no ocular defects, except perhaps retinoblastoma, that are pathognomonic for a specific chromosome aberration. Any ocular malformation can be seen in chromosome disorders. The physician should be alerted to the possibility of a chromosome abnormality when a child has multiple congenital anomalies or a single major anomaly coupled with growth retardation or developmental delay.

When a chromosome abnormality is suspected, a karyotype must be obtained. A blood chromosome study is preferred for the initial evaluation of any patient since T lymphocytes are an easy cell type to obtain and provide the best technical results. The cells must be cultured and require a minimum of 48 to 72 hours' incubation time; hence, even preliminary chromosome results from a leukocyte culture will not be available until 3 to 5 days after the sample has been obtained. Most laboratories require 10 days to 3 weeks for routine chromosome analysis.

If immediate diagnosis is necessary, a bone marrow karyotype can provide results within 4 to 6 hours. If an infant is stillborn or has severe metabolic acidosis, a tissue other than blood such as skin should be obtained for the purpose of establishing a fibroblast culture for chromosome analysis. In instances where chromosomal mosaicism is suspected and leukocyte chromosome analysis is normal, analysis of a second tissue such as skin is advised. Fibroblast cultures involve more complex laboratory procedures and hence are more expensive but, under certain circumstances, may be the only way that diagnosis of a chromosome abnormality can be established.

High-resolution (prometaphase) chromosome studies involve evaluation of more elongated chromosomes and permit detection of smaller duplications and deletions that cannot be visualized on routine metaphase preparations. By using the same staining methods (G- and R-banding) over 850 individual bands can be visualized on prometaphase studies in contrast to about 400 bands visualized in metaphase spreads. High-resolution studies can and should be requested when specific, subtle chromosome abnormalities are suspected.

The following outlines the reasons to establish that a chromosome abnormality is present.

1. Detection of a chromosome abnormality in an infant with multiple anomalies provides a diagnosis. The search for other etiologies such as a teratogen, monogenic disorder, or other syndrome can cease.

2. If a specific phenotype exists for the chromosome abnormality, the physician can evaluate the child for known associated malformations or medical conditions.

3. The parents can be given accurate recurrence risk counseling. Some chromosomal anomalies such as triploidy are always sporadic events. Most aneuploidy syndromes such as trisomy 21, trisomy 18, and trisomy 13 carry a low but slightly increased risk of recurrence compared with the general population risk. Chromosomal duplications or deletions may be de novo events or may be secondary to a balanced chromosomal rearrangement or translocation in one of the parents. De novo structural rearrangements do not present an increased risk for chromosome abnormalities in other offspring; however, parents who carry a balanced rearrangement have a significantly increased risk to have a chromosomally abnormal child.

4. Prenatal testing for chromosome abnormalities is possible. Couples who have had a child with a chromosome abnormality or who are known to be at increased risk to have a child with a chromosome abnormality may desire prenatal diagnosis. Amniocentesis is a safe and reliable procedure in which a needle is inserted into the uterus at 16 to 18 weeks' gestation for the purpose of removing a small amount of amniotic fluid. Results of chromosome analysis on fetal cells cultured from the amniotic fluid are available in 2 to 3 weeks. Chorionic villus sampling (CVS) is a newer method of prenatal testing in which a flexible catheter is introduced transvaginally into the uterus for the purpose of removing a small amount of trophoblastic (placental) tissue. CVS carries a greater risk of pregnancy loss than does amniocentesis but has the advantage of being performed earlier in gestation (9 to 12 weeks).

5. Detection of a balanced translocation or any structural rearrangement in the parent of a child with a chromosome abnormality mandates karyotyping other family members to determine whether they also are translocation carriers.

Although "treatment" per se does not exist for the basic genetic defect in a child with a chromosome abnormality, all of the aforementioned information can be helpful in directing a family to appropriate medical management, developmental therapy, and genetic counseling.

TABLE 11–1.
Ocular Findings in Chromosome Abnormalities

Ocular Finding	Commonly Found in	Rare in
Coloboma (anophthalmia/microphthalmos)	Trisomy 13 Triploidy Cat-eye syndrome (tetrasomy 22q) Deletion 4p16	del 11q25 del 18q
Cyclopia	Trisomy 13 18p –	Triploidy
Aniridia	del 11p13	
Retinoblastoma	del 13q14	

CHROMOSOME ABNORMALITIES IN WHICH OCULAR ANOMALIES OCCUR WITH HIGH FREQUENCY

This section is divided into discussions of the effects of extra chromosomal material (trisomies, triploidy, partial trisomy, or tetrasomy) and deletions (Table 11–1).

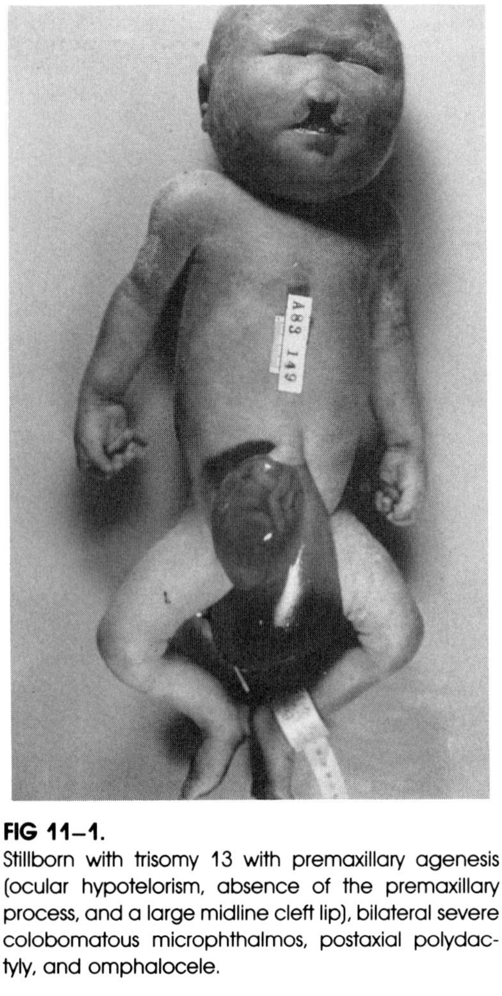

FIG 11–1.
Stillborn with trisomy 13 with premaxillary agenesis (ocular hypotelorism, absence of the premaxillary process, and a large midline cleft lip), bilateral severe colobomatous microphthalmos, postaxial polydactyly, and omphalocele.

Trisomies, Triploidy, Partial Trisomy, or Tetrasomy

Trisomy 13

Trisomy 13, the third most common autosomal trisomy, occurs in approximately 1 in 8,000 to 1 in 12,000 births. Characteristic features are microcephaly, colobomatous malformation of the eye with or without microphthalmos, holoprosencephaly, cleft lip and cleft palate (>50%), and postaxial hexadactyly (extra digit arising next to the fifth digit of the hand and/or feet, >80%) (Fig 11–1).[3] The incidence of ocular anomalies is virtually 100% and almost always is some form of coloboma.[8–12]

The degree of ocular involvement ranges over the entire spectrum of coloboma[13] including an isolated iris coloboma at the more mild end of the spectrum (Fig 11–2,A) and bilateral clinical anophthalmia (Fig 11–2,B) at the severe end of the spectrum. Phenotypes in the midrange of the spectrum include chorioretinal coloboma (Fig 11–3,A and B) and microphthalmos of varying severity (Fig 11–4). Retinal dysplasia in which the retina is poorly differentiated and thrown into folds that appear as rosettes histologically is so common as to be almost invariable in trisomy 13. Intraocular cartilage formation commonly accompanies retinal dysplasia and the more severe colobomatous malformations,[10] but this finding is not specific for trisomy 13 as was once thought.[11] Persistent hyperplastic primary vitreous (PHPV) and retinal detachment

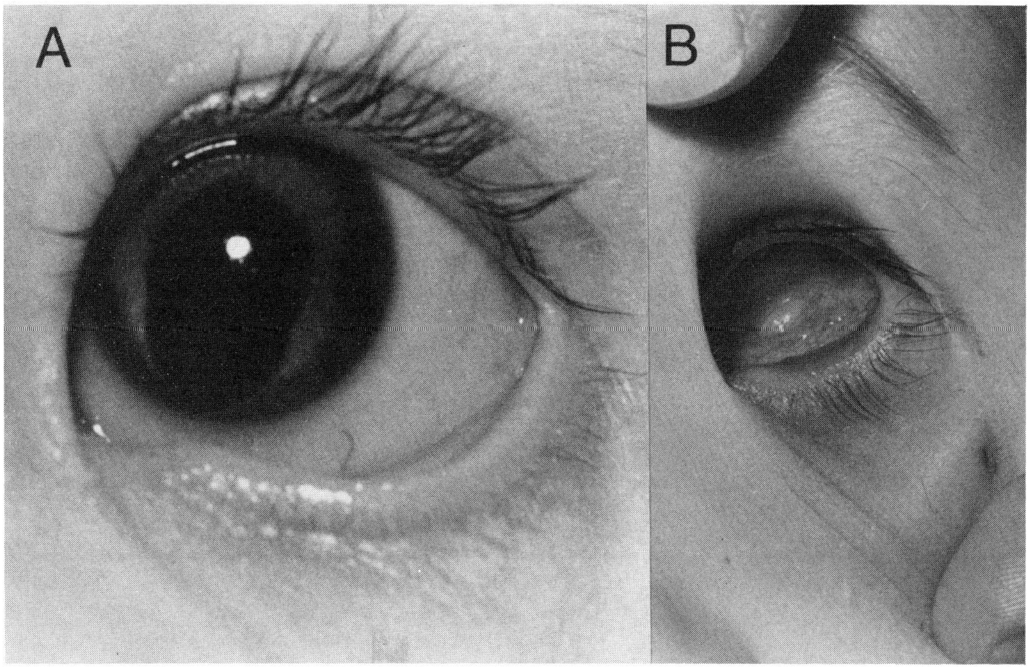

FIG 11–2.
A, typical iris coloboma in which the defect in the pupil is oriented inferionasally. **B**, clinical anophthalmia in which there are no identifiable ocular structures.

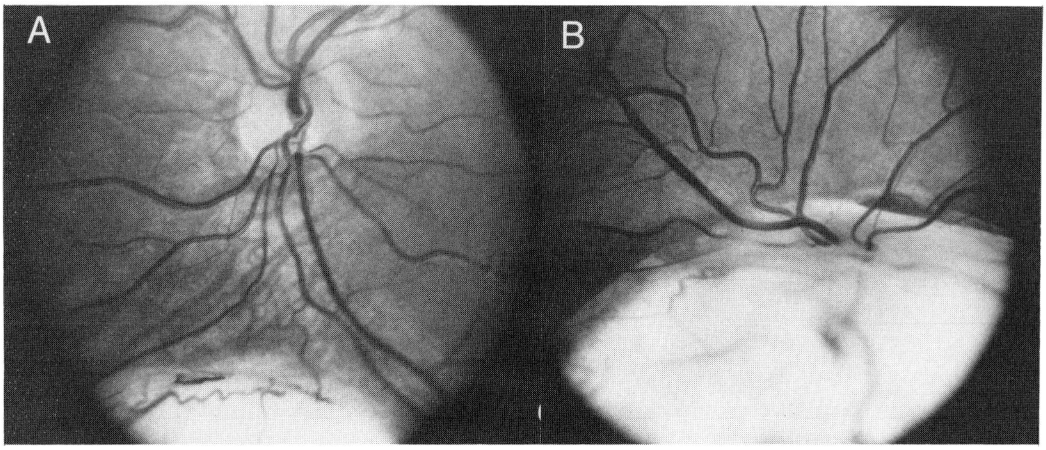

FIG 11–3.
A, chorioretinal coloboma that spares the optic nerve and macula. The position of such a coloboma is always inferionasal to the disc. Vision is preserved. **B**, chorioretinal coloboma that extends through the superior portion of the disc. Such large defects usually include the macula and cause significant visual impairment.

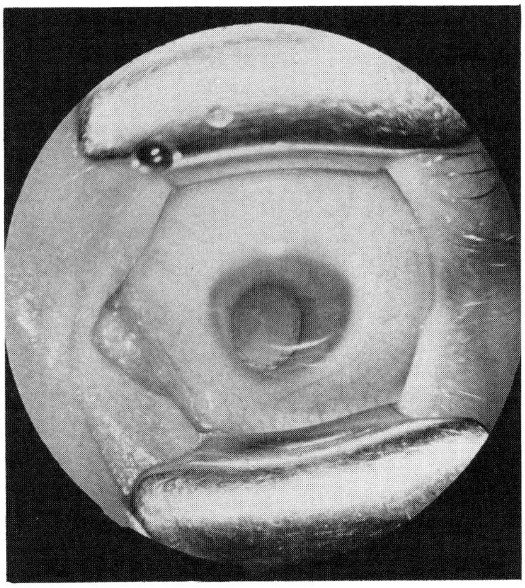

FIG 11–4.
Colobomatous microphthalmos in an eye with an irregularly shaped cornea. The iris coloboma points inferionasally. The white pupillary reflex is caused by a large chorioretinal coloboma and associated retinal detachment.

frequently accompany retinal dysplasia. Lens opacities and incomplete cleavage of the anterior chamber angle are frequent and almost invariably present with more severe ocular malformations. The ocular anomalies seen in infants with trisomy 13 are typically severe and bilateral and prompt requests for immediate evaluation by an ophthalmologist.

The most common central nervous system (CNS) malformation in trisomy 13 is holoprosencephaly. Severe abnormalities in facial morphogenesis usually accompany holoprosencephaly and include cyclopia with a proboscis (Fig 11–5); premaxillary agenesis with ocular hypotelorism, absence of the maxillary process, and a large midline cleft lip (see Fig 11–1); and cebocephaly in which there is a single central nostril and ocular hypotelorism. Infants with holoprosencephaly can have a normal facies as well. Trisomy 13 is the single most common cause of holoprosencephaly[14] and cyclopia.[15]

Other anomalies occurring in trisomy 13 are omphalocele, imperforate anus, camptodactyly of the fingers, scalp defects (aplasia cutis congenita), abnormally shaped ears, ambiguous genitalia in males, and multicystic kidneys. Infants with trisomy 13 characteristically have multiple anomalies, many of which are life threatening. In most instances, the diagnosis of trisomy 13 is suspected clinically. However, atypical presentations may obscure the diagnosis prior to completion of the chromosome studies. About 90% of infants with trisomy 13 do not survive the neonatal period. Those who do survive usually have less severe craniofacial involvement but quite severe mental retardation.

The chromosomal constitution of 85% to 88% of infants with trisomy 13 is free trisomy 13 in which there are three individual copies of chromosome 13. About 12% to 15% are caused by rearrangements, most commonly a 13;14 robertsonian translocation. If free trisomy 13 is found, there is no indication to study the parental chromosomes since there are no known chromosomal variants or find-

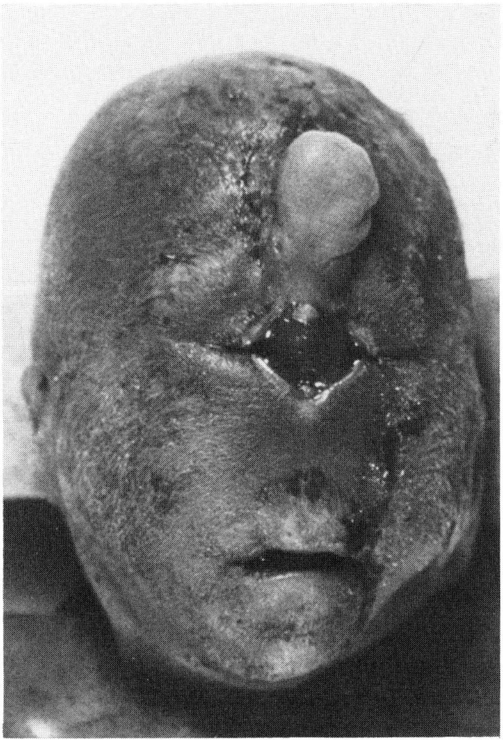

FIG 11–5.
Stillborn with trisomy 13 and cyclopia with a proboscis and severe abnormalities in facial morphogenesis indicative of holoprosencephaly.

ings that predispose to trisomy 13. However, the finding of a robertsonian translocation in the child mandates karyotyping the parents since there is a 40% chance that one of them is a translocation carrier.[16]

For trisomy 13 the recurrence risk is 1%; for a parent with a 13;14 robertsonian translocation, the recurrence risk is also 1% for trisomy 13.

Trisomy 18

Trisomy 18 is the second most common autosomal abnormality and occurs in 1 in 7,000 to 1 in 10,000 births. This chromosomal abnormality also is associated with multiple congenital anomalies and early death, with most infants dying before 2 months of age.[17] Ocular malformations and major CNS anomalies are not as common in trisomy 18 as in trisomy 13.[8,9] Early death is secondary to congenital heart disease or brain stem dysfunction leading to apnea and respiratory failure. Those children with trisomy 18 who survive the neonatal period have profound retardation, often with no independent ambulation, speech development, or independent living skills.

Although the ophthalmologist is likely to be involved in the initial evaluation of an infant with trisomy 13 because of the extensive ocular and craniofacial abnormalities, it is less likely that ophthalmologic evaluation will be requested in the initial assessment of a child with trisomy 18. Short palpebral fissures are common, but significant structural malformations of the globes are rare.[9] Ocular anomalies include microphthalmos, posterior subcapsular cataract, and clouding of the cornea secondary to keratinization of the corneal epithelium. Coloboma and retinal dysplasia[18–20] are reported to occur but generally involve only the posterior pole and are less severe than those seen in trisomy 13. Numerous minor ocular anomalies have been documented on histological examination. These include anisocoria, eccentric pupils, hyperplasia of the retinal layers, hypoplasia of the retinal pigment epithelium, and gliosis and hypoplasia of the optic nerve.[18,20]

Other systemic anomalies in infants with trisomy 18 include microcephaly with characteristic small facies, narrow palpebral fissures, small nose, small mouth, receding chin, abnormally shaped and posteriorly rotated ears, congenital heart disease, short sternum, narrow pelvis, and rocker-bottom feet. The hands are clenched, with the second and fifth fingers overlapping fingers 3 and 4. Esophageal atresia occurs in about 25% of patients and radial hypoplasia in about 10%. Trisomy 18 is one of the few chromosomal syndromes in which dermatoglyphic patterns may be helpful in the initial assessment of patients because of the high frequency of low dermal arches on the fingertips.

Since chromosome 18 is submetacentric, a robertsonian translocation cannot account for this disorder. The recurrence risk is 1% for couples to have another child with trisomy 18.[21]

Triploidy

Triploidy is a chromosomal aberration that occurs frequently in early spontaneous abortuses and stillbirths. Of chromosomally abnormal first trimester spontaneous abortions, about 15% to 20% are triploid.[22] For those triploid conceptuses continuing to term, the incidence of stillbirth is high, although survival beyond the neonatal period has occurred. Surviving infants are usually mosaic for a normal diploid (46) cell line and a triploid (69) cell line.[23,24]

Ocular anomalies are common in triploidy and are typically colobomatous malformations that span the range of involvement from iris coloboma to anophthalmia with any of the intermediate phenotypes (chorioretinal coloboma, microphthalmos with retinal dysplasia and PHPV, and cystic eye).[25] Concomitant ocular anomalies are incomplete development of the angle structures, cataract, and persistent tunica vasculosa lentis.

Holoprosencephaly and cyclopia have been reported in triploidy.[26] Infants who do not have major brain malformations may have a characteristic facies with a flat midface and upturned nose (Fig 11–6).[27] Other common malformations are meningomylocele, om-

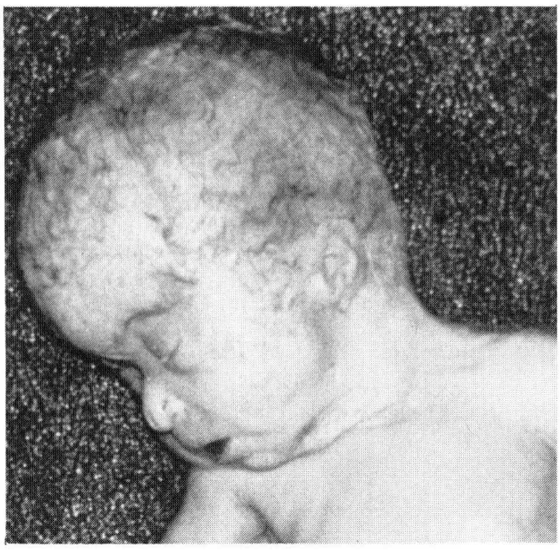

FIG 11–6.
Stillborn with triploidy and characteristic facies with frontal bossing, low nasal root, and depressed nasal tip.

phalocele, syndactyly of digits 3 and 4, ambiguous genitalia, and hydatidiform changes in the placenta.[27] Children who are mosaic often survive the neonatal period and may have few congenital anomalies but can have marked body asymmetry (so-called hemiatrophy), some degree of mental deficiency, and syndactyly of fingers 3 and 4. The ocular involvement is variable, with some having ocular coloboma[24] and others with no ocular anomalies.[25]

The ophthalmologist is likely to be involved in the initial evaluation of infants with triploidy because of the increased incidence of ocular anomalies. The diagnosis may be missed initially in mosaic patients since the lymphocyte karyotype is often normal; in some instances the diagnosis can be established only after a high index of suspicion clinically prompts analysis of a second tissue such as skin. This phenomenon of "tissue-limited mosaicism" in which lymphocyte chromosomes are normal but chromosomes from a second tissue are abnormal is frequent in triploidy.[28] Surviving infants merit ophthalmologic evaluation to diagnose and manage any ocular conditions since the prognosis for children with diploid-triploid mosaicism can be surprisingly good.

Triploidy most commonly results from dispermy (fertilization of a single egg by two sperm).[22] There is no increased risk of recurrence.

Cat Eye Syndrome

In 1965 Schachenmann et al.[29] reported four patients with iris coloboma and a characteristic phenotype who had a small extra chromosome. This subsequently became known as the cat-eye syndrome. The syndrome includes ocular coloboma, characteristic facies with down-slanting palpebral fissures and hypertelorism, preauricular tags or pits, cardiac malformations, anal atresia, and normal or only mildly retarded mental development. The variability of the phenotype and of the chromosomal findings in this syndrome has created controversy.

In a review of 11 patients and an additional 23 from the literature, Schinzel et al.[30] found iris coloboma in 62%, microphthalmos (presumably colobomatous) in 20%, anal atresia in 65%, congenital heart disease in 47%, and preauricular pits or tags in 76%. Some degree of intellectual impairment was seen in most patients, although the range of intellectual abilities was broad. Schinzel et al.[30] found 20 of 24 patients with an intelligence quotient (IQ) of 60 or greater. Not all patients with the cat-eye syndrome have ocular anomalies: some with ocular anomalies have microphthalmos not a "cat eye" (iris coloboma); in others the ocular involvement may be a chorioretinal coloboma that may be missed unless ophthalmologic examination is performed. Hence, the name of the syndrome does not describe the ocular phenotype of all affected individuals.

The precise nature of the additional small marker chromosome present in the cat-eye syndrome has been debated. On the basis of cytogenetic studies, Schinzel et al.[30] concluded that the extra chromosome is a dicentric chromosome 22 and that the syndrome results from partial tetrasomy of chromosome 22 from the terminus of the short arm to band q11 on the long arm (Fig 11–7). Different breakpoints within band 22q11 may account for some of the phenotypic variability.[31] McDermid et al.[32] used a molecular probe

(D22S9) that is localized to 22q11 to study six patients with the cat-eye syndrome. She and her coworkers concluded that, on a gene dosage basis, four copies of 22q11 were present in all their cat-eye syndrome patients with a marker chromosome, which supports the conclusion of Schinzel et al.[30] Reiss et al.[33] reported a boy with many features of the cat-eye syndrome who had 46 chromosomes in which a small interstitial duplication of band q11 of chromosome 22 was detected by high-resolution studies. Such a patient was included in the study of McDermid et al.[32] who showed that three copies of 22q11 were present. Hence, it appears that cat-eye syndrome is caused by partial tetrasomy 22q11 present as an additional marker chromosome or partial trisomy 22q11 caused by an interstitial duplication of band 22q11.

The parents of a child with the cat-eye syndrome should always be karyotyped. Familial transmission of the marker chromosome through a clinically normal or mildly affected parent has occurred, and hence parental karyotypes are warranted when the proband is aneuploid for this marker. As with other chromosome abnormalities, parental karyotypes should be obtained when an interstitial duplication is present.

Deletions

Deletion 13q14

In 1963 Lele et al.[34] first reported the association of a partial deletion of the long arm of chromosome 13 with retinoblastoma. Subsequent reports confirmed the association, but a cause-and-effect relationship was not established until the late 1970s when Yunis and Ramsey[35] determined that despite variation in total size the deleted long arm segment always included band q14. This observation provided the foundation for subsequent research that mapped the retinoblastoma locus to this portion of chromosome 13. This knowledge allowed for extensive and significant research into the understanding of the molecular nature of retinoblastoma (Chapter 22) and the development of a model to explain this and perhaps other embryonal tumors.

The phenotype of patients with a deletion of 13q14 and retinoblastoma varies considerably depending upon the total amount of chromosomal material deleted.[3] Infants with the absence of a major portion of chromosome 13 have a lethal condition with severe microcephaly, termed atelencephaly, and other anomalies that include the absence of thumbs, syndactyly and the absence of some toes, and ambiguous genitalia. Other infants with large but less extensive deletions that include band q14 may have multiple minor anomalies and retinoblastoma without a specific phenotype. These children have significant developmental retardation but may have no abnormalities of craniofacial development other than microcephaly (Figs 11–8,A and 11–9,A). Patients with a small deletion of chromosome 13 that includes band q14 may have retinoblastoma and few or no other phenotypic abnormalities aside from some degree of

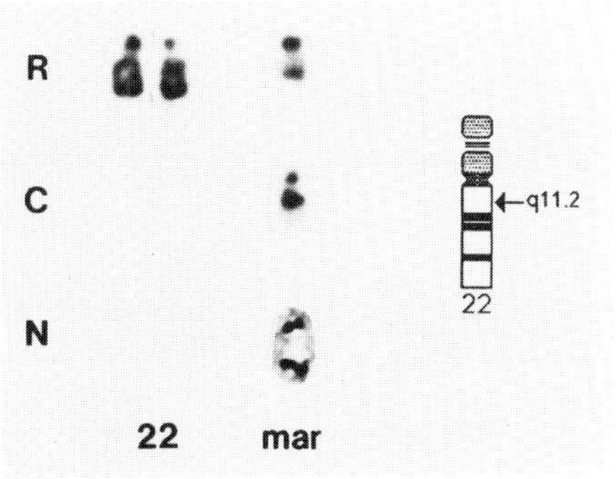

FIG 11–7.
Marker chromosome in cat-eye syndrome. Examples are shown of a marker chromosome (mar) found in a patient with cat-eye syndrome and the karyotype 47, XX+mar. The small marker chromosome and the normal pair of chromosomes 22 are shown after R-banding (R). C-banding (C) shows two C-bands in the marker chromosome, thereby indicating that it is a dicentric chromosome. Nuclear organizing region (NOR) staining (N) shows positive satellites on each end of the marker, which indicates that it is derived from the short arm of acrocentric chromosomes. A diagram of chromosome 22 is shown on the right. The arrow points to the critical band (22q11.2) that is duplicated in patients with cat-eye syndrome.

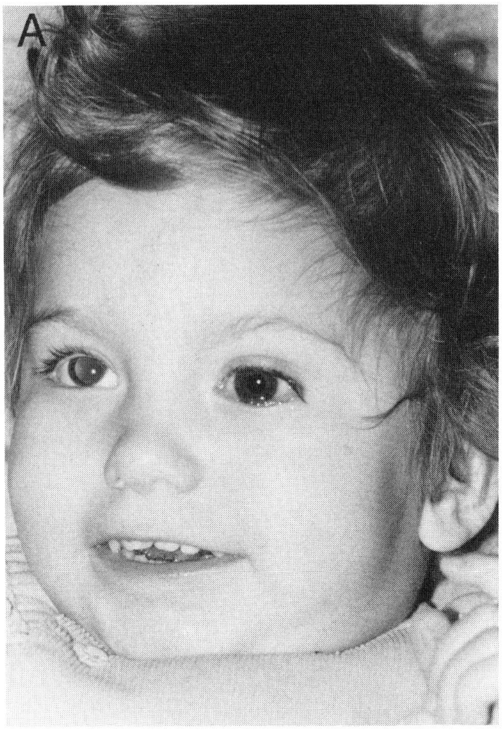

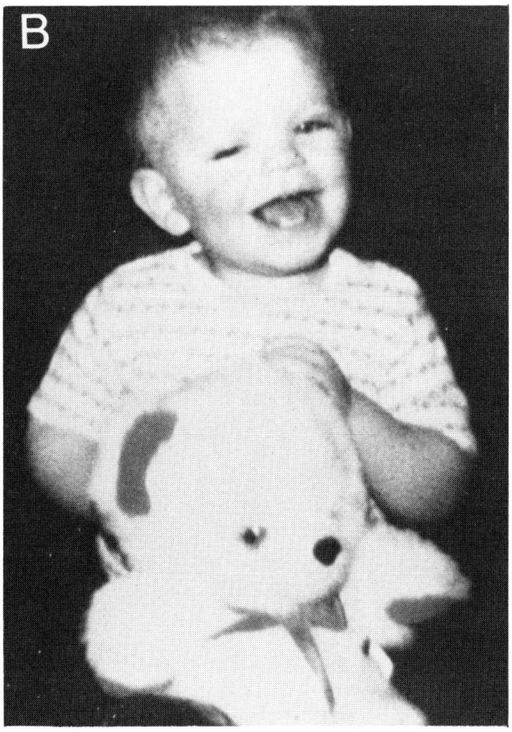

FIG 11–8.
A, 2-year-old girl with bilateral retinoblastoma, Hirschsprung's disease, and developmental delays. Her karyotype is shown in Figure 11–9,A. **B**, 12-month-old boy with bilateral retinoblastoma and some developmental delays. His karyotype is shown in Figure 11–9,B.

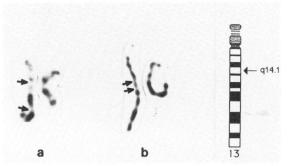

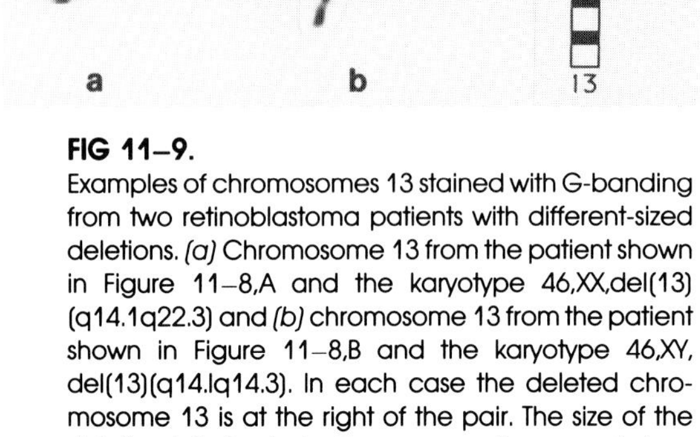

FIG 11–9.
Examples of chromosomes 13 stained with G-banding from two retinoblastoma patients with different-sized deletions. *(a)* Chromosome 13 from the patient shown in Figure 11–8,A and the karyotype 46,XX,del(13)(q14.1q22.3) and *(b)* chromosome 13 from the patient shown in Figure 11–8,B and the karyotype 46,XY, del(13)(q14.lq14.3). In each case the deleted chromosome 13 is at the right of the pair. The size of the deletion is indicated with arrows on the normal chromosome 13. A diagram of chromosome 13 is shown on the right. The arrow points to the critical band (13q14.1) deleted in retinoblastoma.

intellectual impairment (Figs 11–8,B and 11–9,B). Since a visible deletion of a chromosome involves an estimated loss of hundreds if not thousands of genes, it is expected that some degree of intellectual impairment will accompany a visible chromosomal deletion no matter how small.

Interestingly, patients reported with deletion 13q14 and retinoblastoma have about a 65% incidence of bilateral tumors and a 35% incidence of unilateral tumors, which suggests that the same molecular events at the cellular level are a prerequisite for tumorogenesis in them as in patients with a single-gene mutation causing retinoblastoma[36] (see Chapter 22). The natural history of retinoblastoma in patients with the chromosome deletion appears to be the same as for patients with monogenic causes of retinoblastoma.[36] Any infant or young child diagnosed to have this chromosome deletion during the evaluation of multiple anomalies or developmental delay merits close ophthalmologic monitoring during the first 6 to 9 years when the risk for tumor development is highest.

Surveys of children with retinoblastoma consistently reveal that only 2% to 3% have a chromosomal deletion.[36–39] Although most patients with retinoblastoma will not have a chromosome abnormality, high-resolution chromosome studies are warranted in retinoblastoma patients, especially those with no family history of retinoblastoma and those with developmental delay or other congenital anomalies. Occasionally familial retinoblastoma is caused by an inherited chromosomal rearrangement.[40] In the family with a 3;13 balanced translocation reported by Strong et al.,[41] numerous individuals in four generations had retinoblastoma as a result of inheriting the deleted chromosome 13. Although the majority of chromosome deletions causing retinoblastoma are de novo events, such families illustrate that inherited retinoblastoma can sometimes have a chromosomal basis.

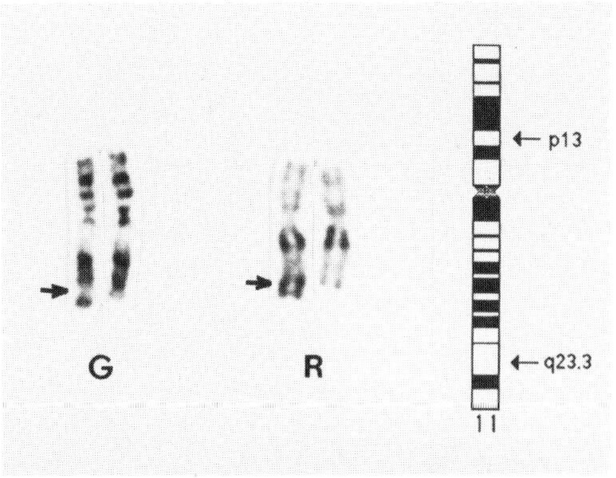

FIG 11–10.
A diagram of chromosome 11 is shown on the right. An arrow points to the critical region, bank p13, deleted in Wilms' tumor–aniridia. Also shown are examples of chromosome 11 from a patient (see Fig 11–12) with the following karyotype: 46,XX,del(11)(q23.3). The deleted chromosome 11 is at the right of each pair stained with G-banding (G) and R-banding (R). The site of the deletion is indicated with an arrow on the normal chromosomes.

Deletion 11p13

In 1964 Miller et al.[42] reported an increased incidence of aniridia in a survey of patients with Wilms' tumor. In 1966 DiGeorge and Harley[43] described three boys with aniridia, Wilms' tumor, undermasculinized genitalia, and mental retardation. This later became known as the aniridia–Wilms' tumor association or syndrome.[44]

In 1978 Riccardi et al.[45] identified an interstitial deletion of the short arm of chromosome 11 in three boys with aniridia, ambiguous genitalia, and mental retardation. One of the three had Wilms' tumor, which established this chromosome deletion as a cause of the aniridia–Wilms' tumor association. High-resolution studies identified band p13 as being deleted in all patients despite variation in total length of the deletion (Fig 11–10).

The phenotype of patients with this chromosome deletion is variable. In a review of 37 patients with this deletion, Turleau et al.[46] determined that all patients had aniridia and all had a severe form with nystagmus, cataracts, and/or glaucoma. Although the data were not complete, she and her colleagues concluded that Wilms' tumor was manifested in only about one third of patients with this chromosome deletion. It has been noted that Wilms' tumor tends to be diagnosed at an earlier age (2.8 years) in children with aniridia compared with those without aniridia (4.4 years).[47] Also there is a higher incidence of bilateral Wilms' tumor in patients with the chromosome deletion (36%) compared with those without the chromosome abnormality (2% to 4.5%).[47] Most males with this deletion have some genital anomalies: cryptorchidism, hypospadias, or ambiguity. Gonadoblastoma has been reported in patients with this deletion who have gonadal dysgenesis. Although present in all patients, mental retardation varied in severity. Turleau et al.[46] concluded that the deletion always includes at least the distal half of 11p13.

Patients with aniridia and severe mental retardation but not Wilms' tumor have been reported.[48] Patients with genital anomalies and Wilms' tumor but normal intelligence and normal eyes have been reported to have the same deletion.[49] Also, patients with aniridia (or iris dysplasia) and Wilms' tumor with no visible chromosome deletion have been reported.[50] It appears that deletion of 11p13 may include either the aniridia or Wilms' tumor locus or both and that submicroscopic deletions also occur.[46]

Attempts to map the gene for autosomal dominant aniridia suggest that two loci exist. Linkage studies have assigned one locus to 2p.[51] A family with dominantly inherited aniridia (without Wilms' tumor and with normal intelligence) and an apparently balanced chromosome translocation with break points at 11p13 supports the data from the 11p deletion patients that a second aniridia locus exists on 11p.[52]

Patients with sporadic aniridia warrant a high-resolution chromosome study to determine whether a deletion of 11p13 is present because of the high risk for both Wilms' tumor and other medical and developmental problems. Just as in other chromosome disorders, the finding of a deletion in the patient warrants karyotyping the parents for evidence of a balanced translocation or rearrangement.[53, 54]

Deletion 4p16 (Wolff-Hirshhorn Syndrome)

Patients with a terminal deletion of 4p have a phenotype characterized by low birth weight, microcephaly, ocular hypertelorism, high arching eyebrows that meet in the midline, short philtrum with beaking of the nose, large mouth with turned-down corners, preauricular pits or tags, and large and simply shaped ears (Fig 11–11,A). Most have hypotonia, severe to profound mental retardation, and seizures that commence after 2 years of age.[55–58]

Scalp defects, congenital heart defects, and cleft lip and/or cleft palate may be present. Hypospadias and cryptorchidism are common. Ocular abnormalies are coloboma (30%) and ectopic pupils, which occasionally are associated with Rieger's anomaly.[59]

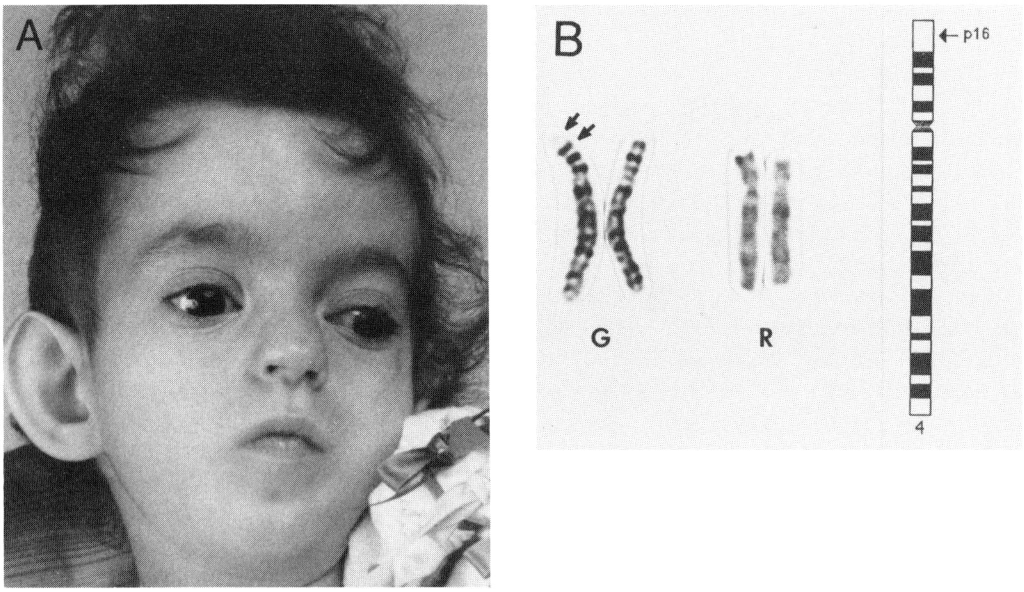

FIG 11–11.
A, 3½-year-old girl with Wolf-Hirshhorn syndrome. Note the ocular hypertelorism, down-slanting palpebral fissures, arching eyebrows, large and simply shaped ear, and broad nasal tip. The metaphase karyotype was normal, but clinical features suggested the diagnosis, and high-resolution studies revealed the expected deletion. **B,** examples of chromosome 4 from the patient in **A,** with the karyotype 46,XX,del(4)(p15.3p16.3). The deleted chromosome 4 is at the right of each pair stained with G-banding (G) and R-banding (R). The size of the deletion is indicated with arrows on the normal chromosome 4. A diagram of chromosome 4 is shown on the right. The arrow points to the critical band (4p16) that is deleted in Wolf-Hirschhorn syndrome.

Terminal deletion of band 4p16 accounts for the phenotype[59] (Fig 11–11,B). The deletion may not be evident on standard metaphase karyotypes, and small deletions are often detected only with high-resolution studies.[60] As in some of the other deletion syndromes discussed here, a high index of clinical suspicion is required before appropriately directed cytogenetic studies can be performed.

About 13% to 15% of patients have inherited deletions secondary to a parental translocation; the other 85% to 87% are de novo events.[57]

OTHER CHROMOSOME ABNORMALITIES

Trisomy 21/Down Syndrome

Trisomy 21 is the most common chromosome abnormality in humans and occurs on the average in 1 in 1,000 infants, with the incidence increasing with advancing maternal age. Children with Down syndrome have characteristic facies, hypotonia, multiple minor congenital anomalies, and a high incidence of congenital heart disease.[61] Characteristic ocular findings are bilateral epicanthal folds (57%), oblique and shortened palpebral fissures (97%), and Brushfield's spots (75%).[62] Epicanthal folds are secondary to a flat nasal bridge and tend to disappear with age. Brushfield's spots are whitish clumps on the surface of the iris just medial to the corneoscleral limbus and are not associated with other ophthalmologic findings.[63] The incidence of these findings varies from series to series, none are specific to Down syndrome, and all occur in individuals with normal chromosomes. Combined with other features, these findings contribute to the characteristic appearance of the face in trisomy 21.

Ophthalmologic disorders causing visual impairment in newborns with Down syndrome are rare. Although older children and adults with Down syndrome have a higher than average incidence of cataracts,[64] it has been debated whether there is an increased incidence of congenital cataracts in Down syndrome.[61] In a recent study of 114 children with Down syndrome, 2 had bilateral congenital cataracts,[62] which suggests that the incidence is increased although the actual risk to any given child is low. Since refractive errors (hyperopia more commonly than myopia) and strabismus (esotropia more commonly than exotropia) occur in 50% or more of Down syndrome patients, routine ophthalmologic examination in older infants and children with Down syndrome is warranted.[61, 65]

The significance of ophthalmologic findings such as an increased number of retinal vessels crossing the margin of the optic nerve,[66] generalized attenuation of fundus pigmentation, and patchy areas of pigment epithelial atrophy[67] is not known. Although common in young adults with Down syndrome, traumatic acute keratoconus and retinal detachment are rare in children. Blepharitis, an almost universal finding in patients with Down syndrome, has been attributed to dry skin, general susceptibility to infection, repeated eye rubbing, and careless hygiene.[65]

Turner Syndrome

Turner syndrome occurs in girls who have only one X chromosome (45,X); mosaicism for 45,X/46,XX; or one normal X chromosome with a structural abnormality of the other X chromosome (deletion of short arm, deletion of long arm, isochromosome, or ring chromosome).[68] About one third of girls with Turner syndrome are diagnosed in the newborn period during evaluation of pedal edema, neck webbing, coarctation of the aorta, or other characteristic features. About one third of patients are diagnosed during childhood for evaluation of short stature, and about one third are diagnosed at puberty during evaluation of amenorrhea.

Although primary ocular abnormalities are rare in this group, a high incidence of strabismus (about 33%), hypermetropia (17% to 40%), ptosis (15% to 30%), and amblyopia (up to 40%) have been reported in large series of patients of all ages when examined carefully.[69, 70] Interestingly, the incidence of red-

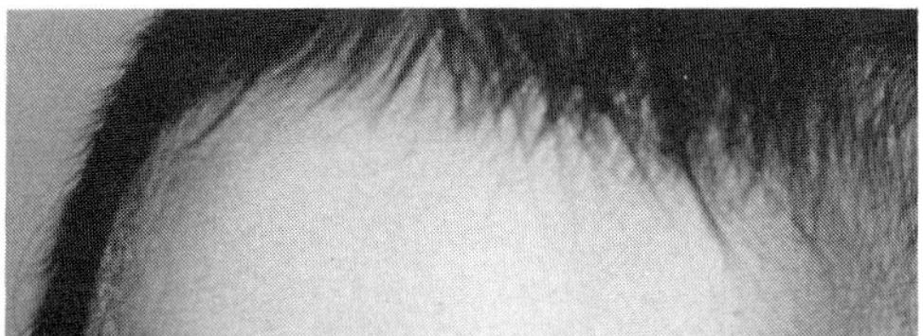

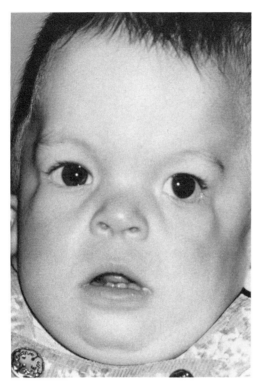

FIG 11–12.
An 8 month-old girl with deletion 11q (shown in Fig 11–10). Note the ocular hypertelorism, exotropia, and bitemporal depressions. The clinical features and ocular findings of this deletion, like many others not discussed in detail here, tend to be variable and nonspecific.

green color deficiency in girls with Turner syndrome (10%) is similar to the incidence in males (8%).[70] As with children with Down syndrome, ophthalmologic follow-up in these patients should be routine.

Deletion Syndromes

Among the well-known deletion syndromes not mentioned before, characteristic ocular abnormalities are not common. Although optic atrophy has been reported in cri du chat syndrome (5p−),[71,72] ptosis in 18p−,[73] nystagmus in 18q−,[73] and ocular hypertelorism in 11q− (Fig 11–12),[74,75] these ocular abnormalities either do not occur with high enough frequency or are not specific enough to suggest the diagnosis of these chromosomal syndromes. Patients with these syndromes tend to have characteristic facial features including variation in the slant of the palpebral fissures, spacing of the eyes, and the presence of ptosis, which allows a tentative clinical diagnosis of these disorders. However, the phenotype may not be as specific as in the disorders described under deletions, thus delaying a definitive diagnosis until obtaining a chromosome analysis.

Other Chromosomal Aberrations

Many children diagnosed to have a chromosome abnormality will not have a recognized clinical syndrome because of the unique nature of their chromosome duplication or deficiency: (1) the break points of many chromosomal duplications or deficiencies do not conform to those of well-described syndromes; (2) some children will have unbalanced translocations in which there is monosomy for a portion of one chromosome and trisomy for a portion of another. Under these circumstances the chromosome imbalance is likely to be unique to each individual since rearrangements with the same break points are unlikely to occur spontaneously in unrelated persons. Hence, many children evaluated for multiple congenital anomalies, growth retardation, or mental retardation have definable chromosome abnormalities but not a recognized clinical "syndrome." Clinicians may find information on other patients reported to have the same or a similar rare aberration in a catalogue[3] or atlas[4] of human chromosomal abnormalities.

CONCLUSION

In many patients with a chromosomal abnormality there is a recognized phenotype that constitutes a "syndrome"; in other patients the chromosome abnormality is unique or rare. Directed cytogenetic studies may be required when certain phenotypes are present; for example, high-resolution studies in patients with retinoblastoma, aniridia, deletion 4p16, and cat-eye syndrome and analysis of a second tissue in patients with triploidy. The detection of a chromosome abnormality in a child provides valuable information that can influence patient management and recurrence risk counseling.

REFERENCES

1. Tijo JH, Levan A: The chromosome number in man. *Hereditas* 1956; 42:1.
2. Therman E (ed): *Human Chromosomes*, ed 2. New York, Springer-Verlag NY, Inc, 1985.
3. Schnizel A: *Catalogue of Unbalanced Chromosome Aberrations in Man*. New York, Walter de Gruyter, 1984.
4. de Grouchy J, Turleau C: *Clinical Atlas of Human Chromosomes,* ed 2. New York, John Wiley & Sons, Inc, 1984.
5. Yunis JJ: *New Chromosomal Syndromes.* Orlando, Fla, Academic Press, Inc, 1977.
6. Gieser SC, Carey JC, Apple DJ: Human chromosomal disorders and the eye, in Renie WA (ed): *Goldberg's Genetic and Metabolic Eye Disease.* Boston, Little, Brown & Co, Inc, 1986, pp 185–240.
7. Harnden D, Klinger HP (eds): *Chromosome Nomenclature: International System for Human Cytogenetic Nomenclature.* New York, S Karger AG, 1985.
8. Taylor AI: Autosomal trisomy syndromes: A detailed study of 27 cases of Edward's syndrome and 27 cases of Patau's syndrome. *J Med Genet* 1968; 5:227.
9. Hodes ME, Cole J, Palmer CG, et al: Clinical experience with trisomies 18 and 13. *J Med Genet* 1978; 15:48.
10. Cogan DG: Ocular pathology of the 13–15 trisomy syndrome. *Arch Ophthalmol* 1964; 72:246.
11. Apple DJ, Holden JD, Stallworth B: Ocular pathology of Patau's syndrome with an unbalanced D/D translocation. *Am J Ophthalmol* 1970; 70:383.
12. Jay M, Jay B: Chromosome 13 and the eye. *Metabolic Ophthalmol* 1977; 1:177.
13. Pagon RA: Ocular coloboma. *Surv Ophthalmol* 1981; 25:223.
14. Cohen MM Jr: An update on the holoprosencephalic disorders. *J Pediatr* 1982; 101:865.
15. Howard RO: Chromosomal abnormalities associated with cyclopia and synophthalmia. *Trans Am Ophthalmol Soc* 1977; 75:505.
16. Hook EB: Unbalanced robertsonian translocations associated with Down's syndrome or Patau's syndrome: Chromosome subtype, proportion inherited, mutation rates and sex ratio. *Hum Genet* 1981; 59:235.
17. Carter PE, Pearn JH, Bell J, et al: Survival in trisomy 18. *Clin Genet* 1985; 27:59.
18. Ginsberg J, Bove K, Nelson R, et al: Ocular pathology of trisomy 18. *Ann Ophthalmol* 1971; 3:273.
19. Mullaney J: Ocular pathology in trisomy 18 (Edward's syndrome). *Am J Ophthalmol* 1973; 76:246.
20. Calerone JP, Chess J, Borodic G, et al: Intraocular pathology of trisomy 18 (Edward's syndrome): Report of a case and review of the literature. *Br J Ophthalmol* 1983; 67:162.
21. Pauli RM, Pagon RA, Hall JG: Trisomy 18 in siblings and maternal chromosome 9 variant. *Birth Defects* 1978; 14:297.
22. Uchida IA, Freeman VCP: Triploidy and chromosomes. *Am J Obstet Gynecol* 1985; 151:65.
23. Jenkins ME, Eisen J, Sequin F: Congenital asymmetry and diploid-triploid mosaicism. *Am J Dis Child* 1971; 122:80.
24. Graham JM Jr, Hoehn H, Lin MS, et al: Diploid-triploid mixoploidy: Clinical and cytogenetic aspects. *Pediatrics* 1981; 68:23.
25. Fulton AB, Howard RO, Albert DM, et al: Ocular findings in triploidy. *Am J Ophthalmol* 1977; 84:859.
26. Lambert JC, Philip P, Charpenter G, et al: Triploidy with cyclopia and identical HLA alleles in the parents. *J Med Genet* 1984; 21:63.
27. Wertelecki W, Graham JM, Sergovich FR: The clinical syndrome of triploidy. *Obstet Gynecol* 1976; 47:69.
28. Pagon RA, Hall JG, Davenport SLH, et al: Abnormal skin fibroblast cytogenetics in four dysmorphic patients with normal lymphocyte chromosomes. *Am J Hum Genet* 1979; 31:54.
29. Schachenmann G, Schmid W, Fraccaro M, et al: Chromosomes in coloboma and anal atresia. *Lancet* 1965; 2:290.
30. Schinzel A, Schmid W, Fraccaro M, et al: The "cat eye syndrome": Dicentric small marker chromosome probably derived from a no. 22 (tetrasomy 22 pter → q11). Report of 11 patients and delineation of the clinical picture associated with a characteristic phenotype. *Hum Genet* 1981; 57:148.
31. Duncan AMV, Hough CA, White BN, et al: Breakpoint localization of the marker chromosome associated with the cat eye syndrome. *Am J Hum Genet* 1986; 38:978.
32. McDermid HE, Duncan AMV, Brasch KR, et al: Characterization of the supernumerary

chromosome in cat eye syndrome. *Science* 1986; 232:646.
33. Reiss JA, Weleber RG, Brown MS, et al: Tandem duplication of proximal 22q: A cause of cat-eye syndrome. *Am J Med Genet* 1985; 20:165.
34. Lele KP, Penrose LA, Stallard HB: Chromosome deletion in a case of retinoblastoma. *Ann Hum Genet* 1963; 27:171.
35. Yunis JJ, Ramsay N: Retinoblastoma and subband deletion of chromosome 13. *Am J Dis Child* 1978; 132:161.
36. Knudson AG Jr, Meadows AT, Nichols WW, et al: Chromosomal deletion and retinoblastoma. *N Engl J Med* 1976; 295:1120.
37. Wilson MG, Ebbin AJ, Towner JW, et al: Chromosomal anomalies in patients with retinoblastoma. *Clin Genet* 1977; 12:1.
38. Vogel F: Genetics of retinoblastoma. *Hum Genet* 1979; 52:1.
39. Dryja TP, Bruns GAP, Gallie B, et al: Low incidence of deletion of the esterase D locus in retinoblastoma patients. *Hum Genet* 1983; 64:151.
40. Rivera H, Turleau C, de Grouchy J, et al: Retinoblastoma-del(13q14): Report of two patients, one with a trisomic sib due to maternal insertion. Gene-dosage effect for esterase D. *Hum Genet* 1981; 59:211.
41. Strong LC, Riccardi VM, Ferrell RE, et al: Familial retinoblastoma and chromosome 13 deletion transmitted via an insertional translocation. *Science* 1981; 213:1501.
42. Miller RW, Fraumeni JF, Manning MD: Association of Wilms' tumor and aniridia, hemihypertrophy and other congenital malformations. *N Engl J Med* 1964; 270:922.
43. DiGeorge AM, Harley RD: The association of aniridia, Wilms' tumor, and genital abnormalities. *Arch Ophthalmol* 1966; 75:796.
44. Fraumeni JF, Glass AG: Wilms' tumor and congenital aniridia. *JAMA* 1968; 206:825.
45. Riccardi VM, Sujansky E, Smith AC, et al: Chromosomal imbalance in the aniridia–Wilms' tumor association: 11p interstitial deletion. *Pediatrics* 1978; 61:604.
46. Turleau C, de Grouchy J, Tournade MF, et al: Del 11p/aniridia complex. Report of three patients and review of 37 observations from the literature. *Clin Genet* 1984; 26:356.
47. Shannon RS, Mann JR, Harper E, et al: Wilms' tumor and aniridia: Clinical and cytogenetic features. *Arch Dis Child* 1982; 57:685.
48. Godde-Salz E, Behnke H: Aniridia, mental retardation and an unbalanced reciprocal translocation of chromosomes 8 and 11 with an interstitial deletion of 11p. *Eur J Pediatr* 1981; 136:93.
49. Turleau C, de Grouchy J, Nihoul-Fekete C, et al: Del 11p13/nephroblastoma without aniridia. *Hum Genet* 1984; 67:455.
50. Riccardi VM, Hittner HM, Strong LC, et al: Wilms tumor with aniridia/iris dysplasia and apparently normal chromosomes. *J Pediatr* 1982; 100:574.
51. Nelson LB, Spaeth GL, Nowinski TS, et al: Aniridia. A review. *Surv Ophthalmol* 1984; 28:621.
52. Simola KOJ, Knuutila S, Kaitila I, et al: Familial aniridia and translocation t(4;11) (q22;p13) without Wilms' tumor. *Hum Genet* 1983; 63:158.
53. Yunis JJ, Ramsay NKC: Familial occurrence of the aniridia–Wilms' tumor syndrome with deletion 11p13-14.1. *J Pediatr* 1980; 96:1027.
54. Hittner HM, Riccardi VM, Francke U: Aniridia caused by a heritable chromosome 11 deletion. *Ophthalmology* 1979; 86:1173.
55. Wolf U, Porsch R, Baitsch H, et al: Deletion of short arms of a B chromosome without "cri du chat" syndrome. *Lancet* 1965; 1:769.
56. Johnson VP, Mulder RD, Hosen R: The Wolf-Hirschhorn (4p −) syndrome. *Clin Genet* 1976; 10:104.
57. Lurie IW, Lazjuk GI, Ussova YI, et al: The Wolf-Hirschhorn syndrome. I. Genetics. *Clin Genet* 1980; 17:375.
58. Wilson MG, Towner JW, Coffin GS, et al: Genetic and clinical studies in 13 patients with the Wolf-Hirschhorn syndrome. *Hum Genet* 1981; 59:297.
59. Wilcox LM, Bercovitch L, Howard RO: Ophthalmic features of chromosome deletion 4p − (Wolf-Hirschhorn syndrome). *Am J Ophthamol* 1978; 86:834.
60. Stengel-Rutkowski S, Warkotsch A, Schimanek P, et al: Familial Wolf's syndrome with a hidden 4p deletion by translocation of an 8p segment. Unbalanced inheritance from a maternal translocation (4;8) (p15.3;p22). Case report, review and risk estimates. *Clin Genet* 1984; 25:500.
61. Pueschel SM, Rynders JE (eds): *Down Syndrome: Advances in Biomedicine and the Behavioral Sciences.* Cambridge, Mass, Ware Press, 1982.
62. Peterson RA: Ocular manifestations, in Pueschel SM (ed): *A Study of the Young Child*

with Down Syndrome. New York, Human Science Press, 1983.
63. Donaldson DD: The significance of spotting of the iris in mongoloids. *Arch Ophthalmol* 1961; 4:26.
64. Robb RM, Marchevsky A: Pathology of the lens in Down's syndrome. *Arch Ophthalmol* 1978; 96:1039.
65. Journel H, Urvoy M, Baudet D, et al: Manifestations oculaires de la trisomie 21. *Ann Pediatr (Paris)* 1986; 33:387.
66. Williams EJ, McCormick AQ, Tischler B: Retinal vessels in Down's syndrome. *Arch Ophthalmol* 1973; 89:269.
67. Ahmad A, Pruett RC: The fundus in mongolism. *Arch Ophthalmol* 1976; 94:772.
68. Hall JG, Sybert VP, Williamson RA, et al: Turner's syndrome. *West J Med* 1982; 137:32.
69. Adhikary HP: Ocular manifestations of Turner's syndrome. *Trans Ophthal Soc UK* 1981; 101:395.
70. Chrousos GA, Ross JL, Chrousos G, et al: Ocular findings in Turner syndrome, a prospective study. *Ophthalmology* 1984; 91:926.
71. Howard RO: Ocular abnormalities in the cri du chat syndrome. *Am J Ophthalmol* 1972; 73:949.
72. Niebuhr E: The cri du chat syndrome. Epidemiology, cytogenetics, and clinical features. *Hum Genet* 1978; 44:227.
73. de Grouchy J: The 18p−, 18q− and 18r syndromes. *Birth Defects* 1969; 5:74.
74. Kaffe S, Hsu LVF, Sachdev RK, et al: Partial deletion of long arm of chromosome 11: del(11)(q23). *Clin Genet* 1977; 12:323.
75. Schinzel A, Auf der Maur P, Moser H: Partial deletion of long arm of chromosome 11 [del(11)(q23)]: Jacobsen syndrome. *J Med Genet* 1977; 14:438.

12 Craniofacial Syndromes and Malformations: Ophthalmic Manifestations*

Marilyn T. Miller, M.D.
Nancy A. Hamming, M.D.

During the past few decades there has been an explosion of interest in congenital anomalies, teratology, genetics, and syndromology. Advances in molecular genetics have identified the changes in DNA sequence responsible for certain genetic diseases. Well-controlled epidemiological studies have been used to implicate environmental agents that may be causative factors for certain malformations. Sophisticated prenatal evaluation allows early detection of a number of genetic and malformation syndromes. Major advances in craniofacial reconstructive surgery offer hope of significant rehabilitation for a previously neglected population—the dysmorphic child or adult. Parents demand information on prevention, early identification, and treatment of malformations from all causes. If a child is born with significant abnormalities, parents now seek risk counseling for future children and the next generation.

The purpose of this chapter is to provide guidelines that will help in the diagnosis and treatment of infants with multiple malformations and counseling of their families. To simplify the task, the major emphasis will be on associated malformations that affect the structures contiguous to the eye (the adnexa) and those of the craniofacial region, with some mention of central nervous system (CNS) anomalies that may be associated with these malformations.

EXAMINATION OF THE DYSMORPHIC CHILD

The Whole Child

No other examining skill is as important in the diagnosis and treatment of patients with craniofacial syndromes as is trained observation of the total patient. If the index of suspicion has not been aroused before retinoscopy and ophthalmoscopy are performed, the diagnosis will rarely be made. Does the child appear dysmorphic? If so, why? Body size and proportion, gait and posture, head size and shape, anomalies of scalp hair, ear position, and skeletal deformities may often be more revealing than a detailed ophthalmic examination. The pieces of the puzzle must be assembled before the final picture becomes obvious, and the ophthalmologist should have

*This study was supported in part by core grant EY1792 and training grant EY7038 from the National Eye Institute, Bethesda, Md.

the skills to identify many of these pieces. Completing the picture is frequently a joint venture requiring the efforts of many disciplines. Information supplied by general references provides a starting point in the literature review.[1-14]

Minor malformations such as flat philtrum, abnormal fissure slant, telecanthus, etc., are considered congenital anomalies that represent failures in normal development but result in no functional or severe cosmetic problems and usually require no specific treatment. Although it is not always easy at times to make the distinction, it is important to attempt to differentiate a minor malformation from a spectrum of normal findings. Even though malformations do occur in otherwise normal individuals and carry no specific threat, they do represent mistakes in normal development and are not normal variants. The presence of three "minor" anomalies markedly increases the chance of an associated major anomaly (one that requires specific treatment).[15]

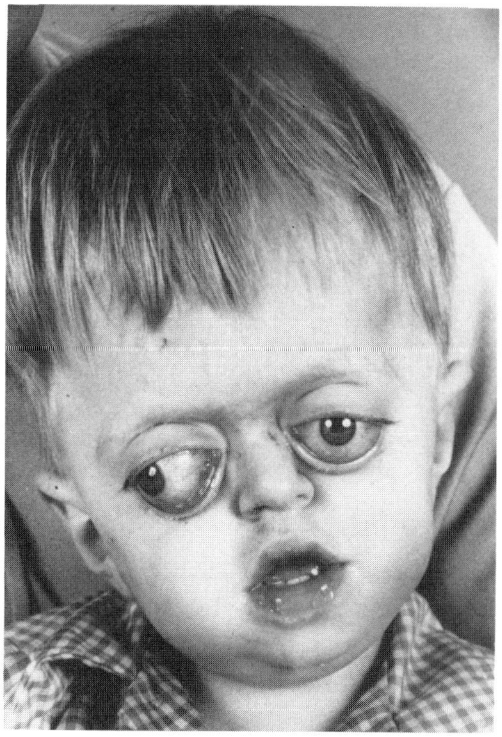

FIG 12–1.
Crouzon syndrome with proptosis and corneal exposure.

Ocular Examination

A routine ophthalmologic examination of the affected infant will reveal the majority of ocular abnormalities, but uncommon types of ocular pathological changes may exist in children with craniofacial syndromes requiring a more careful evaluation. Familiarity with the gestalt of a specific syndrome or common syndrome groups facilitates detection of these less obvious abnormalities. When taking the history, one should inquire about the possibility of prenatal infection, the exposure to teratogenic agents, and the presence of similar anomalies in other family members. Examination of as many family members as possible may be very informative.

ABNORMAL POSITION OF THE EYE AND/OR ORBIT

The general facial configuration and external structure of the orbit are inspected first. The orbital structures should be proportional and symmetrical. The lids are compared for symmetry, horizontal and vertical placement, and movement.

Proptosis

A marked prominence of one or both eyes (proptosis, exophthalmos) may result from retrobulbar masses such as hemangiomas, lymphangiomas, or rarely, a malignant rhabdomyosarcoma. More commonly, the prominent eye is secondary to a congenital shallow bony orbit as seen in the craniosynostosis syndromes. This type of proptosis is also referred to as exorbitism (Fig 12–1).

The diagnosis of proptosis may be confirmed if the examiner sights the infant's eyes and lids from above, over the prominence of the eyebrows. A more anterior protrusion of the orbital contents is observed when compared with the opposite side. The proptotic eye frequently has a widened palpebral fissure. A false diagnosis may occur when there is a slight enophthalmos of the other eye, which gives a normal eye a wider palpebral fissure. Marked enlargement of the eye, as occurs in congenital glaucoma or high myopia, often results in a more prominent eye.

Proptosis caused by anatomic factors in the craniosynostosis syndromes (Table 12–1) such as Crouzon and Apert syndromes differs from proptosis secondary to tumors and pseudotumors. In premature synostosis of the cranial and midfacial sutures, exorbitism results from a reduced volume of the bony orbital space due to numerous factors. Nevertheless, the ophthalmic complaints and derived complications that result from this abnormal position of the eye are similar in both those patients with a retrobulbar mass and those with abnormal bony orbits although the definitive treatment will be different. The severity of the exophthalmos in craniosynostosis patients is not uniform in all cases and frequently increases with age owing to the impaired growth of the bony orbit.

TABLE 12–1.
Craniosynostosis Syndromes

Craniosynostosis syndromes.—A large group of craniofacial syndromes characterized by premature closure of one or more cranial and, at times, facial sutures. This results in abnormal growth patterns and altered shape of the skull. Significant involvement of numerous sutures may lead to increased intracranial pressure.

Ophthalmic features.—Corneal pathological changes secondary to proptosis, papilledema and/or optic atrophy may occur when intracranial pressure is increased. Optic atrophy may also result from local involvement of the optic nerve. Less frequent anomalies include ptosis, cataract, retinal pigmentary changes, and keratoconus.

Etiology.—Isolated craniosynostosis may be caused by a variety of etiologic conditions, but the well-recognized syndromes (Apert, Crouzon, Pfeiffer, Saethre-Chotzen) mostly commonly show an autosomal dominant mode of inheritance (Carpenter syndrome is autosomal recessive).

Systemic features.—Abnormal-shaped skull, midface hypoplasia, oral and dental problems, syndactyly, and other anomalies of the hands and feet that are reported in many syndromes (e.g., Apert, Saethre-Chotzen, Pfeiffer). Mental retardation may occur as a primary finding or secondarily to increased intracranial pressure, but normal intellectual potential exists in many patients.

The most serious complications of severe proptosis are caused by corneal exposure. The lids may not afford adequate protection for the globe, thereby exposing the cornea and causing punctate keratitis (see Fig 12–1). If inadequately managed, perforation of the globe and irreversible damage to the eye may occur and result in serious loss of vision. The progression of exorbitism caused by craniosynostosis syndromes may be slow, thus permitting a response to conservative treatment such as lubricating ointment. But if the exorbitism is severe or rapidly progressive, an emergency tarsorrhaphy may be indicated, although this is not a definitive procedure because the underlying cause (i.e., shallow orbit) has not been removed. Rarely, the eye may be completely dislocated because of the extremely shallow orbit. This constitutes a medical emergency because of the problems of corneal exposure and possible compromise of the blood supply to the eye. The eye may be retroplaced by gently bringing the upper lid over the globe with one's finger.

Although proptosis from tumors is not commonly seen in infancy, it does occur and must be accurately diagnosed before therapy can be undertaken. Orbital tumors may develop from both ectodermal and mesodermal tissues or may be secondary to metastasis from other areas of the body. Dermoid cysts are thought to arise from a congenital nest of primitive ectoderm at the site of a fetal cleft closure. They usually contain connective tissue, sebaceous glands, and hair follicles. Cysts are often located near the orbital rim where they are attached to bone at suture sites. Those located within the orbit produce proptosis and, frequently, vertical or horizontal displacement of the globe. Roentgenographic examination may demonstrate bony erosion in the area where the cyst is attached. Surgical excision is recommended but is often difficult when the dermoid cyst extends through bone into surrounding structures.

Rhabdomyosarcoma is the most common

malignant tumor of the orbit in children. Although the average age of presentation is 6 to 10 years, it may occur in the neonatal period and mimic a congenital anomaly. Rhabdomyosarcoma develops in the orbit more frequently than elsewhere in the body. It produces proptosis with vertical or horizontal displacement, frequently with a palpable mass in the lid or the brow. Diagnosis is made by biopsy. Although surgical exenteration has been used in the past, the present treatment of choice is irradiation and chemotherapy.

Trauma such as that occurring at birth may produce a retrobulbar hemorrhage with proptosis, which must be differentiated from a tumor.

The rare neonatal sequelae of hyperthyroidism occur as the result of maternal Graves' disease during the last trimester of pregnancy. The infant is born with classic hyperthyroidism, including exophthalmos, upper lid retraction, and extraocular muscle involvement.

Abnormal orbits may result in disturbances in ocular movement and, at times, amblyopia. This will necessitate appropriate treatment if good vision is to be preserved.

Hypertelorism

Ocular hypertelorism is a term indicating increased separation between the bony orbits. It is an anatomic description rather than a diagnostic entity. Mild to moderate hypertelorism is found in many syndromes and may be the result of morphokinetic arrest during embryogenesis because the ocular structures in the fetus are normally widely spread.

Moderate hypertelorism is a characteristic of many craniosynostosis syndromes and other craniofacial syndromes (e.g., cerebrohepatorenal syndrome, Smith-Lemli-Opitz syndrome; (Table 12–2). Numerous reports of chromosomal anomalies (e.g., 4p-, 5p-, 21q-, etc.) have described patients with hypertelorism. Very large distances between the orbits are uniformly present in the relatively common condition of median facial clefting syndromes (frontonasal dysplasia).

TABLE 12–2.
Hypertelorism Examples

Smith-Lemli-Opitz syndrome
- Ophthalmic features.—Epicanthus, ptosis, strabismus, occasional cataracts, hypertelorism, optic pallor, small fissures with antimongoloid obliquity, nystagmus, iris deformities, retinal pigment defects, various low-incidence anomalies
- Etiology.—Autosomal recessive
- Systemic features.—Broad nasal tip with anteverted nostrils, low-set ears, micrognathia, genital defects, anomalies of toes

Median facial clefting syndrome (frontonasal dysplasia)
- Ophthalmic features.—Exotropia, lacrimal system anomalies; less frequent anomalies include Duane's syndrome and epibulbar dermoids
- Etiology.—Usually sporadic
- Systemic features.—Increased separation between bony orbits; median cleft nose, lip, and premaxilla; cranium bifidum; widow's peak; mental retardation in some individuals

Hypotelorism

Decreased separation of the orbits (hypotelorism) is frequently associated with severe malformations of the brain such as holoprosencephaly (Fig 12–2). Certain craniofacial and chromosomal (e.g., trisomy 13) syndromes also demonstrate hypotelorism. Patients with severe hypotelorism are usually mentally retarded.

PALPEBRAL FISSURES AND LIDS

Palpebral fissure should be examined for size, shape, slant, and intercanthal distances (Table 12–3). Downward or upward slanting of the fissures are found in many syndromes and are also considered a minor anomaly if they vary from the typical fissure shape in the patient's racial group (Fig 12–3). In mandibulofacial dysostosis (Treacher Collins syndrome), the downward slant is the characteristic position of the fissures, although the frequently present lower lid colobomas may give a false impression of a slant.

The lid fissures of the full-term infant are usually quite narrow, often being widely separated horizontally by prominent epicanthal folds. The term *telecanthus* indicates a disproportionate increase in distance between the medial canthi. It may occur secondarily to an increased distance between the bony orbits (hypertelorism) or as a primary soft-tissue anomaly (primary telecanthus). Telecanthus is particularly noticeable in infants with fetal alcohol[16] and Waardenburg syndromes but is present in a number of other syndromes (Fig 12–4). Measurements between the two medial canthi in infants may vary from 18 to 22 mm. Horizontal measurements of the lid fissures usually range between 17 and 27 mm. These measurements should be symmetrical but will be different in conditions producing orbital asymmetry. An example is plagiocephaly, which is characterized by asymmetrical or unilateral involvement of the sutures.

Epicanthus is the most frequently encountered lid abnormality. A skin fold originating in the upper lid extends over the medial end of the upper lid, the medial canthus, and the caruncle and ends in the skin of the lower lid. It occurs in many normal infants and grad-

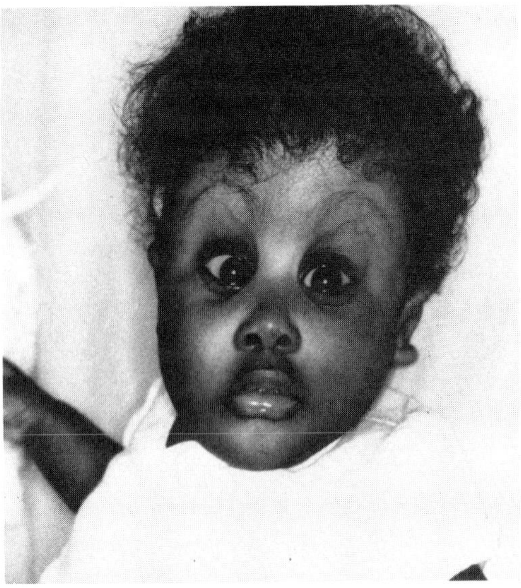

FIG 12–2.
Hypotelorism in dysmorphic child. Computed tomography (CT) of the skull showed major malformations of the brain.

TABLE 12–3.
Examples of Palpebral Fissure Abnormalities

Mandibulofacial dysostosis (MFD, Treacher Collins, Franceschetti-Zwahlen-Klein)
- Ophthalmic features.—Coloboma or notching of the outer part of lower lid, downward slant of the palpebral fissures, missing eyelashes, nasal-to-lid coloboma, astigmatism, strabismus, variety of low-incidence anomalies
- Etiology.—Autosomal dominant with wide expressivity
- Systemic features.—Lack of development of the malar bone and mandible, large mouth, malformations of external and middle ear, atypical hairline, blind fistula between the ears and angles of the mouth

Fetal alcohol syndrome (FAS)
- Ophthalmic features.—Telecanthus, small palpebral fissures, ptosis, strabismus, epicanthal folds, optic nerve hypoplasia, tortuous retinal vessels; less frequent anomalies include anterior segment anomalies, high refractive error, cataract
- Etiology.—Alcohol acting as a teratogen
- Systemic features.—Growth deficiency, mental retardation, flat philtrum, characteristic facial features, cardiac and pulmonary findings

Waardenburg syndrome
- Ophthalmic features.—Primary telecanthus, occasional hypertelorism, lateral displacement of inferior puncta, hypoplasia of iris pigment resulting in heterochromia; less frequent findings include pigmentary changes in retina, dacryocystitis, cataracts, ptosis, high refractive errors, microphthalmos
- Etiology.—Autosomal dominant with wide expressivity
- Systemic features.—White forelock, sensorineural deafness, occasional cleft palate and lips, skeletal anomalies

Neurofibromatosis (von Recklinghausen's disease)
- Ophthalmic features. — Gliomas of optic nerves, lid neurofibromas, orbital tumors
- Etiology.—Autosomal dominant
- Systemic features. — Café au lait spots, multiple tumors of skin and central nervous system

de Lange syndrome (Cornelia de Lange's Brachmann–de Lange syndromes)
- Ophthalmic features.—Confluent eyebrows, long curly eyelashes, occasionally high myopia, optic atrophy, telecanthus
- Etiology.—Mostly sporadic, few chromosomal abnormalities
- Systemic features.—Low birth weight, severe mental retardation, brachycephalic skull, hirsutism of forehead, low-set ears, hypoplastic mandible, small mouth with angles turned down (fish mouth), hand and foot anomalies with thumbs proximately placed, feeble low-pitched cry

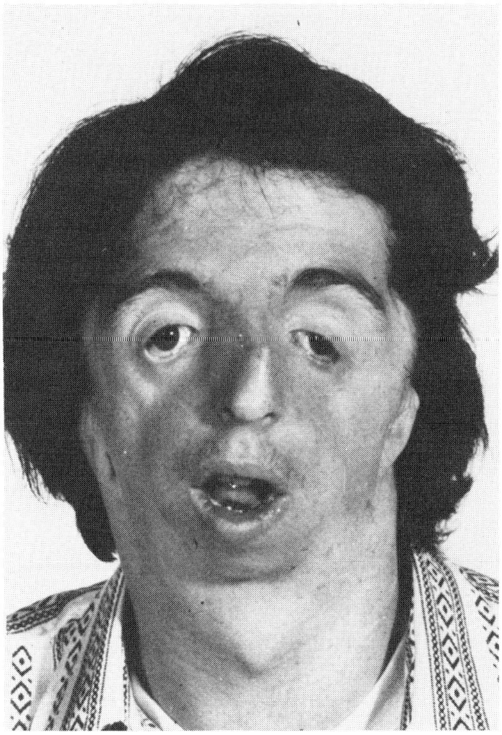

FIG 12–3.
Mandibular facial dysostosis (Treacher Collins syndrome) showing a downward slant of the palpebral fissures and a mild coloboma of the lower lid.

ually disappears as the growth of the bridge of the nose obliterates the excess skin in this area. It is a characteristic finding of certain racial groups. Epicanthus is considered a minor anomaly and reported to occur in many syndromes. Epicanthus inversus is similar except that the predominance of the skin fold arises in the lower lid and runs diagonally upward toward the root of the nose to overlie the medial canthus.

Blepharophimosis describes palpebral fissures that are too narrow horizontally and vertically. There is usually an associated ptosis and frequently strabismus. Lid fissure measurements commonly are reduced to approximately two thirds of normal, whereas the space between the medial canthi is considerably widened (telecanthus). Although it may occur in some craniofacial syndromes, familial blepharophimosis may exist without other anomalies and usually demonstrates an autosomal dominant mode of transmission. Surgical repair improves the appearance but is usually deferred until the child is older.

Inability to elevate the eyelid (ptosis) may occur from edema of the lid, as a component of neurological diseases (e.g., myasthenia gravis, third-nerve palsy), or as a congenital and isolated finding. It may also be secondary to a hemangioma or neurofibroma involving the lid and may be a characteristic of some craniofacial syndromes (e.g., Saethre-Chotzen).

Colobomas or defects in the lid may be complete and involve all layers of the lid; less commonly, an absence of part of the lid is seen. The defects may be so minimal that only a small notch in the lid margin is observable with a decrease in the number of cilia in that area. Possible complications from the coloboma include corneal exposure, corneal ulcer, abnormal tear drainage, and refractive error.

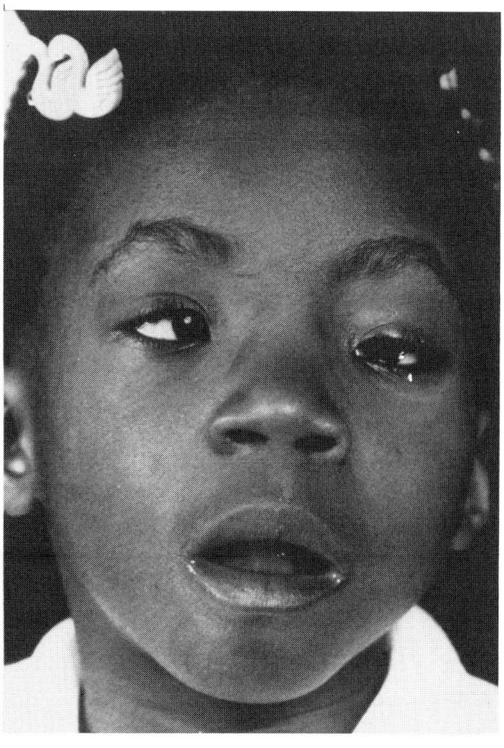

FIG 12–4.
Typical facies of child with fetal alcohol syndrome with telecanthus, asymmetrical ptosis, anteverted nostrils, and flat philtrum.

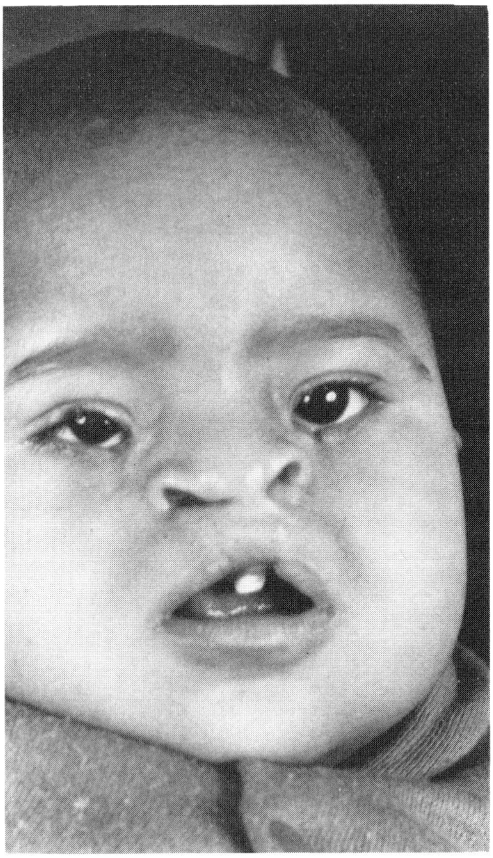

FIG 12–5.
Amniotic band syndrome. The child has colobomas of the upper and lower lids in the right eye and lower lid in the left eye where the amniotic bands were present during embryogenesis. There is also a repaired cleft lip and palate.

In addition to mandibulofacial dysostosis with its characteristic bilateral lower lid coloboma, lid colobomas are observed in Goldenhar syndrome (upper lid), in amniotic bands (Fig 12–5), and as isolated findings.

Treatment of the more severe defects includes primary closure, usually after reconstruction of the underlying bony defect has been undertaken. Reconstruction of the lid is desirable for cosmetic reasons and also to eliminate exposure keratitis.

Eyebrows/Eyelashes

The eyebrows may show disruption in the facial clefting syndrome (Fig 12–6). Confluent eyebrows (synophrys) and long eyelashes are characteristic of de Lange syndrome.

STRABISMUS

A high incidence of strabismus is found in many syndromes of various etiologies.[17] In a few conditions the motility disturbance is a necessary component for diagnosis (e.g., the lateral rectus palsy in Möbius syndrome), but in most syndromes strabismus is reported as a "frequent finding," and little detail is given to its characteristics. Strabismus present in patients with craniofacial anomalies can be considered to occur in three groups.

Association With Poor Visual Acuity

Because ocular motility disturbances frequently occur secondarily to poor visual acuity in one or both eyes, it is not surprising that a number of patients with craniofacial anomalies demonstrate ocular misalignment attributable to the presence of ocular disease. For example, patients with the craniofacial synostosis (Apert and Crouzon) syndromes have an increased incidence of optic atrophy that may contribute to strabismus. Poor vision sec-

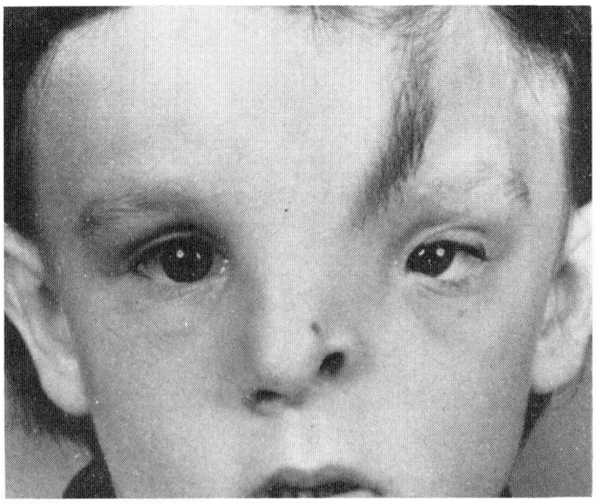

FIG 12–6.
Facial cleft resulting in disruption of the left eyebrow. There has been a repaired upper lid coloboma and a significant astigmatic correction on the left side only.

ondary to ocular dermoids, microphthalmos, anisometropia (difference in refraction between the two eyes), and numerous other types of eye abnormalities associated with many craniofacial syndromes may be the precipitating factor for the occurrence of strabismus.

The disturbed bony orbit and frequent asymmetry of ophthalmic pathology and refraction are causative factors for strabismus or anisometropic amblyopia. When the amblyopia is superimposed on organic defects, the evaluation of potential vision and treatment effectiveness is difficult, especially in a young child.

Characteristic Patterns of Strabismus

Patients with craniosynostosis may demonstrate a variety of horizontal deviations in the primary position, although exotropia is the more frequent. The most consistent finding, however, is a marked V pattern, most frequently with an exotropia on upgaze and a small exotropia, orthotropia, or esotropia on downgaze. Often this is accompanied by a marked overaction of the inferior oblique muscles. In some patients there is a definite limitation of movement seen when testing ocular movements in various fields of action, especially that of the superior rectus muscle. In a number of patients ocular muscles have been noted to be abnormally inserted or unusually small on CT scan or at the time of surgery. (Another unusual motility disturbance in addition to the lateral rectus palsy with Möbius syndrome is Duane syndrome, reported frequently in association with craniofacial malformations particularly ear and vertebral anomalies [e.g., Goldenhar].) In the most common type of Duane syndrome, an apparent lateral rectus palsy is associated with a narrowing of the palpebral fissure of the affected eye on attempted adduction (Fig 12–7).

Nonspecific Ocular Deviation

Many syndromes of congenital anomalies are associated with an increased incidence of strabismus, but the type of deviation may not appear to be in any way characteristic of the syndrome or secondary to any obvious abnormality. More complete motility evaluation, however, may indicate that patients with "nonspecific" ocular deviation actually demonstrate a "specific" deviation that is related to the particular craniofacial malformation.

REFRACTION

Unusual and asymmetrical refractions are very common findings associated with craniofacial anomalies. These refractive errors merit close attention not only to have such children reach their full visual potential but also to treat any amblyopia that might go otherwise unnoticed. At times the refractive errors are due to anomalies in soft tissue around the bony orbit such as colobomas, dermoids, and ptosis, and at other times they appear intrinsic but associated with the syndrome itself. Examples of the latter include the high myopia and retinal problems in Stickler syndrome and also the high myopia associated with fetal alcohol syndrome. Correction of these refractive errors is based on the usually accepted principle, but additional problems occur in these children because they may have abnormal to malplaced ears or nose. Patient assistance from the optician may be necessary to overcome these facial malformations.

INTRINSIC OCULAR MALFORMATIONS

Anophthalmia/Microphthalmos

Anophthalmia is a rare phenomenon in which there is a total absence or a rudiment of the globe, and it usually occurs bilaterally. This can result from a developmental failure of the optic vesicle and is often accompanied by other congenital anomalies such as CNS defects and mental retardation. It has been observed in a number of chromosomal syndromes (e.g., trisomy 13). Since lid formation is not dependent on ocular formation, the lids are present with lashes and lacrimal puncta

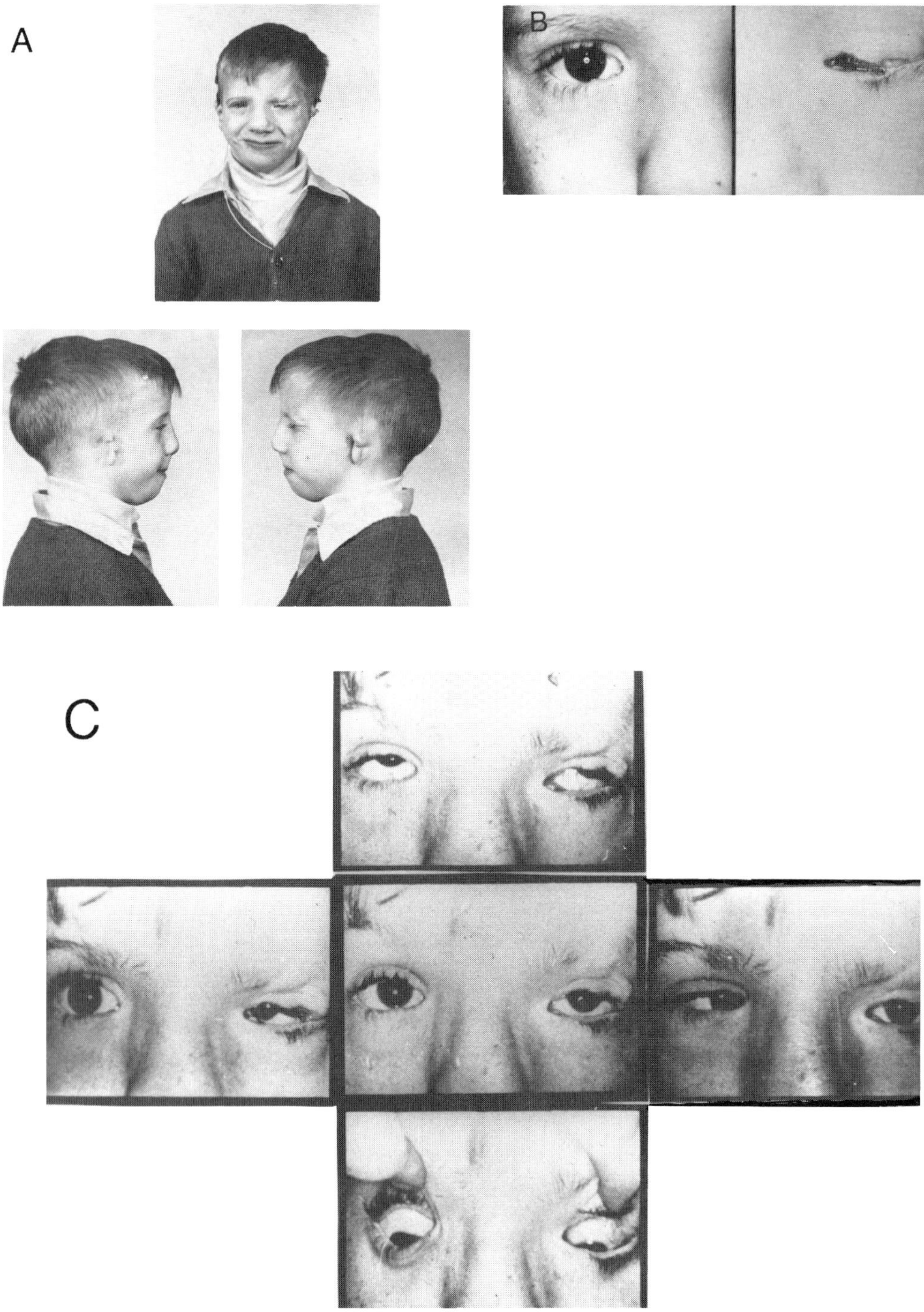

FIG 12–7.
Hemifacial microsomia (Goldenhar variant). **A,** the patient has bilateral ear anomalies with asymmetric facial involvement. **B,** a small lipodermoid is noted at the medial canthal area in the right eye. The left eye shows a lid coloboma. Also present were lipodermoids in that eye. **C,** bilateral Duane syndrome characterized by limitation of abduction and narrowing of the fissure on adduction.

even though the globe may be absent. However, the lids remain closed or may be partially fused and will be sunken without the support of the eye. The lacrimal gland is present and is capable of producing tears. Anophthalmia can occur sporadically, but some cases of familial incidence with varied types of inheritance have been described. Treatment is for the cosmetic deformity.

In an unusual syndrome, cryptophthalmos, the eyelids fail to form their normal cleavage, and uninterrupted skin runs from the forehead to the malar area. The eyelids and eyelashes usually are absent; however, the eye can be palpated beneath the skin and may even be observed to move with the stimulation of a strong light. The anterior segment of the eye is invariably disorganized into fibrovascular tissue adherent to the subcuticular tissue of the lids. The conjunctival sac is absent. Therefore, attempts to separate the lids from the ocular structures are usually unsuccessful, and surgical correction is not advisable in most circumstances. Cryptophthalmos is frequently associated with systemic anomalies (particularly genitourinary) and may show an autosomal recessive mode of inheritance.

Microphthalmos describes a variety of conditions in which the diameter of the neonatal eye is less than two thirds of the normal 16 mm. It is usually associated with hypermetropia, hypoplasia of the macula, and the late occurrence of glaucoma. It has been reported in both recessive and dominant transmission.

Colobomatous microphthalmos occurs when the embryonic cleft of the optic vesicle fails to close. These colobomas typically involve the iris, ciliary body, choroid, or optic nerve and may be transmitted as an autosomal dominant or X-linked trait.

Microphthalmos may also be associated with other ocular and systemic syndromes including intrauterine infections such as rubella and cytomegalovirus, craniofacial anomalies, anterior chamber developmental anomalies, and chromosomal abnormalities, particularly trisomy 13 (Fig 12–8).

Corneal Pathology

Primary corneal involvement in the form of a limbal dermoid is a characteristic finding in Goldenhar syndrome. The dermoids are usually located in the inferotemporal quadrant and occur bilaterally in about 25% of the patients. They occasionally impinge on the visual axis but more commonly interfere with visual acuity by causing astigmatism and predisposing to strabismic and anisometropic amblyopia.

Lipodermoids are also seen in Goldenhar

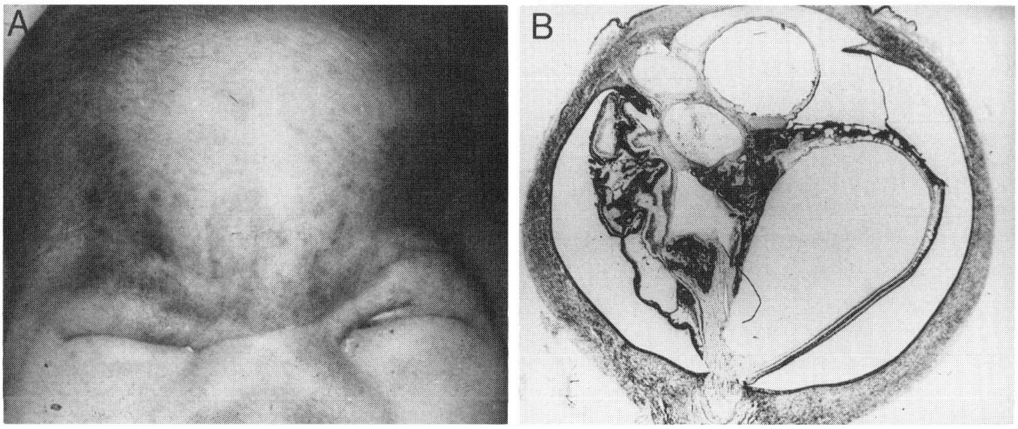

FIG 12–8.
Trisomy 13 showing **(A)** small palpebral fissures, frontal bossing, bilateral microphthalmia; and **(B)** disorganized globes that included retinal dysplasia and cartilage formation.

TABLE 12–4.
Hemifacial Microsomia

Hemifacial microsomia (hemifacial hypoplasia, oculoauricular vertebral, first and second arch syndromes).

Ophthalmic features.—Epibulbar dermoids and lipodermoids, microphthalmos, decreased corneal sensation, anophthalmia, Duane retraction syndrome, upper lid colobomas, cataract, iris anomalies and other low-incidence anomalies.

Etiology.—Occurs sporadically.

Systemic features.—Vertebral anomalies, external- and inner-ear anomalies, branchial pits, mandibular ramus and condyle, macrostomia, involvement of facial nerve muscles and muscle or mastication, and absence of parotid duct. The condition is unilateral in approximately 70% to 80% of the patients.

syndrome, most commonly located some distance from the limbus in the temporal quadrants. Upper lid colobomas are noted in about 25% of the patients but rarely are bilateral and occur on the affected side. The most frequent eye anomalies are microphthalmos, Duane retraction syndrome, changes in corneal sensation, iris anomalies, and occasionally anophthalmia (see Fig 12–7). This condition is unilateral but not invariable in most cases and is often associated with vertebral anomalies and ear and other facial anomalies. Gorlin et al.[10] feel that this is a variant of a larger group of patients that they refer to as hemifacial microsomia (Table 12–4).

In the Riley-Day syndrome (familial dysautonomia), decreased tearing and corneal sensation result in keratitis and often ulceration. Associated findings in this autosomal recessive condition include vasomotor instability, relative indifference to pain, fixed facial expression with characteristic slitlike mouth, skin blotching, and difficulty in swallowing.

Iris

Colobomas of the iris and/or retina may be present in a wide array of syndromes involving craniofacial structures, including mesenchymal dysgenesis (anterior chamber developmental anomalies), chromosomal, first and second branchial arch, Lenz microphthalmos, Waardenburg, Aicardi, and a few oculodermal syndromes.[15] Since the embryonic fissure closes 33 to 40 days postconception, any insult to the embryo during that time or before could be associated with these colobomas. A wide variety of craniofacial malformations and syndromes have been reported with colobomas (Fig 12–9).

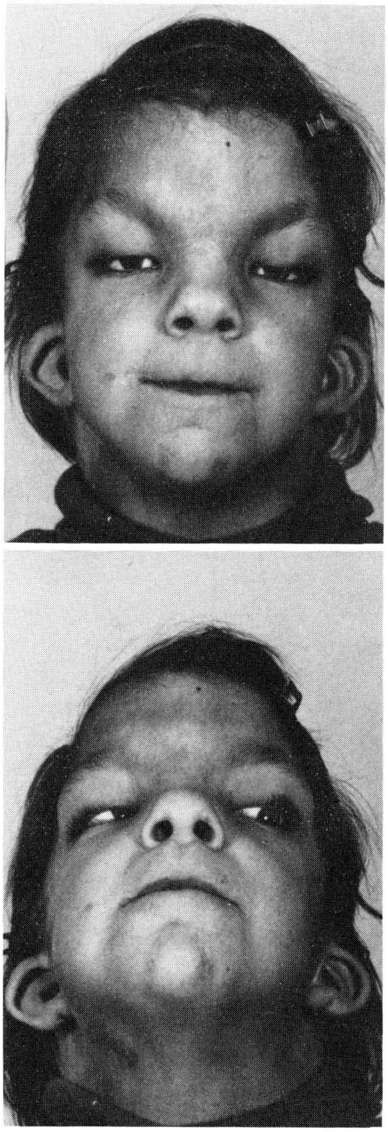

FIG 12–9.
Dysmorphic child with low-set ears, bilateral ptosis, and iris and retina l colobomas. The diagnosis is not established after extensive evaluation. She also had a high astigmatic correction.

Glaucoma

Congenital glaucoma has also been noted in many conditions involving the craniofacial structures (Hallermann-Streiff Stickler, Lowe oculodentodigital, Sturge-Weber, Pierre Robin, Rieger, Turner and Down syndromes; trisomy 13 and 18; rubella; and others as noted in Table 12–5).

Secondary glaucoma can occur in syndromes associated with dislocated or abnormal lenses (Marfan syndrome, homocystinuria, Weill-Marchesani syndrome).

Congenital Cataract

The list of craniofacial syndromes with case reports of cataracts is probably considerably longer than the list of syndromes in which they have never been reported.[19] Most are low-incidence anomalies, but cataracts are frequently found in Hallermann-Streiff syndrome (Fig 12–10), Lowe syndrome, and a number of dermatologic disorders with some craniofacial characteristics (e.g., Cockayne syndrome, Rothmund-Thomson syndrome, Marshall-type ectodermal dysplasia, incontientia pigmenti). In Conradi syndrome, congenital cataract occurs along with changes in the bones including hypoplasia of the malar bone, punctate calcification in vertebral column epiphyses, and saddlenose. Cataracts may occur as an isolated finding with variable types of mendelian inheritance. Cataracts that are frequently associated with deficiencies of enzymes in galactosemia (galactose-1-phosphate uridyl transferase or galactokinase) show an autosomal recessive form of transmission. Electrolytes and amino acid disturbances may occasionally cause cataract formation.

TABLE 12–5.
Some Craniofacial Syndromes Involving Glaucoma

Hallermann-Streiff syndrome (oculomandibulodyscephaly
Ophthalmic features.—Microphthalmos congenital cataracts, spontaneous absorption of lens, microcornea, glaucoma; less frequently blue sclera, uveal coloboma, iridocyclitis, nystagmus, and many low-incidence anomalies
Etiology.—Occurs sporadically
Systemic features.—Dwarfism, mandibular hypoplasia, dyscephaly, beaked nose, hypotrichosis
Lowe's syndrome (oculocerebrorenal syndrome)
Ophthalmic features.—Congenital cataract and glaucoma, malformations of anterior chamber angle and iris, corneal clouding, nystagmus; punctate cataracts in carriers
Systemic features.—Renal aminoaciduria, skeletal anomalies, growth retardation
Etiology.—X-linked recessive
Marshall's syndrome
Ophthalmic features.—Congenital cataract (may spontaneously resorb), myopia, retinal detachment
Systemic features.—Saddle nose, sensorineural deafness, hypoplastic midface, hypohidrosis
Etiology.—Autosomal dominant
Sturge-Weber syndrome
Ophthalmic features.—Glaucoma, choroidal angiomas, angiomas of conjunctiva; less frequently heterochromia of iris, dislocation of lens, etc.
Etiology.—Occurs sporadically
Systemic features.—Cutaneous angiomatosis of the face and ipsilateral leptomeningeal angiomatosis frequently causing seizures, mental retardation, hemiplegia.
Rieger's syndrome (oligodontia and primary mesodermal dysgenesis of the iris)
Ophthalmic features.—Iris adhesions to the posterior surface of cornea; other iris, anterior chamber angle, and corneal defects; primary or secondary telecanthus; strabismus; glaucoma
Systemic features.—Brachycephaly, prognathism, defective dentition, wide spectrum of incidental anomalies
Etiology.—Autosomal dominant, often
Weill-Marchesani syndrome (Marchesani's syndrome)
Ophthalmic features.—Spherophakia; other lens pathology, high refractive error, occasional other types of ocular pathology
Systemic features.—Brachydactyly, small stature, broad skull, dental anomalies
Etiology.—Autosomal dominant or recessive

Sclera

The normal full-term neonate has a glistening white sclera. The overlying conjuctiva and conjunctival vessels superimpose a filmy vascular pattern. A generalized bluish discoloration of the underdeveloped sclera is normal in premature infants. The light blue color is caused by thinness of the sclera, which transmits the darker color of the underlying uveal tissue. Osteogenesis imperfecta may be associated with a similar bluish discoloration of the sclera in the full-term neonate because of inadequately developed scleral collagen. Blue scleras may also be seen in other systemic diseases such as Marfan's syndrome, Ehlers-Danlos syndrome, and Crouzon syndrome.

Retina

Vision may also be impaired by numerous types of retinopathy. For example, pigmentary retinal changes occur in the syndromes of Cockayne, rubella, Stickler, Werner, and Laurence-Moon-Biedl and also in some mucopolysaccharidoses (Table 12–6).

Retinal dysplasia is usually bilateral and associated with microphthalmic eyes. It may occur as part of a group of congenital anomalies, including defects of the CNS, cardiovascular system, and skeletal system of sufficient severity to produce early death of the infant. Trisomy 13 should be ruled out (see Fig 12–8,B). When the dysplasia is advanced, a white retrolental mass may be produced.

A coloboma of the fundus is visible as a defect in the retinal and choroidal layers through which the underlying sclera is visible. A coloboma usually occurs inferonasally, which is the site of the closure of the embryonic fissure. The fissure usually begins to close around the equator and then extends posteriorly toward the optic disc and anteriorly toward the periphery. Any part or all of this region may be involved in the colobomatous defect. The associated craniofacial malformations that have been observed are discussed under iris colobomas.

Optic Nerve

Hypoplasia of the optic disc is a rare anomaly in which part or all of the optic nerve fibers fail to develop and reach the disc. The optic disc is smaller than normal and may be pale, but the retinal vessels usually are normal. A hypopigmented ring around the hypoplastic nerve creates the so-called double-ring sign. This may occur unilaterally or bilaterally. Visual impairment may range from mild to severe.

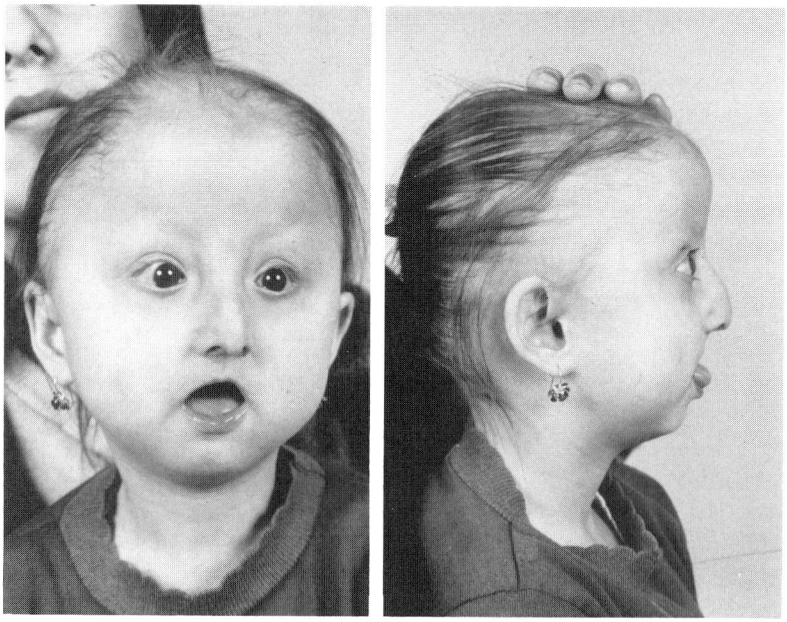

FIG 12–10.
Hallermann-Streiff syndrome. The child had a congenital cataract noted in one eye and no evidence of a lens in the other eye, presumably due to spontaneous absorption. Note the hypotrichosis, mandibular hypoplasia, beaked nose, and endocephaly.

TABLE 12–6.
Examples of Craniofacial Syndromes Involving the Retina

Cockayne syndrome
Ophthalmic features.—Exophthalmos, retinal pigmentary degeneration with optic atrophy, cataract, poor pupillary dilation
Systemic features.—Cachexia, dwarfism, sensorineural deafness, photosensitivity, premature aging, intracranial calcification, progressive neurological signs, mental retardation
Etiology.—Autosomal recessive
Laurence-Moon-Biedl syndrome
Ophthalmic features.—Retinitis pigmentosa, ptosis, nystagmus, epicanthus, strabismus, refractive errors, iris coloboma, occasional optic atrophy
Systemic features.—Obesity, polydactyly, syndactyly, genital hypoplasia, mental retardation
Etiology.—Autosomal recessive

Optic nerve hypoplasia may occur as an isolated finding or in association with other ocular or systemic abnormalities.[20] CT of the brain may also reveal midline abnormalities, a disorder referred to as septo-optic dysplasia (DeMorsier syndrome). Endocrine abnormalities are frequently found in this syndrome. Optic nerve hypoplasia has been reported in a large number of children with fetal alcohol syndrome.

Optic atrophy occurs in a number of craniofacial syndromes, especially those in the craniosynostosis group. If there is enough premature closure of cranial sutures to increase intracranial pressure, papilledema and optic atrophy may result. Local optic nerve damage secondary to changes in the bony anatomy of the optic canal may result in impingement on the nerve and optic atrophy.

OCULAR ANOMALIES ASSOCIATED WITH SKULL AND BRAIN MALFORMATIONS

The Misshapen Skull

A small skull (microcephaly) may result from premature closure of the cranial sutures (craniosynostosis) or failure of normal growth of the brain (primary microcephaly). This is an extremely important distinction to be determined at an early age since aggressive surgical treatment of the synostosed sutures is indicated in the former whereas no specific therapy is available for the baby with the small brain. Intellectual potential is frequently normal in the craniosynostosis group compared with the expected mental retardation in primary microcephaly.

Craniosynostosis may involve one or many sutures, and the resultant skull shape will reflect the location of affected sutures since growth can occur only at open sutures sites. Thus if synostosis of the coronal suture is present, anterior-posterior length will be decreased, and growth around the sagittal suture will give a broad skull (brachycephaly).[1] Figure 12–11,A,B shows possible types of compensating growth that can occur. As mentioned previously, the ophthalmic problems are frequently secondary to the skull changes, with papilledema, optic atrophy, and corneal exposure from proptosis representing the most serious threats to visual function.

Central Nervous System Anomalies

Malformations of the CNS can be associated with orbital, visual, and oculomotor abnormalities. Textbooks in neuro-ophthalmology detail the myriad findings in these syndromes.[21, 22] Because visual and oculomotor pathways are located throughout the brain, eye findings are common. A selected number of CNS abnormalities are discussed below.

Anencephaly

Anencephaly is a condition in which there is an absence or very poor development of the cerebrum and overlying bone and skin. The cerebellum, basal ganglia, brain stem, and spinal cord may also have some abnormalities, although they can be normal. Anencephalic children die shortly after birth.

The retinal ganglion cells and their nerve fibers also do not develop normally, which results in optic nerve aplasia or hypoplasia. Other ocular abnormalities include anophthalmos, microphthalmos, colobomas, and deformed orbits.

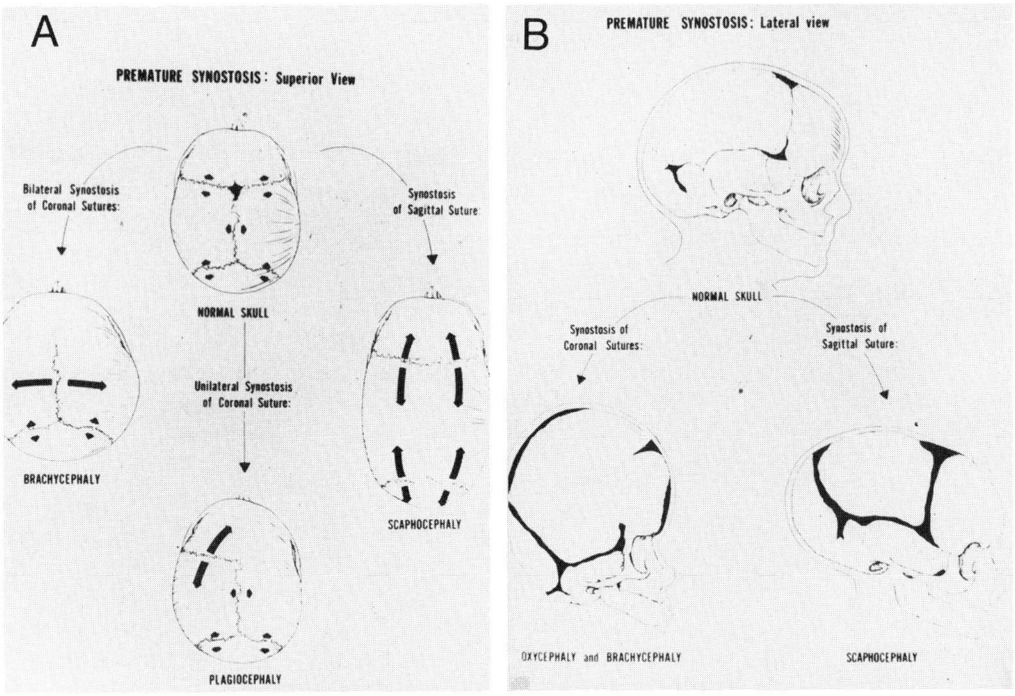

FIG 12–11.
A and B, alterations and skull shape due to premature closure of the sutures. Note that unilateral closure leads to an asymmetrical skull (plagiocephaly).

Microcephaly

CNS findings in microcephaly include the presence of a small brain and skull and poor development of the cerebral cortex. Varying degrees of mental retardation are found together with motor problems and seizure disorders. Autosomal recessive inheritance is common. Microcephaly has also been described in infants who received irradiation in utero.[23]

No one ocular defect is characteristic of microcephaly, but numerous abnormalities have been reported including microphthalmos, nystagmus, epicanthus, microcornea, colobomas, persistent hyperplastic primary vitreous (PHPV), cataract, macular aplasia, pigment degeneration of the retina, and optic atrophy.

Arhinencephaly

In arhinencephalic individuals absence of the olfactory bulbs and tracts is associated with median facial dysplasia including cleft lip and palate. Varying degrees of mental retardation may occur. This is a condition frequently found in trisomy 13.

The position of the orbits is most commonly affected and can vary from hypotelorism (in the most extreme form resulting in cyclopia, or fusion into a median eye) to hypertelorism. Other findings can include anophthalmia, microphthalmos, colobomas, and optic atrophy.

Holoprosencephaly

The prosencephalon is the most anterior of the primitive divisions of the developing embryonic brain. Incomplete division of this structure results in holoprosencephaly, or fusion of the cerebral hemispheres. This abnormality is frequently associated with hypertelorism, arhinencephaly, cleft lip and palate, and mental retardation are common.

Ocular findings are identical to those described under arhinencephaly.

Hydrocephalus

Hydrocephalus may be a congenital or

acquired condition in which there is an increase in cerebrospinal fluid (CSF) that causes elevated pressure and enlargement of the CSF pathways. Hydrocephalus can occur when there is an obstruction (noncommunicating), impaired absorption (communicating), or overproduction of fluid. The causes of hydrocephalus include tumors, congenital malformations, inflammation, and hemorrhage. It is frequently associated with spina bifida. When hydrocephalus occurs in infancy, enlargement of the head is noted, and the fontanelles are tense. Slow development and seizures may occur.

Ocular changes are common in hydrocephalus. A decrease in visual acuity may occur secondarily to damage to the anterior or posterior visual pathways. A rapid rise in intracranial pressure may produce papilledema, but the more common optic nerve appearance is one of pallor or atrophy. Nystagmus and pupillary abnormalities are variable. When hydrocephalus is present in infancy, the enlargement of the skull may be accompanied by the lateral displacement of the orbits. Other characteristic findings in hydrocephalus include retraction of the lids, downward deviation of the eyes ("setting sun" appearance), sixth-nerve palsies, convergence deficiency, and gaze palsies.

Encephalocele

An encephalocele is a protrusion of brain through a defect in the skull. This is frequently associated with spina bifida, hydrocephalus, and cleft lip and palate. Although encephalocele most commonly occurs in the occipital region, it also can be found in the frontal region as well.

An encephalocele located in the nasofrontal region may produce a lateral displacement of the orbits. An orbital encephalocele may present as a mass in the nasal orbit and can be confused with other orbital masses including dermoids. An encephalocele, however, usually demonstrates pulsation and is found in association with a bony defect. A posterior orbital encephalocele usually occurs when there is a defect in the posterior fissures or foramen and is often associated with neurofibromatosis.

Other ocular findings may include anophthalmia, microphthalmos, proptosis, optic atrophy, and colobomas.

Arteriovenous Malformation

An arteriovenous (AV) malformation is a congenital condition in which there is shunting of arterial blood into venous channels. Most AV malformations occur in the supratentorial region. They present clinically as headache, seizures, subarachnoid hemorrhage, hemiplegia, aphasia, hydrocephalus, or cranial nerve palsies.

Ocular findings may include hemianopia. AV malformations of the retina may be associated with intracranial AV malformations in the Wyburn-Mason syndrome.

Arnold-Chiari Malformation

The Arnold-Chiari malformation is a malformation of the brain stem and cerebellum where there is displacement of these structures through the foramen magnum; the cerebellar tissue becomes adherent to the cervical spinal cord. These defects obstruct the flow of CSF and result in hydrocephalus.

Nystagmus may be found and is characteristically a downbeating type. Ocular motor palsies may also be seen. Other ocular findings are those that are typically seen in hydrocephalus.

Tumors

Tumors of the CNS may produce eye problems because of their immediate proximity to structures of the visual and oculomotor pathways or because of the resultant hydrocephalus when obstruction to the CSF pathways occurs. Although many neoplasms may produce ocular signs, several have been chosen for presentation in more detail.

Optic Nerve Glioma.—An optic nerve glioma is often considered to be a congenital hamartoma and usually grows very slowly. It may be confined to the orbital portion of the optic nerve or may involve the intracranial nerve and chiasm as well. Optic nerve gliomas frequently present as a loss of vision or proptosis. They are commonly associated with neurofibromatosis. Treatment is controversial.

Craniopharyngioma.—A benign tumor, craniopharyngioma is caused by displaced remnants of the embryonic craniopharyngeal duct. Because this lesion enlarges near the pituitary gland and optic chiasm and tracts, clinical presentation frequently includes endocrine disturbances and visual field defects. Cranial nerve palsies and see-saw nystagmus may be seen.

Posterior Fossa Tumors.—Posterior fossa tumors including cerebellar astrocytomas, medulloblastomas, ependymomas, and brain stem gliomas, often cause elevated intracranial pressure. Ocular findings are usually secondary to the hydrocephalus and characterized by papilledema, sixth nerve palsies, and nystagmus.

Pinealomas.—Pinealomas are located next to the pretectal area of the brain. Damage to this area may produce the dorsal midbrain syndrome (Parinaud's), which is characterized by a paralysis of vertical gaze, light-near dissociation, and retraction nystagmus. Ptosis, oculomotor paresis, and convergence disorders may also occur.

Phakomatoses.—Phakomatoses comprise a group of disorders characterized by skin lesions and tumors of multiple organs. Syndromes included in this category of diseases are (1) neurofibromatosis (CNS: gliomas and neurofibromas; ocular: optic nerve gliomas, optic atrophy, papilledema, proptosis, lid tumors), (2) tuberous sclerosis (CNS: tumors and cysts; ocular: tumors and cysts of the disc and retina), (3) von Hippel–Lindau (CNS: angiomas and gliomas; ocular: retinal angiomas), and (4) Sturge-Weber (CNS: tumors and calcification; ocular: angiomas, glaucoma). Other syndromes that are sometimes included in this category of disease include ataxia-telangiectasia, Wyburn-Mason, and Klippel-Trenaunay-Weber.

THE DYSMORPHIC CHILD: FURTHER EVALUATION AND TREATMENT

Reconstructive Surgery

Major advances in reconstructive surgery for severe craniofacial malformation have occurred in the last 20 years, primarily under the leadership of Paul Tessier of France. This surgery is frequently extensive in nature and involves en bloc movement of the bony facial structures. It is performed in a number of centers around the world and usually involves a team that includes not only plastic surgeons and neurosurgeons but also many other disciplines. The ophthalmologist is always part of the team, at least in the evaluation and postoperative follow-up of the patient because of the potential involvement of important ocular structures. It is necessary for the ophthalmologist to not only accurately define the status of the visual system preoperatively but also measure certain relationships such as the intercanthal, palpebral fissure, interpupillary distance, etc. Postoperatively the function of the visual system should be re-evaluated and appropriate treatment instituted. Although the orbits are frequently involved in the reconstructive surgery, very few cases of blindness have occurred after these major surgical procedures.[24] The timing of the reconstructive surgery is determined by the team; often there is an optimal time for each type of malformation or syndrome. However, serious problems such as vision-threatening corneal exposure and ulceration may precipitate in a decision by the team to intervene at an earlier time. The ophthalmologist will play a role in this discussion by determining the level of need of intervention since visual function is high on the priority list of important aspects for consideration. Families of children with severe craniofacial malformations should be made aware of the possibilities of reconstructive surgery and referred to the appropriate centers.

Postoperatively, damage may occur by the bandages abrading the cornea or exposure from incomplete protection of the lids due to postoperative edema (Fig 12–12). This may go unnoticed as at times because of a transient or permanent decrease in corneal sensation. There may also be changes in the position of the eye or the canthi, ptosis, and new lacrimal system obstructive symptoms.

Surgical Correction of Strabismus, Ptosis, and Lacrimal Problems

Infants with common forms of strabismus (e.g., congenital esotropia) and no associated neurological problems frequently undergo surgical correction in the first 2 years of life in the hope of achieving better binocular function. However, in children with significant craniofacial anomalies or neurological problems, deferring correction of the ocular misalignment may often be the wisest decision. Strabismus is frequently a low-priority problem compared with life-threatening and serious functional conditions such as compromised airways, increased intracranial pressure, etc. Additionally, reconstructive surgery that involves moving the orbits (e.g., in hypertelorism) may significantly change the degree or type of strabismus, thereby modifying the strabismus surgery indicated. Another consideration is that improved binocular function may not be as attainable in these patients because of their unusual and incomitant form of ocular muscle imbalance, and early surgery is thus of no particular advantage.

Ptosis is not infrequently observed after repositioning the orbit. Although sometimes it may be due to neurological damge, many times it is based on anatomic changes. If a levator resection is done in these patients with postoperative moderate ptosis, a conservative approach is usually indicated because the levator muscles are structurally more normal compared with those in most patients with congenital ptosis.

The lacrimal system frequently is malformed preoperatively; also, it may be effected by the reconstructive surgery and require surgical repair at a later date.

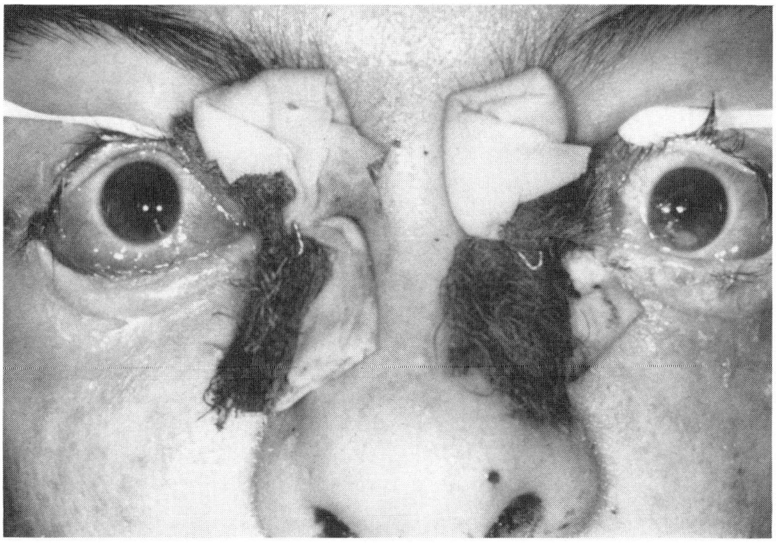

FIG 12–12.
Postoperative reconstructive surgery showing exposure keratitis and ulceration of the cornea due to exposure. The patient had no discomfort because of decreased corneal sensation.

The Dysmorphic Child Without a Definite Diagnosis

Following the initial examination of the dysmorphic child, a specific diagnosis or, at least, a possible syndrome group may have been determined. However, frequently further diagnostic tests and evaluation by other specialists are necessary to establish a secure diagnosis. The pediatric geneticist/syndromologist will contribute more experience in usual conditions and aid in the detection of minor variations of normal structures. CT or magnetic resonance imaging (MRI) will aid in identifying cranial suture closures, CNS malformations, or anomalies of the inner ear or spine, thus assisting in syndrome delineation and therapeutic management. If the anomalies observed are all related to a certain period in development, a teratogenic agent or environmental cause (e.g., hemorrhage in the embryo) should be considered. Multiple malformations involving different systems and different developmental periods are frequently seen with chromosomal anomalies, and detailed chromosomal analysis of the child and both parents is indicated. Involvement of structures derived from a given cell type (e.g., neural crest) gives insight on the type of developmental error but may not be helpful in risk analysis because etiologies can be heterogeneous.

At times, a diagnosis can be suggested by isolating one or more of the malformations and looking up in the general text the different causes of these malformations.[11, 12] For example, Klippel-Feil anomaly and Duane syndrome could be found present in Wildervanck's syndrome, and further evaluation of the inner ear structures would more firmly establish the diagnosis. More in-depth perusal of the literature and future additional testing and observation may be necessary before a valid syndrome identification occurs.

Unfortunately, even in institutions with skilled diagnosticians and facilities for sophisticated evaluation, many dysmorphic children, perhaps up to 50%, do not fall into any clearly recognizable syndrome group. The treatment of these children is symptomatic for the problems detected. It may include special education, reconstructive surgery, hearing aids, etc. A more difficult dilemma is the information that must be given to the parents concerning the natural history of the condition and the risk of a similar condition in future siblings or offspring of the affected child. If there is no suggestion of involvement in the parents or other family members, by examination or history, autosomal dominant diseases are less likely. But risks up to 25% for unrecognized autosomal recessive diseases must often be given for future children of these parents, although a sporadic occurrence may be more probable. In some situations, antenatal diagnosis of future pregnancies may add some information. Even if there is great uncertainty as to future risk, it is necessary that the subject be discussed with the parents at some time. This may not be too soon after the birth of the child because of the strong emotional problems faced by the parents. Skilled physicians anticipate the appropriate time to raise this issue if the parents themselves do not ask specific questions. We are ethically and legally obliged to accept this responsibility.

REFERENCES

1. Bertelson TI: The etiology of the premature synostosis of the cranial sutures. *Acta Ophthalmol (Copenh)* 1958; 36 (suppl 15):359.
2. Waardenburg PJ, Franceschetti A, Klein D: *Genetics and Ophthalmology,* vol 1. Springfield, Ill, Charles C Thomas, Publishers, 1961.
3. Duke-Elder S: Congenital deformities, in *System of Ophthalmology.* vol 3. St Louis, CV Mosby Co, 1964.
4. Francois J: *Heredity in Ophthalmology.* St Louis, CV Mosby Co, 1965.
5. DeMeyer W: The median cleft face syndrome. *Neurology (NY)* 1967; 17:961.
6. Aita JA: *Congenital Facial Anomalies with Neurologic Defects.* Springfield, Ill, Charles C Thomas, Publishers, 1969.
7. Mustarde JC: Congenital deformities in the orbital region. *Proc R Soc Med* 1971; 64:1121.

8. Nema HV: *Ophthalmic Syndromes.* London, Butterworth Publishers, Inc, 1973.
9. Geeraets WJ: *Ocular Syndromes,* ed 3. Philadelphia, Lea & Febiger, 1976.
10. Gorlin RJ, Pindberg JJ, Cohen MM: *Syndromes of the Head and Neck,* ed 2. New York, McGraw-Hill International Book Co, 1976.
11. Miller M, Pruzansky S: Craniofacial anomalies, in Peyman GA, Sanders DR, Goldberg MF (eds): *Principles and Practice of Ophthalmology,* vol 3. Philadelphia, WB Saunders Co, 1980; pp 2354–2422.
12. Cohen MM Jr: *The Patient with Multiple Anomalies.* New York, Raven Press, 1981.
13. Smith DW: *Recognizable Patterns of Human Malformations: Genetic, Embryologic and Clinical Aspects: Major Problems in Clinical Pediatrics,* ed 3. Philadelphia, WB Saunders Co, 1982.
14. Hamming N, Miller MT: The eye, in Fanaroff AA, Martin RJ (eds): *Neonatal-Perinatal Medicine,* ed 4. St Louis, CV Mosby Co, 1987, pp 1200–1231.
15. Marden PM, Smith DW, McDonald MJ: Congenital anomalies in the newborn infant including minor variation. *J Pediatr* 1964; 64:358.
16. Miller MT, Cuttone J, Israel J: Fetal alcohol syndrome. *J Pediatr Ophthalmol Strabismus* 1981; 18:6–15.
17. Miller M, Folk E: Strabismus associated with craniofacial anomalies. *Am Orthopt J* 1975; 25:27–37.
18. Pagon RA: Ocular coloboma. *Surv Ophthalmol,* 1981; 25:223–236.
19. Francois EJ: General anomalies and diseases associated with congenital cataracts, in *Congenital Cataracts.* Springfield, Ill, Charles C Thomas, Publisher, 1963, pp 251–264.
20. Skarf B, Hoyt SC: Optic nerve hypoplasia in children associated with anomalies of the endocrinc and CNS. *Arch Ophthalmol* 1984; 102:62–67.
21. Duke-Elder S: Neuro-ophthalmology, in *System of Ophthalmology,* vol 12. St Louis, CV Mosby Co, 1971.
22. Walsh FB, Hoyt WF: *Clinical Neuro-Ophthalmology.* ed 3, vols 1–3. Baltimore, Williams & Wilkins, 1969.
23. Goldstein L: Radiogenic microcephaly—A surgery of nineteen recorded cases with special reference to ophthalmic defects. *Arch Neurol Psychiatry* 1930; 24:101–115.
24. Whitacker LA, Munro IRF, Sayler KE, et al: Combined report and complications in 793 craniofacial operations. *Plast Reconstr Surg* 1979; 64:198–203.

13 Ocular Size and Shape

Jeffrey S. Schwartz, M.D.
David A. Lee, M.D.
Sherwin J. Isenberg, M.D.

The sagittal diameter of the term newborn eye is approximately 16 to 19 mm at birth. Within the first year of life, normally 95% of ocular growth occurs, which leaves the eye with an axial length between 20 and 21 mm. A small percentage of children, approximately 1.5%, have abnormally smaller or larger eyes with decreased visual function.[1] Attention to these developmental ocular abnormalities is the focus of this chapter (Fig 13–1).

A clear understanding of ocular development is necessary to know why some eyes develop normally and others do not. At approximately 3 weeks' gestational age, a thickening of the neuroectoderm occurs in the forebrain. This is the optic primordia. Following this thickening a depression of the neuroectoderm forms the optic pit. As the neural folds of the embryo close, they create the neural tube. At the same time, the optic pit enlarges to form the optic vesicle. This vesicle initially communicates with the diencephalon through a lumen. As the communication constricts, the optic stalk forms and later develops into the optic nerve. Cellular differentiation begins within the optic vesicles. The inner layer will become the neurosensory retina, while the outer layer forms the pigmented epithelium of the retina, ciliary body, and iris. By day 26, the surface ectoderm adjacent to the optic vesicle begins to thicken and create the lens placode. Eventually the corneal epithelium and conjunctiva will develop from this surface ectoderm.

The neurosensory area of the optic vesicle pushes toward the pigmented epithelial layer to form an optic cup. At the same time the lens placode invaginates to become the lens pit, which continues to deepen and separates from the surface ectoderm to form the lens vesicle complete with a surface ectoderm outer capsule. A layer of tissue forms between the neuroectoderm and the surface ectoderm. This is mesodermal tissue, which differentiates to form all layers of the cornea (except the epithelium), the iris stroma, the ciliary body, choroid, sclera, as well as the aqueous filtration system. Some researchers believe the last is of neuroectodermal origin.

As the optic cup invaginates between the fourth and sixth weeks of gestation, a fissure is formed inferonasally through which the hyaloid artery enters the orbit and ganglion cells exit on the way to the brain. If this fissure is not present in the optic cup, there will be a barrier for ingrowth of neuroectoderm cells and outgrowth of axons into the brain. This fissure normally closes by the sixth week of gestation. It initially closes in the middle of the globe and proceeds anteriorly and posteriorly somewhat like the closing of a zipper. After this closure, the initial development of the eye is complete, and cell differentiation and maturation occur for the continued development of the eye. These initial 6 weeks (until the closure of the embryonic fissure) are by far the most critical period for ocular development. Arrested development during

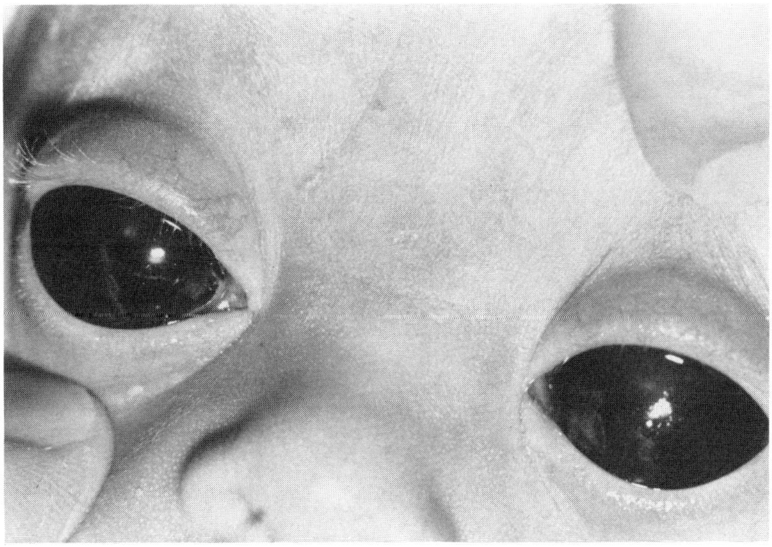

FIG 13–1.
Congenital glaucoma with buphthalmos in both eyes. Corneal diameters measure 17 mm on the right and 21 mm on the left.

this period will lead to severe anatomic abnormalities of the eye as well as greatly impaired visual acuity[2–4] (Table 13–1).

ABNORMALITIES ASSOCIATED WITH SMALL EYES AND ARREST OF DEVELOPMENT

Anophthalmia

Anophthalmia is defined as the absence of the eye. In reality the correct term should be clinical anophthalmia. It is an extremely rare, usually isolated ocular abnormality caused by the failure of optic vesicle outgrowth from the wall of the diencephalon. It is usually a severe form of microphthalmos. In order to make the diagnosis of true anophthalmos, histological serial sectioning is necessary, although magnetic resonance imaging (MRI) or a computed tomography (CT) scan may be helpful. The diagnosis requires serial pathological sections of the orbit to rule out the possibility of a severely microphthalmic eye being present in the orbit.

TABLE 13–1.
Ocular Anomalies Associated With Arrest in Development

Onset of Arrest (Postconception) (wk)	Defect Caused
2	Anophthalmia, cyclopia
3	Congenital cystic eye, nonattachment of the retina
4	Congenital aphakia, congenital cataracts
6	Typical colobomas
8–32	PHPV, Bergmeister's papilla, Mittendorf's dot
32–40	Primary infantile glaucoma

PHPV = persistent hyperplastic primary vitreous.

Mann divided anophthalmia into three types.[5] The first is primary anophthalmia, which results from isolated failure of the optic pit to invaginate. This can occur in an otherwise normal child. She also described secondary anophthalmia that results from complete suppression of forebrain development. This is a lethal condition. A third type of anophthalmia is consecutive or degenerative anophthalmia. In this case there is initial development of ocular structures and secondary degeneration.

Clinical anophthalmia has been associated with several genetic diseases including trisomy 13 and Kleinfelter syndrome. Most cases occur sporadically, although various hereditary linkages have been recorded including autosomal dominant, autosomal recessive, and X-linked recessive transmissions.[6]

In laboratory animals, anophthalmia was noted in 1901 by Stemann.[5] He showed that the application of minute trauma at a specific time in development could induce a specific abnormality, including anophthalmia. Since that time, many researchers have caused anophthalmia in a laboratory setting in rats as well as other mammals by using toxins or drugs or by creating artificial deficiencies of needed compounds.[7] Some of these deficiencies included vitamin A, galactose, adenine, and leucine; some of the toxins included actinomycin, alcohol, arsenic, aminothiazine, chloroquine, Congo red, hydrazine, Niagria sky blue, and metaamphetamine.

Cyclopia and Synophthalmia

Cyclopia and synophthalmia are regional developmental anomalies of the upper face. They constitute a lethal condition in which a single eye or ocular structures appear in the midportion of the face. They are associated with dramatic systemic deformities of both the face and brain. Cyclopia refers to a condition in which only a single median eye occurs. In synophthalmia the ocular rudiment is composed of the mirror image portions of the two incomplete eyes joined in the midline and residing in the upper middle face. Histopathologic sections of fetuses with cyclopia and synophthalmia revealed the eyes not to be grossly malformed but to have colobomas. It is the associated nonocular components of this entity that cause incompatibility with life.[2,8]

Congenital Cystic Eye

Congenital cystic eye results from a failure of the optic vesicle to invaginate.[2] It describes an abnormality or arrest in development that occurs between weeks 2 and 4 of gestation. It is an extremely rare condition that is only properly diagnosed by pathological sectioning of the orbit. The clinical appearance suggests an absent eye that is replaced by a small, thin-walled cyst. The cyst may have a bluish appearance and is usually centrally placed within the orbit. Frequently, patients with microphthalmos and a cyst were thought to have a congenital cystic eye, but Weiss and coworkers[9] showed that a CT scan can distinguish easily between the two.

Congenital Aphakia

Congenital aphakia, or complete absence of the lens, occurs when the surface ectoderm fails to react to the stimulus of the optic vesicle to thicken and invaginate.[10] This leads to complete failure of the ectodermal portion of the lens to develop. It is extremely rare. Congenital aphakia has two subgroups. True congenital aphakia was first described by Baker[11] in 1887, and the mechanism proposed was defects in the inducer neuroectoderm or the target tissue, and the ectoderm, itself. The second and more common type of congenital aphakia is called secondary or apparent aphakia. It is due to early degeneration and absorption of the lens that had already begun to form. It is marked by the presence of lens remnants or by a totally aphakic eye with possible microphthalmos and other ocular malformations. Clinically, the lens may be represented by a wrinkled remnant of the lens capsule. The possible etiology may be some primary fault in the lens fibers or temporary change in their environment that causes degeneration.[10]

Colobomas

The term *coloboma* implies the absence of a tissue and the Greek root means curtailed. Clinically, it refers to any developmental notch, gap, or hole in the eye. Colobomas may be divided into two types, typical and atypical. Typical colobomas result from a failure or arrest of the normal embryonic fissure closure during weeks 4 to 6 of gestation. The embryonic fissure is a temporary cleft in the inferior wall of the optic cup. Closure of the fissure starts normally at the 15-mm stage at approximately 6 weeks. It begins centrally and proceeds anteriorly and posteriorly. Defective closure of the embryonic fissure produces typical colobomas. This was first observed clinically in 1907 by von Szily.[12] Clinically, typical colobomas occur in the inferior nasal border of the eye. A coloboma in any other area is considered atypical.

Most colobomas arise sporadically, but they are occasionally transmitted as an autosomal dominant trait with incomplete penetrance. Colobomas occur when the inner layers of the cup that normally approximate at the margin of the fissure do not fuse to form the usual confluent neurosensory layer. The outer layer also may fail to fuse, which allows the inner layer of the optic cup to evert through the unclosed margin to produce chorioretinal defects. Colobomas usually occur in well-differentiated retinas but may occur with retinal dysplasia. Visual impairment depends on the extent of the ocular malformation.[13–15]

Typical Colobomas

Iris Colobomas.—Colobomas of the iris occur inferiorly in the area of the embryonic fissure. They usually do not involve the ciliary body. Clinically they appear as keyhole shaped or triangular, with the triangle-oriented base located inferiorly at the pupillary margin. The margins are lined with uveal pigment. They are often associated with defects of the lens and zonules as well as opacities of the lens capsule. The iris sphincter is usually present and active except in the area of the notch. The general appearance of the rest of the iris is typically normal. Visual acuity is usually good unless there is choroidal or optic disc involvement. Some patients have high myopia as well as astigmatism. In cases that involve the choroid, there is often a separation of the choroid and pupillary defects by a bridge of normal tissue. Frequently small strands of mesodermal persistent pupillary membrane are present in the iris defect. Mann explained colobomatous defects as "localized failure of a portion of the ectodermal margin of the optic cup or there is undue persistence of fetal mesoderm producing a secondary inhibition of growth of the ectoderm in contact with it"[5] (Fig 13–2).

Lens (Zonular) Colobomas.—Colobomas of the lenses are usually isolated notches in the inferior nasal lens margin. They are

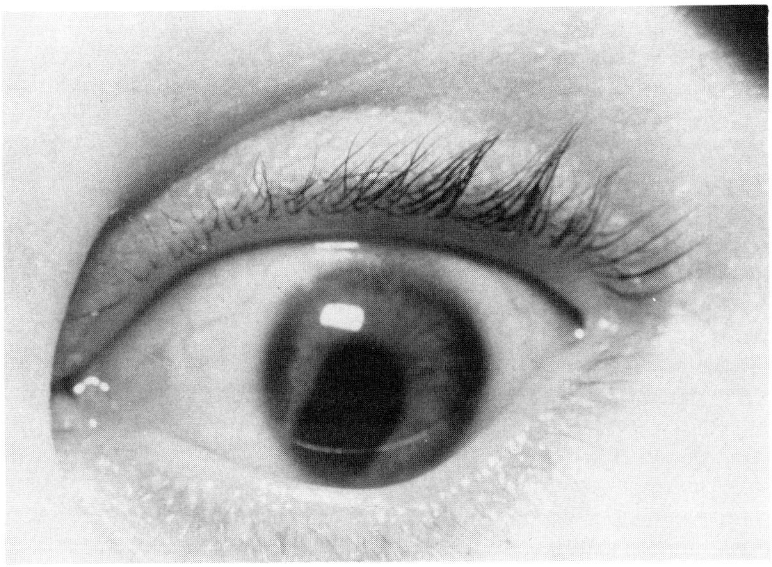

FIG 13–2.
Typical iris coloboma involving the inferior nasal quandrant.

sometimes associated with iris abnormalities and may be either unilateral or bilateral. Notching of the lens margin may take the form of a single concavity or flattening of the lens. There may be slight thickening of the lens diameter in the area of notching. Usually there is an associated lack of lens zonules. Vision is usually good, but there may be significant refractive error if the coloboma is sufficiently large and involves many zonules. Infrequently one sees ectopia lentis or spherophakia as well as localized lens opacities associated with iris colobomas.[5, 15]

Retinal and Choroidal Colobomas.—Occurring inferonasally, retinal and choroidal colobomas occur in an area in which both the neurosensory and the retinal pigment epithelium precursors fail to become confluent. The choroid fails to differentiate at the site because its differentiation is dependent on an intact pigment epithelium. Thus, the defect is actually a chorioretinal coloboma that represents an area of the bare sclera without an overlying differentiated retina or choroid.[15] Clinically it appears as a glistening white defect with distinct margins, often rimmed by irregular pigment clumps. The floor of the defect is usually uneven and bulges posteriorly. Frequently a bridge of normal retina extends between the normal and the abnormal areas. People may live symptom free with chorioretinal colobomas, but approximately 42% of such patients sometime in their lifetime will develop retinal detachments or hemorrhages.[16]

Optic Disc Colobomas.—Not uncommon, optic disc colobomas are caused by failed closure of the most proximal portion of the optic stalk. They can vary in size and involve the entire disc or just the inferior nasal portion. They are frequently associated with an inferior conus. The clinical appearance is of an enlarged disc that is vertically oval and excavated. The retinal vessels have an abnormal origin. The inferior conus may be large and accompanied by a staphylomatous defect, with posterior bowing of the fundus inferior to the defect. The posterior staphyloma may be severe, with bulging of up to 4 mm or more. This may be considered an early form of colobomatous cyst. Clinical and visual symptoms in cases of fundus and optic nerve colobomas depend on the extent and location of the lesion and whether or not other intraocular abnormalities are also present. When the macula is not involved, one may simply find a scotoma corresponding to the site of the defect, with normal or near-normal visual acuity. A coloboma of the optic nerve may cause some decrease in vision, even when the macula is spared. Sometimes amblyopia develops. The primary cause for colobomatous defects may be faulty, aberrant induction along the fusion line of neuroectodermal tissue that results in multiple secondary intraocular changes including retinal dysplasia, rosette formation, or aberrant differentiation of adjacent tissue.

Occasionally a severe coloboma may be associated with an orbital cyst. This cyst is thin-walled, without evidence of internal differentiated ocular structures. Frequently in the presence of an orbital cyst, microphthalmos develops. An enlarging cyst may displace an accompanying microphthalmic eye and result in the appearance of clinical anophthalmia.[2, 5, 13, 15, 17]

Typical colobomas may be isolated or associated with other ocular or systemic abnormalities. Any coloboma, whether iris, chorioretinal, or disc, may be unilateral or bilateral. When bilateral they tend to be asymmetrical and may be associated with more systemic abnormalities. The next section discusses colobomas associated with genetic patterns as well as other systemic abnormalities.

Autosomal Inherited Isolated Coloboma

Dominant Inheritance.—Colobomas from autosomal dominant inheritance are isolated anomalies in the absence of other systemic malformations. Pedigrees have been described in the literature that illustrate the variable expression of the gene.[13] The pedigrees encompass a spectrum from iris coloboma to clinical anophthalmia, with various degrees of colobomatous abnormalities in between. Penetrance of this gene is variable and has been estimated to be between 20% and 30%.[15]

Recessive Inheritance.—Autosomal recessive isolated ocular colobomas have been suggested in the literature. Francois[13] in 1968 as well as Kronberg[18] in 1949 and McMillan[19] in 1921 described cases that appear to have an autosomal recessive inheritance pattern. Although complete information on the examination of the parents was not available, the records give credence to the possibility of autosomal recessive inheritance patterns. Kronberg's work demonstrates this type of pattern in a family with consanguinity.

Inherited Colobomas Associated With Multiple System Disease

Lenz Syndrome.—Lenz microphthalmos syndrome is an X-linked recessive disorder in which the entire spectrum of ocular colobomas have been demonstrated. Other ocular abnormalities include microphthalmos and frequently congenital cataracts. In addition to the ocular coloboma, the syndrome is manifested by a normal retina and the following nonocular abnormalities: characteristic facies, dysmorphic ears, narrow shoulders, short structure, and low birth weight. Frequently renal abnormalities as well as mental retardation are seen. The diagnosis is based on physical findings and family history.[4, 15]

Aicardi Syndrome.—Aicardi syndrome is an X-linked dominant disorder lethal to males. Thus only females have been found to have this disorder. They have optic disc colobomas with associated chorioretinopathy, microphthalmos, and persistent pupillary membranes. In addition there are associated vertebral anomalies, mental retardation, and absence of the corpus callosum.[15, 20]

Goltz Syndrome.—Goltz focal dermal hypoplasia is associated with colobomatous malformations. Most of the patients reported are female. A proposed X-linked dominant gene that is lethal to males has been suggested. Approximately 40% of affected patients have ocular abnormalities including microphthalmos, colobomas, aniridia, pupillary irregularities, lens subluxation, pigmentary changes of the retina, corneal clouding, strabismus, nystagmus, blepharoptosis, ectropion, photophobia, and lacrimal duct blockage.[7, 21] Multisystem involvement includes abnormalities of skin that are noted at birth and consist of asymmetrical linear streaks of hyperpigmentation, atrophy, and telangiectasia. There are also skin nodules of the posterior portion of the thigh, groin, and iliac crest area. Focal subepidermal herniation of fat has been noted. Physical and mental development are retarded; there is facial and structural asymmetry. Skeletal anomalies include syndactyly, polydactyly, absent digits, microcrania, and spine and pelvic deformities.[7, 15, 21, 22]

Meckel Syndrome.—Meckel syndrome is a lethal autosomal recessive disorder in which a full spectrum of ocular coloboma is seen as well as retinal dysplasia. Nonocular findings include microcephaly, occipital encephalocele, postaxial polydactyly, and polycystic disease of the kidneys, liver, and pancreas.[4, 15]

Warburg Syndrome.—An autosomal recessive abnormality, Warburg syndrome consists of appreciable central nervous system (CNS) and ocular abnormalities. Ocular abnormalities include corneal leukomas, retinal dysplasia, congenital nonattachment of the retina, as well as colobomatous defects. CNS abnormalities include hydrocephalus with dilated ventricles, microcephaly, absent cerebral gyri, polymicrogyria, and occasionally encephaloceles. Patients with this syndrome have profound mental retardation and a poor prognosis for life.[15]

CHARGE Association.—A new aggregation of symptoms has been described that has been given the mnemonic CHARGE: C = coloboma; H = heart defect; A = atresia choanae; R = retarded growth and development; G = genital hypoplasia; E = ear anomalies and deafness. The CHARGE association is diagnosed on the basis of any four of the six cardinal features. Most people with this diagnosis have an ocular coloboma. Recent studies show all types of inheritance patterns as well as sporadic cases. The majority of cases appear to be sporadically inherited and might be attributed to arrest of development between the fifth and sixth weeks of gestation.[15, 23]

Chromosomal Abnormalities Associated With Colobomas

Ocular colobomas are common in trisomy 13, triploidy, cat-eye syndrome, 4P deletion, and trisomy 18.[15]

Trisomy 13, Patau Syndrome.—Trisomy 13 occurs in approximately 1 in 10,000 live births.[4] In addition to uveal colobomas, these children have other ocular abnormalities including cataracts, hypertelorism, shallow orbital ridges, absence of eyebrows, epicanthal folds, corneal clouding, retinal dysplasia, persistent hyperplastic primary vitreous (PHPV), optic atrophy, intraocular connective tissue, and sometimes microphthalmos or even anophthalmia. Systemic abnormalities include severe CNS anomalies including holoprosencephaly (developmental failure of cleavage of the forebrain), cebocephaly (monkeylike deformity and appearance of the head) and arhinencephaly (congenital absence of the olfactory portions of the brain). They also have scalp defects and focal dermal hypoplasia. Clinically they show a sloping forehead, a broad nose, and frequently a cleft palate and cleft lip. The heart may have atrial or ventral septal defects or both. They tend to have renal anomalies, polycystic kidneys, and hydronephrosis. They may have polydactyly, clenched fists, and "rocker-bottom" feet. The proposed etiology is nondysjunction of chromosome 13 during meiosis or an unbalanced translocation. Severely affected individuals die within 1 month of birth. Less than 5% survive more than 3 years. The colobomas themselves tend to occur anteriorly along the fetal fissure, usually involving the iris or lens and occasionally the anterior choroid.[4, 7]

Triploidy.—An individual with triploidy has 69 chromosomes rather than the normal 46. There are three of each autosome, usually because of an extra set of maternal chromosomes. Triploidy is extremely rare among healthy newborns but is estimated to occur in approximately 1% of all conceptions.[4] Most are spontaneously aborted and account for 20% of all fetuses with abnormal chromosome constitution aborting in the early stages of pregnancy. Their incidence in pregnancies carried to term is approximately 1 in 10,000.[4] The frequency and percentage increase with increasing maternal age as well as in delayed fertilization (late in the menstrual cycle). Predisposing factors to this may include heat, shock, hypoxia, and hormonal therapy during pregnancy. Hydatidiform change in the placenta is associated in 75% of the cases. Ocular findings include hypertelorism in half of these fetuses, typical colobomas in one third, and microphthalmos in one third. They may also have microcornea, blepharophimosis, clinical anophthalmia, or ectopic pupils. Systemic abnormalities include marked CNS malformations, cranial-facial abnormalities, syndactyly, ventral and atrial septal defects, genital defects, renal dysplasia, and omphalocele (protrusion of part of the intestine through a defect in the abdominal wall). Some individuals may have triploidy, but not involving all of their chromosomes. They have a mosaic of diploid and triploid cells, thus increasing their chances of survival beyond birth. These children tend to have some of the aforementioned ocular and systemic manifestations listed above.[4, 7, 20]

Cat-Eye Syndrome.—A triad of uveal coloboma, imperforate anus, and renal malformations, cat-eye syndrome obtains its name from the vertical iris colobomas. The findings of the small, extra submetacentric chromosome composed of chromatin fragments originating from chromosomes 22 and either 13 or 14 may explain this abnormality. These extra fragments are mitotically unstable and may retard cell division during embryogenesis. Additional findings other than the aforementioned triad include preauricular skin tags, fistulas, congenital heart disease, antimongoloid lid slant, and skeletal abnormalities.[4, 20, 24]

Wolff Syndrome.—Children with Wolff syndrome (P4 deletion) tend to be severely retarded with microcephaly. They may have grand mal seizures with minor motor seizures, hypotonia as well as congenital heart disease, simian creases of the palms, cryptorchism (failure of testicular development) and hypospadias (abnormal urethral orifices on the undersurface of the penis). The ocular findings in addition to iris colobomas include antimongoloid lid fissures, prominent epicanthal folds, hypertelorism, blepharoptosis, and strabismus.[4, 7, 20]

Trisomy 18 (Edwards Syndrome).—Trisomy 18 is one of the more common malformation syndromes in humans and occurs in 1 of 8,000 live births.[4] The majority of these children die in the nursery, but some may live 15 years or more. The ocular manifestations include uveal coloboma, usually located at the proximal end of the embryonic cleft and involving the optic nerve and/or retina. Other ocular findings include hypertelorism, hyperplastic supraorbital ridges, blepharophimosis, prominent epicanthal folds, thick lower lids, blepharoptosis, microphthalmos, corneal opacities, congenital glaucoma, and optic nerve anomalies. These children also have multiple systemic abnormalities that account for their high mortality rate, including mental retardation, growth failure, a protruding occiput, micrognathia, misshapen low-set ears, microstoma, cardiovascular abnormalities, psychomotor retardation, flexion deformities of the fingers, rocker-bottom feet, and sometimes myelomeningoceles.[4, 20]

Other causes of coloboma with chromosomal abnormalities include the following: 11Q−, 13Q−, 18P−, 18Q−, 18R, 13R, trisomy 17, Kleinfelter's syndrome (XXX), XYY syndrome, Turner's syndrome (XO), Kleideshat syndrome (5P−), and trisomy 8. These abnormalities all have a low incidence of typical colobomas. Also of note is 13Q−, which has been associated with retinoblastoma. The linkage of the two has not been fully evaluated or understood at this time.[15, 22]

Colobomas Associated With Multiple System Disorders of Unknown Etiology

Colobomas may also be part of multisystem disorders. Some of the more common disorders associated with typical colobomatous malformation are described in the following sections.

Rubinstein-Taybi Syndrome.—The Rubinstein-Taybi syndrome consists of the characteristic systemic signs and symptoms of mental retardation, broad thumb and broad great toe, antimongoloid lid fissures, a characteristic beaked nose, undescended testes, hypoplasia of the maxilla, narrow palate, inguinal hernias, genu valgum (knock-knees), and short stature. The ocular findings include colobomas of the iris, lens, and choroid as well as glaucoma, esotropia, and cataract.[7, 15, 21]

Goldenhar Syndrome.—In 1952 Goldenhar reported a triad of anomalies occurring in the same patient. They included epibulbar dermoid, accessory auricular appendages, and an aural fistula. Since that time many patients have been identified with these same findings, and Goldenhar's name has been associated with them. The syndrome tends to be unilateral and is associated with mandibular facial dysostosis. It is thought to be a manifestation of first and second brachial arch arrest. Its inheritance pattern is sporadic, with over 90% of cases showing no family history. One family was described by Krause as having an autosomal dominant pattern.[25] Ocular abnormalities in addition to coloboma of the optic nerve include the following: dermoids, antimongoloid slant, anophthalmia, cryptophthalmos, microphthalmos, iris defects, stenosis of the lacrimal ducts, dacrocystitis, dry eye, corneal anesthesia, neurotrophic ulcers, microcornea, and Duane's retraction syndrome. Systemic manifestations include vertebral anomalies, cardiovascular defects, auricular anomalies including appendages, hydrocephalus, mental retardation, parotid duct abnormalities, renal defects, and urethral, rectal, and oral abnormalities.[4, 7, 15, 26]

Linear Sebaceous Nevus Syndrome.—Also known as epidermal needle nevus syndrome or nevus sebaceous of Jadassohn, the linear sebaceous nevus syndrome is characterized by mental retardation, seizures, and epithelial hamartomas of the scalp, forehead, and midface. At birth, sebaceous nevi appearing as yellowish lesions with an abundance of sebaceous glands and immature hair follicles are found. At puberty and afterward, these lesions progress from the waxy plaques of childhood to nevoid tumors in adulthood. They are rarely associated with colobomatous microphthalmos.[15, 20, 22]

Other Coloboma-Associated Syndromes.—Other systemic diseases or syndromes with which colobomas have been associated or described include the following: Laurence-Moon-Biedel syndrome is an autosomal recessive disorder characterized by mental retardation, polydactylism and visual disturbances. Stickler syndrome is an autosomal dominant syndrome that is characterized by high myopia, vitreoretinal degeneration, retinal detachments, cleft palate, micrognathia, and skeletal abnormalities. Incontinentia pigmenti syndrome (Bloch-Sulzberger disease) is an X-linked dominant syndrome characterized by hypopigmented skin lesions, alopecia, tooth anomalies, small stature, and ocular abnormalities. Ellis-van Creveld syndrome is an autosomal recessive disorder characterized by thoracic dysplasia, short-limb dwarfism, postaxial polydactyly, and occasional ocular abnormality. Crouzon disease is an autosomal dominant disorder characterized by craniofacial dysostosis. Kartagener syndrome is an autosomal recessive disorder characterized by complete situs inversus associated with bronchiectasis and chronic sinusitis. Tuberous sclerosis is an autosomal dominant disorder characterized by adenoma sebaceum, epilepsy, and mental retardation.[15]

Atypical Colobomas

A colobomatous defect located anywhere but in the inferior nasal region of the eye must be considered atypical because it cannot be explained by abnormal closure of the embryonic fissure. Three examples of atypical colobomas are worthy of further discussion.

Optic Pits.—Congenital defects in the nerve head, optic pits vary in shape: slit, triangular, oblong, round, or polygonal. They have varying depths of 1 to 8 mm, and their diameters tend to be more than 30% of the disc diameter. Clinically they appear gray to gray-olive or gray-yellow, occasionally with bluish tinting. Often tissue lies within or over the pit, which may appear pulsatile because of blood vessels running through it. The incidence varies in different studies from between 1 in 7,000 live births to one in 65,000 live births, with the accepted number being approximately 1 in 11,000.[17] Seventy percent of these occur in the temporal part of the optic disc. Most fundi also show abnormal pericapillary pigmentation associated with these pits. They may occur bilaterally or unilaterally. Visual field defects have been described and are noted to be variable and include an enlarged blind spot, nasal step, arcuate and paracentral scotomas, and generalized field constriction. Also associated with optic pits is serous maculopathy. On a fluorescein angiogram, the macula shows late hyperfluorescence. Temporally located optic pits have often been associated with serous retinal detachment of the macula, and sometimes a macular hole may be present. Studies report that 40% to 60% of patients with optic pits develop macular edema or detachment at some time. The etiology of the subretinal fluid in dog studies by Brown and Shields suggests that it arises from liquefied vitreous humor that gains entrance into the subretinal space through the pit.[27]

Histopathologic examination of the optic pit reveals a depression or herniation of rudimentary or degenerative neuroectodermal tissue that contains pieces of neurosensory retina, retinal pigment epithelium, and glial tissue. The defect is usually surrounded by a connective tissue capsule that lies in conjunction with the meninges. Apple and colleagues suggested that the embryonic fissure surrounds the developing optic nerve and therefore any defect or pit of the nerve head is actually a typical coloboma due to failed or incomplete closure of the fissure.[17]

Atypical Iris Colobomas.—Occurring much less commonly than typical ones, atypical iris colobomas may occur in any quadrant, can be solitary or multiple, and range in size from a small notch to sector iridectomies or even aniridia. Often remnants of the anterior hyaloid system and the pupillary membrane are associated with them. Atypical iris colobomas may be associated with aniridia, anterior polar cataracts, and nystagmus. Most cases are uncomplicated and sporadic.[2, 5]

Macular Colobomas.—A macular coloboma may actually be described as macular dysplasia because it is unlikely that this is a true developmental anomaly. Probably it represents scarring, pigmentation, and atrophy following intrauterine inflammation. It tends to be bilateral, causes severe loss of vision, and has some familial association in certain cases. Clinically it appears as a round to oval white lesion with a craterlike depression and pigmented borders. It may be associated with an inflammatory scar elsewhere in the retina. Possible causes for macular colobomas include congenital toxoplasmosis or congenital syphilis.[2]

Persistent Hyperplastic Primary Vitreous

PHPV is caused by arrest or abnormality in development of the vitreous humor between 2 and 8 months of gestational age. The primary vitreous begins development at 3 weeks of gestational age starting with protoplasmic bridging between the surface ectoderm of the lens plate and neuroectoderm of the optic vesicle. These adhesions are formed by the basement membrane of the two ectodermal surfaces. As these two surfaces separate, mesodermal cells invade the space. At the 10-mm (6-week) stage, vasoformative mesodermal cells enter the optic cup through the fissure and lead to formation of the hyaloid vascular system. The artery runs forward to the lens and eventually forms the tunica vasculosa lentis, the primary blood supply to the lens. When the fissure closes, these vessels must then enter the eye through the optic disc. The vessels continue to grow, fill the vitreous cavity, and freely anastomose. Two types of cells are noted around the vessels: fibroblasts, which are responsible for collagen fiber production, and mononuclear macrophages. At the 13-mm (6.5-week) stage, secondary vitreous development begins and continues on to the 40-mm (10-week) stage. The secondary vitreous is an avascular substance that slowly compresses the primary vitreous and causes eventual atrophy until the hyaloid system is condensed to a mere remnant, Cloquet's canal. At term, normally all the vessels of the hyaloid system have disappeared. If they have not, a condition of PHPV results.

Partial remnants of the fetal hyaloid system are common, and although they could be considered mild PHPV, they occur too frequently without other complications to be considered as such. Frequently a small dot is seen on the posterior lens surface that represents a remnant of the tunica vasculosa lentis and is called Mittendorf's dot. Sometimes a glial sheath anterior to the optic nerve head is seen; this is called Bergmeister's papilla.

True PHPV is defined as idiopathic persistence and proliferation of normally transient vasculature of the primary vitreous that leads to the formation of a retrolenticular mass and subsequent visual loss. This usually occurs unilaterally in an otherwise healthy, normal infant. The most common initial sign is leukokoria (white pupil). The differential diagnosis of a white pupil includes retinoblastoma, which must be ruled out. Two clinical findings that help distinguish PHPV from retinoblastoma are that PHPV is associated with microphthalmos and that on dilation the eyes are noted to have elongated and enlarged ciliary processes. Other findings on clinical examination include a retrolental opacity, a funnel-shaped mass of fibrovascular tissue that is usually richly vascular. Multiple hemorrhages have been noted in the vitreous face secondary to this fibrovascular mass. The pupil sometimes dilates poorly, and there may also be an ectropian uvea. The lens at birth is usually clear but with time may become cataractous because of rupture of the posterior capsule and swelling of the lens, which may lead to secondary angle-closure glaucoma. The natural course of PHPV is that after the development of angle-closure glaucoma an unrelenting, absolute glaucoma occurs, with recurrent massive vitreal hemorrhaging, retinal detachment, and eventual deterioration to atrophy and phthisis bulbi. Few eyes have escaped this sequence without surgical intervention. Most of these eyes were enucleated to rule out tumor, relieve pain, or improve an unsightly appearance. Jensen in Denmark examined 14 eyes after enucleation and found the tissue to be composed exclusively of mesodermal components staining positive with periodic acid–Schiff (PAS), Alcian blue, and Hale staining. They had the same microscopic properties as normal vitreous collagen.[28]

The natural course of fully developed PHPV suggests an extremely poor prognosis for such eyes without early surgical intervention. Whether early surgical intervention improves vision has not been determined, but any chance for useful vision is increased by early intervention. The basic surgical approach is twofold: (1) to aspirate all of the lens remnants and (2) to remove the retrolental membrane in order to open a clear pupillary space. After surgery, the child should be fitted with an aphakic contact lens, and amblyopia should be managed with occlusion therapy.[2, 29–31]

Cryptophthalmos

Cryptophthalmos literally means hidden eye. In cryptophthalmos, a sheath of skin continuous with the skin of the periorbital region overlies the eye. The skin overlying the orbit may be attached to the globe as its anterior surface and substitute for the normal underlying corneal epithelium. Cryptophthalmos is usually bilateral and asymmetrical in a third of the cases. The globe is usually microphthalmic. The anterior chamber is usually small or nonexistent, and no trabecular meshwork or canal of Schlemm is usually seen. The lens may be absent. The iris may be absent or totally adherent to the cornea. From an embryological standpoint cryptophthalmos is a combined ectodermal and mesodermal abnormality in development. Cryptophthalmos frequently occurs in association with other ocular abnormalities and systemic anomalies. The proposed mechanism for this development includes (1) primary failure of mesodermal and ectodermal differentiation, which causes an absence of the eyelid folds; (2) intrauterine inflammation producing fusion of the eyelids to the globe; and (3) normal eyelid fold development with maldifferentiation of the conjunctiva that results in a symblepharon.[32]

The general appearance is that the eyelids are replaced by skin extending from the forehead to the cheek. The eyebrows, lashes, glands, and puncta are incompletely developed or nonexistent. The globe appears shrunken and may in fact be microphthalmic. A systemic syndrome called cryptophthalmos syndactyly syndrome includes cryptophthalmos with syndactyly (webbing or fusion of the fingers or toes), brachycephaly (disproportionate shortness of the head), and renal anomalies. Cryptophthalmos can clinically appear in three forms. Complete cryptophthalmos is the most common type; here skin replaces the eyelids, covers the orbit, and adheres to the underlying globe. There may be some response to a bright light stimulus by constriction of the orbicularis oculi muscles. The second form is partial cryptophthalmos. Twenty percent of cases occur this way, and usually the lateral portion of the eyelid is uninvolved. The third type is known as congenital symblepharon syndrome in which the upper eyelids fuse with the globe and the superior cornea is covered with stratified squamous epithelium cells. François described an autosomal recessive pattern in 15% of patients with cryptophthalmos with frequent examples of associated parental consanguinity.[21,31,33]

ABNORMALITIES ASSOCIATED WITH SMALL EYES AND NO SPECIFIC ARREST OF DEVELOPMENT

Microphthalmos

Microphthalmos is a relatively common ocular developmental anomaly and occurs in approximately 1 per 2,000 live births.[1] It refers to an eye that is smaller than normal or reduced in volume. A normal adult eye has an axial length of 20.5 to 24.5 mm. A microphthalmic eye, from a clinical standpoint, includes any adult eye with an axial length of 20 mm or less; in babies an eye measuring less than 16 mm should also be included. Microphthalmos covers a range of entities from clinical anophthalmia at the most severe end of the spectrum to a mild reduction of the anterior posterior dimension, with normal visual acuity as the most mild form. Microphthalmos may be isolated or may be associated with other ocular abnormalities or systemic diseases and syndromes. Unlike the other entities discussed earlier in this chapter, a single kind of arrest in development will not explain microphthalmos, although an arrest in development at almost any time could cause it. Microphthalmos includes the entire spectrum of developmental abnormalities and is frequently associated with several of the disease entities already discussed. Microphthalmic patients may maintain good visual acuity with a full visual field and no problems ever noted. The earlier in development the eye experiences an arrest, the more severe the resulting microphthalmos can be, with associated ocular abnormalities, and the worse the visual prognosis is. In a prospective study of greater than 50,000 pregnancies in the United States, the frequency of microphthalmos was found to be 0.22 per 1,000 live births[22] (Fig 13–3, Table 13–2).

Isolated Microphthalmos.—Isolated microphthalmos without associated ocular or systemic abnormalities is frequently mild and allows for good visual function. Reports of autosomal dominant, autosomal recessive, and X-linked inheritance patterns have been made, but approximately 75% occur sporadically.[22,34]

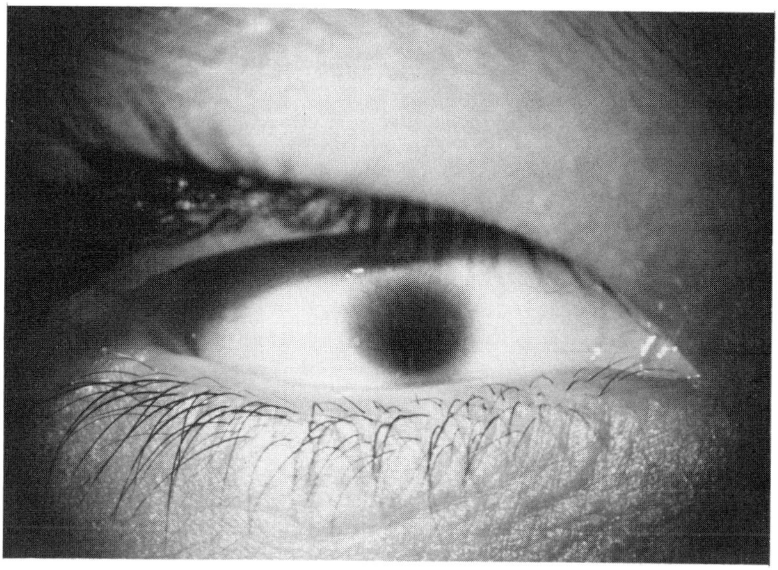

FIG 13–3.
Microphthalmia may be isolated or may be associated with other ocular or systemic abnormalities.

TABLE 13–2
Classification of Microphthalmos

- I. Isolated microphthalmos
  - A. Nanophthalmos
  - B. Inherited
  - C. Idiopathic
- II. Microphthalmos associated with ocular disease
  - A. With congenital cataracts
  - B. With PHPV
  - C. With coloboma
    - 1. Coloboma with cyst
    - 2. Coloboma without cyst
- III. Microphthalmos associated with systemic and/or ocular disease
  - A. Colobomatous microphthalmos
    - 1. Monogenic syndromes
      - a. X-linked
        - (1) Lenz microphthalmos
        - (2) Goltz focal dermal hypoplasia
        - (3) Incontinentia pigmenti syndrome
        - (4) Aicardi syndrome
      - b. Autosomal recessive
        - (1) Meckel syndrome
        - (2) Warburg syndrome
        - (3) Sjögren-Larsson syndrome
        - (4) Humeroradial synostosis
        - (5) Laurence-Moon-Biedl syndrome
        - (6) Ellis-van Creveld syndrome
        - (7) Kartagener syndrome
      - c. Autosomal dominant
        - (1) Basal cell nevus syndrome
        - (2) Congenital contractural arachnodactyly
        - (3) Stickler syndrome
        - (4) Crouzon syndrome
        - (5) Tuberous sclerosis
    - 2. Chromosomal abnormalities
      - a. Triploidy
      - b. Trisomy 8, 13, 17, 18, XXX, XYY
      - c. Duplications 4q, 7q, 9p, 9q, 13q, 22q
      - d. Deletions 4p, 4r, 11q, 13q, 18q, 18r, XO
    - 3. Unknown etiology
      - a. CHARGE association
      - b. Cat-eye syndrome
      - c. Rubinstein-Taybi syndrome
      - d. Goldenhar syndrome
      - e. Linear sebaceous nevus syndrome
  - B. Noncolobomatous microphthalmos
    - 1. Monogenic syndromes
      - a. X-linked
      - b. Autosomal recessive
        - (1) Fanconi syndrome
        - (2) Diamond-Blackfan syndrome
      - c. Autosomal dominant
    - 2. Chromosomal abnormalities
      - a. Duplication 10q
    - 3. Unknown etiology
      - a. Hallermann-Streiff syndrome
      - b. Oculodentodigital syndrome
      - c. Cryptophthalmos syndactyly syndrome

(Continued.)

TABLE 13–2 (cont.)

4. Infectous etiology
   a. Congenital rubella
   b. Epstein-Barr virus
   c. Cytomegalovirus
   d. Varicella
   e. Herpesvirus

Nanophthalmos.—Nanophthalmos refers to a microphthalmic eye with normal intraocular structures. The eye is small, with a small cornea, shallow anterior chamber, narrow angle, and high lens volume–to–eye volume ratio. The patients are noted to have a thick sclera and uvea. It is a rare, usually sporadic disease, with different studies suggesting an autosomal dominant or recessive pattern. Individuals with the entity tend to develop uveal effusions and episodes of angle-closure glaucoma that are difficult to treat and may actually be worsened by miotics.[35] Eyes with nanophthalmos are noted to be very hyperopic; a shallow anterior chamber along with a large lens-to-eye volume ratio makes these eyes predisposed to episodes of angle-closure glaucoma. Surgery in nanophthalmic eyes has an extremely high rate of complications and possibly disastrous results. These episodes of angle closure have been reported to be best treated with laser iridotomy.[36] The proposed etiology of nanophthalmos is an arrest of ocular development after closure of the embryonic fissure. The small dimensions of the eye are not associated with other gross developmental anomalies.

Microphthalmos With Cyst.—A very severe malformation, macrophthalmos with cyst accompanies a fundus coloboma. The cyst represents an actual herniation of embryonic neuroectoderm through the incompletely closed embryonic cleft. It is adjacent to the globe and may be in direct communication through a channel within the coloboma (Figs 13–4 to 13–6). It may vary in size from that of a small ectasia or appendage of the eye to

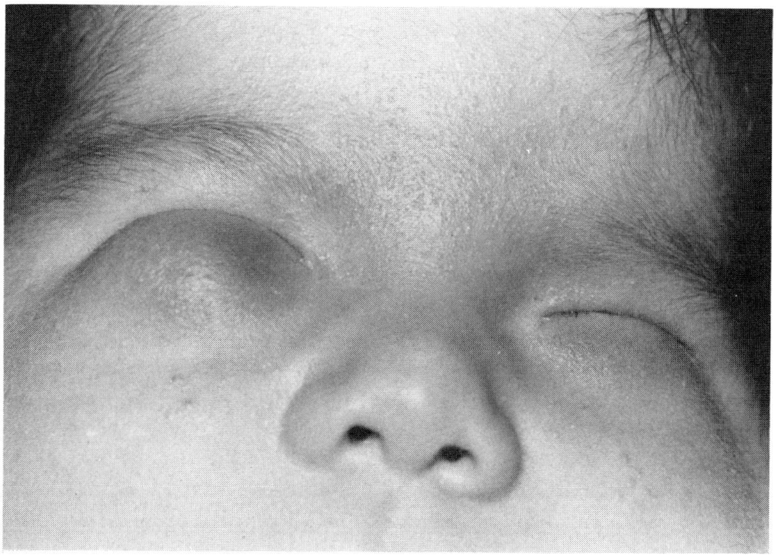

FIG 13–4.
Bilateral microphthalmia with cyst. Note the discoloration and mass below the right eye; this represents the cyst.

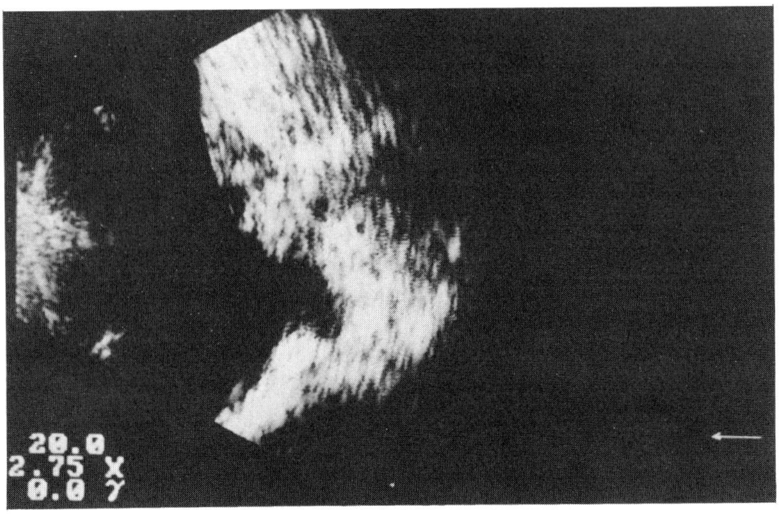

FIG 13–5.
Two-dimensional ultrasound of patient in Figure 13–4 that demonstrates a cyst as a posterior protrusion of the orbital wall.

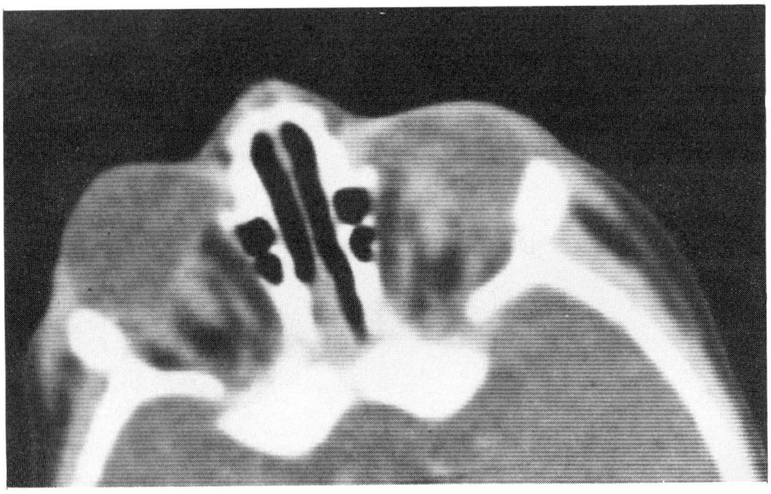

FIG 13–6.
CT scan of the patient in Figure 13–4 that demonstrates bilateral microphthalmia with cyst.

a mass much larger than the globe itself. Occasionally a cyst may be large enough to displace the globe out of the visible orbit and may lead to an inaccurate diagnosis of anophthalmia or congenital cystic eyeball. The diagnosis of microphthalmos with cyst can be made on clinical examination by recognizing the cyst visually. In some cases the cyst is not visible, and the fundus may be examined by indirect ophthalmoscopy to show a deep coloboma in the posterior pole that by its depth suggests a cyst. Ultrasonography also is useful in diagnosing microphthalmos with cyst. The best and most accurate way of making the diagnosis and assessing this condition is by CT scan. With this technique the cyst appears as a thin-walled, homogeneous area similar to density to the vitreous humor. The cyst should be contiguous with the globe. The CT scan may be the only way to rule out a congenital cystic eye in an individual in whom the actual globe is displaced. Histologically the cyst consists of collagenous connective tissue with a similar appearance to sclera that is lined by neuroectodermal tissue. These individuals may have other ocular abnormalities that include microcornea, iris coloboma, anterior segment and corneal abnormalities, cataract, very poor vision, and incomplete angle differentiation. The retina may be involuted or detached and may show rosette formation.[9]

Microphthalmos with cyst is usually unilateral and sporadic, but occasional bilateral cases are reported (Figs 13–7 and 13–8). These are frequently associated with major systemic abnormalities, mostly cardiac and CNS. Microphthalmos with cyst has a poor visual prognosis. Because most cases appear to be unilateral, there is little to be done to improve vision because of severe refractive amblyopia. When the cyst enlarges, it may be excised or

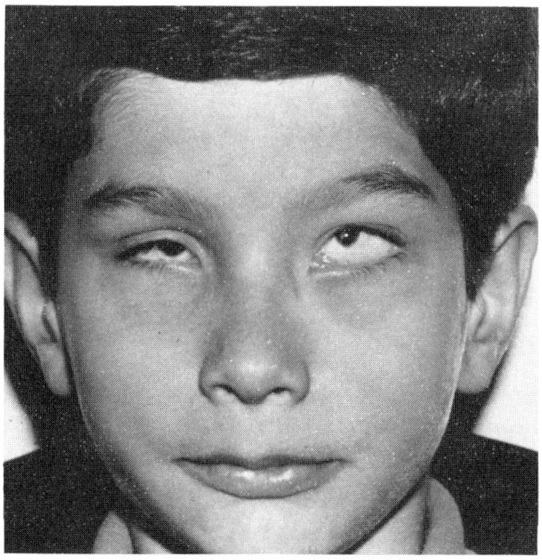

FIG 13–7.
Bilateral microphthalmia. The smaller left eye is displaced forward by a cyst. (Courtesy of Avery Weiss, M.D.)

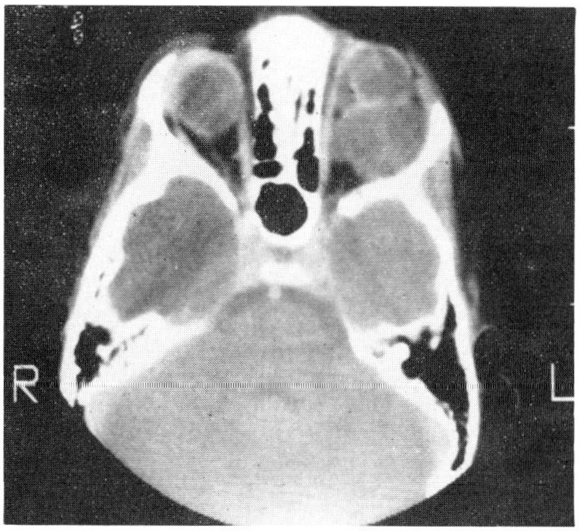

FIG 13–8.
CT scan of the patient in Figure 13–7 that demonstrates microphthalmia in the right eye and microphthalmia with a cyst in the left eye. (Courtesy of Avery Weiss, M.D.)

aspirated with a needle. A prosthesis may be placed over it for cosmetic appearance, or it may be removed in total with the globe. It has been recommended that prior to enucleation aspiration of the cyst be performed to make the surgery easier.[9, 22, 37]

Microphthalmos With PHPV.—Occurring secondarily to developmental arrest after closure of the embryonic fissure, the microphthalmos is not usually severe, although the visual prognosis is poor for reasons discussed in the previous section. Occasionally an enlarged or buphthalmic eye may develop secondarily to the glaucoma associated with PHPV.

Basal Cell Nevus Syndrome.—An autosomal, dominantly inherited disorder, basal cell nevus syndrome is characterized by multiple basal cells, bony abnormalities, mental retardation, and odontogenic cysts of the jaw. Children with this syndrome tend to have a broad facial appearance and may have hypertelorism. Associated multiple ocular anomalies have included microphthalmos, coloboma, congenital cataract, and strabismus as well as glaucoma. Sometimes medulloblastomas have been reported in these children.[7, 21, 22]

Hallermann-Streiff Syndrome.—The Hallermann-Streiff is probably an autosomal dominant disorder that includes malformation of the skull and face with characteristic birdlike facies, dental abnormalities, hypotrichosis, dwarfism, and motor and occasional mental retardation. Ocular abnormalities include microphthalmos, cataract, nystagmus, strabismus, and optic disc colobomas. Occasionally blue sclera, underdeveloped iris, and degenerative retinal disease have been reported.[7, 22]

Other less common causes of microphthalmos with coloboma and other nonocular findings include Sjögren-Larsson syndrome, characterized by coloboma, microphthalmos, and mental retardation; humeroradial stenosis, characterized by coloboma, microphthalmos, microcephaly, occipital meningocele, and abnormalities in movement of the elbow; congenital contractural arachnodactyly, characterized by coloboma (usually uveal), microphthalmos, marfanoid habitus, and joint contractures; Lenz microphthalmos syndrome; CHARGE association; epidermal nevus syndrome; Rubinstein-Taybi syndrome; as well as the chromosomal aberrations listed in Table 13–2.

Noncolobomatous Microphthalmos.—Noncolobomatous microphthalmos includes some unusual entities such as Fanconi's syndrome, which is characterized by microphthalmos with congenital hypoplastic anemia, increased skin pigmentation, short stature, skeletal abnormalities, and mental retardation; Diamond-Blackfan syndrome, characterized by microphthalmos with congenital hypoplastic anemia; and oculodentodigital syndrome, which includes microphthalmos, enamel hypoplasia of the teeth, visual anomalies, small palpebral fissures, epicanthal folds, and glaucoma.[22]

Treacher Collins Syndrome.—In addition to microphthalmos, Treacher Collins syndrome includes malar hypoplasia (receding chin), downslanting palpebral fissures, and ear malformations. In addition to this there are lower lid colobomas, mandibular hypoplasia, macrostomia, high palate, and anomalies of the skeleton or gastrointestinal tract.[7, 21]

Congenital Rubella Syndrome.—Resulting from maternal rubella during the first trimester of pregnancy, congenital rubella syndrome may result in ocular findings of cataract, microphthalmos, congenital glaucoma, iris abnormalities, and a salt-and-pepper pigmentary retinopathy. The virus has been known to survive within the lens up to 3 years after birth. The following nonocular findings also occur in congenital rubella syndrome: low birth weight, congenital heart disease, patent ductus arteriosus, CNS abnormalities, thrombocytopenia purpura, diabetes mellitus, osteomyelitis, dental abnormalities, pneumonitis, and hepatomegaly.[2, 7, 22]

ABNORMALITIES ASSOCIATED WITH LARGE EYES

Congenital Glaucoma

After closure of the fetal fissure and formation of the vitreous cavity, the anterior chamber still remains a small, slitlike opening, and the angle is composed of undifferentiated mesodermal cells. At approximately 4 months' gestational age, differentiation begins in the anterior chamber as widening occurs and greater separation between the cornea and iris develops. Cleavage of the angle begins to occur. This mechanism may be secondary to unequal growth rates of the two types of tissues composing the primitive angle. Starting from the fourth month and extending to the eighth month of gestation, collagen and elastic fibrils are seen to form at the base of the fissure to create the trabecular meshwork. Iris processes form as a bridge between the uveal meshwork and the iris root in normal angle cleavage. Failure of this normal development of the angle structures is considered the underlying cause for congenital or infantile glaucoma.

Primary infantile glaucoma is an uncommon, developmental defect of the trabecular meshwork and anterior chamber that manifests itself in the neonatal period, with increasing ocular pressures due to obstruction of aqueous humor outflow. Infantile glaucoma is believed to have an incidence of 1 in 10,000 live births.[38] Although most cases appear sporadic in nature, there may be a recessive inheritance pattern responsible for this.

Two theories may explain the abnormality causing infantile glaucoma. The first holds that there is an imperforate membrane consisting of mesodermal tissue known as Barkan's membrane that covers the trabecular meshwork. This membrane results from improper reabsorption and leads to incomplete angle cleavage. The second holds that abnormal development or failure of proper rearrangement of chamber angle structures results in trabecular dysgenesis. Infantile glaucoma presents initially at birth 25% of the time, 60% at 6 months of age, and 80% during the first year of life. Approximately 75% of infantile glaucoma patients have bilateral disease.[39]

A child with infantile glaucoma exhibits epiphora, photophobia, and blepharospasm. These initial symptoms may occur weeks before any other manifestations of infantile glaucoma are seen. Following this, corneal edema and clouding is noted. The later in life initial corneal edema occurs, the better the prognosis for good future visual acuity. Corneal edema is secondary to increased intraocular pressure and the inability of the corneal endothelium to keep the corneal stroma and epithelium relatively dehydrated and transparent. In early childhood the collagen fibers of the eye are more elastic than in later life. Therefore increased intraocular pressure over a long period causes progressive enlargement of the cornea as well as the entire globe. This enlargement is known as buphthalmos, literally "ox eye." Also associated with enlargement of the cornea are tears that may occur in Descemet's membrane. Initially these tears are seen in the peripheral cornea and run parallel to the limbus. Later they become horizontal and extend into the visual axis. The common term for these tears is *Haab's striae*. Tears in Descemet's membrane are an unusual finding; other than infantile glaucoma, their only other common cause in childhood is birth trauma. In birth trauma the tears tend to occur in one eye, usually the left eye rather than bilaterally. They tend to be oriented vertically, and the left eye is involved more frequently because of the normal position of the head at delivery. On examining a child with congenital glaucoma, the physician may notice an anterior chamber deepened to the point that the angle structures are visible without a gonioscopy lens. In addition, cupping and atrophy of the optic nerve occurs, which leads to permanent visual loss (see Fig 13–1).[38–40]

A more detailed description of findings, etiology, diagnosis, and treatment of infantile glaucoma is found in Chapter 19 of this text.

Buphthalmia

In the previous section the term buphthalmos was introduced. It refers to an enlarged globe secondary to increased intraocular pressure in an eye in which collagen filaments have not yet become rigid and may stretch. Buphthalmia is a rare, autosomal recessive trait not associated with glaucoma or increased intraocular pressure that has sometimes been associated with pedigrees of families with Sturge-Weber syndrome and von Recklinghausen syndrome.[5] Sturge-Weber syndrome is one of the phakomatoses characterized by a congenital cutaneous angioma (nevus flammeus) in the distribution of the trigeminal nerve, ipsilateral meningeal angioma with intracranial calcifications and neurological signs, and angioma of the choroid occasionally with secondary glaucoma. Von Recklinghausen syndrome (neurofibromatosis) is also one of the phakomatoses characterized by café au lait spots, fibroma molluscum, and plexiform neurofibromas. Ocular findings in addition to buphthalmia include proptosis of the globe, lid abnormalities, and Lisch nodules of the iris.

Megalocornea

Megalocornea is defined as a cornea with

a diameter of 13 mm or greater; it must be congenital and stationary. The enlargement is not associated with increased intraocular pressures or optic nerve head cupping. Two subdivisions of megalocornea have been described: the first is simple megalocornea, and the second is called anterior megalophthalmos.

In simple megalocornea there is a proposed autosomal dominant transmission. It is a stationary, bilateral enlarged cornea, usually 12 mm or greater at birth and 13 mm or greater in adulthood. Other than the enlargement of the cornea, the eye is normal histologically. There are no associated ocular abnormalities or systemic abnormalities.

Anterior megalophthalmos occurs more frequently than simple megalocornea and has an X-linked inheritance pattern. It is bilateral, symmetrical, and nonprogressive. The cornea may be clear or have a mosaic dystrophy, and there is no corneal thickening. Ocular abnormalities include a deep anterior chamber with iris hypoplasia and an angle that is wide open with excess mesenchymal tissue and pigmentation of the trabecular meshwork. Some of these patients have lens subluxations leading to secondary glaucoma. They also tend to develop cataracts in the fifth decade of life. Occasionally systemic skeletal, neurological, or dermatologic abnormalities are associated with anterior megalophthalmos.[41,42]

Keratoglobus

Keratoglobus is a rare, bilateral, autosomal recessive malformation of the cornea that is characterized by a markedly thinned cornea. The thinning is mostly peripheral to as much as one third its normal thickness. The corneal diameter is usually normal, with a protruding appearance and keratometry readings of 50 to 60 D. Because of the extreme thinness of the cornea it is predisposed to rupture with minor trauma. For this reason children with this abnormality should avoid contact sports. Occasionally there are spontaneous breaks in Descemet's membrane that lead to acute hydrops of the cornea. The globe, other than the corneal changes, is totally normal. Biglan proposed that keratoglobus may be part of the Ehlers-Danlos syndrome because it is frequently associated with blue scleras, hyperextendability of hand and ankle joints, hearing loss, and dental abnormalities.[41–43]

CONCLUSION

Anomalies in the size and shape of the eye in the newborn are relatively common, occurring in approximately 1.5% of all newborns.[31] Most are associated with arrest of normal development. If this occurs before 2 weeks' gestational age when the optic vesicle is formed, anophthalmia, cyclopia, congenital cystic eye, or nonattachment of the retina may occur. If arrest occurs at the fourth week, congenital aphakia or cataracts may abound. If arrest is between 4 and 6 weeks during closure of the embryonic fissure, typical colobomatous abnormalities are found. During the 2nd to 8th months of gestation the primary vitreous humor is formed. If it does not resorb at birth, a child may be found to have PHPV, Bergmeister's papilla, Mittendorf's dot, or a persistent pupillary membrane. Arrest during the last 2 months of gestation may lead to congenital glaucoma secondary to anomalous anterior chamber angle cleavage. Microphthalmos may accompany nearly all of these abnormalities and may vary from mild to severe. When a patient is seen with microphthalmos, it is essential to evaluate ocular function and look for other anatomic abnormalities. Special attention should be given to systemic abnormalities that are frequently associated with microphthalmos.

REFERENCES

1. Singh YP, Gupta SL: Congenital ocular abnormalities of the newborn *J Pediatr Ophthalmol Strabismus* 1986; 17:162.
2. Apple DJ, Rabb MF: *Ocular Pathology—Clinical Applications and Self Assessment.* St Louis, CV Mosby Co, 1985, p 10.
3. Mann I: *The Development of the Human Eye.* Philadelphia, JB Lippincott, 1964, p 1.
4. Smith ME: *Fundamentals & Principles of*

Ophthalmology. San Francisco, American Academy of Ophthalmology, 1984, p 106.
5. Mann I: *Developmental Abnormalities of the Eye*. Philadelphia, JB Lippincott, 1957, p 60, 94, 113, 235, 315.
6. Al-Ghadyan AA, Kazi GQ, Cotlier E: Anophthalmos and first brachial arch defects. *Ophthalmic Paediatr Genet* 1985; 6:169.
7. Spaeth GL, Nelson LB, Beaudon AR: Ocular tetratology, in Duane TD, Jaeger EA (eds): *Biomedical Foundations of Ophthalmology,* vol 1. Philadelphia, Harper & Row, Publishers, Inc, 1986.
8. Torczynski E, Jakobiec FA: Cyclopia & synophthalmia: A model of embryonic interactions, in Duane TD, Jaeger EA (eds): *Biomedical Foundations of Ophthalmology,* vol. 1. Philadelphia, Harper & Row, Publishers, Inc, 1986.
9. Weiss A, Martinez C, Greenwald M: Microphthalmos with cyst: Clinical presentation and computed tomographic findings. *J Pediatr Ophthalmol Strabismus* 1985; 22:6.
10. Worgul BU: Lens, in Duane TD, Jaeger EA (eds): *Biomedical Foundations of Ophthalmology,* vol 1. Philadelphia, Harper & Row, Publishers, Inc. 1986.
11. Baker WH: Congenital aphakia. *NY Med J* 1887; 46:595.
12. von Szily, A: Die Ontogenese der Iris Kolobom. *Klin Monatsbl Augenheilkd* 1907; 45:422.
13. Francois, J: Colobomatous malformations of the ocular globe. *Int Ophthalmol Clin* 1968; 97:797.
14. Man I: *Developmental Abnormalities of the Eye*. Philadelphia, JB Lippincott, 1957, p 74.
15. Pagon RA: Ocular colobomas. *Surv Ophthalmol* 1981; 25:223.
16. Jesberg DA, Schepens CL: Retinal detachment associated with coloboma of the choroid. *Arch Ophthalmol* 1961; 65:165.
17. Apple DJ, Rabb MF, Walsh PM: Congenital anomalies of the optic disc. *Surv Ophthalmol* 1982; 27:3.
18. Kronberg B: Microphthalmia associated with a variety of congenital anomalies in three siblings, *NY Med J* 1949; 47:78.
19. McMillan L: Anophthalmos and maldevelopment of the eyes: Four cases in the same family. *Br J Ophthalmol* 1921; 5:121.
20. Renie WA: *Goldberg's Genetic & Metabolic Eye Disease*. Boston, Little, Brown & Co, Inc, 1986.
21. Edwards W: Facial and orbital dysplastic syndromes, in Duane TD, Jaeger EA (eds): *Biomedical Foundations of Ophthalmology,* vol 1. Philadelphia, Harper & Row, Publishers, Inc, 1986.
22. Bateman JB: Microphthalmos. *Int Ophthalmol Clin* 1984; 24:87.
23. Mitchell JA: Dominant CHARGE association. *Ophthalmic Paediatr Genet* 1985; 6:31.
24. Murphree AL: Chromosomes: Structure, function & clinical syndromes, in Duane TD, Jaeger EA (eds): *Biomedical Foundations of Ophthalmology,* vol 3. Philadelphia, Harper and Row, Publishers, Inc, 1986.
25. Krause U: The syndrome of Goldenhar affecting two siblings. *Acta Ophthalmol* 1970; 48:494.
26. Baum JL, Feingold M: Ocular aspects of Goldenhar's syndrome. *Am J Ophthalmol* 1973; 75:250.
27. Brown GC, Shields JA, Rutty BE, et al: Congenital pits of optic nerve head: I. Experimental studies in collie dogs. *Arch Ophthalmol* 1979; 97:1341.
28. Jensen OA: Persistent hyperplastic primary vitreous cases in Denmark. *Acta Ophthalmol* 1968; 46:418.
29. Federman JL, Shields JA, Altman B, et al: The surgical and nonsurgical management of PHPV. *Ophthalmology* 1984; 97:632.
30. Karr DJ, Scott WE: Visual acuity results following treatment of PHPV. *Arch Ophthalmol* 1986; 104:662.
31. Maumenee AE: PHPV: Results of surgery. *Trans Am Acad Ophthalmol* 1974; 78:911.
32. Nelson LB, Folberg R: Ocular developmental anomalies, in Duane TD, Jaeger EA (eds): *Biomedical Foundations of Ophthalmology,* vol 3. Philadelphia, Harper & Row, Publishers, Inc, 1986.
33. Waring GO, Shields JA: Partial unilateral cryptophthalmos with syndactyly, brachycephaly, and renal anomalies. *Am J Ophthalmol* 1975; 79:437.
34. Cennamo G, Magli A, Corrino C: Genetic and ultrasound study of hereditary pure microphthalmos. *Ophthalmic Paediatr Genet* 1985; 6:33.
35. Ryan EA, Zwann J, Chylack LT: Nanophthalmos with uveal effusions. *Ophthalmology* 1982; 89:1013.
36. Singh OS, Simmons RJ: Nanophthalmos, a prospective on identification and treatment. *Ophthalmology* 1982; 89:1006.

37. Foxman S, Cameron JD: The clinical implications of bilateral microphthalmos with cyst. *Am J Ophthalmol* 1984; 97:632.
38. DeLuise VP, Anderson DA: Primary infantile glaucoma. *Surv Ophthalmol* 1983; 28:1.
39. Kolker AE, Hetherington J: *Becker and Schaffer's Diagnosis and Therapy of the Glaucomas.* St Louis, CV Mosby Co, 1983, p 317.
40. Bardelli AM, Hadjistilienou T, Frezzotti R: Etiology of congenital glaucoma. *Ophthalmic Paediatr Genet* 1985; 6:25.
41. Waring GO, Rodriques MM: Congenital and neonatal corneal abnormalities, in Duane TD, Jaeger EA (eds): *Biomedical Foundations of Ophthalmology,* vol 1. Philadelphia, Harper & Row, Publishers, Inc, 1986.
42. Harley RD: *Pediatric Ophthalmology,* ed 2. Philadelphia, WB Sanders Co, 1983, p 468.
43. Biglan AW, Brown SI, Johnson BL: Keratoglobus and blue sclera. *Am J Ophthalmol* 1977; 83:225.

14 Abnormalities of the Eyelids

J. S. Crawford, M.D.
R. C. Pashby, M.D.

The rudiments of the eyelids appear very early in fetal development (16 mm) as two folds in the ectoderm. The upper lid, which is two parts (median and lateral), grows downward from the frontonasal process, and the lower lid grows upward from the maxillary process. The folds of ectoderm become skin on the outside and conjunctiva on the inside. The mesoderm grows in and forms the tarsal plate and the connective tissue of the substance of the lid. At about the eighth week of gestation, the eyelids fuse together, beginning at the inner canthus. At the end of the fifth month, the lids begin to separate, starting at the nasal side. This process is completed during the sixth month.

When this normal progression of lid development is interrupted, a wide range of congenital anomalies occurs. In some cases, restoring the eyelid to as normal function and appearance as possible presents a considerable challenge to the ophthalmologist.

ABNORMALITIES OF THE LID FOLDS

Cryptophthalmos

Cryptophthalmos (ablepharia) is a rare congenital anomaly in which there is a total ablepharia due to the complete failure of the lid folds to develop. The skin passes continuously from the forehead over the eye to the cheek. The extent of the condition varies. Figure 14–1,A shows the absence of an upper lid. The skin has not separated from the cornea. The lower lid is present, but there is a very poor lower fornix. The epithelium, which normally becomes differentiated into the cornea and conjunctiva, is transformed into integument, so skin passes continuously from the forehead over the eye and down to the lower lid border. It is very difficult to create a conjunctival sac to hold a prosthesis. The patient shown in Figure 14–1,A had a pedicle flap brought down from the forehead to create an upper lid as seen in Figure 14–1,B. The skin defect in the forehead was then closed with a free skin graft.

Microblepharia

Microblepharia is a developmental, vertical shortening of the lids. It is a rare anomaly in which the lids are normally formed but are not quite long enough to allow the eye to close in sleep. This may result in lagophthalmos (where eyelids cannot be completely closed), which in turn may lead to corneal problems as a result of exposure.

Any congenital anomaly associated with increased vertical diameter of the orbit may give rise to a condition that simulates microblepharia.

Coloboma

A coloboma is a defect in the lid border. Typically, the defect is triangular, with its base at the lid margin. The notch may be quadrilateral or irregular. Upper lid colobomas, which constitute the majority of these defects, usually affect the medial half of the lid, whereas

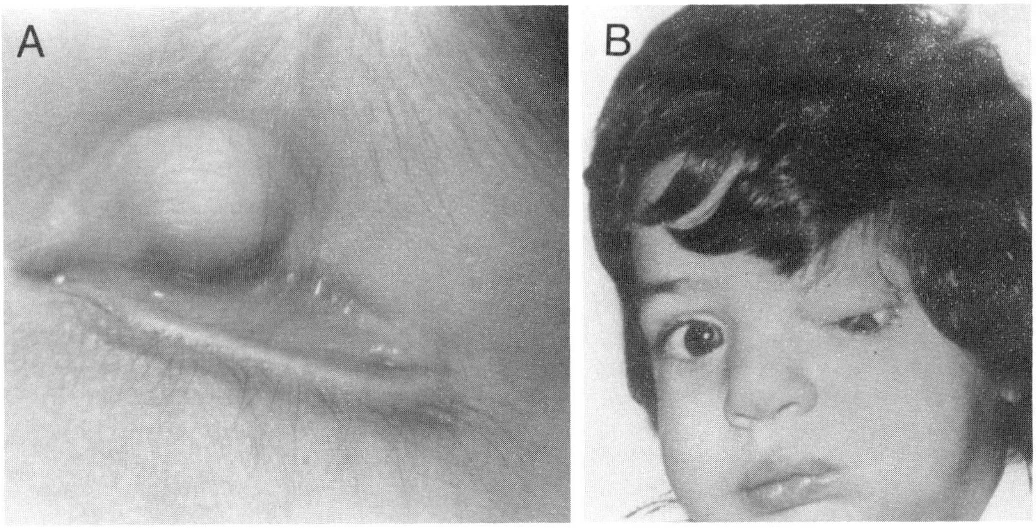

FIG 14–1.
A, ablepharia or absence of the upper lid. The skin has not separated from the cornea. The lower lid is present but there is a very poor lower fornix. **B,** a pedicle flap has been brought down from the forehead to create an upper lid.

lower lid lesions affect the lateral half. There may be several colobomas on the same lid. They may occur in one lid, the same lids on each eye, or all four lids. The degree of severity determines the surgical techniques used in their repair. Early treatment offers very satisfactory results.

A coloboma may occur in isolation or be associated with other developmental anomalies such as cleft palate, harelip, various types of mandibulofacial dysostosis, dermoids, or lipodermoids. The defect may be triangular or rectangular.

Successful repair of any coloboma is based on the principle of anchoring the lid to firm tissue, either adjacent tarsus or periosteum. A small coloboma (up to 25% of the lid margin) may be closed in the upper or lower lids directly after freshening the margins or excising a wedge of tissue to include the defect (Fig 14–2, A–D).

Larger colobomas (25% to 50% of the lid margin) require a relaxation cantholysis of the upper or lower arm of the lateral canthal tendon to provide relaxation and permit direct closure. If sufficient relaxation has not been obtained, an incision is made along the side of the face, with one vertical incision above and one below the horizontal incision so as to form a Z flap (Fig 14–3).

Meticulous closure of the skin margins is required. This is done by using 8-0 silk and polyglactin 910 (Vicryl) or polyglycolic acid (Dexon) sutures to approximate the tarsal borders. In large colobomas, the edges of the defect are covered with palpebral conjunctiva, which connects the lid to the bulbar conjunctiva. The medial stump has a thickened edge that is thought to be caused by contracture of the muscle tissue. In many such cases, the cornea thickens, and opacities develop (Fig 14–4, A–C).

For a large, shallow defect of the upper lid involving more than half of the lid margin, the skin and muscle are reflected from that tarsus, and a T-shaped incision is made (Fig 14–5, A and B). The arms of the T are overlapped and sutured (Fig 14–5,C). Since this method causes shortening of the upper lid, a wedge or full thickness of tissue should be removed from the lower lid to maintain symmetry (Fig 14–5,D and E). This operation was described by Erbakan.[1]

The lower lid defects seen in Treacher

Collins syndrome present a problem because of the shortage of conjunctiva and skin (Fig 14–6, A). If there is a great shortage of skin in the lower lid, a skin graft can be taken from behind the ear and placed in the lower lid, as seen in Figure 14–6,B. When the defect is not as large, it can be corrected by the method shown in Figure 14–6,C, as described by Jackson.[2]

Treacher Collins Syndrome

Children with Treacher Collins syndrome (mandibulofacial dysostosis, Franceschetti-Klein syndrome; Fig 14–6, A) have antimongoloid slanting palpebral fissures, malar hypoplasia, lower eyelid coloboma, partial to total absence of lower eyelashes, malformation of the auricles, external ear canal defects, conductive deafness, cleft palate, and continuation of scalp hair onto the cheek.

Goldenhar Syndrome

Goldenhar syndrome is also known as first and second branchial arch syndrome, oculoauricular vertebral dysplasia, and hemifacial microsomia. The predominant defects result from errors of development of the first and second branchial arches, sometimes accom-

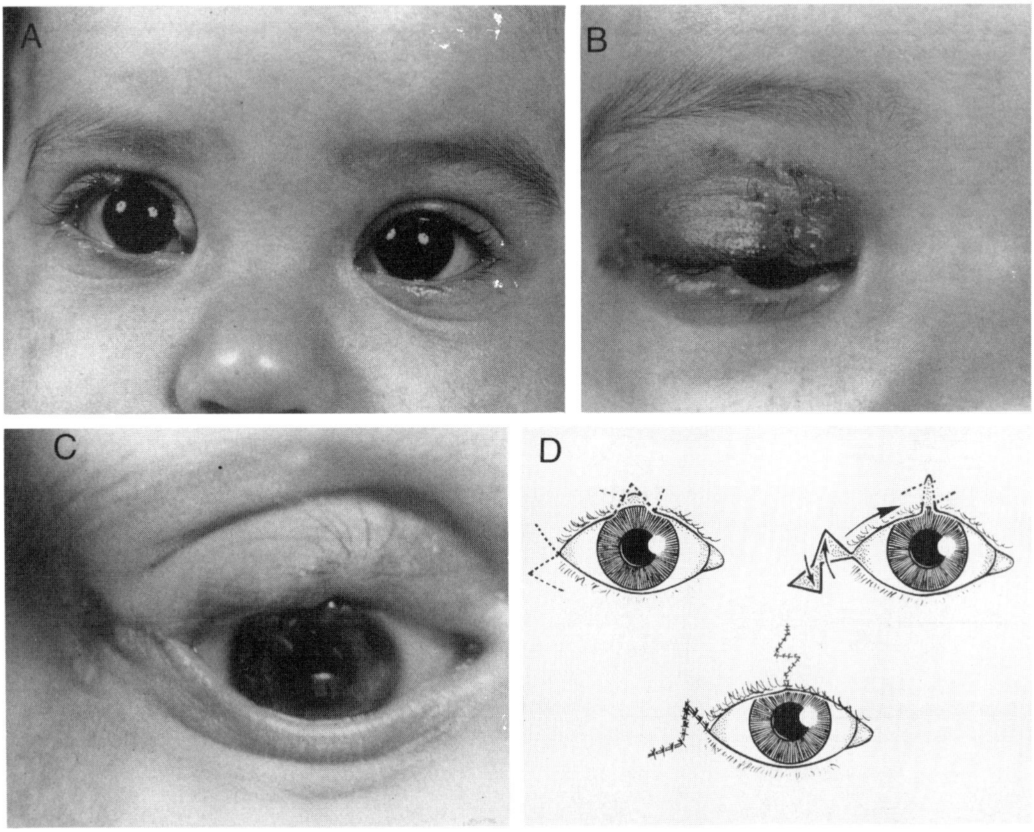

FIG 14–2.
A, a coloboma of slightly less than half the upper lid. **B**, the day after repair. **C**, 3 months postoperatively. **D**, the edges of the coloboma are freshened and then closed directly, thus shortening the upper lid. A Z-plasty is performed at the outer canthus. A triangle of skin is brought up into the upper lid, thereby shortening the lower lid and lengthening the upper. (From Crawford JS, Morin JD (eds): *The Eye in Childhood.* New York, Grune & Stratton, 1983. Used with permission.)

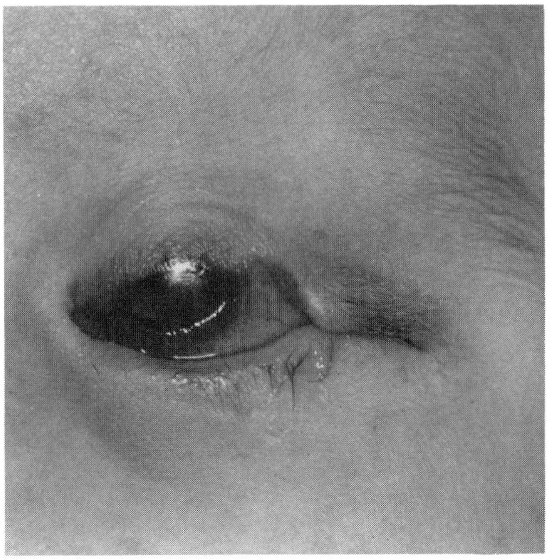

FIG 14–3.
A coloboma of more than half the upper lid. The skin over the medial two thirds is fused to the sclera and the upper cornea. (From Crawford JS, Morin JD (eds): *The Eye in Childhood.* New York, Grune & Stratton, 1983. Used with permission.)

panied by vertebral and ocular anomalies. The malar, maxillary, and/or mandibular regions are hypoplastic, especially the ramus and condyle of the mandible and temporomandibular joint. There is a lateral cleftlike extension of the corner of the mouth, and the facial musculature may be hypoplastic. Eye anomalies consist of epibulbar dermoid, lipodermoid, notch in the upper lid, strabismus, and microphthalmos.

Epicanthus

Four recognized types of epicanthus have been described by Carl Johnson[3]: in epicanthus supraciliaris the epicanthal fold arises in the region of the eyebrow and runs toward the tear sac (Fig 14–7, A); in epicanthus palpebralis the epicanthal fold arises from the upper lid above the tarsal region and extends to the lower border of the orbit (Fig 14–7,B); in epicanthus tarsalis the epicanthal fold arises from the tarsal region and loses itself in the

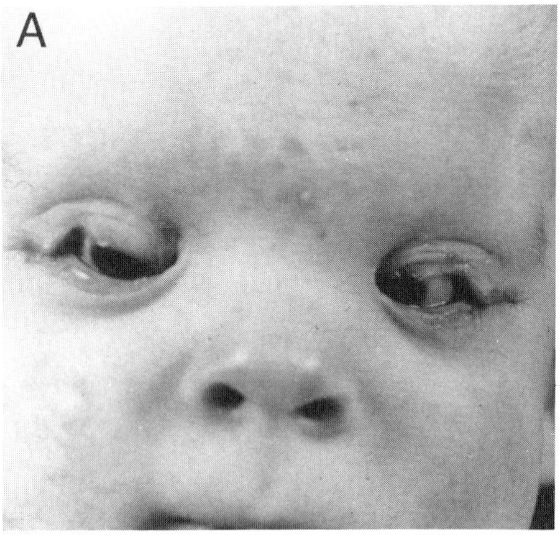

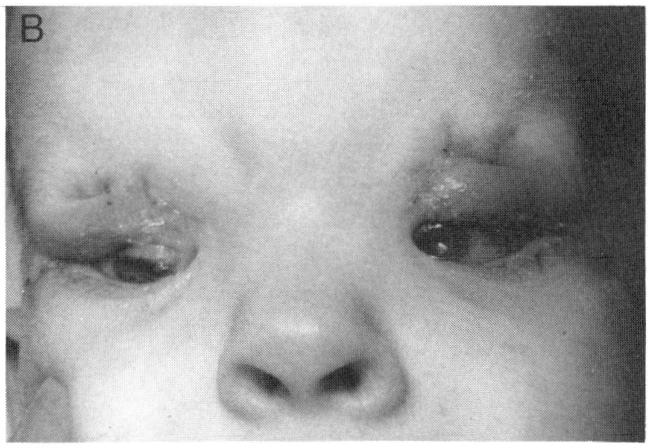

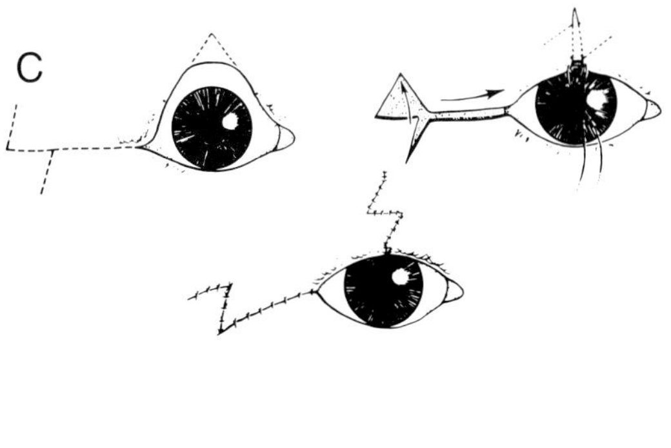

FIG 14–4.
A, large coloboma with skin over the medial two thirds of the lid fused to the sclera. **B,** after repair. **C,** an incision is made along the side of the face, with one vertical incision above and one below the horizontal incision so as to make a Z flap. The skin is moved medially, and a triangle of skin from the lower lid is swung up into the upper lid to fill the defect.

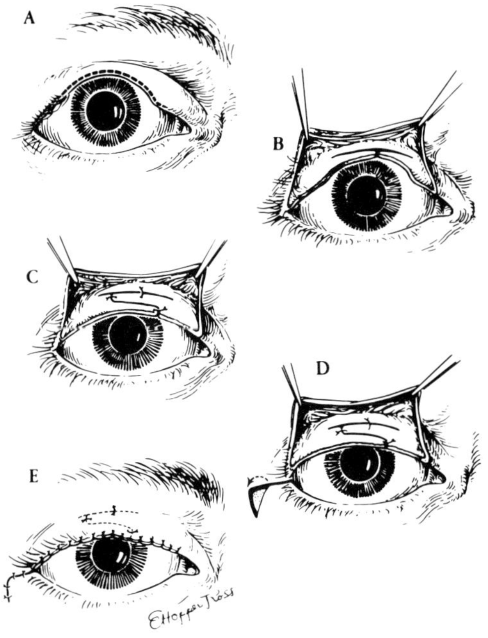

FIG 14–5.
Treatment of a large shallow defect of the upper lid: **A** and **B,** skin and muscle reflected from the tarsus and T-shaped incision. **C,** the arms of the T overlapped and sutured. **D,** a triangular piece of skin removed from the outer canthus to shorten the lower lid. **E,** the skin sutured back into the normal position. (From Crawford JS, Morin JD (eds): *The Eye in Childhood.* New York, Grune & Stratton, 1983. Used with permission.)

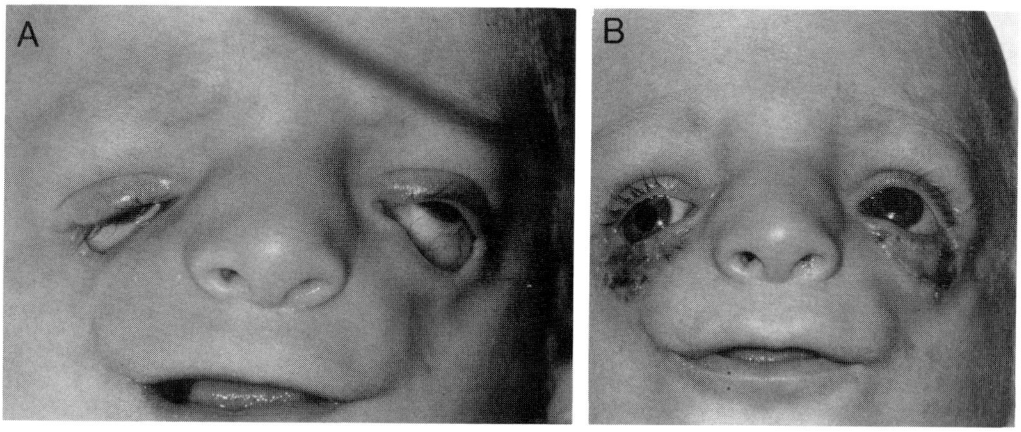

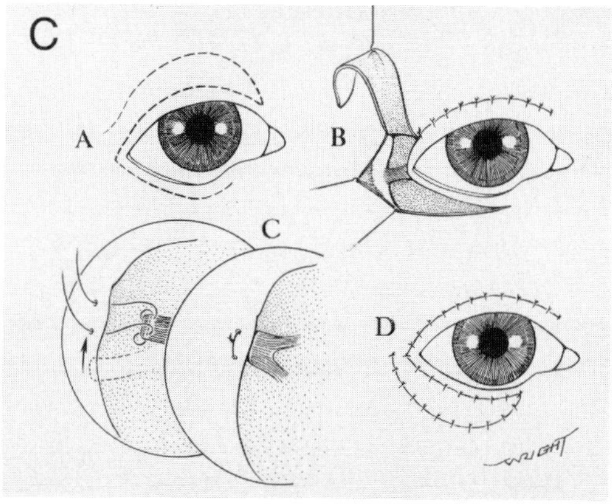

FIG 14–6.
A, a young patient with Treacher Collins syndrome. **B,** after skin graft. **C,** repair of lids in a child with Treacher Collins syndrome where the outer side of the lower lid is too low. An incision is made across the lower lid. A flap is raised in the upper lid of a length sufficient to reconstruct the lower lid defect. This full-thickness graft is subcutaneous tissue, tarsal plate, and conjunctiva. The lateral canthal ligament is cut from its attachment and reattached from the orbital rim in its proper position.

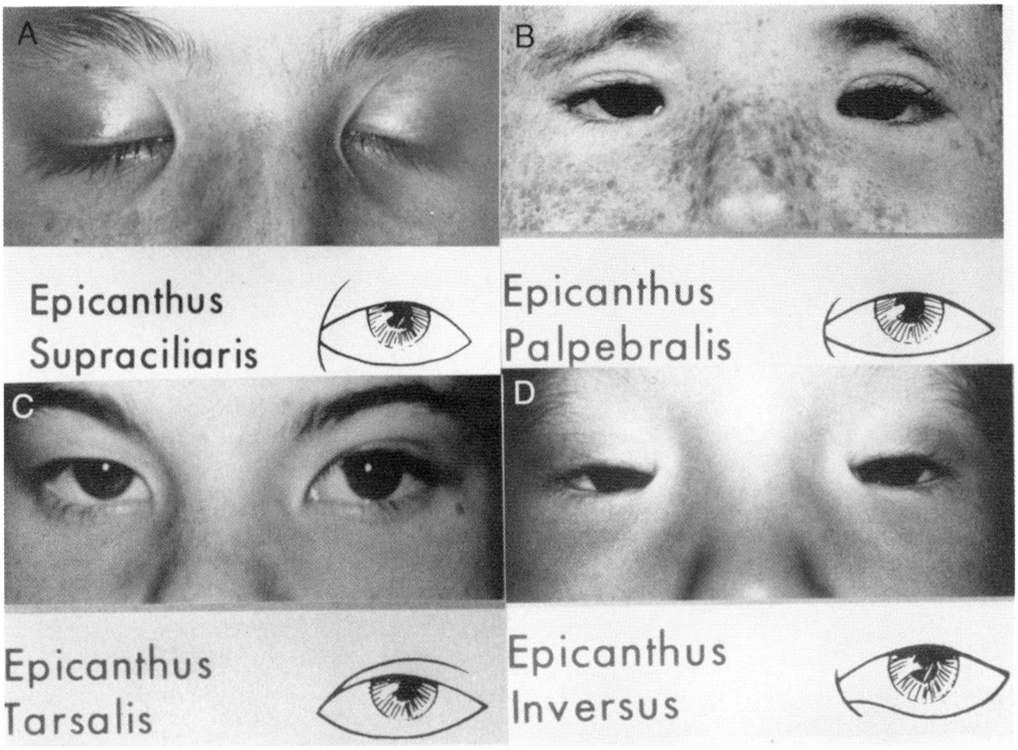

FIG 14–7.
A, epicanthus supraciliaris. **B,** epicanthus palpebralis. **C,** epicanthus tarsalis. **D,** epicanthus inversus. (From Crawford JS, Morin JD (eds): *The Eye in Childhood.* New York, Grune & Stratton, 1983. Used with permission.)

skin close to the inner canthus (Fig 14–7,C); and in epicanthus inversus the fold arises in the lower lid and extends upwards, partially covering the inner canthus (Fig 14–7,D). Epicanthus inversus is always associated with some degree of blepharophimosis (see later) and ptosis with poor levator function.

Epicanthus represents a shortage of skin in the medial canthal region, and treatment should be directed toward increasing the amount of skin in the area to relieve the lines of tension. The V-Y operation of Verwey usually gives disappointing results. However, a satisfactory correction is achieved when using the Roveda[4] operation, which is a modification of the V-Y procedure and consists of a series of small skin flaps that eliminate the skin fold (Fig 14–8).

Congenital Ptosis and Abnormalities of the Levator Palpebrae Superioris

Most (62% to 88%) surgical cases of ptosis are classified as congenital,[5,6] and most patients with congenital ptosis have no family history of any similar condition. Ptosis may be unilateral or bilateral and may occur with a normal superior rectus or with superior rectus weakness. Many cases of congenital blepharoptosis are associated with a weakness of the ipsilateral superior rectus muscle, which is developmental and not innervational.

There is a synkinetic group of ptosis cases that includes Marcus Gunn jaw-winking syndrome and misdirected third-nerve ptosis. From 4% to 6% of congenital ptosis cases are associated with Marcus Gunn syndrome, which is characterized by ptosis, with up and down movements of the lid associated with the opening and closing of the mouth or moving the jaw from side to side. This anomaly is first noticed by the mother when the baby is sucking. The problem is almost always unilateral, and the amount of lid movement varies from minimal to large and conspicuous and affects the patient's appearance adversely.[7]

The surgical treatment involves excising a large section of the levator muscle and then suspending the lid from the frontalis muscle with autogenous fascia lata. The most symmetrical result is obtained by doing a similar procedure on the other lid; however, most surgeons place fascia lata in the normal lid without excising the levator muscle. Since there is more swelling in the lid from which the levator has been excised, that lid should be raised higher than the normal lid; if this is not done, it will be lower when the swelling has subsided. The most symmetrical result is achieved by excising a section of levator at one operation and then putting the fascia in both lids 1 month or more later. The surgery is done after 3.5 years of age when autogenous fascia can be obtained and before the child starts to school at the age of 5 years.

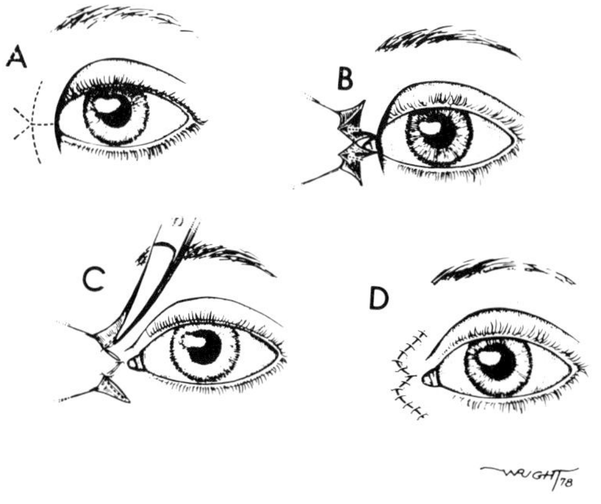

FIG 14–8.
Roveda's operation. A line is drawn parallel to and about 5 to 6 mm medially to the edge of the epicanthal fold. At the midpoint of the curve, a horizontal line is drawn from the medial canthal angle to the curved line that has been drawn previously. Two arms of the Y are drawn to a distance of 5 to 7 mm toward the nose. **A,** the angle between these two lines is 90 degrees. **B,** the curved line is incised, and then the skin is cut in the Y. The skin is undermined in all directions. **C,** the two small triangular flaps of skin are trimmed off. The two triangular flaps are advanced medially to fill the spaces previously occupied by the excised triangular flaps. **D,** the wound, which is now W shaped, is closed with 6-0 cat gut sutures in children or nylon sutures in adults. (From Crawford JS, Morin JD (eds): *The Eye in Childhood.* New York, Grune & Stratton, 1983. Used with permission.)

Congenital ptosis is frequently associated with the following syndromes: blepharophimosis, congenital fibrosis, Dubowitz's, epicanthus inversus, Freeman-Sheldon, Marcus-Gunn Möbius' anomalad, and Saethre-Chotzen. Occasionally, it is associated with fetal alcohol syndrome, fetal trimethadione, Noonan syndrome, Robinstein-Taybi syndrome, and misdirected third-nerve ptosis.

Ptosis Associated With Third-Nerve Palsy

In patients with third-nerve palsy, the only extraocular muscles that continue to function are the external rectus and the superior oblique. The eye is pulled outward and downward, and ptosis of the upper lid is present. The patient has a negative Bell's phenomenon, and therefore, care must be taken in correcting the ptosis. Frontalis suspension surgery is required because of the paralysis of the levator muscle. Unless the eye is straightened and carefully watched for corneal exposure problems, it may be better not to carry out any ptosis surgery.

Turner Syndrome

Turner syndrome involves gonadal dysgenesis in females. Patients have short stature and neck webbing. Sexual maturation does not occur. Eye defects are rare, but there may be bilateral congenital ptosis associated with epicanthus, strabismus, or cataracts.

Apert Syndrome

Children with Apert syndrome (syndactylic oxycephaly) have a short anterior-posterior diameter of the skull with a high full forehead and flat occiput. They have flat facies,

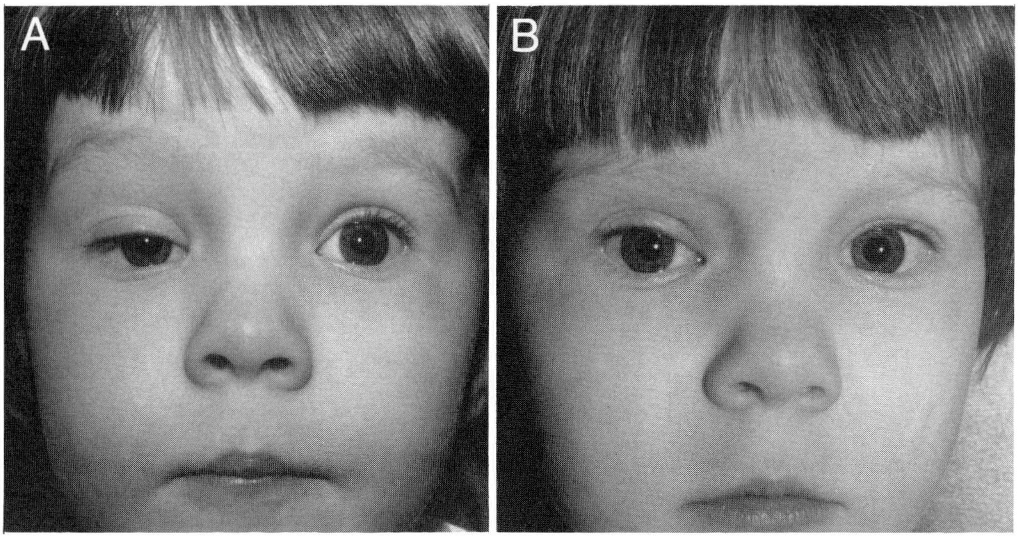

FIG 14–9.
A, a young girl with a 3-mm ptosis of the right upper lid with a 12-mm levator excursion. **B**, following Müller's muscle resection (Gavaris' technique).

shallow orbits, hypertelorism, strabismus, down-slanting palpebral fissures, a small nose, and maxillary hypoplasia.

Horner Syndrome

A small ptosis is usually present with Horner syndrome. The other signs include a small pupil, enophthalmos, and lack of sweating (anhydrosis) on the affected side. The ptosis may not be large enough to require repair. Good results can be obtained by a müllerectomy (Fasanella-Servat or Gavaris' operations).

Abnormalities of the Levator Palpebrae Superioris

Two studies have been carried out to examine the pathology of ptosis; Berke and Wadsworth[6] used light microscopy to examine levator tissue removed at surgery and Hornblass and coworkers[8] used electron microscopy to study levator muscle specimens. They noted that in cases where there was no levator function, there were no striated muscle fibers. Berke and Wadsworth found a definite correlation between the amount of ptosis and the number of striated muscle fibers and concluded that true congenital ptosis results from a developmental anomaly of the levator muscle.

Ptosis of the upper eyelid is judged by the amount the lid or lids are low, for example, how much the lower lid is below the cornea, and also by the extent of the excursion of the lid (indicating the function of the levator muscle). If the ptosis is small and the excursion is good, shortening of Müller's muscle is all that is required (Fig 14–9,A and B). When the ptosis is greater but the levator function is good, levator resection is needed (Fig 14–10,A and B). When there is a large ptosis with poor levator function, the lid is suspended from the frontalis muscle by using fascia lata. Usually the fascia is placed in both eyelids to achieve a symmetrical result (Fig 14–11,A and B). Beard[5] and Crawford[9] provide more detailed explanations of treatment.

Ptosis of the Lower Eyelids

Ptosis of the lower eyelid is a rare condition that occurs in some cases of Down syndrome, in variations of the Treacher Collins syndrome, and occasionally in normal children. It results in a dry cornea.

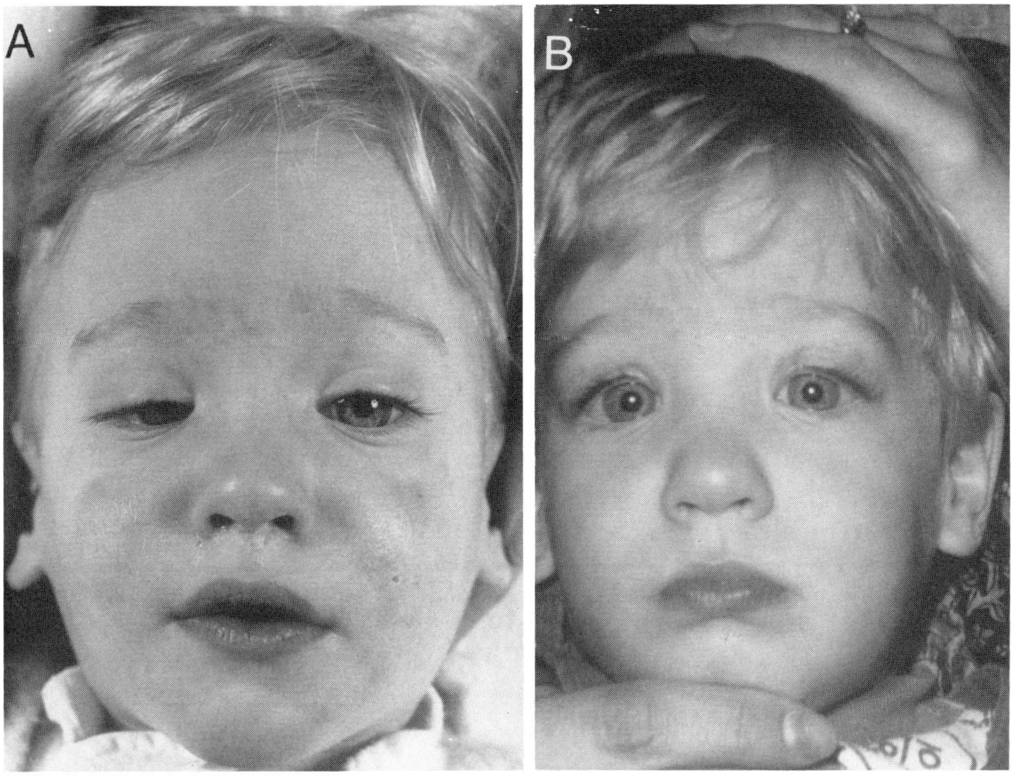

FIG 14–10.
A, large ptosis of the right upper lid with good levator function. **B,** after right levator resection.

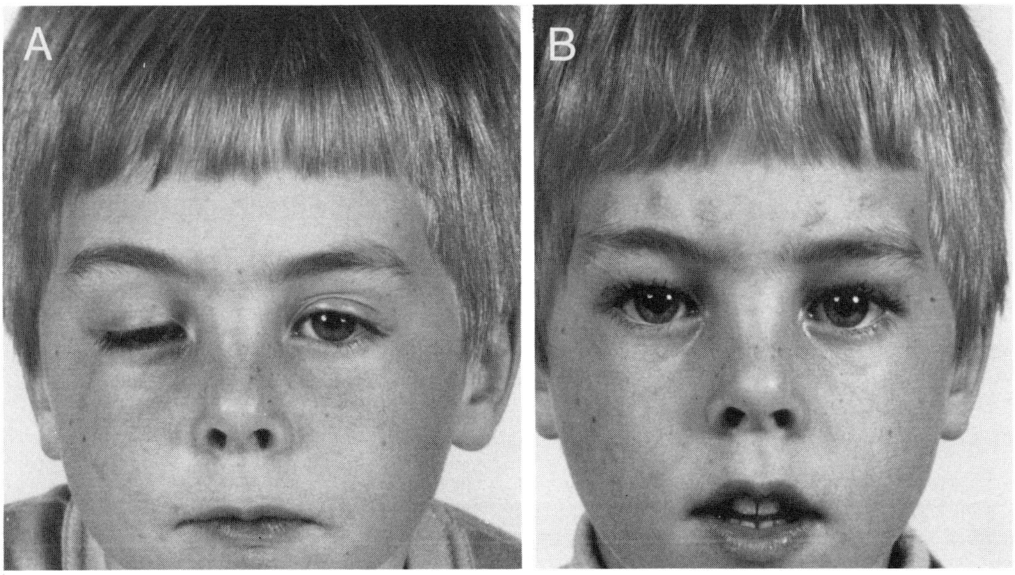

FIG 14–11.
A, a young boy with a large ptosis of the right upper lid with only 3 mm of levator excursion. **B,** postoperative results. Both upper lids have been suspended from the frontalis muscles to obtain a symmetrical lagophthalmos.

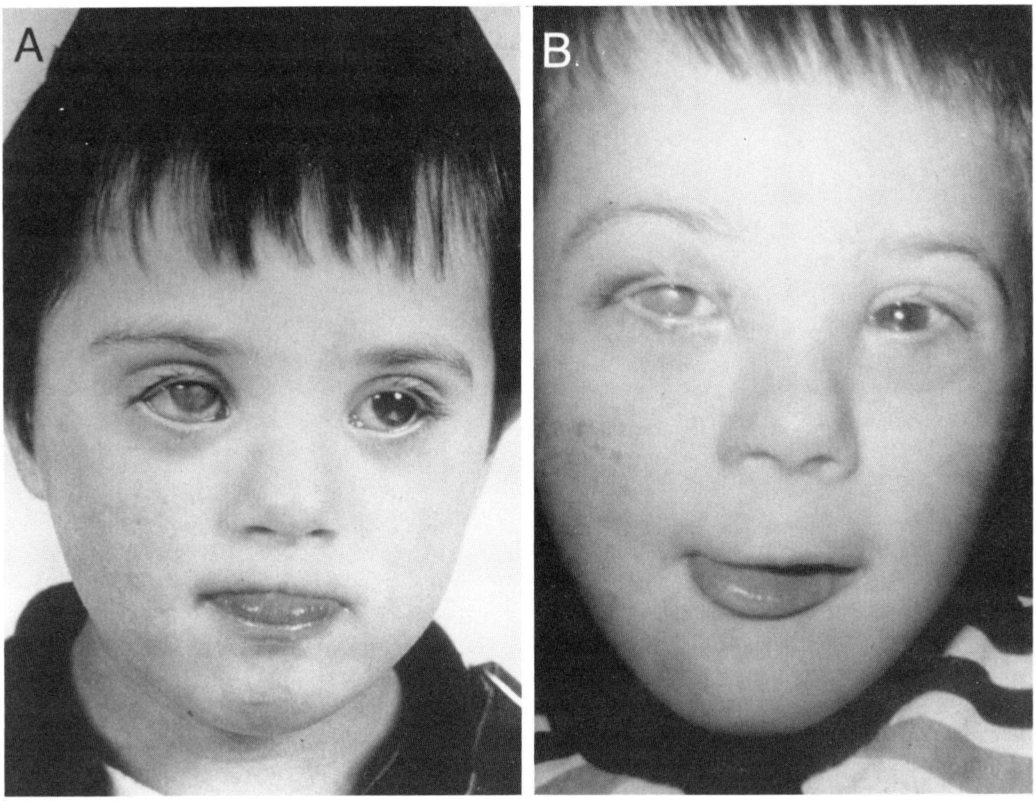

FIG 14–12.
A, a child with Down syndrome with ptosis of the lower lids. **B**, the lower lid is held up by fascia fastened medially through a hole in the nasal bone and laterally through a hole in the lateral orbital rim.

If there is adequate skin, the lower lids may be held up with a strip of fascia that is attached medially through a hole in the bone, similar to that made for transnasal wiring, or it may be attached to the medial canthal ligament. The fascia is run laterally in front of the tarsus and brought up and through a hole drilled in the lateral orbital wall. It is pulled up until the lid is in the proper position and then sutured to itself (Fig 14–12,A and B). If there is insufficient skin, a graft from behind the ear may have to be used.

Blepharmophimosis

Blepharmophimosis is a narrowing of the palpebral aperture that is often associated with epicanthus inversus, ptosis, and telecanthus. It is frequently transmitted as an autosomal dominant trait but can occur without a family history of it. Three types of blepharophimosis are recognized[3, 10]: type 1, the classic triad of epicanthus inversus, ptosis, and telecanthus (Fig 14–13); type 2, ptosis, telecanthus, absent epicanthal folds, and skin shortage (Fig 14–14) in the lids that cause a degree of lagophthalmos; and type 3, the same as type 2 but with the addition of low placed lateral canthal tendons and mild hypertelorism. Telecanthus is defined as increased width between the medial canthi, normal interpupillary distance, and no radiological evidence of abnormal width of nasal bones. Hypertelorism is defined as increased width between the eyes as measured by increased interpupillary distances. There is radiological evidence of excessive nasoethmoid bones and increased interorbital width.

The surgical repair of blepharophimosis varies with the type and severity of the abnormality.[11] The treatment for type 1 consists of medial canthal and ptosis surgery. Often a two-stage procedure is used, with medial canthal surgery done first (as described before for epicanthus treatment) and ptosis surgery performed 6 months later. Both procedures can be completed at the same time, but revision surgery may be required at a later date. At The Hospital for Sick Children, Toronto, we prefer Roveda's technique[4] to the Mustarde Z-Z–plasty, or the V-to-Y–plasty described by Callahan[12] and Spaeth.[13] The amount of correction with Roveda's repair is equal to the others, and the scars are cosmetically more acceptable. The ptosis can be corrected by levator resection if levator function is good. More frequently, a bilateral fascia lata frontalis suspension procedure is used because levator function is usually poor to minimal.

Treatment for type 2 blepharophimosis may require retroauricular skin grafts to the lids, with later repair of medial canthus and ptosis. The dilemma faced here is how long one can temporarily close the lids to allow the skin grafts to heal without causing amblyopia. Type 3 repair requires correction of hypertelorism. Today, the surgery is usually performed by a craniofacial surgeon, and the orbits are moved closer together. Repair of epicanthus and ptosis may have to be done later. When the craniofacial surgery is performed, care must be taken not to interrupt the nasolacrimal drainage apparatus since this might lead to later epiphora or chronic dacryocystitis. Silicone tube intubation may be needed at surgery.

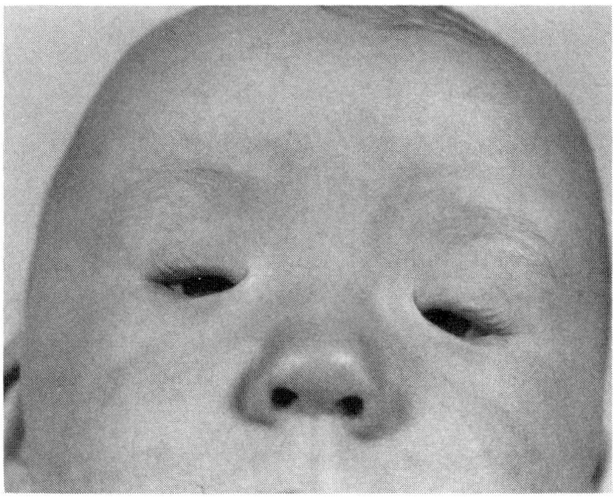

FIG 14–13.
Blepharophimosis, type 1. This child has a narrow palpebral aperture, ptosis, epicanthus inversus, and telecanthus.

CONGENITAL LID RETRACTION

Lid retraction may be a problem in patients with thyroid disease or overcorrected ptosis and occurs occasionally as a congenital condition without antecedent disease. In such cases, the patients must be medically assessed to determine the etiology.

Surgery is indicated when corneal exposure problems arise and also for cosmetic reasons. The methods for correcting retracted lids include Berke's levator tenotomy. However, we have found that a more predictable result is obtained by using a scleral graft (usually fresh sclera).[14] The graft should be 2 to 3 mm wider (vertically) and 2 mm longer than the amount by which the lid must be lowered (Fig 14–15,A and B).

CONJUNCTIVAL PROLAPSE

Prolapse of the conjunctiva of the upper lid is extremely rare. It may be either unilateral or bilateral and may be present from birth or a few days later. The etiology of this condition is obscure. Blechman and Isenberg[15] studied the surgical anatomy of a case of congenital eyelid eversion. At surgery they found adipose tissue beneath the tendon of the levator palpebrae and extending anteriorly to the tarsus because the orbital septum was not attached inferiorly. The defect was repaired. In this case, nonattachment of the orbital septum may have induced eversion of the upper lids.

Lid eversion may be present when there is very little or no birth trauma. The lid or lids are everted, the conjunctiva is prolapsed (Fig 14–16,A and B), and the tissues are edematous and partially strangulated. Occasionally the problem follows a levator resection or a fascia lata repair of ptosis.

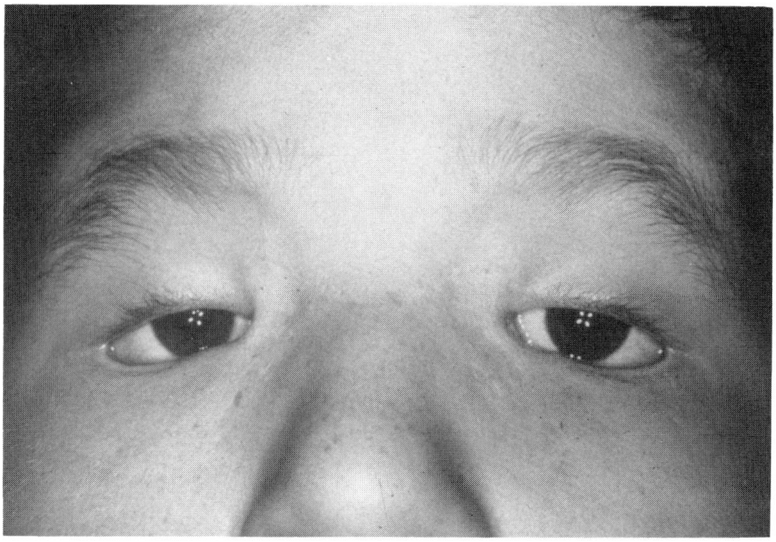

FIG 14–14.
Blepharophimosis, type II. This type does not have epicanthal folds but does have ptosis and telecanthus.

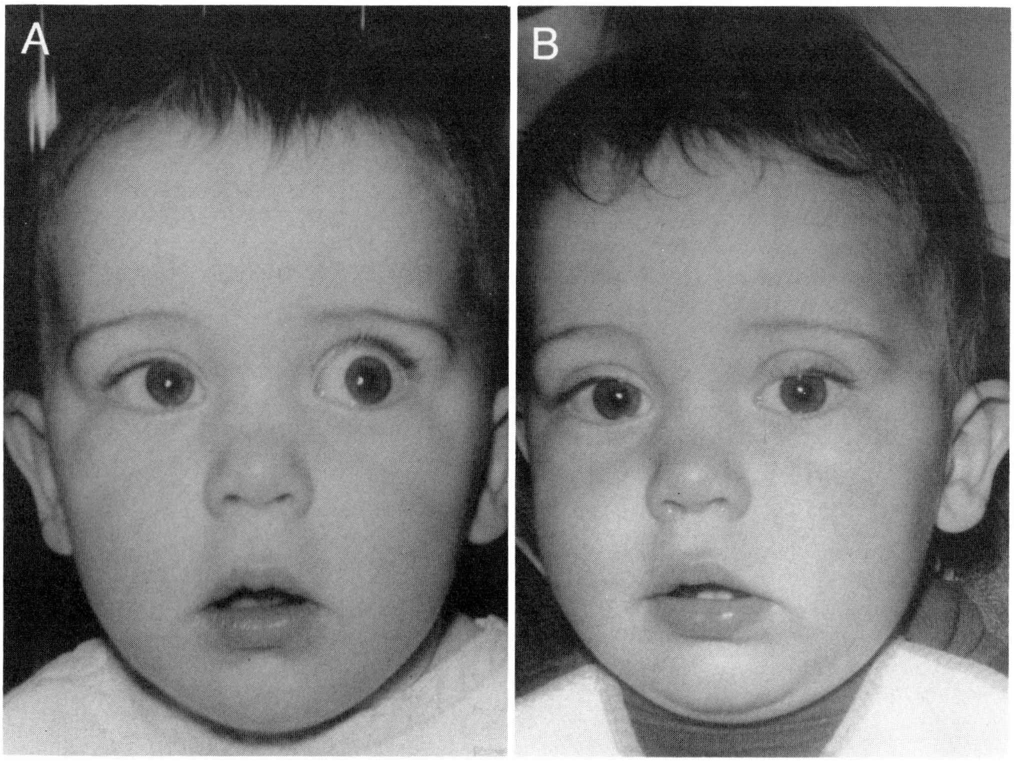

FIG 14–15.
A, congenital retraction of left upper lid. **B,** correction by insertion of fresh scleral graft.

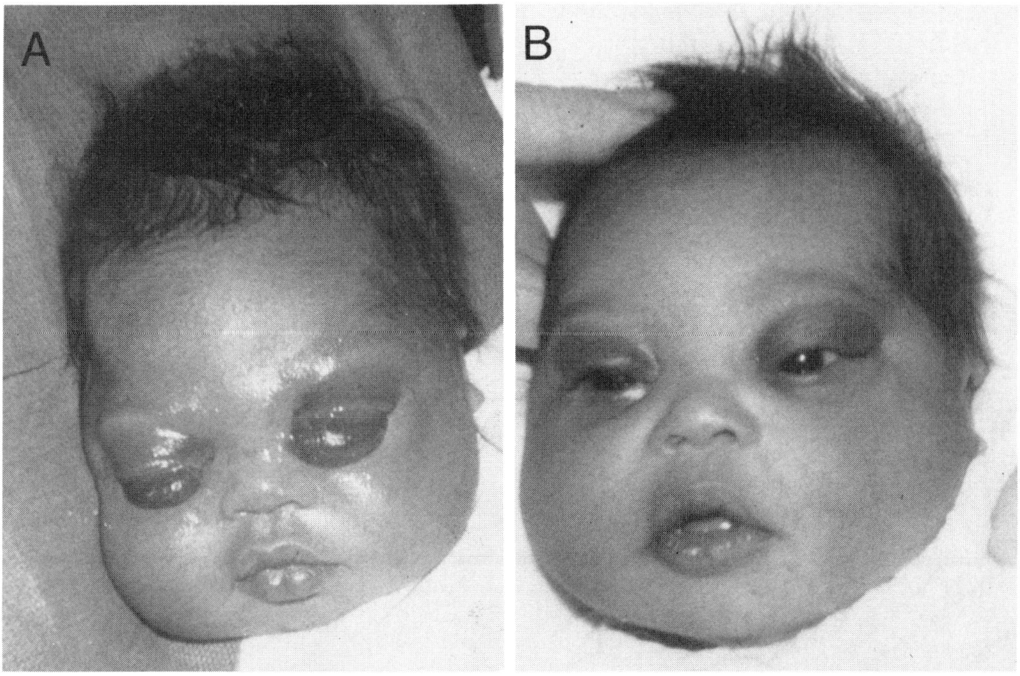

FIG 14–16.
A, bilateral congenital prolapse of conjunctiva. **B,** after replacement of prolapsed conjunctiva to normal position and the lid borders temporarily sutured together.

To repair the condition, the conjunctiva is replaced by using a muscle hook or the handle of a Bard-Parker knife. Some surgeons have suggested holding the lids in this position by using adhesive tape, but my experience has been that lid borders should be temporarily sutured together as temporary tarsorrhaphies. Double armed 4-0 silk sutures are used. They are passed through a small piece of plastic or a small button and into the skin of the upper lid and emerge through the gray line. The two needles are then passed through the gray line of the lower lid and again brought out through the skin about 0.25 in. from the border and tied over another piece of plastic or button. Two such sutures are placed so as to hold the conjunctiva in its proper position. The sutures are left in place for about 48 hours and then removed. A tight patch is applied to the lids. The eyelids are held in this position until the fluid has drained from under the conjunctiva. Occasionally the problem occurs following ptosis surgery in older children. In this case, it may be necessary to place several gut sutures through the conjunctiva in the upper fornix, bring them out through the lid, and tie them on the skin surface.

ABNORMALITIES OF MARGINAL DIFFERENTIATION

Distichiasis

Distichiasis (Fig 14–17) is a rare condition. The name means two rows of lashes, but this is a misnomer because the normal lid has more than one row of lashes. Sometimes a few extra lashes are seen, or a complete extra row is visible on the lid margin in or near the meibomian gland orifices. The greater the number of extra lashes, the more likelihood there is of epiphora, photophobia, and chronic infection. Frequently, congenital nasolacrimal obstruction is suspected. Often the offending lashes are light colored and difficult to visualize in an uncooperative child. In our series at The Hospital for Sick Children, we have treated 13 patients with distichiasis, three of whom had a family history of lymphedema of the lower extremities. The average age at diagnosis and treatment was 4 years. Referral was delayed by the inability to see the offending lashes.

Various treatment modalities have been tried. One author (JSC) has had success with carefully splitting the lid at the gray line and resecting the posterior lid margin, including the abnormal lash follicles. There have been no problems with the lid margin. The other author (RCP) prefers the technique described by Anderson and Harvey[16] in which the lid margin is split to a depth of 4 mm between the normal lash follicles and the abnormal distichiasis follicles. The anterior lid lamella is retracted and cryotreatment is applied in a double–free-thaw cycle to −20°C to the posterior lamella. Thermocouple monitoring of the posterior lamella is important. An iceball may form at 0°C, and the temperature may go well below −20°C, which is potentially damaging to other lid structures. The offending lashes are then epilated, and the anterior lamella is recessed 1 mm by tacking it to the tarsus with a 6-0 plain gut suture.

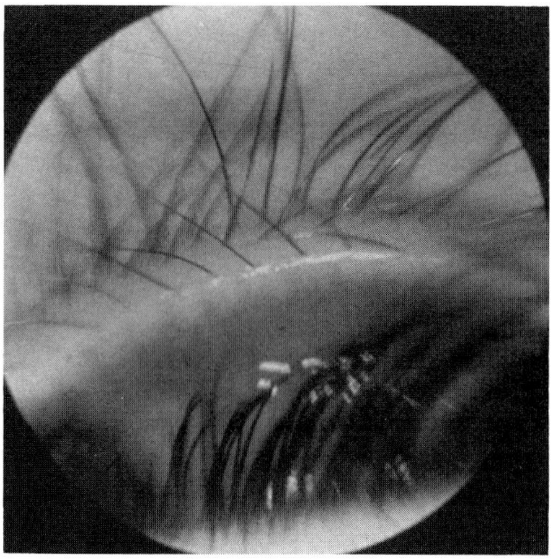

FIG 14–17.
Congenital distichiasis with two rows of lashes. The extra row on the lid margin comes out of or near the meibomian gland orifices.

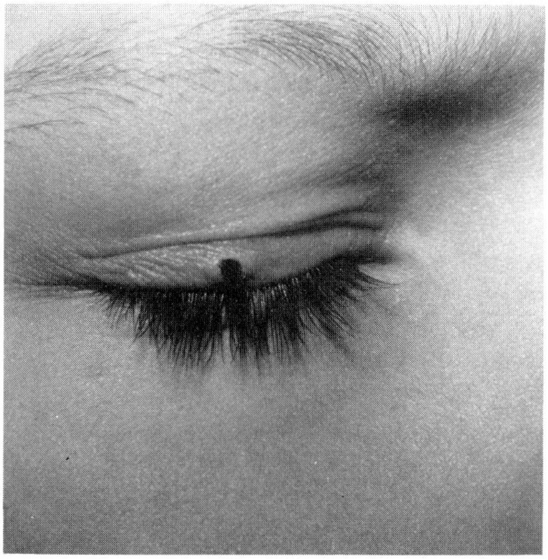

FIG 14–18.
Eyelashes growing from the center of the tarsus through a hole in the lid.

Trichiasis

Trichiasis is an acquired condition, usually seen after lid trauma or as a result of diseases such as Stevens-Johnson syndrome. Other eyelash anomalies that may be seen are hypotrichosis, or underdevelopment of the lashes, and hypertrichosis, or increased length or number of lashes. Distichiasis (two rows), tristichiasis (three rows), and tetrastichiasis (four rows) all fall under the heading of polytrichia. We have seen one case in which eyelashes grew anteriorly through the lid skin and exited 4 mm above the lash line. The abnormal area, including a small portion of tarsus with the follicles, was simply excised (Fig 14–18).

Congenital Alopecia

Congenital alopecia is a rare condition in which the lashes are absent, as is the hair on the rest of the body.

Ankyloblepharon

Ankyloblepharon is the partial or complete fusion of the lids. In ankyloblepharon filiforme (Fig 14–19) the lids are joined by fine bands, which may be simply cut. If the adhesion is more complete, the lid margins may be divided by scissors. A new lid margin can be formed by advancing the conjunctival surface slightly beyond the skin surface and suturing it in place with 6-0 plain gut sutures. If the fusion involves the medial ends of the lids, the lacrimal puncta may be involved. It may then be necessary to attempt to dissect and marsupialize the canaliculi.

ABNORMALITIES OF LID DIFFERENTIATION

Epiblepharon

Epiblepharon is an extra fold of skin at the margin of the lower lid (Fig 14–20). Usually it decreases during the first 2 years of life as the facial contour develops. Occasionally, the epiblepharon turns lashes on the medial half of the lid against the cornea, and in rare cases they may irritate the cornea and require surgical correction. This condition can be cured by excising the skin fold and suturing the superior border of the incision to the deep tissues prior to closing the skin (Fig 14–21,A–C).

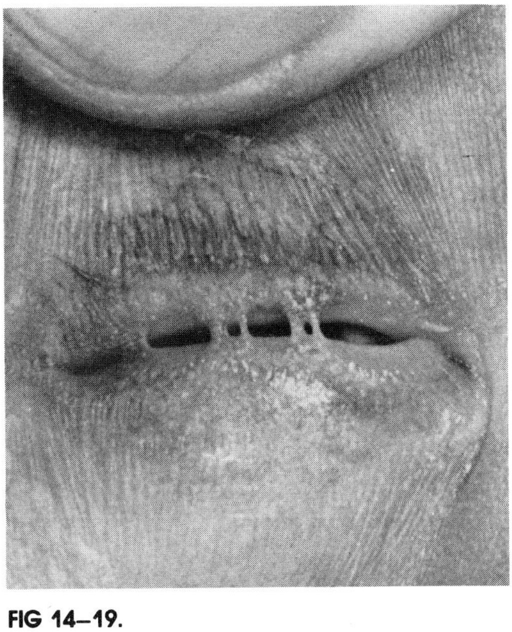

FIG 14–19.
Ankyloblepharon filiforme.

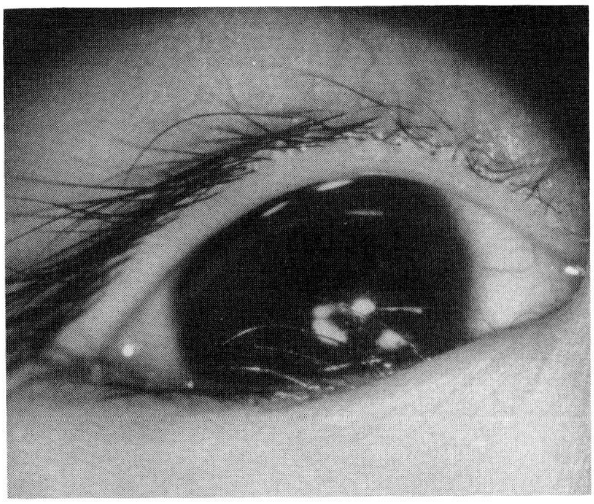

FIG 14–20.
Epiblepharon.

Congenital Entropion

Congenital entropion (Fig 14–22,A and B) is a very rare condition in children. Unlike senile entropion, which is caused by weakness of the preseptal orbicularis fibers, congenital entropion is caused by hypertrophy of the pretarsal fibers, specifically the fibers of the muscles of Riolan. In this condition, the lid margin may be inverted along its entire length or along the medial two thirds. The problem may be caused by a relative shortness of the conjunctiva, or by hypertrophy of the pretarsal and preseptal orbicularis muscles, or both. Surgical correction is required only if the lashes abrade the cornea.

The extreme form of congenital entropion is the horizontal tarsal kink, which is characterized by a fixed, inward rotation of the distal tarsal margin and causes the lashes to abrade the cornea (Fig 14–23, A and B). In this condition there is a permanent bend in the tarsus of about 135 degrees, the cause of which is unknown. This form of entropion is an ocular emergency. If correction is not carried out early, permanent corneal scarring results (Fig 14–24). The bend in the tarsus must be corrected, but this cannot be done by simple excision of skin and orbicularis.

Biglan and Buerger[17] suggest a partial horizontal splitting procedure as advocated by Wies[18] and later applied to the upper lid by Ballen.[19] This procedure was modified in one of our patients. The skin incision was made in the eyelid fold, and the tarsus was cut horizontally (Fig 14–25,A). The incision was not carried through the conjunctiva as in the Wies' operation. Three everting sutures were placed through the edges of the incision above, brought out through the skin below, and tied over plastic or rubber pegs (Fig 14–25,B), thereby turning the distal margin to a normal position. These sutures were left in place for about 2 weeks (Fig 14–25,C).

Congenital Ectropion

Congenital ectropion, or eversion of the edge of the eyelid, is relatively rare and is usually associated with mongolism. In the newborn, treatment consists of bland ointment if the conjunctiva becomes dry and infected. Surgery may be indicated. When there is excess lid tissue, simple lateral excision of the full thickness of the lid with direct closure

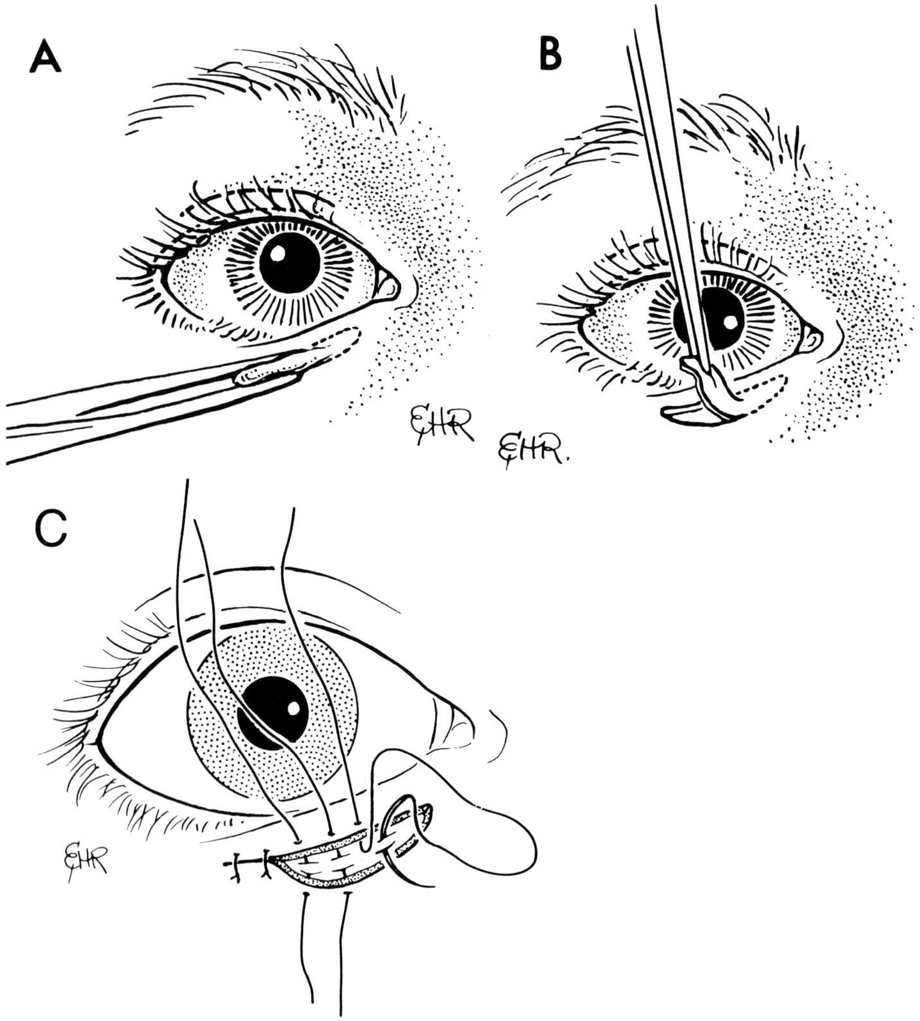

FIG 14–21.
A, repair of epiblepharon. Forceps pinch the skin so that the lid margin is everted adequately. **B**, removal of an ellipse of skin after marking. A small ellipse of orbicularis is also excised. **C**, closure with interrupted 6-0 plain gut suture. (From Crawford JS, Morin JD (eds): *The Eye in Childhood.* New York, Grune & Stratton, 1983. Used with permission.)

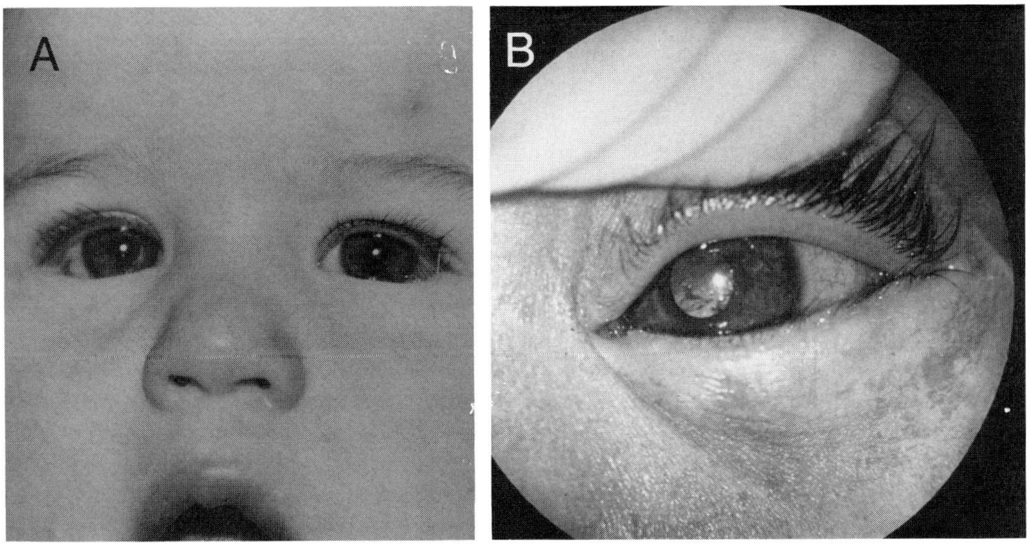

FIG 14–22.
A, congenital entropion. **B**, the lid margins are inverted along their entire length.

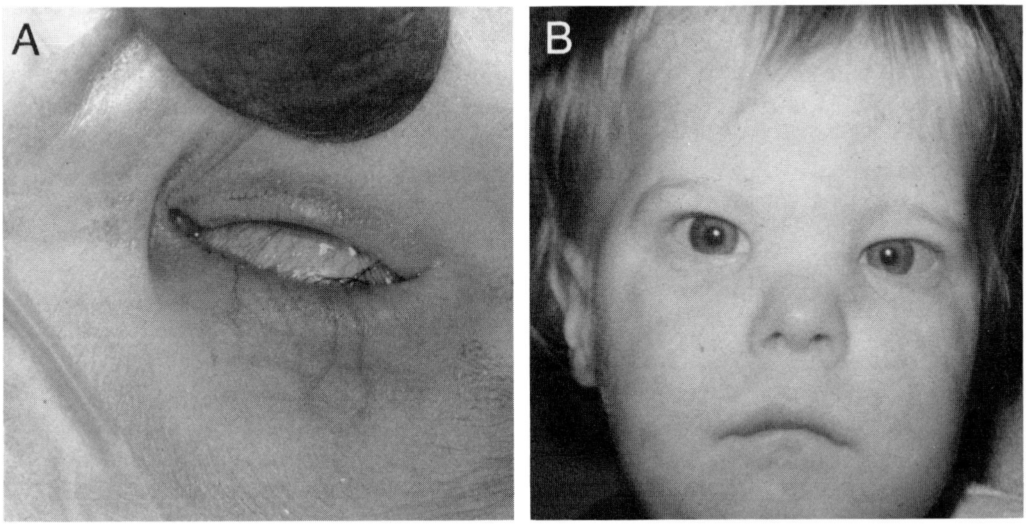

FIG 14–23.
A and **B**, horizontal tarsal kink.

should be sufficient (Fig 14–26,A). If there is no effective lateral canthal tendon, a full-thickness wedge can be removed from both the upper and lower lids laterally, and the posterior margins can be joined to form a new lateral canthus. A strip of periosteum is elevated from the lateral orbital rim, and the tarsus is anchored to it. Another method is to rotate flaps of tarsus laterally and attach them to the periosteum.

Ectropion may occur with blepharophimosis if the amount of skin is insufficient to allow the lids to close completely. In this case, full-thickness retroauricular skin grafts combined with temporary tarsorrhaphies are used to compensate for the deficiency.

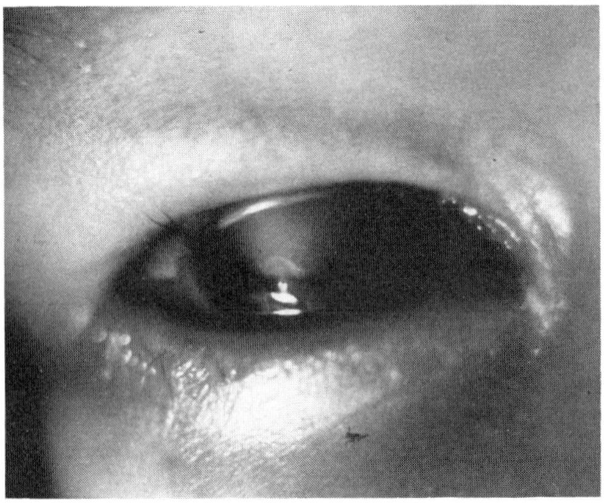

FIG 14–24.
Corneal scarring in a child where the horizontal tarsal kink was not corrected early enough.

Symblepharon

Symblepharon is an adhesion between the palpebral conjunctiva and the bulbar conjunctiva or cornea. Congenital symblepharon is rare (Fig 14–27, A and B). Usually the condition results from trauma, radiation, burns, severe inflammation, or infection. Stevens-Johnson syndrome and ocular pemphigoid are two of the more frequent conditions that cause the more severe adhesions.

The symblepharon can be excised and the raw edges covered by using either conjunctiva from the other eye or mucous membrane from the mouth. If the symblepharon is attached to the cornea, a lamellar graft is needed to cover the defect on the cornea.

Linear Sebaceous Nevus Anomalad

Linear sebaceous nevus anomalad, or nevus sebaceous of Jadassohn (Fig 14–28,A,B), is usually found in an otherwise normal individual. However, it has been reported in conjunction with seizures and mental deficiency. The skin involvement consists of nevus sebaceous with hyperpigmentation and hyperkeratosis. The lesions are most common in the midface extending from the forehead down over the lids to the nasal area. They tend to be linear in distribution and may be present on the trunk and limbs. Occasionally the cornea is involved. Colobomas of the lids and lipodermoids of the conjunctiva may occur.

Tumors

Papillomas

Papillomas (Fig 14–29) are benign tumors of the surface epithelium that are caused by an upward proliferation of skin and result in an elevated, irregular lesion with an undulating surface. Nevus verrucosus consists of a single lesion that is present at birth or appears early in life. Nonspecific papillomas are divided into wide-based simple or sessile papillomas and narrow-based pedunculated, fibroepithelial, or skin tags. Simple excision is usually adequate.

Angiomatous Tumors

Hemangiomas are common in children (Fig 14–30). They range from the small strawberry mark (hemangioendothelioma) to a large cauliflower-shaped mass. Twenty percent of strawberry hemangiomas are present at birth, and almost all are visible within the first month of life. In the vast majority of cases, hemangiomas regress spontaneously by the age of 7 years; however, a sudden dramatic increase in size may occur before this regression. Ultrasound and computed tomography (CT) scan are needed to rule out any orbital involvement. We feel that intervention in the normal course of these lesions is indicated if vision is being threatened by globe distortion, displacement, or occlusion. At present, our preferred treatment is intralesional injection of 40 mg triamcinolone and 6 mg betamethasone sodium phosphate as described by Kushner.[20] Repeated intralesional injections may be required, but it is suggested that at least 3- to 4-month intervals be observed. It is also suggested that the pediatrician be consulted before any injection because of the systemic effects of the steroids. Systemic steroid treatment may be indicated but often involves side effects. Radiation, cryotherapy, sclerotic agents, and surgical excision have been tried with less success.

Astigmatic anisometropic ambylopia has

been documented by Robb[21] and Stigmar and colleagues,[22] with a direct correlation between the axis of astigmatism and the location of the hemangioma.

Port wine hemangiomas (nevus flammeus) seldom cause any problem. Cavernous hemangiomas are rare in children and occur mostly in the orbit.

Lymphangiomas

Lymphangiomas are seen much less frequently than hemangiomas. If they occur in the lids, there is often an associated conjunctival or facial lesion. Pathological studies show vascular spaces filled with clear fluid rather than blood, as in hemangiomas. These lesions may increase in size when the child has an upper respiratory infection. Complete surgical excision is most difficult and frustrating because of the difficulty in completely removing the tumor without damage to normal lid structures. If hemorrhage occurs into a lymphangioma a "chocolate cyst" may ensue. B scan ultrasonography can often show the

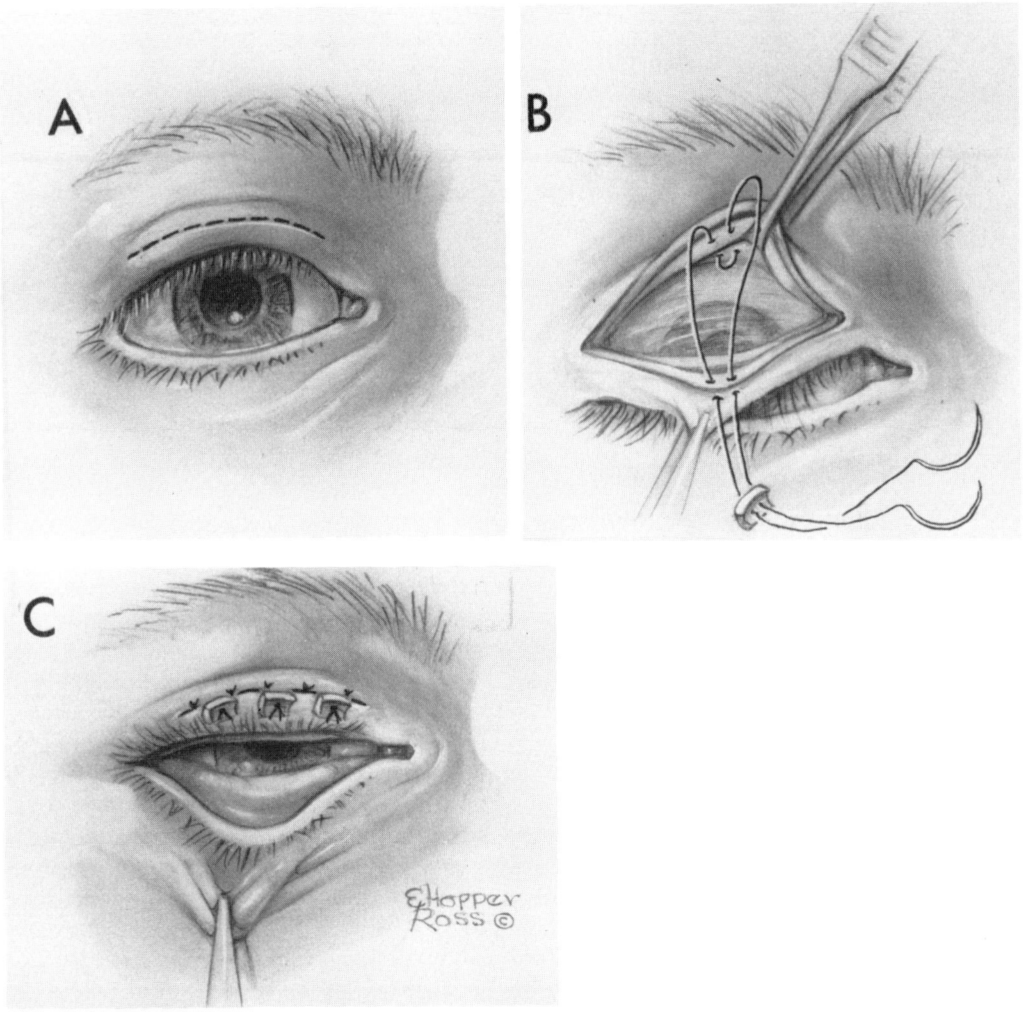

FIG 14–25.
Repair of horizontal tarsal kink. **A**, skin incision through skin above the center of the tarsus. **B**, three everting sutures placed through the edge of the tarsus above, brought out through the skin below the wound, and tied over small pieces of plastic. **C**, the lid margin is returned to its normal position.

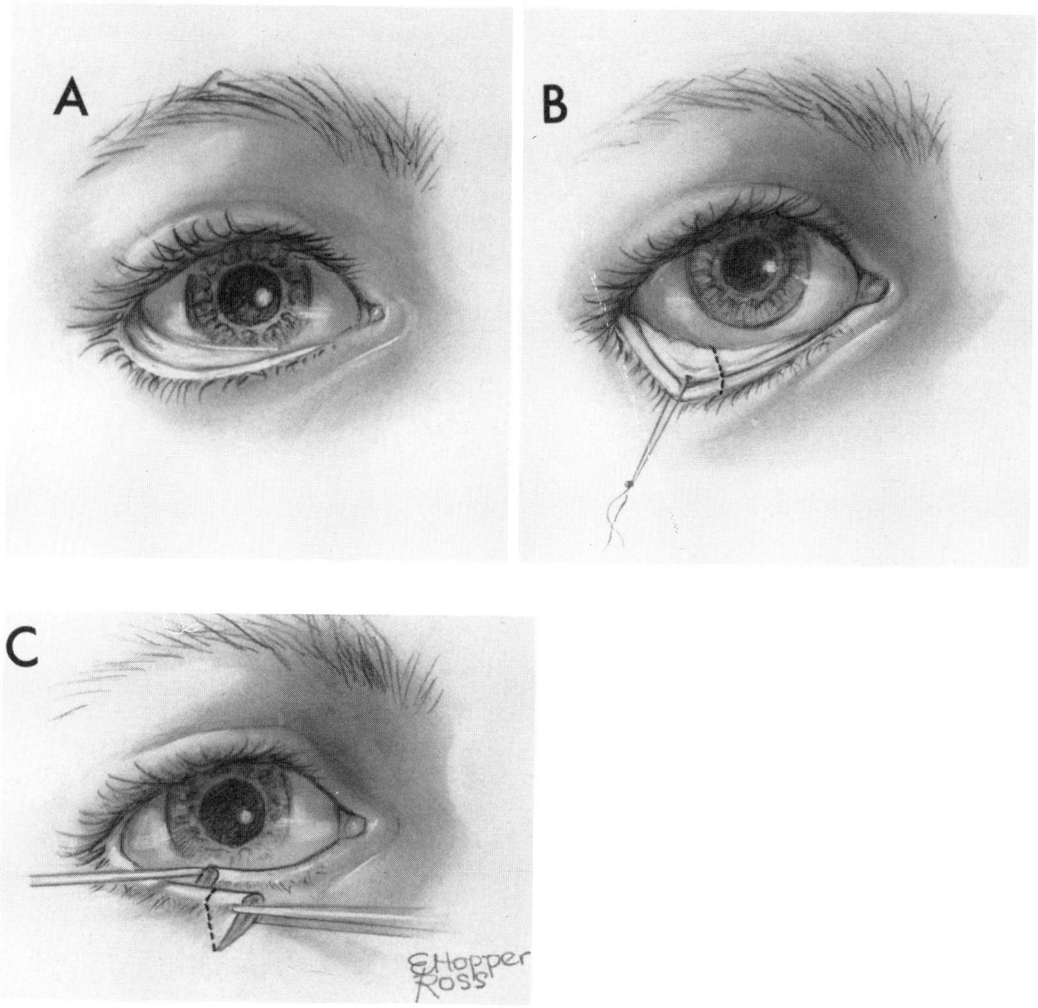

FIG 14–26.
A, congenital ectropion due to horizontal lid laxity. B, and C excision of full-thickness wedge from lower lid with direct closure.

cystic spaces. Tapping the tumor and withdrawing fluid may decrease the size of the lesion and allow diagnosis by fluid analysis.

Nevus

Nevus, a hamartomatous tumor, is a congenital flat or elevated, circumscribed lesion. It may be pigmented early in life or not become pigmented until puberty or early adulthood. Figure 14–31 shows a "kissing" nevus that was barely visible at birth but became an increasing cosmetic problem as the child grew. Usually a nevus can simply be watched. When surgery is required, it varies from simple excision to a more extensive procedure requiring plastic repair, depending on the size and location of the nevus.

Neurofibroma

Neurofibroma (Fig 14–32) is a phacomatosis that is manifested as multiple tumors proliferating within the nerve sheaths of cranial, spinal, sympathetic, and peripheral nerves. Neurofibromas usually appear in later childhood and are rarely seen in the first year of life. Surgical removal of lid involvement is extremely difficult, and repeated procedures are often required. The upper lid is usually the lid involved. Neurofibroma is extremely rare in the first year of life.

The skin may show areas of hyperpigmentation or hypopigmentation with café au lait spots in 94%, and about 75% of affected individuals have six or more spots measuring 1.5 cm or more, most commonly on the trunk.

Dermoid Cysts

Dermoid cysts usually develop in the tem-

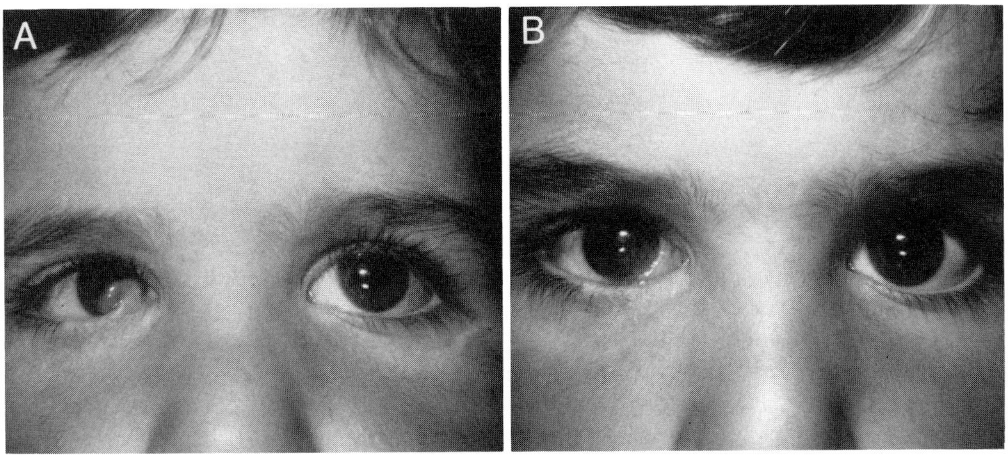

FIG 14–27.
A, and **B,** symblepharon. This child had a forceps injury at birth. She was not brought for treatment until the age of 3 years. The symblepharon was dissected from the cornea, and a lamellar graft was placed to cover the defect.

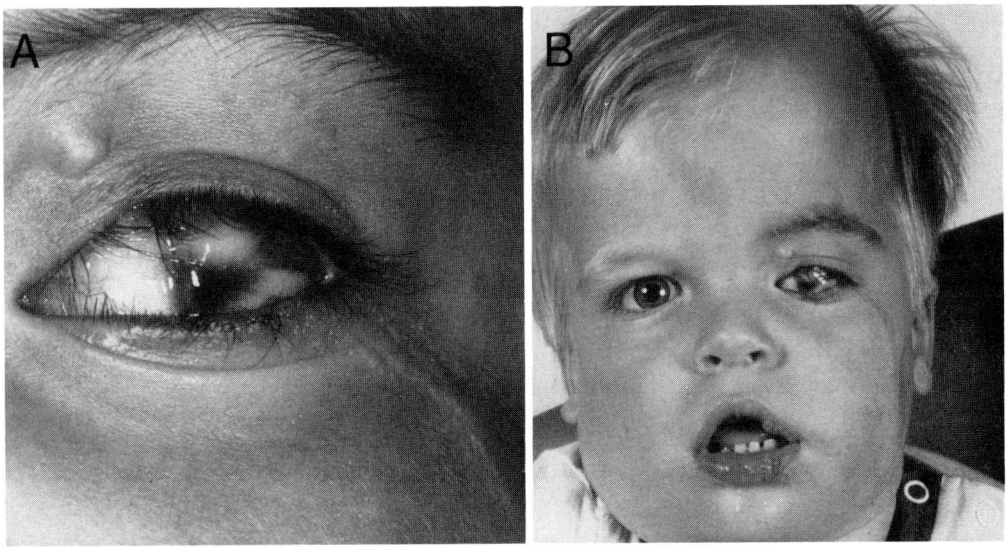

FIG 14–28.
A, and **B,** linear sebaceous nevus anomalad. There is hyperpigmentation in the brow with hyperkeratosis in the upper lid, lower lid, and cheek. The cornea is also involved.

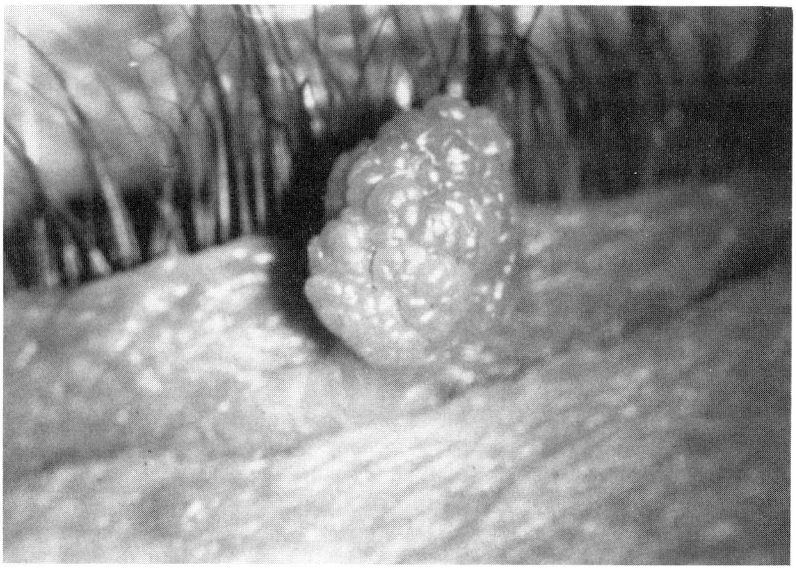

FIG 14–29.
Papilloma on the lid margin.

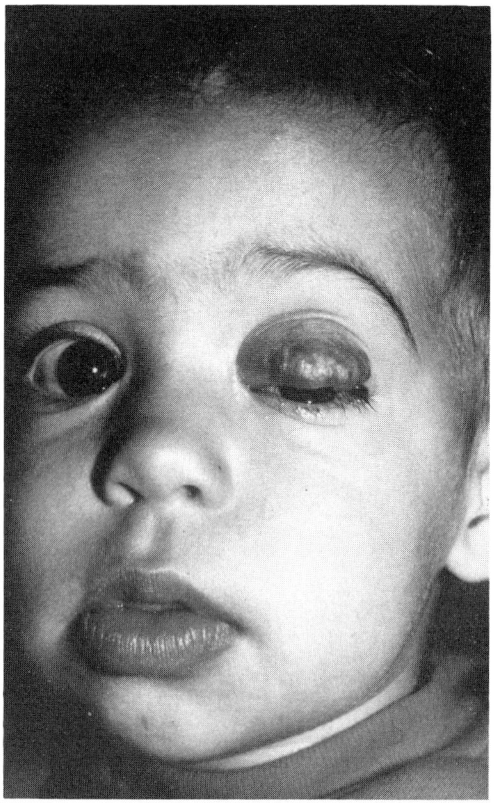

FIG 14–30.
Infantile hemangioma first noted at 2 weeks of age. The patient is 2 years old.

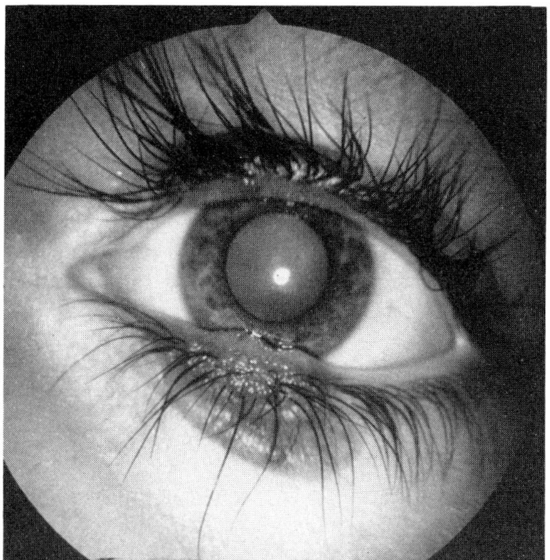

FIG 14–31.
Nevus on lower lid with a small nevus on upper lid (kissing nevus).

poral aspects of the upper lid (Fig 14–33). They are seen less frequently on the nasal side (Fig 14–34). The cyst is formed if an ectodermal remnant is cut off from the surface during development. It has a wall of stratified squamous epithelium, with epithelial appendages (hair follicles, sebaceous glands, sweat glands) in thc wall that linc thc cavity with kcratin, hair shafts, and debris. Usually it is firmly anchored to the periosteum, and compressive bone changes may be seen on x-ray film. During surgery, attempts should be made to remove the entire cyst because its contents incite tissue reaction if spilled. Irrigation with saline in the area should be done if the cyst ruptures. Preoperative x-ray, ultrasound, and CT scan help the surgeon to diagnose the problem and determine the exact location and extent of the cyst. Often the use of a retinal cryoprobe to fixate and freeze the cyst will allow safer and easier dissection.

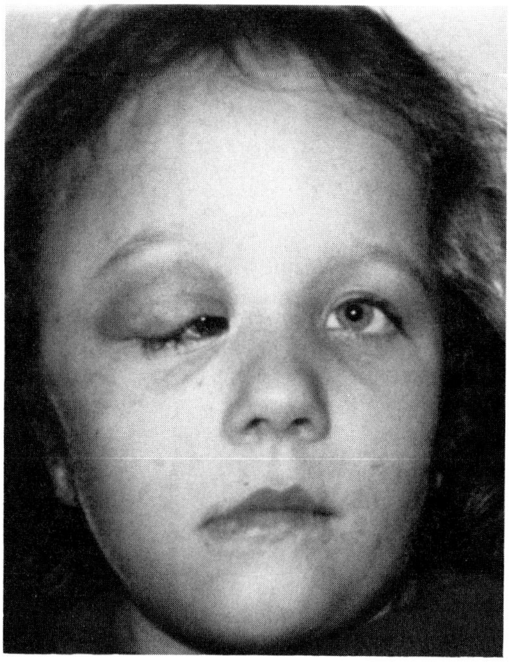

FIG 14–32.
A 9-year-old girl with a neurofibroma in right upper lid that appeared during the first year of life. She has von Recklinghausen's disease.

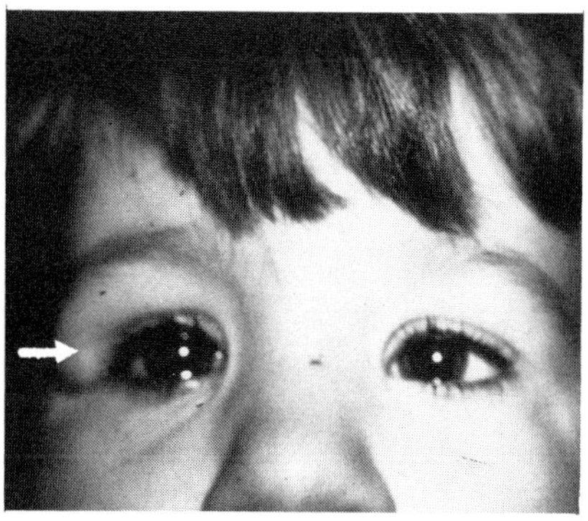

FIG 14–33.
Dermoid cyst in outer side of the right upper lid.

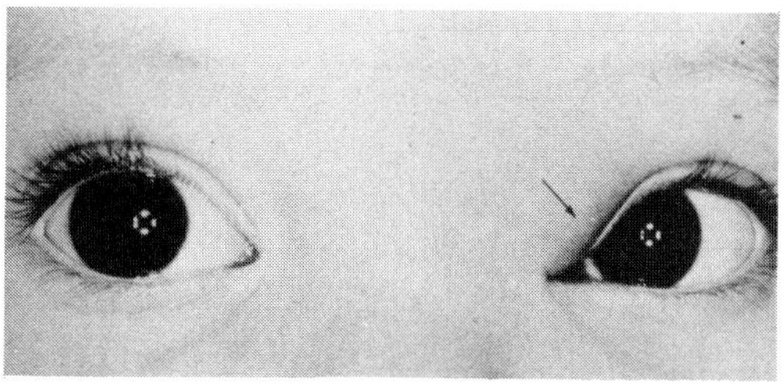

FIG 14–34.
Dermoid cyst in the upper nasal area of the lid.

Rhabdomyosarcoma

Rhabdomyosarcoma is the most common malignant tumor of the orbit in children. About 10% of all rhabodomyosarcomas in children occur in the orbit. They are extremely rare in the first year of life. Orbital rhabodomyosarcoma is commonly heralded by a rapid development of exophthalmos that is frequently associated with ptosis of the upper lid. Pain is not a prominent feature. The differential diagnosis of rhabdomyosarcoma includes benign orbital masses such as infantile hemangioma, lymphagioma, dermoids, and leiomyoma.

REFERENCES

1. Erbakan S: Plastic repair of eyelid margin. *Am J Ophthalmol* 1961; 51:835–837.
2. Jackson IT: Reconstruction of lower eyelid defect in Treacher Collins syndrome. *Plast Reconstr Surg* 1981; 67:365–368.
3. Johnson CC: Epicanthus and epiblepharon. *Arch Ophthalmol* 1978; 96:1030–1033.

4. Roveda JM: Epicanthus et blepharophimosis. Notre technique de correction. *Ann Oculist (Paris)* 1967; 200:551–555.
5. Beard C: *Ptosis*, ed 3. St Louis, CV Mosby Co, 1981.
6. Berke RN, Wadsworth JAC: Histology of levator muscle in congenital and acquired ptosis. *Arch Ophthalmol* 1955; 53:413–428.
7. Doucet TW, Crawford JS: The quantification, natural course, and surgical results in 57 eyes with Marcus Gunn (jaw-winking) syndrome. *Am J Ophthalmol* 1981; 92:702–707.
8. Hornblass A, Adachi M, Wolintz A, et al: Clinical and ultrastructural correlation in congenital and acquired ptosis. *Ophthalmic Surg* 1976; 7:69–76.
9. Crawford JS: *Pediatric Ophthalmology and Strabismus*, Transactions of the New Orleans Academy of Ophthalmology. New York, Raven Press, 1986.
10. Johnson CC: Operations for epicanthus and blepharophimosis: An evaluation and a method of shortening the medial canthal ligament. *Am J Ophthalmol* 1956; 41:71–79.
11. Callahan A: Surgical correction of the blepharophimosis syndromes. *Trans Am Acad Ophthalmol Otolaryngol* 1973; 77:687–695.
12. Callahan A: *Ptosis Associated with Congenital Defect. Symposium on Surgery of the Orbit and Adnexa,* Transactions of the New Orleans Academy of Ophthalmology. St Louis, CV Mosby Co, 1974.
13. Spaeth EB: Further considerations of the surgical correction of blepharophimosis [epicanthus]. *Am J Ophthalmol* 1956; 41:61–79.
14. Crawford JS: Easterbrook M: The use of bank sclera to correct lid retraction. *Can J Ophthalmol* 1976; 11:304–308.
15. Blechman B, Isenberg S: An anatomical etiology of congenital eyelid eversion. *Ophthalmic Surg* 1984; 15:111–113.
16. Anderson RL, Harvey JT: Lid splitting and posterior lamella cryosurgery for congenital and acquired distichiasis. *Arch Ophthalmol* 1981; 99:631–634.
17. Biglan AW, Buerger GF Jr: Congenital horizontal tarsal kink. *Am J Ophthalmol* 1980; 89:522–524.
18. Wies FA: Spastic entropion. *Trans Am Acad Ophthalmol Otolaryngol* 1955; 59:593–596.
19. Ballen PH: A simple procedure for the relief of trichiasis and entropion of the upper lid. *Arch Ophthalmol* 1964; 72:239–240.
20. Kushner BJ: Intralesional corticosteroid injection for infantile adnexal hemangioma. *Am J Ophthalmol* 1982; 93:496–506.
21. Robb RM: Refractive errors associated with hemangiomas of the eyelids and orbit in infancy. *Am J Ophthalmol* 1977; 83:52–58.
22. Stigmar G, Crawford JS, Ward CM, et al: Ophthalmic sequelae of infantile hemangiomas of the eyelids and orbit. *Am J Ophthalmol* 1978; 85:806–813.

15 Tearing Abnormalities

Richard M. Robb, M.D.

ALACRIMA

Absence of the secretion of tears in infancy may represent only a physiological delay in the onset of normal reflex tearing, which usually appears shortly after birth but may be delayed for several weeks.[1] Tearing associated with crying is usually later in appearance, often between 2 and 4 months of age.[2,3] It also may be delayed in onset without any adverse effect on the eyes. A few cases of more severe and evidently permanent deficiency of reflex and psychic tearing have been reported in otherwise healthy individuals, usually in association with some photophobia and irritation of the eyes.[4–6] Corneal sensation is intact, but the tears are viscous, and there are punctate erosions of the corneal epithelium, which can be seen with a slit lamp. In one frequently cited case this congenital alacrima was unilateral and was associated with severe epidermalization and vascularization of the cornea.[7] Other rare cases have been associated with nuclear aplasia of various cranial nerves.[8]

Infantile alacrima also occurs as a manifestation of systemic disease in the Riley-Day syndrome (familial dysautonomia).[9,10] In this generalized disorder of autonomic and sensory function there is both a deficiency of tears and insensitivity of the cornea, a combination that may result in exposure keratitis and even corneal ulceration and perforation in severe cases[11–13] (Fig 15–1).

Systemic signs and symptoms include blotching of the skin, emotional instability, cyclic vomiting, hyporeflexia, and indifference to pain.[10] The condition is inherited in an autosomal recessive pattern and is found almost exclusively in families of Ashkenazic Jewish ancestory.[14] The deficiency of tears appears to be the result of altered parasympathetic innervation of the lacrimal gland since systemic treatment with bethanecol (Urecholine) increases lacrimation to normal levels.[15] The pupils also exhibit supersensitivity to dilute solutions of parasympathomimetic drugs: they constrict to 2.5% methacholine or 0.06% pilocarpine, neither of which induces miosis of the normal pupil.[16–18] Such pupillary reactivity supports the diagnosis of Riley-Day syndrome but is not pathognomonic.[19]

Congenital alacrima is said to have been present in some early reports of congenital ectodermal dysplasia,[8] but more recent descriptions of this condition do not mention defective tearing as a prominent feature.[20–22]

EXCESS TEARING

Although nearly all cases of overflow tearing in infancy are due to an obstruction of drainage rather than excessive tear production, there are a few notable exceptions. Silver nitrate applied topically as prophylaxis for ophthalmia neonatorum can cause tearing and redness of the conjunctiva for several days. Tearing and photophobia are occasionally

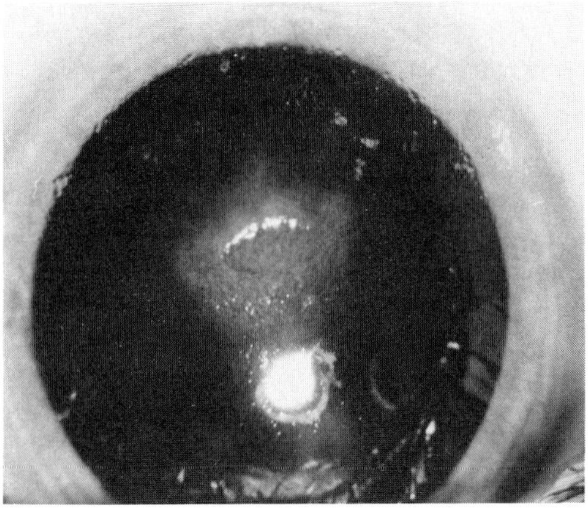

FIG 15–1.
Superficial corneal ulceration in patient with Riley-Day syndrome. (Courtesy of Sumner Liebman, M.D.)

signs of infantile glaucoma, a condition further characterized by elevated ocular pressure and an enlarged, hazy cornea. Excess lacrimation can also be produced by the paradoxical gustatory-lacrimal reflex, a rare abnormal linkage between the salivary and lacrimal glands. In the presence of this linkage, stimuli that produce salivation such as chewing and sucking also cause abnormal lacrimation in one or both eyes. The phenomenon can be acquired after trauma to the facial or greater superficial petrosal nerves, but it also occurs as a congenital lesion associated with lateral rectus muscle paralysis.[23, 24] In the latter case the abduction deficit and profuse tearing have usually been noted at the time of breast or bottle feeding in infancy.

CONGENITAL NASOLACRIMAL DUCT OBSTRUCTION

Obstruction of the nasolacrimal duct has been found in 5% to 6% of unselected newborn infants.[3, 25] The obstruction is the result of incomplete opening of the duct, which forms embryologically in an invagination of the surface ectoderm along the side of the nose between the inner canthus of the eyelids and the inferior turbinate of the nasal cavity. The usual obstruction is at the lower end of the duct (Fig 15–2) where the epithelium of the lacrimal duct and the mucosa of the nose abut each other and form an imperforate membrane.[26, 27] In the presence of such an obstruction tears well up and overflow the eyelids, and a variable amount of mucopurulent discharge develops (Fig 15–3). Less commonly there is impatency of the lacrimal puncta at the margin of the eyelids or absence of the canaliculi proximal to the lacrimal sac, which

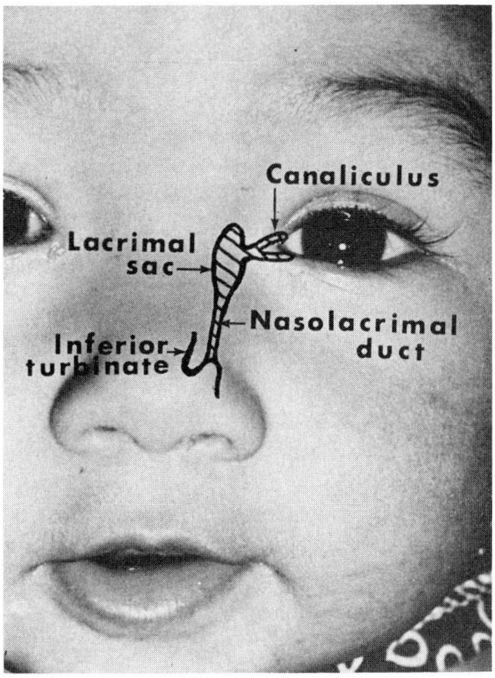

FIG 15–2.
Outline of lacrimal drainage system from the lacrimal puncta at the inner margin of the eyelids to the opening of the nasolacrimal duct in the nasal cavity beneath the inferior turbinate.

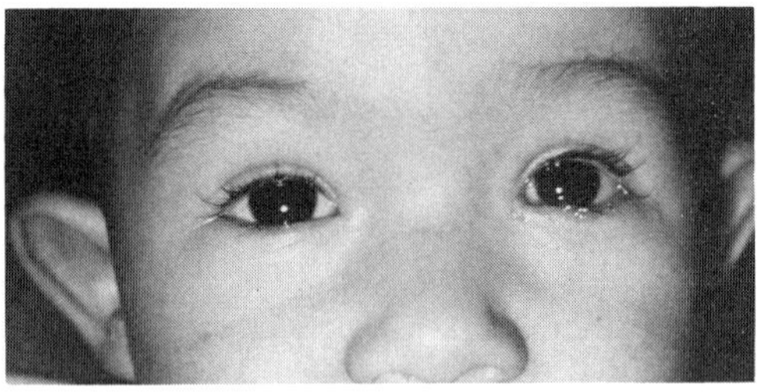

FIG 15–3.
Infant with obstruction of the left nasolacrimal duct that is causing tears to well up and overflow the eyelids.

causes an overflow of tears without purulent discharge. In none of these obstructions is there inflammation or redness of the conjunctiva such as one sees in neonatal conjunctivitis due to infectious agents or chemical irritation.

Although the prophylactic use of silver nitrate in the eyes of newborn infants has been considered a possible cause of nasolacrimal duct obstruction, this seems unlikely in view of the location and character of the usual distal obstruction. Moreover, a controlled study of 145 newborn infants randomized to receive either 1% silver nitrate or 1% tetracycline prophylaxis revealed no significant difference in the incidence of nasolacrimal duct obstruction between the two groups.[28]

The diagnosis of nasolacrimal duct obstruction is usually evident from overflow of tears, but in questionable cases fluorescein dye can be instilled in the conjunctival cul de sac and its disappearance time assessed.[29] If the dye fails to disappear in several minutes, an obstruction in the lacrimal drainage system can be presumed.

Fortunately, nasolacrimal duct obstruction clears spontaneously with time in most infants. Between 90% and 95% of congenitally obstructed ducts will open by 1 year of age,[30–32] with only local massage over the lacrimal sac combined with topical antibiotic drops or ointment as needed for discharge.[33,34] Massage over the sac usually results in retrograde expression of discharge onto the eye by way of the canaliculi. This serves to decompress the sac but does not alter the distal obstruction. Occasionally purulent material in the sac can be pushed downward through the duct into the nose, breaking through the duct obstruction with a sudden popping sensation. Unfortunately this curative maneuver can be accomplished only rarely.

Probing of the nasolacrimal duct will also clear the obstruction, and this can be done whenever the tearing and discharge become troublesome enough to warrant surgical resolution. Since the rate of spontaneous clearing declines after 1 year of age and since most parents tire of dealing with the discharge by that time, there is no reason to delay probing beyond the end of the first year. On the other hand, if the tearing and discharge are copious and irritating, probing may be indicated before then. The procedure can be done under topical or general anesthesia,[35,36] the latter being the author's preference for children over 6 months of age. In either case one canaliculus is dilated, and the lacrimal probe is passed through the canaliculus into the lacrimal sac, from which point it can be directed down along the nasolacrimal duct (Fig 15–4) to enter the nasal cavity under the inferior turbinate. At the distal end of the duct a membranous obstruction is usually encountered and can be broken with gentle pressure, whereupon the probe advances suddenly into the nose. The probe is then withdrawn and saline is irrigated through the system to demonstrate its patency. Only a small amount of fluid (approximately 1 mL) is needed to establish that

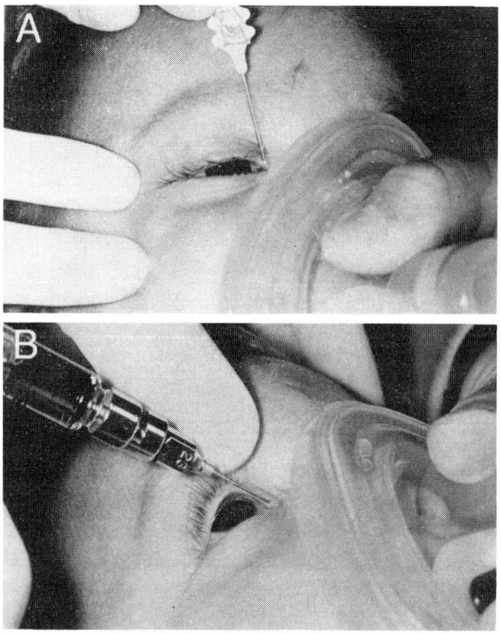

FIG 15–4.
Probing of the lacrimal drainage system under brief general anesthesia. **A**, the lacrimal probe is passed into the nasal cavity by breaking membranous obstruction at the lower end of the duct. **B**, saline is irrigated through the duct via a cannula passed into the lacrimal sac.

the duct is open; larger amounts increase the risk of aspiration in anesthetized patients.

Properly performed probings are successful in over 90% of patients.[36–38] There appears to be little difference in the success rate whether the probing is done before or after 1 year of age.[36, 38] One or two repeat probings are recommended if symptoms persist after an initial probing that was felt to pass successfully into the nose.[36–38] Various additional maneuvers[39–41] including silicone intubation of the nasolacrimal duct[42, 43] and fracture of the inferior turbinate have been suggested to establish and maintain the patency of the lacrimal drainage system if simple probing does not work, but these are not often required. A small number of cases for which probing has been unsuccessful because of abnormal bony obstruction can be resolved with a dacryocystorhinostomy.[38]

CONGENITAL DACRYOCYSTOCELE

This uncommon variant of congenital nasolacrimal duct obstruction is characterized by distention of the lacrimal sac with a clear mucoid material at birth.[30, 44, 45] A bluish lump, sometimes mistaken for a hemangioma, is present at the inner canthus (Fig 15–5). Functional blockage of retrograde flow through the canaliculi prevents regurgitation of the sac contents back onto the surface of the eye. Tearing may not be a prominent feature since tear production is at a reduced level in the neonatal period.[1] Occasionally the duct obstruction gives way spontaneously or with pressure over the lacrimal sac, which results in a gush of mucoid material into the nasal cavity, but this happens in the minority of cases. Decompression of the sac via a canaliculus within a few days is recommended to avoid secondary infection,[30, 45] and at the same time the nasolacrimal duct can be probed to open the obstruction at its distal end. This probing can usually be done under topical anesthesia in the newborn period, but special care is required to find the communication between the distended sac (in an enlarged lacrimal fossa) and the duct. Once the duct has been opened, the lacrimal sac returns to its normal size and configuration.

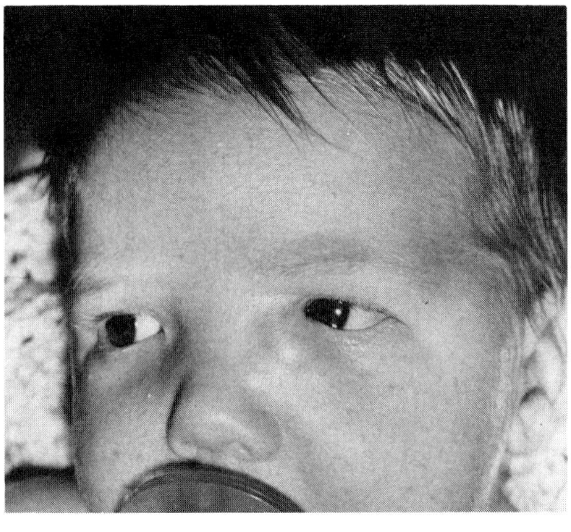

FIG 15–5.
Newborn infant with dacryocystocele on the left. The swollen lacrimal sac was decompressed by probing through the canaliculi and nasolacrimal duct shortly after birth.

REFERENCES

1. Sjogren H: The lacrimal secretion in newborn premature and fully developed children. *Acta Ophthalmol (Copenh)* 1955; 33:557–560.
2. Darwin C: *The Expression of the Emotions in Man and Animals.* London, John Murray, 1872, p 153.
3. Cassady JV: Dacryocystitis of infancy. *Am J Ophthalmol* 1948; 31:773–780.
4. Duke-Elder WS: Keratitis sicca. *Br J Ophthalmol* 1930; 14:691–694.
5. Sjogren H, Eriksen A: Alacrima congenita. *Br J Ophthalmol* 1950; 34:691–694.
6. Keith CG, Boldt DW: Congenital absence of the lacrimal gland. *Am J Ophthalmol* 1986; 102:800–801.
7. Smith RS, Maddox F, Collins BE: Congenital alacrima. *Arch Ophthalmol* 1968; 70:45–48.
8. Duke-Elder S: Congenital deformities, in *System of Ophthalmology, vol 3.* St Louis, CV Mosby Co, 1963, p 914.
9. Riley CM, Day RL, Greeley DM, et al: Central autonomic dysfunction with defective lacrimation. *Pediatrics* 1949; 3:468–476.

10. Riley CM: Familial autonomic dysfunction. *JAMA* 1952; 149:1532–1535.
11. Dunnington JH: Congenital alacrima in familial autonomic dysfunction. *Arch Ophthalmol* 1954; 52:925–931.
12. Liebman SD: Ocular manifestations of Riley-Day syndrome. *Arch Ophthalmol* 1956; 56:719–725.
13. Liebman SD: Riley-Day syndrome (familial dysautonomia). *Arch Ophthalmol* 1957; 58:188–192.
14. Brunt PW, McKusick VA: Familial dysautonomia. *Medicine (Baltimore)* 1970; 49:343–374.
15. Axelrod FB, Branom N, Becker M, et al: Treatment of familial dysautonomia with bethanechol (Urecholine). *J Pediatr* 1972; 81:573–578.
16. Smith AA, Dancis J, Breinin G: Ocular responses to autonomic drugs in familial dysautonomia. *Invest Ophthalmol* 1965; 4:358–361.
17. Goldberg MF, Payne JW, Brunt PW: Ophthalmologic studies of familial dysautonomia. *Arch. Ophthalmol* 1968; 80:732–743.
18. Epstein RL: Inborn metabolic disorders and the eye, in Peyman GA, Sanders DR, Goldberg MF (eds): *Principles and Practice of Ophthalmology*. Philadelphia, WB Saunders Co, 1980, p 1761.
19. Riley CM, Moore RH: Familial dysautonomia differentiated from related disorders. *Pediatrics* 1966; 37:435–446.
20. Weech AA: Hereditary ectodermal dysplasia (congenital ectodermal defect). *Am J Dis Child* 1929; 37:766–790.
21. Gregory IDR: Congenital ectodermal dysplasia. *Br J Ophthalmol* 1955; 39:44–47.
22. Marshall D: Ectodermal dysplasia. *Am J Ophthalmol* 1958; 45:143–156.
23. Lutman FC: Paroxysmal lacrimation when eating. *Am J Ophthalmol* 1947; 30:1538–1585.
24. Jampel RS, Titone C: Congenital paradoxical gustatory-lacrimal reflex and lateral rectus paralysis. *Arch Ophthalmol* 1962; 67:123–126.
25. Gerry D, Kendig EL: Congenital impatency of the nasolacrimal duct. *Arch Ophthalmol* 1948; 39:193–204.
26. Cassady JV: Developmental anatomy of nasolacrimal duct. *Arch Ophthalmol* 1952; 47:141–158.
27. Sevel D: Developmental and congenital abnormalities of the nasolacrimal apparatus. *J Pediatr Ophthalmol Strabismus* 1981; 18:13–19.
28. Hick JF, Block DJ, Ilstrup DM: A controlled study of silver nitrate prophylaxis and the incidence of nasolacrimal duct obstruction. *J Pediatr Ophthalmol Strabismus* 1985; 22:92–93.
29. Zappia RJ, Milder B: Lacrimal drainage function. 2. The fluorescein dye disappearance test. *Am J Ophthalmol* 1972; 74:160–162.
30. Petersen RA, Robb RM: The natural course of congenital obstruction of the nasolacrimal duct. *J Pediatr Ophthalmol Strabismus* 1978; 15:246–250.
31. Paul TO: Medical management of congenital nasolacrimal duct obstruction. *J Pediatr Ophthalmol Strabismus* 1985; 22:68–70.
32. Nelson LB, Calhoun JH, Menduke H: Medical management of congenital nasolacrimal duct obstruction. *Ophthalmology* 1985; 92:1187–1190.
33. Crigler LW: The treatment of congenital dacryocystitis. *JAMA* 1923; 81:23–24.
34. Kushner BJ: Congenital nasolacrimal system obstruction. *Arch Ophthalmol* 1982; 100:597–600.
35. Robb RM: Treatment of congenital nascolacrimal system obstruction. *J Pediatr Ophthalmol Strabismus* 1985; 22:36–37.
36. El-Mansoury J, Calhoun JH, Nelson LB, et al: Results of late probing for congenital nasolacrimal duct obstruction. *Ophthalmology* 1986; 93:1052–1054.
37. Baker JD: Treatment of congenital nasolacrimal system obstruction. *J Pediatr Ophthalmol Strabismus* 1985; 22:34–35.
38. Robb RM: Probing and irrigation for congenital nasolacrimal duct obstruction. *Arch Ophthalmol* 1986; 104:378–379.
39. Walter JR, Bogdasarian R: The management of persistent congenital occlusion of the nasolacrimal duct after unsuccessful probing. *J Pediatr Ophthalmol Strabismus* 1978; 15:251–252.
40. Havins WE, Wilkins RB: A useful alternative to silicone intubation in congenital nasolacrimal duct obstruction. *Ophthalmic Surg* 1983; 14:666–670.
40. Wesley RE: Inferior turbinate fracture in the treatment of congenital nasolacrimal duct obstruction and congenital nasolacrimal duct anomaly. *Ophthalmic Surg* 1985; 16:368–371.
42. Kraft SP, Crawford JS: Silicone tube intuba-

tion in disorders of the lacrimal system in children. *Am J Ophthalmol* 1982; 94:290–299.
43. Dortzbach RK, France TD, Kushner BJ, et al: Silicone intubation for obstruction of the nasolacrimal duct in children. *Am J Ophthalmol* 1982; 94:585–590.
44. Harris GJ, DiClementi D: Congenital dacryocystocele. *Arch Ophthalmol* 1982; 100:1763–1765.
45. Weinstein GS, Biglan AW: Congenital lacrimal sac mucoceles. *Am J Ophthalmol* 1982; 94:106–110.

16 Strabismus and Eye Movement Disorders*

Steven M. Archer, M.D.
Eugene M. Helveston, M.D.

Disorders of ocular motility that present in the first year of life are rarely diagnosed in the neonatal period. In some disorders such as congenital estropia, there is legitimate controversy as to whether or not the condition is indeed connatal. Other disorders that are almost certainly connatal, such as Duane syndrome, also are not diagnosed in the neonatal period. This is due in part to the difficulty of performing a motility examination and in part to the shortage of precise guidelines as to what constitutes normal ocular motility in the neonate. Expectations of the neonate's oculomotor system are minimal on the part of parents and clinicians, that is, a wide range of strabismus patterns are accepted as normal in the context of the neonate's immaturity. Indeed, a relatively imprecise system may well suit the limited needs of the neonate. Between birth and roughly 6 months of age, however, there is a rapid maturation of visual function. The visual acuity improves dramatically,[1-8] and stereopsis has been shown in several different laboratory settings to have its onset during this period.[9-12] This places increasing demands on the oculomotor system for steady foveal fixation and precise binocular alignment. It is during this period of required oculomotor maturation that developmental aberrations (e.g., sensory nystagmus, perhaps congenital esotropia) and adaptations to frank defects (e.g., head turn in Duane syndrome) become manifested.

*Supported in part by grant EY-06645 from the National Institutes of Health, Bethesda, Md.

The purpose of this chapter is, first, to give some preliminary guidelines as to what can be accepted as normal ocular motility findings in an infant of a given age. The second object is to describe the various abnormalities of ocular motility that occur in infancy and the manner in which they deviate from the normal course of development. In many instances, treatment of these entities will be briefly discussed. However, a detailed discussion of the surgical management of these problems is beyond the scope of this chapter. For this information, the interested reader may refer to the standard strabismus texts and atlases.

THE NORMAL NEONATE

Ocular Motility Examination

In examining the ocular motility of a neonate, the first requirement is that the baby must be in an awake, alert, and responsive state. This can usually be acomplished if several points are observed. Infants are most responsive when they are hungry and are best examined just prior to the next scheduled feeding. Subdued lighting is very helpful in getting the baby to open his eyes spontaneously since many neonates behave as if they are photophobic. A gentle bouncing of side-to-side rocking movement accompanied by the sound of human voice will often initiate attentiveness, which is signaled widening of the palpebral fissures and mydriasis (reversal of the sleep miosis). Occasionally, these efforts must be prolonged (as much as 10 minutes) but are usually eventually successful.

Once the neonate is attentive, it is necessary to document fixation behavior. This serves two functions: (1) it demonstrates adequate alertness of the infant, and (2) it confirms where the infant is fixating. These criteria must be met before assessment of the ocular alignment can be made. It is possiblc to demonstrate refixation behavior in most neonates; one of us (SMA) was able to do so in 983 of 1,000 consecutive normal neonates examined in a newborn nursery.

Although the central retina in a full-term infant appears to be relatively mature by electroretinographic,[13,14] ophthalmoscopic,[15] and psychophysical[16,17] criteria, its histological immaturity[14,18–20] may leave some doubt as to whether a neonate can have fixation behavior. Whether or not neonates foveate, our clinical observation has been that they steadily and repeatedly direct the same point relative to the pupillary axis toward the fixation target; this appears to correspond to some region of the central part of the retina. Similar conclusions have been drawn from photographic studies of neonatal fixation.[21]

Fixation is best proved by first waiting until the infant appears to be fixating on the examiner's face. This can be recognized by observing centering of the corneal reflex of the examiner's face on the child's cornea. The examiner then moves his face to one side (taking care not to provide auditory cues or to elicit a vestibulo-ocular response by rotating the infant) and observes the infant making refixation saccades and recentering the reflex of the examiner's face on the cornea of the fixating eye. This can be repeated to the opposite side and as often as necessary to convince the examiner that the observed eye movements are indeed refixation responses and not random eye movements that coincide with the examiner's head movement. However, the refixation saccades are so characteristic and robust that many repetitions are seldom necessary. In recognizing refixation behavior in a neonate there are two points that must be kept in mind. First, infants usually do not show smooth pursuit movements before 3 months of age[22]; the neonate responds to target movement with one or more saccades to bring the target back into fixation.[23,24] Second, these refixation saccades have a very long latency of up to 1 second in a newborn. The latency for voluntary saccades decreases to 300 to 400 ms by 4 months of age and approaches an adult latency of about 200 ms by 12 months.[12]

Evaluation of alignment in the neonate is best accomplished by assessing the corneal reflexes. In the traditional Hirschberg test, the corneal reflexes produced by a penlight are used to judge alignment. In the neonate, the penlight is ineffective as a fixation stimulus and more often than not will produce eyelid closure. The corneal reflex of the examiner's face should be substituted for the penlight. A face is the ideal fixation stimulus[25] and produces a well-localized and clearly visible image on the steep cornea of the neonate. Neonates often do not respond well to cover testing. It is interesting that they seem distressed by occlusion of one eye at a time when a large manifested deviation frequently precludes single binocular vision. When a neonate does tolerate cover testing, there is often a long delay between the time the fixating eye is occluded and the unoccluded eye takes up fixation. At several months of age, traditional Hirschberg, Krimsky, and cover testing become more satisfactory.

Horizontal ductions and versions can be tested to some extent while verifying refixation behavior; however, vestibular stimulation by rotation of the neonate at arm's length is a better way of accomplishing this. The development of vestibular nystagmus is discussed later under the heading Nystagmus.

Normal Neonatal Alignment

Exodeviation is probably the normal state of alignment for a neonate, which may con-

TABLE 16–1
Ocular Alignment in Neonates*

Orthotropia	29.9
Exotropia	51.5
Intermittent exotropia	15.0
Esotropia	0.3
Intermittent esotropia	0.7
Eso- to exodeviation	2.6

*Values are percentages of examinable infants.

tribute to the common misapprehension that the neonate's eyes move independently when in fact, neonatal eye movements are quite conjugate.[23, 24] In being exodeviated, the eyes may simply be assuming their anatomic positions in the divergent orbits.[26] After birth, the eyes tend toward a progressively more convergent position and orthotropia.

Nixon and co-workers examined the ocular alignment in 1,219 neonates and found the majority of them to be either straight or exodeviated.[27] As part of an ongoing phase of this study we have examined an additional 2,771 infants to date. Our findings in these infants (Table 16–1) and the findings of other independent investigators[28] have shown an even greater proportion of neonates with exodeviation but have otherwise confirmed the results of Nixon and colleagues[1]. The exodeviations seen in the neonate (Fig 16–1) behave similarly to the exotropia that is pathological when seen in older children. In more than half of the neonates with exotropia, the deviation is larger than 25 p.d.; however, the amount of deviation can be quite variable during the course of the examination. Many of the exotropic neonates repeatedly alternate fixation spontaneously. Follow-up examination of infants with exodeviation at birth shows a progressive decrease in the number of infants with exotropia. The vast majority of these infants are orthotropic by 6 months of age.

Previous photographic studies that found exotropia in neonates[29–32] have been criticized because of the possibility that a large angle κ produced the appearance of exotropia.[21] Indeed, when not attending to anything in particular, neonates assume a symmetrically divergent eye position that is indistinguishable from a large angle κ. Largely because of this problem of verifying fixation, our attempts to analyze commercial photos of neonates taken in the nursery have yielded no useful information. However, when the examiner is interactively checking fixation as described earlier, the line of sight and consequently the angle κ for the fixating eye can be readily judged (see Fig 16–1). Any infant with symmetrical divergence is always interpreted as having a positive angle κ or inattentiveness and not an exodeviation.

The relatively small number of neonates who have esodeviations or who vary between esotropia and extropia are of particular interest. Most of these esodeviations are small and variable. On follow-up, virtually all of these infants have been found to have normal motility. We have also seen two infants with large concomitant esodeviations at birth that would

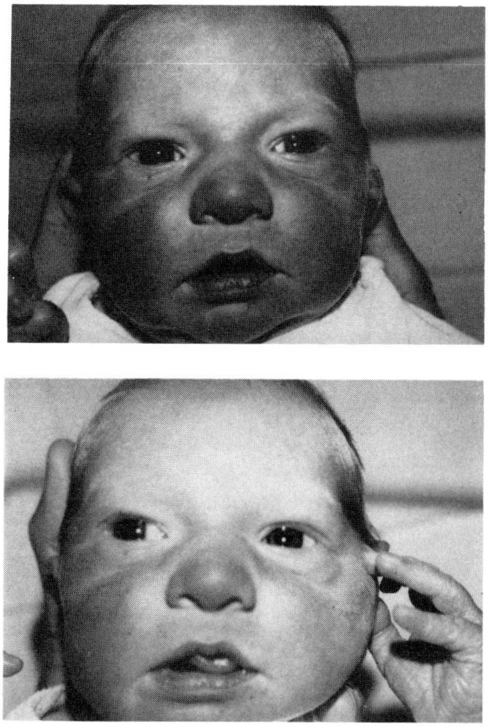

FIG 16–1.
A typical neonate with exotropia and spontaneous alternation of fixation. Note that while a small positive angle κ (displacement of light reflex from pupillary axis in the fixating eye) is present, it does not begin to account for the amount of exodeviation observed.

have been characteristic of congenital esotropia had they not resolved by 2 months of age.

Laboratory studies have yielded a variety of conclusions regarding the neonate's ability to converge.[29, 31, 33, 34] It is of interest because an inability to converge might explain the exodeviations noted under our examination condition of near fixation (although most of the deviations are sufficiently large that the eyes must be exotropic at any distance). From clinical observations, however, it is clear that at least some neonates are able to converge their eyes. Those infants characterized as having intermittent esotropia or varying between esotropia and exotropia have demonstrated the mechanical capacity for convergence during the course of the examination. Most infants have brief (1- to 4-second) episodes of convergence spasm in which both eyes make simultaneous adduction movements. Since fixation is not maintained with either eye during these episodes, this is not categorized as esotropia. These episodes become less frequent with increasing age but can be seen up to 4 months. That some neonates can converge in response to visual stimuli is suggested by the behavior of those neonates classified as having intermittent exotropia. Many of these neonates can be observed, while maintaining fixation with one eye, to adduct the exodeviated eye until it also appears to be fixating. Most neonates classified as varying between esodeviation and exodeviation exhibit similar behavior except that they continue to converge past the point of alignment.

Several transient supranuclear disturbances of motility have been described in otherwise normal neonates. These will be discussed under the heading of "Supranuclear Disturbances."

CONCOMITANT STRABISMUS

Congenital Esotropia

There are several distinct syndromes of concomitant esotropia in infancy[35] (Table 16–2). The discussion in this section will be largely restricted to the "essential" form of congenital esotropia. Congenital esotropia is the most common pathological strabismus diagnosed in infancy. Since the presence of esodeviation at birth is not adequately documented in most cases, it has been suggested that the term *congenital esotropia* be replaced with the noncommittal term *infantile esotropia*[36] or even *congenital-infantile esotropia*.[37] However, it is possible that there are neurological factors leading to the development of esotropia that are connatal, even if the esotropia itself is not. Indeed, some congential heart defects (such as the tetralogy of Fallot) may be asymptomatic at birth; cyanosis develops later in response to increasing demands imposed by extrauterine life. These defects might not be classified as congenital heart disease if the stethoscope did not make it relatively easy to identify these infants at birth. On the other hand, while this is currently an important area of research, the contributions of connatal and developmental factors leading to esotropia remain obscure. Therefore, by convention, we will continue to use *congential esotropia,* the traditional term introduced by Costenbader[38] and championed by Parks.[39]

On questioning the parents of an infant with esotropia, the ophthalmologist frequently obtains the history that the child's eyes were crossed from birth. This history must always be suspect. We have learned through clinical experience and during our prospective study of alignment in the newborn that many parents of normal infants believe that their child's eyes have turned in since birth. Four reasons for this are described: (1) the normal brief episodes of convergence spasm have been noted; (2) the infant has an exotropia, and the parents refer to the adduction of the nonfixating eye when it takes up fixation

TABLE 16–2
Concomitant Esotropia in Infancy

Essential esotropia
Esotropia with abduction nystagmus (Ciancia syndrome, nystagmus blockage syndrome)
Refractive accommodative esotropia
Esotropia associated with abnormal neurological status
Secondary (sensory) esotropia

as "turning in"; (3) an exotropia has been noted, and the parents do not distinguish between "wall-eyed" and "cross-eyed"; and (4) many neonates have prominent epicanthal folds that give the impression of esotropia (pseudostrabismus).

Anecdotal experience suggests that the manifested deviation of congenital esotropia is acquired during the first few months of life. The few infants in whom we have documented the onset of esotropia have followed a course similar to the following case.

Case 1.—A 2-month-old infant was examined in follow-up to his brief postnatal exposure to oxygen. He was 9 weeks premature, weighed 1,630 gm at birth, and was one of a set of quadruplets. At the time of this initial examination his ocular alignment varied from orthotropic to 35 p.d. of *exotropia*. His fundus examination findings were normal. He was seen again at 6 months of age with alignment varying from orthotropia to 40 p.d. of esotropia. The diagnosis of congenital esotropia was made 2 weeks later when he was seen with a constant esotropia of 30 to 45 p.d., cross-fixation, and a cycloplegic retinoscopy of −0.75 D in both eyes.

In Nixon and colleagues' study of 1,219 newborn infants,[27] the attempt to identify congenital esotropia at birth did not yield a single neonate with the characteristic findings of congenital esotropia. On the basis of the number of infants examined and the published incidence of congenital esotropia[40, 41] (approximately 1%) it was concluded on statistical grounds that congenital esotropia was unlikely to be identifiable at birth. This is probably correct but not conclusive. Subsequent examination and follow-up that we have obtained suggest that the incidence of congenital esotropia in this population may be somewhat lower than 1%. The findings of Nixon et al. also do not exclude the possibility of esotropia being present at birth in a small subset of infants with congenital esotropia.

Infants with the congenital esotropia syndrome (Fig 16–2) are characterized by (1) moderate- to large-angle esotropia (30 to 50 p.d.), (2) onset before 6 months of age with confirmation by a reliable observer by 1 year of age, (3) deviation unattributable to accommodative factors, (4) no neurological abnormality other than the esotropia, and (5) alternation or amblyopia. Other characteristics that are usually not noted during early infancy but may subsequently be found include (6) frequent vertical strabismus (oblique muscle overaction, dissociated vertical deviation) and (7) frequent association with latent nystagmus.

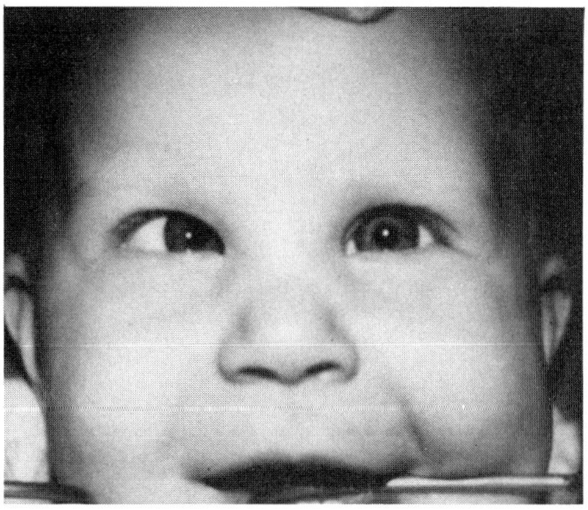

FIG 16–2.
Congenital esotropia in an 8-month-old infant.

A large esodeviation in a normal infant is sufficiently uncommon that referral for a complete ophthalmologic examination is justifiable at any age. However, because we have seen uneventful resolution of esotropia at ages up to 2 months, it may be reasonable to delay referral until this age. Prompt referral for esotropia persisting after 2 months of age is mandatory. While it may be preferable to delay surgical treatment until after 6 months of age for anatomic reasons,[42] early referral excludes other more ominous causes of esotropia (see the section on sensory strabismus later) and permits early diagnosis and treatment of any associated amblyopia.

There is general agreement in this country that the management of essential congenital esotropia is surgical; however, there is still controversy regarding many of the specifics such as the timing of surgery, the number of muscles to be operated upon, bimedial recession vs. recess-resect, etc. It is sufficient to say that while mechanical straightening of the eyes can be satisfactorily accomplished by a variety of surgical means, the functional results are limited by subnormal binocular vision.[35]

Congenital Exotropia

Exotropia in the infant is a somewhat amorphous entity. Even very large angle exotropia may not be pathological in a neonate (Fig 16–3,A). Indeed, the most common form of exotropia that usually presents in older children may have its origin as an exophoria or intermittent exotropia in infancy.[43–45] However, there are occasional patients who develop a constant, large-angle exotropia during the first year of life (Fig 16–3,B) for whom the term *congenital exotropia* seems appropriate.[45] These patients have some similarity to those with congenital esotropia—they may have associated inferior oblique overaction and dissociated vertical deviation, and the functional result from surgical treatment is likely to be subnormal binocular vision.[46, 47]

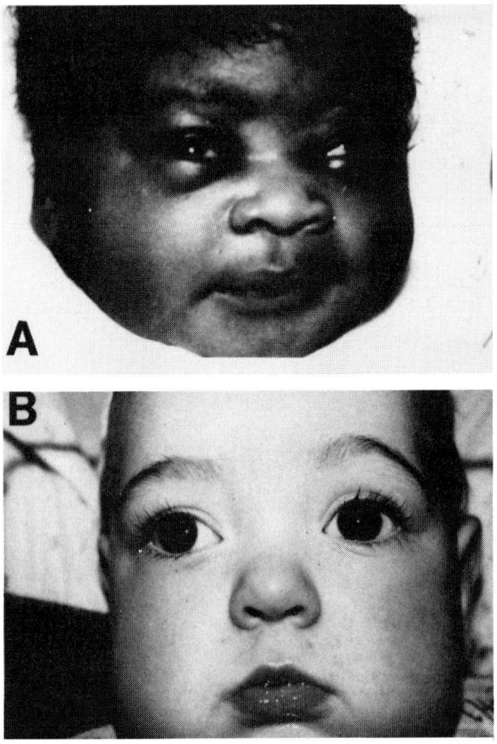

FIG 16–3.
A, even large-angle exotropia in a neonate is benign. Two weeks later this infant was orthotropic. **B,** exotropia in an infant older than 6 months is pathological and should be taken as seriously as esotropia.

Guidelines as to which infants with exotropia should be referred for ophthalmologic evaluation are unclear. Exotropia of any magnitude may be nonpathological in a neonate. This benign neonatal exotropia may persist as long as 6 months; however, the angle of deviation becomes progressively less with time. We recommend that infants with any detectable exotropia after 6 months of age be referred; those whose deviation persists as a large-angle exotropia may warrant referral at a younger age.

Accommodative Esotropia

Typically, accommodative esotropia has its onset between 2 and 3 years of age. However, accommodative ability is probably present to some degree in neonates, and most infants are able to accommodate accurately by 6 months of age.[48–50] The reflex synergism between accommodation and convergence has been shown in infants as young as 2 months of age.[51] Therefore, it is not surprising that refractive esotropia (Fig 16–4) has been reported in infants under 1 year of age.[52, 53] For this reason, cycloplegic refraction must be performed on all infants with esotropia in order to identify any refractive component. In infants under 1 year old, adequate cycloplegia for this purpose is obtained 40 minutes after instillation of 1 drop of 0.5% cyclopentolate in each eye. In infants with heavily pigmented irides, an additional drop of cyclopentolate along with a drop of 2.5% phenylephrine and a drop of 1% tropicamide may be needed for adequate cycloplegia and mydriasis.

For infants in whom hyperopia exceeding +2.00 D is found, accommodative factors must be excluded as the cause of esotropia. This can be accomplished on a short-term basis by means of loaner glasses or daily instillation of 1 drop of 0.06 to 0.125% echothiophate. Occasionally, these measures will completely correct the esotropia, and long-term therapy

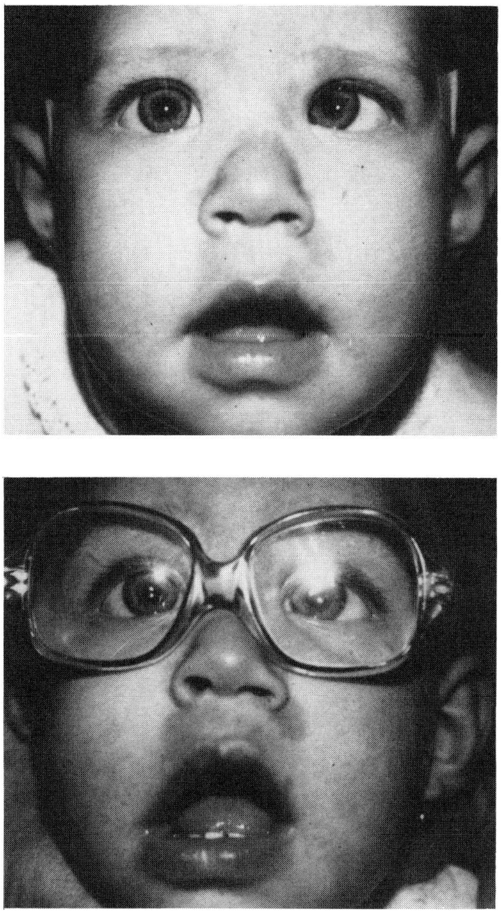

FIG 16–4.
Refractive acommodative esotropia in a 10-month-old infant. Note how the eyes straighten with the hyperopic spectacle correction.

with glasses prescribed for the full cycloplegic refraction is instituted. In most instances, however, antiaccommodative treatment in an esotropic child under 1 year of age turns out to be a negative therapeutic test.

Sensory Strabismus

Development and maintenance of ocular alignment requires binocular sensory feedback to the controlling motor mechanisms. With unilateral disruption of vision during infancy a sensory strabismus frequently ensues. Bilateral visual impairment may also result in strabismus, but nystagmus is usually the more striking finding (discussed under the section on sensory nystagmus). In an infant, sensory strabismus is equally likely to be an esotropia or an exotropia.[54] The causes of visual impairment in infancy are numerous. In some, such as retinoblastoma, strabismus is often the presenting sign.[55] The requirement for urgent treatment in these cases provides a strong argument for prompt and complete ophthalmologic evaluation of all infants with acquired strabismus.

We have observed an unusual type of "strabismus," which is presumed to be due in part to sensory loss, in which an "esodeviation" of the *sound* eye developed after enucleation of the other eye in early infancy.[56] In these patients, a marked head turn toward the remaining eye with preference for fixation in adduction occurred. These patients developed nystagmus when the remaining eye was abducted and presented a picture compatible with the nystagmus compensation syndrome (the distinction between conjugate gaze null point and convergence forms of nystagmus compensation is difficult in the absence of one eye). The patients responded well to recession of the medial rectus and resection of the lateral rectus muscles. On long term follow-up, a fine nystagmus persists with a null point when the remaining eye is in the primary position. We and others[57] have also observed this clinical picture without enucleation in infants with one blind eye, usually due to severe microphthalmos.

PARALYTIC STRABISMUS

Congenital Abducens Palsy

Permanent congenital sixth-nerve palsy is unusual, except as part of a syndrome with other characteristic findings (e.g., Duane Möbius). Transient neonatal sixth-nerve palsy (Fig 16–5), on the other hand, occurs relatively frequently.[58–60] Reisner et al. described lateral rectus paresis in 35 of 6,360 neonates.[60] All cases but one had resolved by 6 weeks of age. Nixon et al. found 3 of 1,219 infants with sixth-nerve palsy, all cases of which resolved.[27] The etiology of transient neonatal sixth-nerve palsy is not clear. An unusually traumatic delivery could not be implicated in Reisner and colleagues' series, but the uniform time course of recovery suggests that some event associated with labor and delivery is responsible. Perhaps in support of the speculation that transient neonatal sixth-nerve palsy may play a role in the development of congenital esotropia,[60] one of Nixon and colleagues' infants with sixth-nerve palsy developed findings typical of nystagmus blockage syndrome. This resolved, however, and the infant eventually became orthotropic.

Duane Retraction Syndrome

Duane retraction syndrome is the most common permanent cause of abduction defects in infants. It is characterized by limited abduction with narrowing of the palpebral fissure and enophthalmos on adduction. An upshoot or downshoot of the affected eye may occur in adduction. Duane syndrome may occur unilaterally (1:3 right vs. left) or bilaterally (about 20%).[61–64] It may be associated with Goldenhar syndrome[62, 65, 66] and other branchial cleft abnormalities. It also may be associated with other phenomena believed to be due to anomalous innervation such as crocodile tears (gustolacrimal reflex)[64, 67] and Marcus Gunn jaw winking.[68]

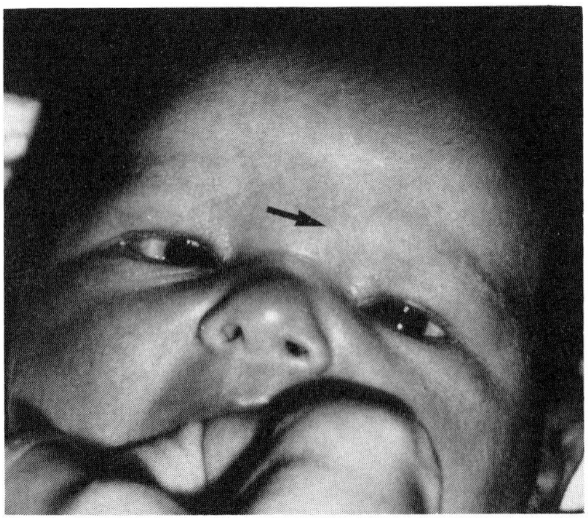

FIG 16–5.
Benign left abducens palsy in a neonate seen in Nixon and colleagues' series.[27] The eyes are in left gaze, as indicated by *arrow*. The palsy resolved without sequelae.

In most cases, the defect in Duane retraction syndrome is an abnormal synkinesis between the medial and lateral rectus muscles.[69–76] In several clinicopathologic reports from patients with documented Duane syndrome, it was found that the abducens nucleus and nerve were absent[77] and the lateral rectus muscles of the affected eyes were innervated by a branch of the inferior division of the oculomotor nerve.[78, 79]

In Duane syndrome, the eyes may be straight or exotropic in the primary position. Most commonly though, there is a moderate esotropia. The infant subsequently develops a head turn toward the side of the defect that permits alignment of the eyes. The development of the head turn roughly coincides with the expected age of onset for stereopsis. This is evident in the following case report in which an infant with Duane syndrome was identified prospectively and then followed closely for the onset of head turn.

> Case 2.—An otherwise normal 8-week-old son of a pediatric ophthalmology fellow was examined for intermittent esotropia. He was found to have a small variable esotropia and an abduction defect of the left eye. He was closely observed until, at 3 months of age, retraction of the left eye during adduction became apparent, which confirmed the diagnosis of Duane syndrome. Subsequently, at 4 months of age, he developed a head turn to the left that produced orthophoria.

In Duane syndrome, treatment is usually not required during infancy, but surgery may be indicated in the preschool child for an objectionable head turn with esotropia in primary position, retraction, or upshoot or downshoot in adduction.

Möbius Syndrome

Möbius syndrome (Fig 16–6) is a congenital condition resulting from palsy of the sixth and seventh cranial nerves, usually bilaterally. There is generally a moderate-angle esotropia. Vertical eye movements may be

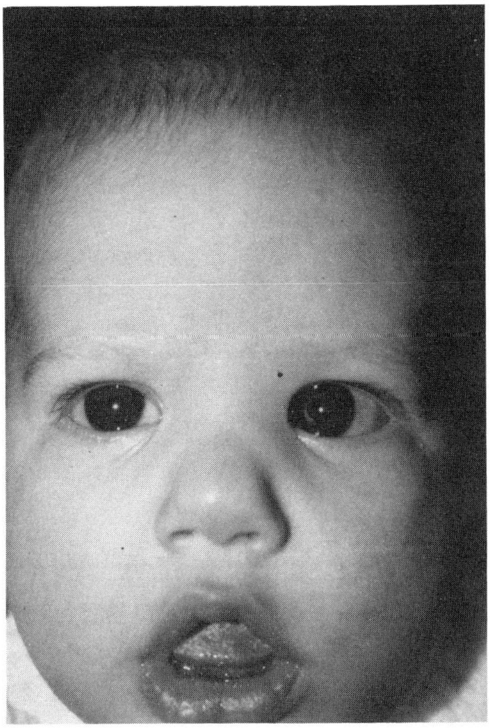

FIG 16–6.
Möbius syndrome. Note the small-angle esotropia, flattened nasolabial folds, and atrophic tongue.

present, but the only apparent horizontal movement is convergence. There is associated flattening of the nasolabial folds and hemiatrophy of the tongue. In infancy, poor feeding associated with the tongue atrophy is frequently a problem. Clinicopathologic studies of Möbius syndrome patients have shown hypoplasia of the affected cranial nerve nuclei in some cases and degenerative changes in others.[80]

Acquired Abducens Palsy

Acquired abducens palsy in childhood may be due to hydrocephalus, trauma, tumors in the posterior fossa or nasopharynx, inflammatory disease (e.g., Gradenigo syndrome), or vascular malformations.[81, 82] Management in these cases is directed at diagnosis and treatment of the underlying etiology. Amblyopia may develop and require treatment while waiting for recovery of lateral rectus function. Measures to prevent secondary contracture such as patching the sound eye or botulinum toxin injection of the antagonistic medial rectus muscle[83] may be helpful during this period. Residual lateral rectus palsy may be treated with a recess-resect or a muscle transposition procedure, depending on the degree of remaining lateral rectus function.

There is also a benign sixth-nerve palsy in childhood[84] that can occur in infancy.[85–87] This is frequently preceded by a febrile illness and may be recurrent. Complete resolution is the rule; however, a concomitant esotropia may remain after lateral rectus function has returned to normal. It has been postulated that benign sixth-nerve palsy in childhood has an immunologic basis similar to the parainfectious neuropathy seen in Guillian Barré syndrome.[85]

Oculomotor Palsy

Congenital oculomotor palsy, in our experience and that of others,[88] is often associated with other neurological abnormalities, although it may occur as an isolated defect.[89, 90] It typically presents as an exotropia and hypotropia of the affected eye (Fig 16–7) present from birth. Involvement is usually unilateral, although bilateral cases do occur. There is variable involvement of the medial, superior and inferior rectus and, less obviously, the inferior oblique. Blepharoptosis and pupillary involvement are also usually present. Although hypoplasia of the oculomotor nucleus has been reported in congenital oculomotor palsy,[91] the frequent signs of aberrant regeneration and lack of contralateral superior rectus or levator involvement in these patients suggest that injury to the oculomotor nerve itself is the more usual etiology.

Treatment in these cases is problematic. Amblyopia is frequent (usually in the paretic eye but occasionally in the nonparetic eye) and requires appropriate occlusion therapy. The strabismus can be managed with various combinations of lateral rectus recession, medial rectus resection, superior oblique tendon transfer, and horizontal rectus muscle upshift.

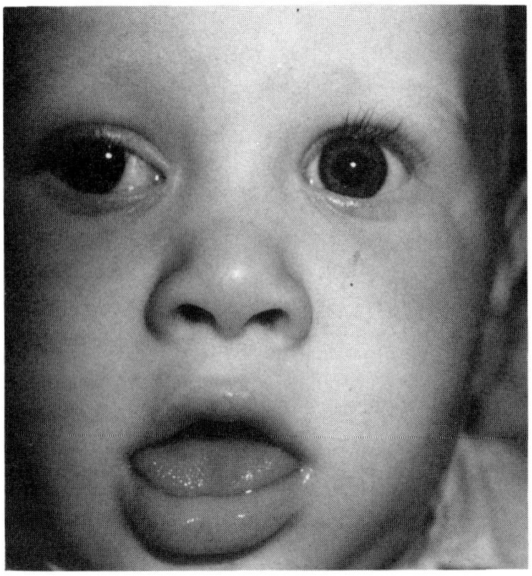

FIG 16–7.
Congenital right oculomotor palsy. Note the exotropia, hypotropia, and slight blepharoptosis.

The blepharoptosis may require levator resection or a frontalis sling.

Congenital syndromes, presumably involving anomalous innervation of extraocular muscles supplied by the oculomotor nerve, have also been described. Simultaneous contraction of the lateral rectus muscles ("perversion of the extraocular muscles") is a rare syndrome characterized by exotropia, absent adduction of the affected eye, and simultaneous bilateral abduction on attempted gaze to the side opposite the affected eye.[92–95] Electromyographic evidence suggests that this syndrome is similar to Duane's syndrome; however, the oculomotor nerve provides much less innervation to the medial rectus than it provides to the lateral rectus via an anomalous branch.[94] A vertical retraction syndrome has also been described[96, 97] that, at least in some cases, appears to be due to anomalous innervation involving the oculomotor nerve.[98]

Cyclic oculomotor paresis[99, 100] is a condition that is present from birth and consists of complete unilateral oculomotor palsy. Every 2 to 3 minutes, however, the blepharoptosis improves, the pupil constricts, and the eye adducts. After a few seconds the paresis returns. The condition usually persists throughout life.

Superior Oblique Palsy

Isolated superior oblique palsy in children is a relatively common entity and generally presumed to be congenital; however, it is rarely diagnosed in the neonatal period. The patient is usually brought to the physician's attention because of the compensatory torticollis that develops in later infancy. Additional diagnostic findings that are usually present at this time are hypertropia of the affected eye, inferior oblique overaction, and a positive Bielschowsky head tilt test response. In most cases the etiology of congenital superior oblique palsy is obscure.

Due to the relationship of utricular activity to cyclovertical muscle activity,[101, 102] the hypertropia due to superior oblique palsy is largely absent in a supine or prone position. Therefore, compensatory torticollis does not develop until after the infant has assumed an upright posture (sitting and walking) and the onset of stereopsis has provided a reward for maintaining binocular alignment. For treatment purposes, it is important to distinguish torticollis due to superior oblique palsy from congenital muscular torticollis, which, in contrast, has an onset at birth or shortly thereafter.[103] For diagnostic purposes, ocular torticollis due to superior oblique palsy can be eliminated by patching the palsied eye[104] or by placing the patient in a supine position,[105] except in long-standing conditions in which secondary musculoskeletal abnormalities have developed.[106] Hiatus hernia is an unusual nonocular cause of abnormal head movement and posture in infants and children (Sandifer syndrome)[107] that must occasionally be considered in the differential diagnosis of torticollis.

Neuromuscular Ophthalmoplegias

Neonates may show ocular involvement in two forms of myasthenia gravis. Transitory neonatal myasthenia develops in 12% of infants born to mothers with generalized myasthenia gravis and is due to a circulating factor transmitted from the mother. The most common manifestation is feeding difficulty. Ophthalmoplegia (usually just blepharoptosis) is noted in only about 15% of infants with this condition.[108] Congenital myasthenia occurs in infants born to nonmyasthenic mothers. In the neonatal period this condition is characterized by a weak cry and some general weakness. With the exception of blepharoptosis, the ophthalmoplegia that becomes the predominant feature in childhood is usually not present in the neonatal period.[109] Familial infantile myasthenia presents with respiratory and feeding difficulty at birth but does not have extraocular muscle involvement.

External ophthalmoplegia may be a feature of foodborne and wound botulism occurring in children and adults.[110,111] Infantile botulism, on the other hand, in which *Clostridium botulinum* organisms colonize the intestinal tract and produce toxin that is absorbed systemically, is generally not reported to produce external ophthalmoplegia other than blepharoptosis.[112,113] Internal ophthalmoplegia is common in all three types of botulism.

While external ophthalmoplegia is known to develop in a number of congenital myopathies, ophthalmoplegia (other than blepharoptosis) present in the neonatal period has been described in relatively few conditions. These include myotubular myopathy,[114,115] congential fiber-type disproportion,[116] and a fatal mitochondrial cytochrome deficiency.[117]

SUPRANUCLEAR DISTURBANCES

Neuropathologic vs. Benign

Skew deviation is a vertical divergence of the eyes that is usually found in association with brain stem or cerebellar disease. However, in 242 otherwise normal consecutive neonates, Hoyt et al. found 22 instances of skew deviation.[118] The skew deviation resolved by 3 days of age in most of these infants. Seven of these neonates were said to have had an associated horizontal strabismus; 5 developed congenital esotropia. In contrast, we have not seen a case that we would classify as skew deviation in 2,771 neonates. Many of these infants have large exotropias and asymmetrical lid positions that make vertical deviations difficult to judge. Because an infant spontaneously looks in various gaze positions, we have often seen what appeared to be a hyperdeviation or hypodeviation of the abducted eye. However, once good fixation with one eye is obtained, there is no evident vertical deviation of the nonfixating eye when judgment is based on the corneal reflex and care is taken to ignore the relative lid positions.

The "setting-sun" sign consists of tonic downward deviation of the eyes along with lid retraction. In infants, the most commonly associated neuropathology is hydrocephalus or kernicterus. It has also been described with or without lid retraction as a transient finding after obstetrical trauma[119] and in otherwise healthy neonates.[118,120] We have seen tonic downward deviation with and without lid retraction relatively frequently in healthy neonates. In contrast to infants with Parinaud's syndrome, elevation of the eyes can be demonstrated by utilizing the oculocephalic reflex. They can also be induced to fixate in the primary position (this eliminates any associated lid retraction) when appropriately stimulated; with lapses in attentiveness the tonic downward deviation returns.

Opsoclonus is a rapid, chaotic to-and-fro movement of the eyes. It has been described in infants with encephalitis[121,122] and hydrocephalus[123] and in association with other unexplained neurological findings (e.g., mental retardation, truncal ataxia, unexplained poor vision).[124] Opsoclonus may also be the presenting sign in infants with occult neuroblastoma[125,126]; therefore, it is mandatory that infants with opsoclonus have appropriate radiological and urinary vanillylmandelic acid evaluation. Opsoclonus has also been described as a transient finding in otherwise normal neonates.[118,127] Prospectively, Hoyt identified eight infants with transient opsoclonus in 242 consecutive neonates.[127] We have not seen what we would describe as opsoclonus in an otherwise healthy neonate.

Internuclear ophthalmoplegia (INO) is characterized by deficient adduction of the eye ipsilateral to a lesion involving the medial longitudinal fasciculus (MLF). It has been described in otherwise normal premature infants[128] and is presumably due to immaturity of the MLF. When present, INO is better demonstrated by caloric testing than by perotatory stimulation.

Double Elevator Palsy

Congenital double elevator palsy (Fig 16–8) consists of an apparent paralysis of the superior rectus and inferior oblique muscles of one eye that is not adequately explained by the passive duction findings.[129–131] There is a hypotropia of the affected eye in primary position when fixating with the uninvolved eye; a head posture with chin elevation frequently develops to allow binocular vision. Varying degrees of pseudoptosis and true ptosis of the ipsilateral portion of the eyelid are frequently present. Treatment of double elevator palsy is by surgical transposition of the medial and lateral rectus muscles.

Neuroanatomic considerations make it unlikely that a single nuclear or infranuclear lesion could account for the findings. A supranuclear etiology is likely in those cases where elevation of the affected eye can be produced by Bell's phenomenon.[131] Congenital anomalies[132] or fibrosis[133] involving the inferior rectus can produce a clinical picture similar to double elevator palsy and must be excluded by passive duction testing. In those cases where restrictive factors produce a clinical picture similar to double elevator palsy, surgery directed at relieving the restriction, usually recession of the inferior rectus muscle, is the appropriate treatment.

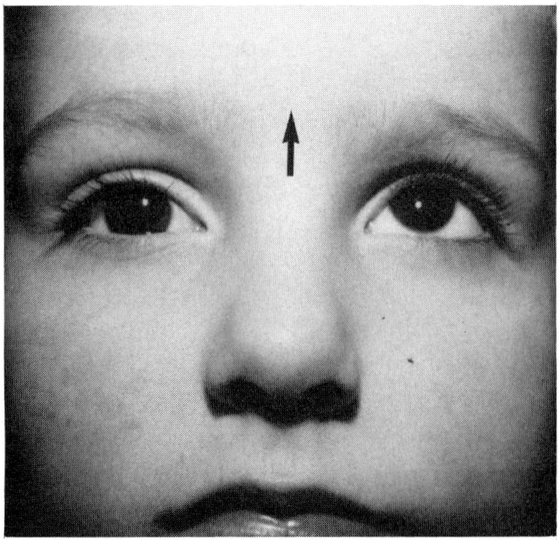

FIG 16–8.
Right double elevator palsy. The child is looking upward, as indicated by *arrow*.

Congenital Ocular Motor Apraxia

Congenital ocular motor apraxia is a rare condition in which there is a congenital defect in the supranuclear mechanism responsible for producing voluntary saccades.[134, 135] In early infancy, these children are sometimes thought to be blind[135, 136] because they have no way of tracking visual targets—they cannot produce refixation saccades, and smooth pursuit movements are not normally present in the neonate. At several months of age with improved motor control of the head, the infant develops a strategy for fixating on objects by using the vestibulo-ocular reflex and smooth pursuit movements that are now functional. This produces the head thrusts that are characteristic of this disorder as the infant turns his head toward and beyond the object to be fixated on. Fixation is then maintained by smooth pursuit and vestibulo-ocular reflexes as the child returns his head to the primary position. As the child grows older, he generally develops some ability to initiate voluntary saccades, usually in association with exaggerated blinking.

MECHANICAL STRABISMUS

Brown Syndrome

The major finding in Brown syndrome (Fig 16–9) is an inability to elevate the eye that is most pronounced in adduction.[137] Restriction of eye movement in this field on passive duction testing is required to confirm the diagnosis. Historically it was believed that congenital cases were due to an anomaly of the

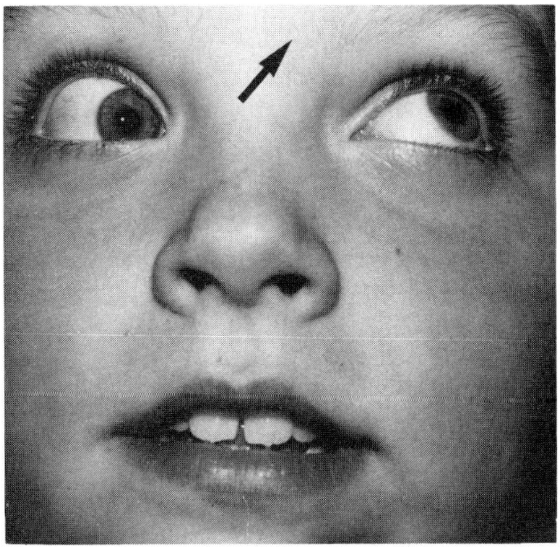

FIG 16–9.
Right-sided Brown syndrome. The child is looking up and to the left, as indicated by *arrow*.

superior oblique tendon or sheath; however, it is now well understood that mechanical limitation of elevation in adduction results from a variety of etiologies. In mild cases, findings may only be present on attempted upgaze; these children usually present for diagnosis after 5 years of age, if at all. In more severe cases there is hypotropia of the affected eye in the primary position that may be noted in infancy. In order to obtain binocular vision, these patients may develop a chin-up head position (with or without head tilt). Treatment, when necessary, consists of superior oblique tenotomy or recession with or without an ipsilateral inferior oblique weakening procedure. Neither surgical technique nor results obtained are widely agreed upon.

Congenital Fibrosis Syndrome

Congenital fibrosis syndrome[137, 138] (Fig 16–10) is inherited as an autosomal dominant disorder in which the muscle fibers of most or all of the extraocular muscles are replaced by fibrous elements.[139–143] There is typically a fixed hypodeviation of both eyes, blepharoptosis, a head posture with chin elevation, and spastic convergence on attempted lateral gaze or upgaze. Treatment is bilateral inferior rectus recession, bimedial recession, and bilateral frontalis suspension of the upper lids which are performed when the child is in the toddler or preschool years.

Absent and Anomalous Extraocular Muscles

Rarely, congenital absence of an extraocular muscle can produce the clinical picture of a profound palsy of that muscle.[144] This most frequently involves the superior oblique muscle[145–150] and should be suspected in cases of congenital superior oblique palsy with associated amblyopia, horizontal strabismus, facial asymmetry, or marked underaction of the superior oblique. Cases involving an absence of the inferior rectus,[151–158] medial rectus,[159–161]

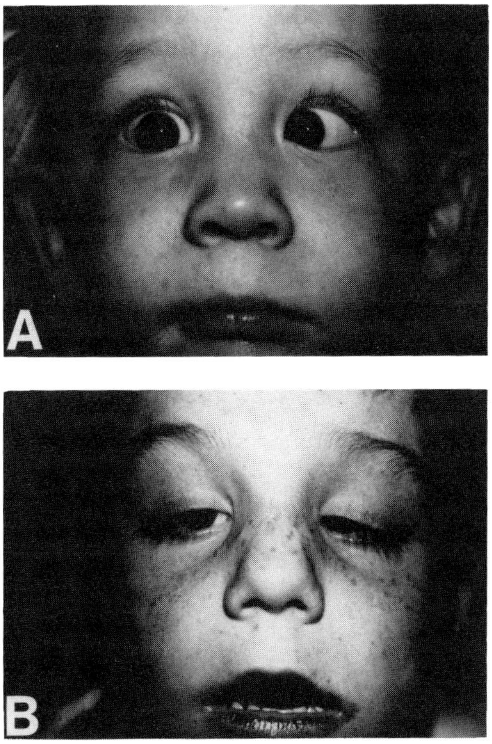

FIG 16–10.
A, congenital fibrosis syndrome in a 12-month-old infant. This child eventually required bilateral inferior rectus recessions and bilateral medial rectus recessions. The levator function remained good, which is atypical for this condition. **B**, a more typical appearance of congenital fibrosis syndrome in an older child.

lateral rectus,[160, 162] and superior rectus[163] have also been reported.

Strabismus is frequently seen in cases of craniosynostosis and is presumably due to abnormal anatomic relationships between the extraocular muscles, the orbit, and the eye.[164, 165] Exotropia is more common than is esotropia, particularly when there is associated hypertelorism. Many of these patients have an apparent superior oblique palsy with marked inferior oblique overaction, a *V* pattern, and superior oblique underaction.[165–168] Asymmetrical cases in which there is a large hypertropia in primary position may present for diagnosis in infancy. The craniosynostoses are also associated with congenitally absent or anomalous extraocular muscles.[169–174]

NYSTAGMUS

Physiological Nystagmus

Vestibular nystagmus is efficiently produced in an infant by rotating the infant at arm's length with the head inclinded 30 degrees forward.[175] This normally produces nystagmus with a tonic deviation of the eyes toward the direction in which the examiner is rotating and a repetitive fast component returning the eyes toward midline. Most neonates will give at least a single fast component if rotated long enough; however, the tonic phase is predominant. Consistent with previous reports,[176, 177] we have found that sustained nystagmus can be elicited in only about half of all normal alert neonates and, in these, often with some difficulty. It is interesting to find the saccadic component of vestibular nystagmus missing in an infant who could produce only saccades and no smooth pursuit when following the examiner's face only moments earlier. By 4 weeks of age, both the slow and fast phases of vestibular nystagmus are easily elicited in essentially all normal infants.

Optokinetic nystagmus occurs when viewing contours that pass continuously in one direction. Although smooth pursuit movements are not present when following a target,[23, 24] both the smooth pursuit and saccadic return phases of horizontal optokinetic nystagmus are present in the neonate.[178] In the clinical examination of infants, vertical optokinetic nystagmus is often more easily observed as the lids follow the vertical movements of the eyes; however, vertical optokinetic nystagmus usually cannot be elicited in infants less than 1 month of age.[179]

Sensory Nystagmus

Sensory nystagmus in infancy occurs with bilateral disruption of central vision such as occurs with cataracts, macular colobomas or chorioretinal scars, albinism, achromatopsia, Leber's amaurosis, and many other conditions. Clinically, the nystagmus usually appears to be pendular with the major component in the horizontal axis,[180] although this is not helpful as a distinguishing feature in that irregular or jerk-type nystagmus may also occur.[181] In the most severe visual impairment, the excursions are very large[180] and often described as "searching nystagmus."

Sensory nystagmus may develop if the visual defect is congenital or acquired during the first 2 years of life.[180] When the visual defect is present from birth, the onset of nystagmus is not immediate but, rather, parallels the course for development of the fixation reflex in normal infants. However, in the absence of visual feedback, the attempt to develop the fixation reflex results in the abnormal eye movements. An example in which the time course for the onset of sensory nystagmus was well documented is given in the following case.

Case 3.—A diagnosis of Peters anomaly was made in a newborn girl with bilateral central corneal opacities and iridocorneal adhesions. The pupils were completely occluded by the opacities. There was no fixation or nystagmus, and the eyes were in an exodeviated position. She was followed with the hope that some clearing at the periphery of the opacities would improve her treatment options until, at 2 months of age, she began to develop searching nystagmus. She would orient toward a bright light, and the eyes remained in a moderately exodeviated position. Her searching nystagmus was well developed 2 weeks later when optical iridectomies were performed that resulted in clear peripheral visual axes in both eyes. By 4 months of age the searching eye movements had essentially ceased, and the exodeviation had been replaced by a variable esodeviation up to 40 p.d. At the age of 5 months the red reflex through the iridectomies remained clear in both eyes, and there was no nystagmus. She showed refixation behavior (albeit with abnormal fixation movements) with the right eye but not the left, and a variable esodeviation persisted.

The development of sensory nystagmus may be reversed if central vision can be restored in a timely fashion, as demonstrated in this and other cases.[182–184] With longer delays in visual rehabilitation the nystagmus becomes irreversible. In this regard, the plasticity of the oculomotor system during development resembles the problem of amblyopia in the sensory limb of the visual system. There exists a critical period during which the infant is susceptible to the development of sensory nystagmus and during which treatment may be effective in reversing the nystagmus.

The sensory nystagmus discussed to this point is that seen with binocular visual impairment. However, monocular nystagmus can occur with a unilateral vision defect in the ipsilateral eye. We have observed this most commonly in children with unilateral optic nerve hypoplasia or unilateral high myopia. It can also occur with optic nerve glioma,[185–192] amblyopia,[193] or media opacities. The nystagmus is typically small amplitude, pendular, and primarily vertical.[194]

Congenital Motor Nystagmus

Congenital motor nystagmus is a primary defect of the efferent (motor) limb that occurs in the absence of any abnormalities of the afferent (sensory) limb of the visual system, except perhaps for secondary amblyopia. Clinically, it typically appears as a conjugate horizontal jerk nystagmus, but a wide variety and complexity of characteristics can be seen.[181] As with congenital esotropia, the condition is said to be present at birth, but its presence is not usually documented prior to several weeks of age or later. In the course of our study we have not seen nystagmus in an otherwise normal neonate. With an estimated prevalence of 1:6,550, however,[195] we have not yet examined enough neonates to make a statistical statement as to whether the condition is unlikely to be connatal.

Infants with congenital motor nystagmus may exhibit head shaking. This may be a compensatory response to the nystagmus that results in improved acuity in some patients.[196–199] In addition, there are three other factors that may be used to minimize the nystagmus and improve acuity. These include simply keeping both eyes open, placing the eyes in a specific gaze position, and convergence or adduction of the eyes. It is clinically useful to subclassify congenital motor nystagmus on the basis of which of these factors is predominant in a particular case.

Latent nystagmus is a nystagmus of both eyes that is present only under monocular viewing conditions. It is characteristically a horizontal jerk nystagmus with the fast component beating toward the fixating eye and a decelerating-velocity, exponential slow phase toward the occluded eye.[200] With both eyes unoccluded, some of these patients continue to have nystagmus with the same waveform characteristics (but diminished in amplitude).[200] Manifested latent nystagmus is the peculiar term that has been applied to this situation. Latent nystagmus is very commonly associated with congenital esotropia.

With null-point nystagmus, there is a particular gaze position that results in dampening of the eye movements.[201] Typically this is a lateral-gaze position but may also be a vertical or rotary position. In order to maximize visual acuity, the infant will assume a head position that allows him to place his eyes in this position (Fig 16–11).

Esotropia may develop as part of the nystagmus compensation syndrome.[202–204] In these patients, dampening of the nystagmus occurs with adduction, and the eyes assume a con-

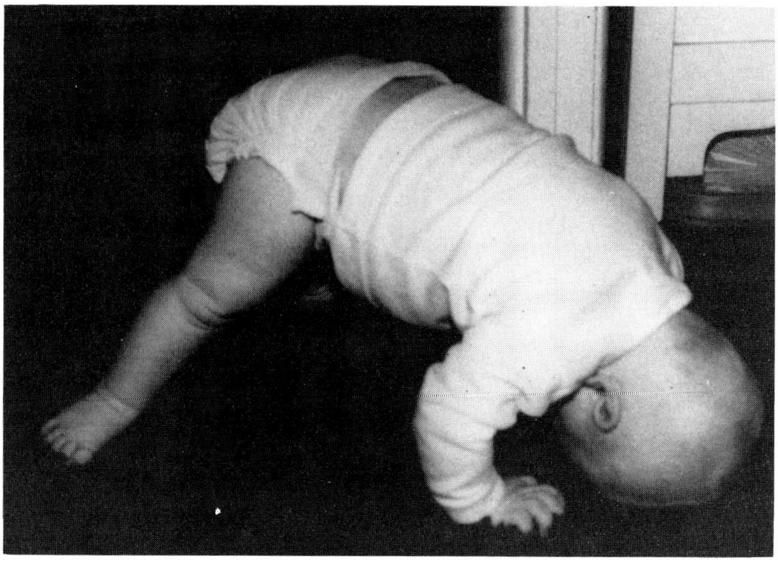

FIG 16–11.
Abnormal head posture due to congenital null-point nystagmus in a 6-month-old infant. When not assuming this unusual posture for activities requiring good visual acuity (e.g., watching television), this infant exhibited a simple head turn, which is the more usual manifestation of null-point nystagmus.

vergent position in order to maximize visual acuity. Rather than abduct the fixating eye to look at a new target, these infants tend to exhibit cross-fixation. The difficulty in getting these infants to abduct their eyes sometimes leads to a misdiagnosis of abducens palsy or Duane syndrome. However, full abduction can be demonstrated with the oculocephalic reflex.

It may be possible to distinguish between some of these groups of patients on the basis of the waveform found on electronystagmography.[200] Clinically, however, there can be considerable overlap. For example, most patients with null-point nystagmus will also have increased nystagmus with one eye occluded and improved acuity with convergence for near vision. Patients have been described in whom the primary mechanism of compensation for the nystagmus switches between convergence and gaze position.[205] The overlap of these clinical groups is also reflected in that congenital motor nystagmus may be treated with extraocular muscle surgery designed to produce a conjugate gaze shift,[201, 206] an induced exodeviation to produce convergence,[207] or a combination of both.[208, 209]

Acquired Nystagmus

Acquired nystagmus in infants, as in adults, may result from a variety of neurological disorders that require appropriately aggressive work-up. Spasmus nutans, however, is a benign form of acquired nystagmus that is peculiar to infants. Spasmus nutans comprises the triad of nystagmus, head nodding, and abnormal head posture. The onset usually occurs between 4 and 12 months of age.[210] It is self-limited, with resolution usually beginning several months after onset and complete within 1 to 2 years. The nystagmus is typically high frequency, pendular, and mostly horizontal. Marked asymmetry of the nystagmus between the two eyes is the rule and may even appear to be monocular at some point in the course of the disorder.

There have been reports of serious organic lesions producing nystagmus that could be mistaken for spasmus nutans.[185–192, 211] The lesion most commonly presenting in this manner has been a glioma of the optic nerve or chiasm. These cases generally have a presentation that is not entirely typical of spasmus nutans, or there are other neurological or constitutional signs suggesting more serious pathology. Nontheless, caution is advised in making the diagnosis of spasmus nutans. Careful follow-up is mandatory, and any atypical finding or other neurological sign should prompt appropriate radiological studies.

REFERENCES

1. Fantz RL, Ordy JM, Udelf MS: Maturation of pattern vision in infants during the first six months. *J Comp Physiol Psychol* 1962; 55:907.
2. Teller DY, Morse R, Borton R, et al: Visual acuity for vertical and diagonal gratings in human infants. *Vision Res* 1974; 14:1433.
3. Banks MS, Salapatek P: Contrast sensitivity function of the infant visual system. *Vision Res* 1976; 16:687.
4. Atkinson J, Braddick O, Moar K: Development of contrast sensitivity over the first three months of life in the human infant. *Vision Res* 1977; 17:1037.
5. Dobson V, Mayer DL, Lee CP: Visual acuity screening of preterm infants. *Invest Ophthalmol Vis Sci* 1980; 19:1498.
6. Gwiazda J, Brill S, Mohindra I, et al: Preferential looking acuity in infants from two to fifty-eight weeks of age. *Am J Optom Physiol Opt* 1980; 57:428.
7. Marg E, Freeman DN, Peltzman P, et al: Visual acuity development in human infants: Evoked potential measurements. *Invest Ophthalmol Vis Sci* 1976; 15:150.
8. Sokol S: Measurement of infant visual acuity from pattern reversal evoked potential. *Vision Res* 1978; 18:33.
9. Held R, Birch EE, Gwiazda J: Stereoacuity of human infants. *Proc Natl Acad Sci USA* 1980; 77:5572.
10. Fox R, Aslin RN, Shea SL, et al: Stereopsis in human infants. *Science* 1980; 207:323.
11. Petrig B, Julesz B, Kropfl W, et al: Development of stereopsis and cortical binocularity in human infants: Electrophysiological evidence. *Science* 1981; 213:1402.
12. Archer SM, Helveston EM, Miller KK, et al: Stereopsis in normal infants and infants with congenital esotropia. *Am J Ophthalmol* 1986; 101:591.
13. Horstein GPM, Winkelman JE: Electrical activity of the retina in relation to histological differentiation in infants born prematurely and at full-term. *Vision Res* 1962; 2:269.
14. Winkelman JE, Horsten GPM: The ERG of premature and full-term born infants during the first days of life. *Ophthalmologica* 1962; 143:92.
15. Isenberg SJ: Macular development in the premature infant. *Am J Ophthalmol* 1986; 101:74.
16. Lewis TL, Maurer D, Kay D: Newborns' central vision: Whole or hole? *J Exp Child Psychol* 1978; 26:193.
17. Lewis TL, Maurer D: Central vision in the newborn. *J Exp Child Psychol* 1980; 29:475.
18. Hollenberg MJ, Spira AW: Human retinal development: Ultrastructure of the outer retina. *Am J Anat* 1973; 137:357.
19. Abramov I, Gordon J, Hendrickson A, et al: The retina of the newborn infant. *Science* 1982; 217:265.
20. Hendrickson AE, Yuodelis C: The morphological development of the human fovea. *Ophthalmology* 1984; 91:603.
21. Slater AM, Findlay JM: The measurement of fixation position in the newborn baby. *J Exp Child Psychol* 1972; 14:349.
22. Hoyt CS, Nickel BL, Billson FA: Ophthalmological examination of the infant. Developmental aspects. *Surv Ophthalmol* 1982; 26:177.
23. Dayton GO, Jones MH, Steele B, et al: Developmental study of coordinated eye movements in the human infant. II. An electrooculographic study of the fixation reflex in the newborn. *Arch Ophthalmol* 1964; 71:871.
24. Dayton GO, Jones MH: Analysis of characteristics of fixation reflex in infants by use of direct current electrooculography. *Neurology NY* 1964; 14:1152.
25. Goren CC, Sarty M, Wand-Wu PYK: Visual following and pattern discrimination of face-like stimuli by newborn infants. *Pediatrics* 1975; 56:544.
26. Réthy I: Development of the simultaneous fixation from the divergent anatomic eye-position of the neonate. *J Pediatr Ophthalmol* 1969; 6:92.
27. Nixon RB, Helveston EM, Miller K, et al: Incidence of strabismus in neonates. *Am J Ophthalmol* 1985; 100:798.

28. Friedrich D, de Decker W: Study of the development of strabismus during the first six months of life. Presented at the Sixth International Orthoptic Congress, Harrogate Great Britain, July 1987.
29. Ling BC: A genetic study of sustained visual fixation and associated behavior in the human infant from birth to six months. *J Genet Psychol* 1942; 61:227.
30. Salapatek P, Kessen W: Visual scanning of triangles by the human newborn. *J Exp Child Psychol* 1966; 3:155.
31. Wickelgren LW: Convergence in the human newborn. *J Exp Child Psychol* 1967; 5:74.
32. Wickelgren LW: The ocular response of human newborns to intermittent visual movement. *J Exp Child Psychol* 1969; 8:469.
33. Slater AM, Findlay JM: Binocular fixation in the newborn baby. *J Exp Child Psychol* 1975; 20:248.
34. Aslin RN: Development of binocular fixation in human infants. *J Exp Child Psychol* 1977; 23:133.
35. von Noorden GK: Infantile esotropia: A continuing riddle. *Am Orthoptic J* 1984; 34:52.
36. Costenbader FD: Infantile esotropia. *Trans Am Ophthalmol Soc* 1961; 59:397.
37. Helveston EM, Ellis FD, Schott, J, et al: Surgical treatment of congenital esotropia. *Am J Ophthalmol* 1983; 96:218.
38. Costenbader FD: The management of convergent strabismus, in Allen JH (ed): *Strabismus Ophthalmic Symposium.* St Louis, CV Mosby Co, 1950, p 343.
39. Parks MM: Operate early for congenital strabismus, in Brockhurst RJ, Boruchoff SA, Hutchinson TB, et al (eds): *Controversy in Ophthalmology.* Philadelphia, WB Saunders Co, 1977, p 424.
40. Graham PA: Epidemiology of strabismus. *Br J Ophthalmol* 1974; 58:224.
41. Friedman Z, Neumann E, Hyams SW, et al: Ophthalmic screening of 38,000 children, age 1 to 2 1/2 years, in child welfare clinics. *J Pediatr Ophthalmol Strabismus* 1980; 17:261.
42. Swan KC, Wilkins JH: Extraocular muscle surgery in early infancy: Anatomical factors. *J Pediatr Ophthalmol Strabismus* 1984; 21:44.
43. Costenbader FD: The physiology and management of divergent strabismus, in Allen JH (ed): *Strabismus Ophthalmic Symposium.* St Louis, CV Mosby Co, 1950, p 353.
44. Jampolsky A: Management of exodeviations, in Haik GM (ed): *Strabismus: Symposium of the New Orleans Academy of Ophthalmology.* St Louis, CV Mosby Co, 1962, p 143.
45. Parks MM: Comitant exodeviations in children, in Haik GM (ed): *Strabismus: Symposium of the New Orleans Academy of Ophthalmology.* St Louis, CV Mosby Co, 1962, p 46.
46. Williams F, Beneish R, Polomeno RC, et al: Congenital exotropia. *Am Orthoptic J* 1984; 34:92.
47. Moore S, Cohen RL: Congenital exotropia. *Am Orthoptic J* 1985; 35:68.
48. Haynes HM, White BL, Held R: Visual accommodation in human infants. *Science* 1965; 148:528.
49. Braddick O, Atkinson J, French J, et al: A photorefractive study of infant accommodation. *Vision Res* 1979; 19:1319.
50. Banks MS: The development of visual accommodation during early infancy. *Child Dev* 1980; 51:646.
51. Aslin RN, Jackson RW: Accommodative-convergence in young infants: Development of a synergistic sensory-motor system. *Can J Psychol* 1979; 33:222.
52. Pollard ZF: Accommodative esotropia during the first year of life. *Arch Ophthalmol* 1976; 94:1912.
53. Baker JD, Parks MM: Early onset accommodative esotropia. *Am J Ophthalmol* 1980; 90:11.
54. Sidikaro Y, von Noorden GK: Observations in sensory heterotropia. *J Pediatr Ophthalmol Strabismus* 1982; 19:12.
55. Ellsworth RM: The practical management of retinoblastoma. *Trans Am Ophthalmol Soc* 1969; 67:463.
56. Helveston EM, Pinchoff B, Ellis FD, et al: Unilateral esotropia after enucleation in infancy. *Am J Ophthalmol* 1985; 100:96.
57. Kushner BJ: Ocular causes of abnormal head postures. *Ophthalmology* 1979; 86:2115.
58. Benson PF: Transient unilateral external rectus muscle palsy in newborn infants. *Br Med J* 1962; 1:1055.
59. Paine RS: Neurologic condition in the neonatal period. *Pediatr Clin North Am* 1961; 8:577.
60. Reisner SH, Perlman M, Ben-Tovim N, et al: Transient lateral rectus muscle paresis in the newborn infant. *J Pediatr* 1971; 78:461.

61. Kirkham TH: Duane's syndrome and familial perceptive deafness. *Br J Opthalmol* 1969; 53:335.
62. Pfaffenbach DD, Cross HH, Kearns TP: Congenital anomalies in Duane's retraction syndrome. *Arch Ophthalmol* 1972; 88:635.
63. Isenberg S, Urist MJ: Clinical observations in 101 consecutive patients with Duane's retraction syndrome. *Am J Ophthalmol* 1977; 84:419.
64. Maruo T, Kusota N, Arimoto H, et al: Duane's syndrome. *Jap J Ophthalmol* 1979; 23:453.
65. Pieroni D: Goldenhar's syndrome associated with bilateral Duane's syndrome. *J Pediatr Ophthalmol* 1969; 6:16.
66. Velez G: Duane's retraction syndrome associated with Goldenhar's syndrome. *Am J Ophthalmol* 1970; 70:945.
67. Ramsay J, Taylor D: Congenital crocodile tears: A key to the aetiology of Duane's syndrome. *Br J Ophthalmol* 1980; 64:518.
68. Isenberg S, Blechman B: Marcus Gunn jaw winking and Duane's retraction syndrome. *J Pediatr Ophthalmol Strabismus* 1983; 20:235.
69. Breinin GM: Electromyography: A tool in ocular and neurologic diagnosis. II. Muscle palsies. *Arch Ophthalmol* 1957; 57:165.
70. Sato S: Electromyographic study on retraction syndrome. *Jpn J Ophthalmol* 1960; 4:57.
71. Blodi FC, Van Allen MW: Duane's syndrome: A brainstem lesion. *Arch Ophthalmol* 1964; 72:171.
72. Huber A, Esslen E, Klöti R, et al: Zum problem des Duane syndromes. *Albrecht von Graefes Arch Klin Exp Ophthalmol* 1964; 167:169.
73. Zauberman H, Magora A, Chaco J: An electromyographic evaluation of the retraction syndrome. *Am J Ophthalmol* 1967; 64:1103.
74. Scott AB, Wong GY: Duane's syndrome: An electromyographic study. *Arch Ophthalmol* 1972; 87:140.
75. Strachan IM, Brown BH: Electromyography of extraocular muscles in Duane's syndrome. *Br J Ophthalmol* 1972; 56:594.
76. Huber A: Electrophysiology of the retraction syndromes. *Br J Ophthalmol* 1974; 58:293.
77. Matteuci P: I difetti congenit di abduzione con particolare riguardo alla patogenesi. *Rass Ital Ottal* 1946; 15:345.
78. Hotchkiss MG, Miller NR, Clark AW, et al: Bilateral Duane's retraction syndrome: A clinical-pathologic case report. *Arch Ophthalmol* 1980; 98:870.
79. Miller NR, Kiel SM, Green WR, et al: Unilateral Duane's retraction syndrome (type I). *Arch Ophthalmol* 1982; 100:1468.
80. Towfighi J, Marks K, Palmer E, et al: Möbius syndrome: Neuropathologic observations. *Acta Neuropathol* 1979; 48:11.
81. Robertson DM, Hines JD, Rucker CW: Acquired sixth nerve paresis in children. *Arch Ophthalmol* 1970; 83:574.
82. Harley RD: Paralytic strabismus in children: Etiologic incidence and management of the third, fourth, and sixth nerve palsies. *Ophthalmology* 1980; 86:24.
83. Scott AB, Kraft SP: Botulinum toxin injection in the management of lateral rectus paresis. *Ophthalmology* 1985; 92:676.
84. Knox DC, Clark DB, Schuster FF: Benign sixth nerve palsies in children. *Pediatrics* 1967; 40:560.
85. Bixenman WW, von Noorden GK: Benign recurrent VI nerve palsy in childhood. *J Pediatr Ophthalmol Strabismus* 1981; 18:29.
86. Reinecke RD, Thompson WE: Childhood recurrent paralysis of the lateral rectus. *Ann Ophthalmol* 1981; 13:1037.
87. Metz HS: Benign sixth nerve palsy of childhood. *Am Orthoptic J* 1983; 33:42.
88. Balkan R, Hoyt CS: Associated neurologic abnormalities in congenital third nerve palsies. *Am J Ophthalmol* 1984; 97:315.
89. Victor DI: The diagnosis of congenital unilateral third-nerve palsy. *Brain* 1976; 99:711.
90. Miller NR: Solitary oculomotor nerve palsy in childhood. *Am J Ophthalmol* 1977; 83:106.
91. Norman MG: Unilateral encephalomalacia in cranial nerve nuclei in neonates: Report of two cases. *Neurology NY* 1974; 24:424.
92. Burian HM, Cahill JE: Congenital paralysis of medial rectus muscle with unusual synergism of the horizontal muscles. *Trans Am Ophthalmol Soc* 1952; 50:87.
93. Znajda JP, Krill AE: Congenital medial rectus palsy with simultaneous abduction of the two eyes. *Am J Ophthalmol* 1969; 68:1050.
94. Wilcox LM Jr, Gittinger JW Jr, Breinin GM: Congenital adduction palsy and synergistic divergence. *Am J Ophthalmol* 1981; 91:1.
95. Jimura T, Tagami Y, Isayama Y, et al: A case of synergistic divergence associated with Horner's syndrome. *Folia Ophthalmol Jpn* 1983; 34:477.
96. Scassellati-Sforzolini G: Una sindroma molto

rara: Diffeto congenito monolaterale della elevazione con retrazione del globe. *Riv Otoneurooftal* 1958; 33:431
97. Khodadoust AA, von Noorden GK: Bilateral vertical retraction syndrome: A family study. *Arch Ophthalmol* 1967; 78:606.
98. Pruksacholawit K, Ishikawa S: Atypical vertical retraction syndrome: A case study. *J Pediatr Ophthalmol* 1976; 13:215.
99. Burian HM, Van Allen MW: Cyclic oculomotor paralysis. *Am J Ophthalmol* 1963; 55:529.
100. Loewenfeld IE, Thomspon HS: Oculomotor paresis with cyclic spasms. A critical review of the literature and a new case. *Surv Ophthalmol* 1975; 20:81.
101. Miller EF II: Counterrolling of the human eyes produced by head tilt with respect to gravity. *Acta Otolaryngol Stockh* 1962; 54:479.
102. Szentagothai J: Pathways and synaptic articulation patterns connecting vestibular receptors and oculomotor nuclei, in Bender MB (ed): *The Oculomotor System.* New York, Harper & Row, Publishers, Inc, 1964, pp 211–215.
103. Chandler FA, Alfons A: "Congenital" muscular torticollis. *JAMA* 1944; 125:476.
104. Manzitti E, Ciancia AD: Torticollis ocular. *Arch Oftalmol Buenos Aires* 1954; 29:525.
105. Caputo A: Sit-up test. Presented at American Association of Certified Orthoptists meeting, San Fransisco, October 1985.
106. Ruedmann AD Jr: Scoliosis and vertical muscle balance. *Arch Ophthalmol* 1956; 56:389.
107. Sutcliffe J: Torsion spasms and abnormal postures in children with hiatus hernia, Sandifer's syndrome. *Prog Pediatr Radiol* 1969; 2:190.
108. Fenichel GM: Clinical syndromes of myasthenia in infancy and childhood. *Arch Neurol* 1978; 35:97.
109. Millichap JG, Dodge PR: Diagnosis and treatment of myasthenia gravis in infancy, childhood, and adolescence. *Neurology NY* 1960; 10:1007.
110. Miller NR, Moses H: Ocular involvement in wound botulism. *Arch Ophthalmol* 1977; 95:1788.
111. Terranova W, Palumbo JN, Breman JG: Ocular findings in botulism type B. *JAMA* 1979; 241:475.
112. Pickett J, Berg B, Chaplin E, et al: Syndrome of botulism in infancy: Clinical and electrophysiologic study. *N Engl J Med* 1976; 295:770.
113. Johnson RO, Clay SA, Arnon SS: Diagnosis and management of infant botulism. *Am J Dis Child* 1979; 133:586.
114. Schochet SS Jr, Zellweger H, Ionasescu V, et al: Centronuclear myopathy: Disease entity or a syndrome? *J Neurol Sci* 1972; 16:215.
115. Bender AN, Bender MB: Muscle fiber hypertrophy with intact neuromuscular junctions—a study of a patient with congenital neuromuscular disease and ophthalmoplegia. *Neurology NY* 1977; 27:206.
116. Owen JS, Kline LB, Oh SJ, et al: Ophthalmoplegia and ptosis in congenital fiber type disproportion. *J Pediatr Ophthalmol Strabismus* 1981; 18:55.
117. Boustany RN, Aprille JR, Halperin J, et al: Mitochondrial cytochrome deficiency presenting as a myopathy with hypotonia, external ophthalmoplegia, and lactic acidosis in an infant and as fatal hepatopathy in a second cousin. *Ann Neurol* 1983; 14:462.
118. Hoyt CS, Mousel DK, Weber AA: Transient supranuclear disturbances of gaze in healthy neonates. *Am J Ophthalmol* 1980; 89:708.
119. Lebensohn JE: Parinaud's syndrome. From obstetrical trauma with recovery. *Am J Ophthalmol* 1955; 40:738.
120. Biglan AW: Setting sun sign in infants. *Am Orthoptic J* 1984; 34:114.
121. Smith JL, Walsh FB: Opsoclonus-ataxic conjugate movements of the eyes. *Arch Ophthalmol* 1960; 64:244.
122. Cogan DG: Opsoclonus, body tremulousness, and benign encephalitis. *Arch Ophthalmol* 1968; 79:545.
123. Shetty T, Rosman NP: Opsoclonus in hydrocephalus. *Arch Ophthalmol* 1972; 88:585.
124. Bienfang DC: Opsoclonus in infancy. *Arch Ophthalmol* 1974; 91:203.
125. Solomon GE, Chutorian AM: Opsoclonus and occult neuroblastoma. *N Engl J Med* 1968; 279:475.
126. Sandok BA, Kranz H: Opsoclonus as the initial manifestation of occult neuroblastoma. *Arch Ophthalmol* 1971; 86:235.
127. Hoyt CS: Neonatal opsoclonus. *J Pediatr Ophthalmol* 1977; 14:274.
128. Donat IFG, Donat JR, Lay KS: Changing response to caloric stimulation with gestational age in infants. *Neurology NY* 1980; 30:776.

129. White JW: Paralysis of the superior rectus and inferior oblique muscles of the same eye. *Arch Ophthalmol* 1942; 27:366.
130. Metz HS: Double elevator palsy. *Arch Ophthalmol* 1979; 97:901.
131. Barsoum-Homsy M: Congenital double elevator palsy. *J Pediatr Ophthalmol* 1983; 20:185.
132. McNeer KW, Jampolsky A: Double elevator palsy caused by anomalous insertion of the inferior rectus. *Am J Ophthalmol* 1965; 59:317.
133. von Noorden GK: Congenital hereditary ptosis with inferior rectus fibrosis. *Arch Ophthalmol* 1970; 83:378.
134. Cogan DG: A type of congenital motor apraxia presenting jerky head movements. *Trans Am Acad Ophthalmol Otolaryngol* 1952; 56:853.
135. Cogan DG: Congenital ocular motor apraxia. *Can J Ophthalmol* 1966; 1:253.
136. Gittinger JW Jr, Sokol S: The visual-evoked potential in the diagnosis of congenital ocular motor apraxia. *Am J Ophthalmol* 1982; 93:700.
137. Brown HW: Congenital structural muscle anomalies, in Allen JH (ed): *Strabismus Ophthalmic Symposium.* St Louis, CV Mosby Co, 1950, pp 219–233.
138. Heuck G: Über angeborenen vererbten Beweglichkeitsdefekts der Augen. *Klin Monatsbl Augenheilkd* 1879; 17:253.
139. Holmes WJ: Hereditary congenital ophthalmoplegia. *Trans Am Ophthalmol Soc* 1956; 53:245.
140. Laughlin RC: Congenital fibrosis of the extraocular muscles. *Am J Ophthalmol* 1956; 41:432.
141. Crawford JS: Congenital fibrosis syndrome. *Can J Ophthalmol* 1970; 5:331.
142. Harley RD, Rodrigues MM, Crawford JS: Congenital fibrosis of the extraocular muscles. *Trans Am Ophthalmol Soc* 1978; 76:197.
143. Apt L, Axelrod RN: Generalized fibrosis of the extraocular muscles. *Am J Ophthalmol* 1978; 85:822.
144. Duke-Elder S, Wybar K: Squints of peripheral origin, in Duke-Elder S (ed): *System of Ophthalmology,* vol 6. St Louis, CV Mosby Co, 1973, p 736.
145. Kaufmann H, Kluxen M: Ein Fall von Aplasie des Musculus obliquus superior. *Klin Monatsbl Augenheilkd* 1972; 160:710.
146. Schellenback R: Agenesie des Musculus obliquus superior. *Klin Monatsbl Augenheilkd* 1972; 160:708.
147. Mejeer F: Über eine seltene Anomalie des M. obliquus superior. *Klin Monatsbl Augenheilkd* 1974; 165:928.
148. Mumma JV: Surgical procedure for congenital absence of the superior oblique. *Arch Ophthalmol* 1974; 92:221.
149. Helveston EM, Giangiacomo JG, Ellis FD: Congenital absence of the superior oblique tendon. *Trans Am Ophthalmol Soc* 1981; 79:123.
150. Yoshimura Y, Nemoto R, Nemoto K, et al: Congenital dysplasia of superior oblique muscle simulating superior oblique muscle palsy: A case report. *Folia Ophthalmol Jpn* 1983; 34:2429.
151. Stieren E: Congenital absence of both inferior recti muscles. *Am Med* 1903; 5:581.
152. McDannald CE: Report of a case of sursumvergence due to congenital absence of the inferior rectus muscle. *Arch Ophthalmol* 1914; 43:515.
153. Posey WC: Anomalies of eye muscles. *Trans Am Acad Ophthalmol Otolaryngol* 1921; 26:83.
154. Casten VG: Isolated congenital absence of the inferior rectus muscle. *Arch Ophthalmol* 1940; 24:55.
155. Pietrowa N: A case of congenital strabismus treated surgically. *Klin Oczna* 1958; 28:209.
156. Giller H: Congenital absence of the inferior rectus muscle. *Arch Ophthalmol* 1962; 68:182.
157. Cooper EL, Greenspan JA: Congenital absence of the inferior rectus muscle. *Arch Ophthalmol* 1971; 86:451.
158. Mets MB, Parks MM, Freeley DA, et al: Congenital absence of the inferior rectus muscle: A report of three cases and their management. *Binocular Vision* 1987; 2:77.
159. Girard LJ, Neely RA: Agenesis of the medial rectus muscle: Correction of a case by transplantation of slips from the vertical recti. *Arch Ophthalmol* 1958; 59:337.
160. Wong GY, Jampolsky A: Agenesis of three horizontal muscles. *Ann Ophthalmol* 1974; 6:909.
161. Murphy BF, Annable WL: Congenital absence of the medial rectus muscle with review of previous case reports. *Binocular Vision* 1987; 2:87.
162. Sandall GS, Morrison JW Jr: Congenital ab-

sence of lateral rectus muscle. *J Pediatr Ophthalmol Strabismus* 1979; 16:35.

163. Steinheim A: Blepharoptosis congenita und Defect der Musculus recti superioris. *Klin Monatsbl Augenheilkd* 1877; 15:99.
164. Laitinen L, Miettinen P, Sulamaa M: Ophthalmological observations in craniostenosis. *Acta Ophthalmologica* 1956; 34:121.
165. Miller M, Folk E: Strabismus associated with craniofacial anomalies. *Am Orthoptic J* 1975; 25:27.
166. Muir J: Strabismic manifestations in Apert's syndrome. *Am Orthoptic J* 1981; 31:60.
167. Murphree AL, Edelman PM: Strabismus associated with congenital anomalies. *Am Orthoptic J* 1982; 32:22.
168. Robb RM, Boger WP III: Vertical strabismus associated with plagiocephaly. *J Pediatr Ophthalmol Strabismus* 1983; 20:58.
169. Weinstock FJ, Hardesty H: Absence of superior recti in craniofacial dysostosis. *Arch Ophthalmol* 1965; 74:152.
170. Cuttone J, Brazis P, Miller M, et al: Absence of the superior rectus muscle in Apert's syndrome. *J Pediatr Ophthalmol Strabismus* 1979; 16:349.
171. Caputo AR, Lingua RW: Aberrant muscular insertions in Crouzon's disease. *J Pediatr Ophthalmol Strabismus* 1980; 17:239.
172. Diamond GR, Katowitz, JA, Whitaker LA, et al: Variations in extraocular muscle number and structure in craniofacial dysostosis. *Am J Ophthalmol* 1980; 90:416.
173. Pinchoff BS, Sandall G: Congenital absence of the superior oblique tendon in craniofacial dysostosis. *Ophthalmic Surg* 1985; 16:375.
174. Miller NR: *Clinical Neuro-Ophthalmology*. Baltimore, Williams & Wilkins, 1985, p 785.
175. Eviatar L, Eviatar A: Neurovestibular examination of infants and children. *Adv Otorhinolaryngol* 1978; 23:169.
176. Mitchell T, Cambon K: Vestibular response in the neonate and infant. *Arch Otolaryngol* 1969; 90:556.
177. Eviatar L, Miranda S, Eviatar A, et al: Development of nystagmus in response to vestibular stimulation in infants. *Ann Neurol* 1979; 5:508.
178. Dayton GO, Jones MH, Aiu P, et al: Developmental study of coordinated eye movements in the human infant. I. Visual acuity in the newborn human: A study based on induced optokinetic nystagmus recorded by electrooculography. *Arch Ophthalmol* 1964; 71:865.
179. McGinnis JM: Eye movement and optic nystagmus in early infancy. *Genet Psychol Monogr* 1930; 8:374.
180. Cogan DG: *Neurology of the Ocular Muscles*. Springfield, Ill, Charles C Thomas, Publishers, 1956, pp 189–192.
181. Dell'Osso LF, Daroff RB: Congenital nystagmus waveforms and foveation strategies, *Doc Ophthalmol* 1975; 39:155.
182. Enoch JM, Wilson GE: Remission of nystagmus following fitting contact lenses to an infant with aniridia. *Am J Ophthalmol* 1968; 66:333.
183. von Noorden GK: Oculomotor effects on vision—Clinical aspects, in Lennerstrand G, Bach-y-Rita P, (eds): *Basic Mechanisms of Ocular Motility and their Clinical Implications*. Oxford, Pergamon Press, Inc, 1975, p 419.
184. Allen ED, Davies PD: Role of contact lenses in the management of congenital nystagmus. *Br J Ophthalmol* 1983; 67:834.
185. Udvarhelyi GB, Khodadoust AA, Walsh FB: Gliomas of the optic nerve and chiasm in children: An unusual series of cases. *Clin Neurosurg* 1966; 13:204.
186. Donin JF: Acquired monocular nystagmus in children. *Can J Ophthalmol* 1967; 2:212.
187. Kelly TW: Optic glioma presenting as spasmus nutans. *Pediatrics* 1970; 45:295.
188. Schulman JA, Shults WT, MacAndrew Jones J Jr: Monocular vertical nystagmus as an initial sign of chiasmal glioma. *Am J Ophthalmol* 1979; 87:87.
189. Antony JH, Ouvrier RA, Wise G: Spasmus nutans: A mistaken identity. *Arch Neurol* 1980; 37:373.
190. Halpern J: Spasmus nutans. *Arch Neurol* 1980; 37:737.
191. Koenig SB, Naidich TP, Zaparackas Z: Optic glioma masquerading as spasmus nutans. *J Pediatr Ophthalmol Strabismus* 1982; 19:20.
192. Lavery MA, O'Neill JF, Chu FC, et al: Acquired nystagmus in early childhood: A presenting sign of intracranial tumor. *Ophthalmology* 1984; 91:425.
193. Smith JL, Flynn JT, Spiro H: Monocular vertical oscillations of amblyopia. *J Clin Neuro Ophthalmol* 1982; 2:85.
194. Yee RD, Jelks GW, Baloh RW, et al: Uniocu-

lar nystagmus in monocular visual loss. *Ophthalmology* 1979; 86:511.
195. Hemmes GD: *Hereditary Nystagmus.* Doctorate thesis, Ulrecht, abstracted in *Am J Ophthalmol* 1927; 10:149.
196. Cogan DG: Congenital nystagmus. *Can J Ophthalmol* 1967; 2:4.
197. Gresty MA, Halmagyi GM, Leech J: The relationship between head and eye movement in congenital nystagmus with head shaking: Objective recordings of a single case. *Br J Ophthalmol* 1978; 62:533.
198. Metz HS, Jampolsky A, O'Meara DM: Congenital ocular nystagmus and nystagmoid head movements. *Am J Ophthalmol* 1972; 74:1131.
199. Carl JR, Optican LM, Chu FC, et al: Head shaking and vestibulo-ocular reflex in congenital nystagmus. *Invest Ophthalmol Vis Sci* 1985; 26:1043.
200. Dell'Osso LF, Schmidt D, Daroff RB: Latent, manifest, and congenital nystagmus. *Arch Ophthalmol* 1979; 97:1877.
201. Anderson, JR: Causes and treatment of congenital eccentric nystagmus. *Br J Ophthalmol* 1966; 37:271.
202. Franceschetti A, Monnier M, Dieterle P: Analyse du nystagmus congénital par la méthode electro-nystagmographique (ENG). *Bull Schweiz Akad Med Wiss* 1952; 8:403.
203. Ciancia AO: La esotropia con limitacion bilateral de la abduccion en el lactante. *Arch Oftalmol Buenos Aires* 1962; 37:207.
204. Adelstein FE, Cüppers C: Zum Problem der echten und der scheinbaren Abducenslähmung (das sogenannte "Blockierungssyndrom"). *Augenmuskellähmungen Büch Augenarzt* 1966; 46:271.
205. Isenberg S, Yee RD: The ETHAN syndrome. *Ann Opthalmol* 1986; 18:358.
206. Kestenbaum A: Nouvelle operation du nystagmus. *Bull Soc Ophtalmol Fr* 1953; 6:599.
207. Cüpers C: Probleme der oiperativen Therapie des ocularen Nystagmus. *Klin Monatsbl Augenheilkd* 1971; 159:145.
208. Roggenkamper P: Combination of artificial divergence with kestenbaum operation in cases of torticollis caused by nystagmus, in Reinecke RD (ed): *Strabismus II.* Orlando, Fla, Grune & Stratton, 1984, pp 329–333.
209. Economopoulos NK, Damanakis AG: Modification of the Kestenbaum operation for correction of nystagmic torticollis and improvement of visual acuity with the use of convergence. *Ophthalmic Surg* 1985; 16:309.
210. Norton EWD, Cogan DG: Spasmus nutans. A clinical study of twenty cases followed two years or more since onset. *Arch Ophthalmol* 1954; 52:442.
211. Sedwick LA, Burde RM, Hodges FJ III: Leigh's subacute necrotizing encephalomyelopathy manifesting as spasmus nutants. *Arch Ophthalmol* 1984; 102:1046.

17 Corneal Abnormalities

George R. Beauchamp, M.D.
Gary A. Varley, M.D.

Congenital corneal abnormalities are particularly important in a fragile, developing visual system (Chapter 4). Establishment of the fixation reflex (in the first 6 weeks of life) is critical to further visual system development. Congenital corneal opacities, managed after development of the fixation reflex would normally occur, may result in dense amblyopia. Further, the cornea is responsible for about two thirds of the total refractive power of the eye; even a clear cornea, if abnormally shaped, may yield major changes in refractive quality and power and contribute to amblyopia. Finally, some abnormalities in corneal development may be associated with an underlying systemic syndrome. Thus, recognition and appropriate management of corneal abnormalities may facilitate normal visual development and recognition of otherwise unsuspected systemic abnormalities.

The normal neonatal anterior segment has several characteristics of incomplete development. The anterior chamber is shallow. The cornea is smaller than adult size and may have a faint "ground-glass" haze. Presumably the haze derives from some combination of incompletely formed and irregularly spaced collagen fibrils. Such normal findings must be systematically differentiated from pathological conditions.

Embryogenesis of the newborn eye has been reviewed (Chapter 2). Certain aspects of corneal development deserve emphasis, however. Anterior segment development occurs early, with separation of the lens vesicle from overlying surface ectoderm by day 33 of gestation.[1] In recent years, the importance of neural crest cells in ocular development has been emphasized.[2–4] The corneal endothelium and stroma are derivatives of neural crest; thus derive implications for other syndromes of neural crest maldevelopment and dysmorphogenesis. The forming cornea consists of cells, collagen, noncollagenous structural proteins, and extracellular ground substance containing complex carbohydrates. The interaction of these elements is dictated by genetic and (local) environmental factors. Despite new information, the events of ocular anterior segment morphogenesis at the biologic level of the cell are incompletely understood.

ABNORMALITIES IN CORNEAL SIZE AND SHAPE

The corneal diameter at birth is approximately 85% of adult size.[5] At birth, both horizontal and vertical diameters are approximately 10 mm.[6] Newborn corneal diameters less than 9 or 10 mm are considered indicative of microcornea,[5,7] while diameters greater than 11 or 12 mm (in the absence of congenital glaucoma) are considered evidence for megalocornea.[6]

Microcornea

The diagnosis of primary microcornea is made by measuring corneal diameter and ax-

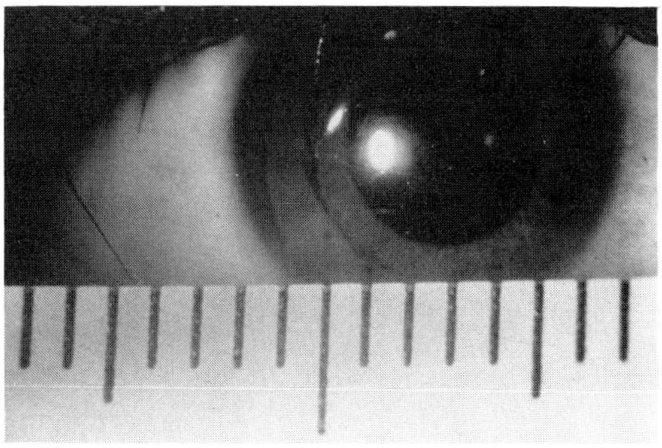

FIG 17–1.
Microcornea. The cornea measures approxiamtely 9 mm horizontally.

ial length (Fig 17–1). Axial length is used to differentiate this condition (where the length is normal) from nanophthalmos and microphthalmos (wherein the entire eye is small).[8] Thus, microcornea may occur as an isolated abnormality in an otherwise normal eye[8, 9] or in association with other ocular and systemic abnormalities. The inheritance pattern is either autosomal dominant[9–11] or autosomal recessive.[7, 12] Associated ocular conditions include cataract, subluxated lenses, glaucoma, and aniridia.[7–11] Associated systemic conditions are craniofacial dysmorphism, sinus abnormalities, syndactyly, mental retardation, dwarfism, hypospadias, Ehlers-Danlos syndrome, and undescended testes.[8, 13, 14] Management is directed at recognition and treatment of associated ocular and systemic abnormalities and correction of refractive errors. The visual outcome may be very good.

Megalocornea

Megalocornea is a symmetrical, inherited, nonprogressive condition characterized by enlargement of the anterior segment of the eye with horizontal corneal diameters greater than 11 or 12 mm (Fig 17–2).[6, 15] The posterior segment is normal.[15] Many anterior structures are normal as well: corneal thickness, curvature, endothelial density, endothelial morphology, anterior chamber angles, intraocular pressure, and axial length.[15, 16] Normal corneal endothelial density yields a greater than normal total endothelial cell population, which suggests a process of total corneal hyperplasia.[17] Although all modes of inheritance have been described, X-linked recessive is most common.[16, 18] Ocular findings associated with megalocornea include astigmatic refractive errors, iris stromal atrophy, pupillary miosis, cataracts, iris and lens instability (iridodonesis, phacodonesis), or frank lens subluxation resulting from stretched or ruptured zonules.[17, 19] Less common corneal abnormalities associated with megalocornea are arcus juvenilis,[18] posterior embryotoxon,[16] nebular central opacities,[17] and mosaic corneal dystrophy (crocodile shagreen).[17, 18, 20] Associated systemic abnormalities include lamellar ichthyosis, Marfan syndrome, craniosynostosis, dwarfism, facial hemiatrophy, Down syndrome, and multiple skeletal abnormalities.[16, 19, 21–23] Corneal enlargement associated with congenital glaucoma is not megalocornea. Enlarged corneas in congenital glaucoma are differentiated by diminished endothelial cell density consistent with a distension process and the presence of clinical signs of glaucoma.[17] Management derives from recognition of associated ocular systemic abnormalities and correction of refractive errors if present. Normal visual acuity is common.

Keratoglobus

Keratoglobus is a rare bilateral condition characterized by globular corneal shape. Inheritance has been reported as either auto-

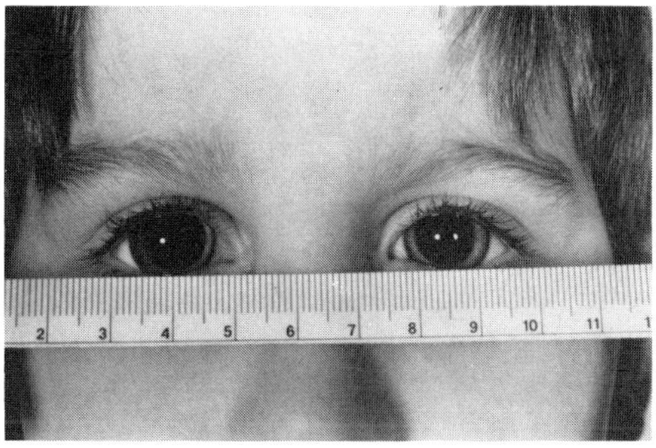

FIG 17–2.
Megalocornea. The corneas measure approximately 14 mm horizontally.

somal dominant or autosomal recessive.[24,25] Despite one reported acquired case, it is generally a developmental abnormality.[26] Increased anterior curvature results in increased corneal refractive power (up to 50 D or more).[6] The cornea may resemble megalocornea; however, the keratoglobus cornea is uniformly thinned (especially in the periphery). The condition has been genetically related to keratoconus yet is clinically distinguishable from it.[27] Additional abnormalities associated with keratoglobus include blue scleras, hearing defects, brittle bones, hyperextensible joints, and abnormal teeth.[24,25,28] Histopathology reveals an absent Bowman's layer; thinned, scarred, and vascularized corneal stroma; diffusely thickened Descemet's membrane with occasional breaks; and scleral thinning.[24] Rupture of the globe with mild trauma is a significant risk.[25] Acute hydrops (corneal swelling with opacity) has been reported in a child with unilateral keratoglobus and vernal keratoconjunctivitis.[29] Appropriate management corrects refractive errors and protects the eyes from the increased susceptibility of rupture by blunt trauma. The diagnosis of congenital glaucoma may mistakenly be made, presumably based on the appearance of bulging corneas.[24] Normal visual acuity occasionally may be obtained.

Cornea Plana

Cornea plana is a rare condition that may be confused with microcornea. The corneal curvature is below normal (flatter), with consequent shallowing of the anterior chamber. At the fourth and fifth gestational months the corneal curvature increases beyond that of sclera, coincident with formation of a dense collagenous limbal ring. Failure of this phase of corneal and limbal development is postulated to contribute to cornea plana.[30] Shallow corneal curvature results in significant hyperopia (up to 20 D), often with accompanying astigmatism.[31] Decreased corneal transparency may result from corneal distortion or collagen maturation defects, and cornea plana with opacification has been reported in Ehlers-Danlos syndrome.[32] Both autosomal dominant and autosomal recessive inheritance patterns have been reported. Other ocular anomalies include coloboma of the iris or choroid, congenital cataract, and the late development of glaucoma.[33]

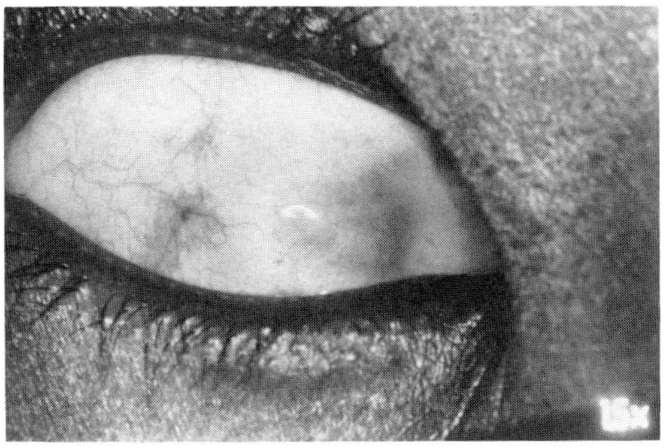

FIG 17–3.
Sclerocornea: opacified cornea with an absence of normal landmarks.

ABNORMALITIES IN CORNEAL DEVELOPMENT THAT LEAD TO A VISUALLY OPAQUE CORNEA

Sclerocornea

Sclerocornea is a developmental corneal abnormality with nonprogressive absence of normal corneal transparency. Limbal definition is poor, which makes definition between cornea and sclera difficult (Fig 17–3). Ninety percent are bilateral.[34] Sclerocornea may be peripheral only or total; the degree is variable. Vascularization may be superficial or deep. While some cases are sporadic, others suggest an autosomal dominant or autosomal recessive inheritance pattern.[34] Histopathology of involved corneal stroma demonstrates morphology resembling sclera. Corneal collagen fibers are larger than normal and irregularly arranged. The lamellar organization is disrupted, with resultant loss of optical clarity.[35] Abnormalities in Descemet's membrane and endothelium may exist.[34,36] Sclerocornea may occur as a primary abnormality but is associated with cornea plana in up to 80% of cases.[37,38] Other ocular abnormalities associated with sclerocornea include microphthalmos, coloboma, posterior embryotoxon, glaucoma, nystagmus, esotropia, Rieger's anomaly, Axenfeld's anomaly, aniridia,[39] and cataract.[37,38] Somatic abnormalities associated with sclerocornea are mental retardation; deafness; and anomalies of skin, face, ears, cerebellum, and testes.[37] It has been associated with many syndromes: Hallermann-Streiff,[36,39] Hurler,[35] Smith-Lemli-Opitz,[40] Mieten,[41] Melnick-Needles,[42] Lobstein,[43] and Dandy-Walker cyst.[44] Peripheral sclerocornea is compatible with good vision; however, total sclerocornea results in poor visual acuity and an extremely poor prognosis for penetrating keratoplasty. Visual prognosis for unilateral total sclerocornea is extremely guarded; keratoplasty is therefore controversial at best, perhaps not warranted.

Posterior Corneal Defects

Anterior segment development is complex, and the mechanisms responsible for tissue migration, proliferation, and cell death/remodeling are poorly understood. Since the posterior cornea is derived from neural crest and the separation of the lens vesicle occurs concurrently with neural crest migration into the cornea,[2] abnormalities in the posterior cornea, anterior chamber angle, and iris represent focal neurocristopathies (Fig 17–4). Some investigators have classified corneal endothelial disorders on the basis of abnormalities in neural crest cell migration, proliferation, and final differentiation.[4]

Posterior Keratoconus

Posterior keratoconus is a rare developmental anomaly with two variations, neither related to anterior keratoconus.[45] Posterior keratoconus generalis is characterized by increased curvature of the entire posterior surface; the net effect is central corneal thinning. In posterior keratoconus circumscriptus, the area of increased posterior of cornea curvature is localized, with focal corneal thinning with or without stromal scarring. This abnormality is usually congenital, unilateral, and nonprogressive. However, acquired (traumatic) and bilateral cases have been reported.[46–48] Without significant stromal scarring there is usually little effect on visual acuity since the posterior part of the cornea is not the major refractive surface of the eye. Ocular abnormalities associated with posterior keratoconus include choroidal and/or retinal sclerosis, aniridia, ectropion uvea, iris atrophy, glaucoma, anterior lenticonus, ectopia lentis, coloboma,[49] and anterior lenticular opacities (cataract).[45,47,50–53] Recognized systemic abnormalities include short stature,[49,54] vertebral abnormalities,[49] brachymorphism with short limbs,[54] cleft lip and palate,[49,53] genitourinary abnormalities,[53] webbed neck,[54] stiff-legged gait,[53,54] broad nose,[53,54] mongoloid slant,[53,54] hypothyroidism,[54] and mental retardation.[49,54] Chromosomal abnormalities have been reported in some cases.[49,55] Whether posterior keratoconus represents a very mild form of Peters' anomaly (see the following) is unknown. The majority of posterior keratoconus patients require no treatment since the abnormal posterior corneal surface has

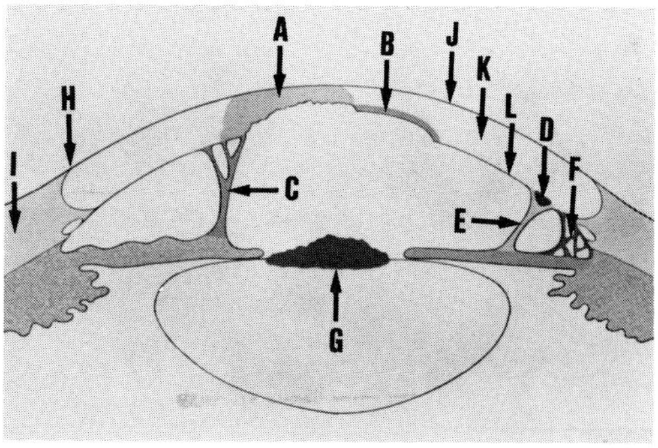

FIG 17–4.
Composite of selected anterior segment anomalies. Arrows point to central corneal opacity with edema *(A)*; central posterior corneal defect with opacity *(B)*; iris process to edge of posterior corneal defect *(C)*; prominent, anteriorly displaced Schwalbe's line *(D)*; iris process *(E)* inserting to *D*; anomalous corneoscleral angle *(F)*; anterior polar lens opacity *(G)*; limbus *(H)*; sclera *(I)*; corneal epithelium of Bowman's membrane *(J)*; corneal stroma *(K)*; and corneal endothelium of Descement's membrane *(L)*. (From Waring GO III, Rodriguez MM, Laibson PR: Anterior chamber cleavage syndrome: A stepladder classification. *Surv Ophthalmol* 1975; 20:3. Used with permission.)

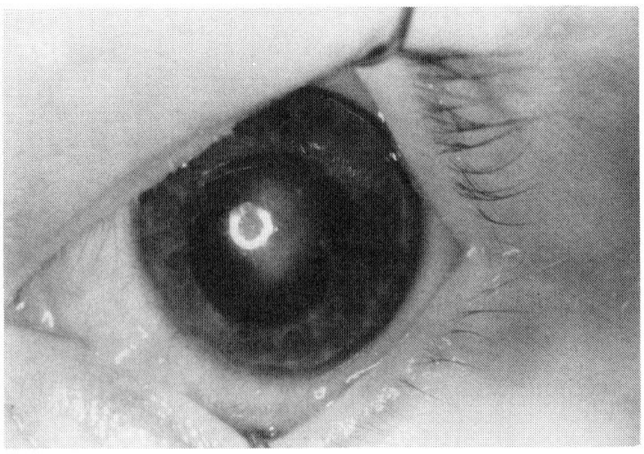

FIG 17–5.
Peter's anomaly. Iris processes insert to edge of posterior corneal defect with opacity.

little effect on visual acuity.[56] However, if significant corneal scarring is present, penetrating keratoplasty may be indicated.

Peter's Anomaly

Peter's anomaly is a rare congenital ocular malformation characterized by a central corneal stromal opacity, with defects in the posterior cornea and variable iris-corneal or lens-corneal adhesions[57] (Fig 17–5). The peripheral part of the cornea is usually normal. Most cases are sporadic, but autosomal recessive and dominant inheritance patterns have been described.[58, 59] In some instances, chromosomal abnormalities have been documented.[59–61] The anomaly has been reported as a feature of the fetal alcohol syndrome.[62] It may be associated with other ocular abnormalities such as glaucoma, cataract,[63] microcornea, aniridia,[64] microphthalmos, cornea plana, sclerocornea, and colobomas.[63, 65, 66] If lens-corneal adhesion is present, there may be posterior segment abnormalities such as persistent hyperplastic primary vitreous (PHPV). Recognition of lens-corneal adhesion may be difficult with a dense opacity (leukoma); however, a ring or doughnut pattern to the leukoma is suggestive of this abnormality.[64] Most patients are otherwise normal, but systemic abnormalities have been reported: hydrocephalus,[67] pulmonary hypoplasia,[68] cleft lip and palate,[63, 69] cardiac[60, 70] and genitourinary[70] malformations, and craniofacial dysostosis.[71] Management of this malformation is very difficult. Definitive therapy is penetrating keratoplasty with or without removal of the lens. Difficulties in transplanting infant corneas have led some to suggest a large sector iridectomy.[72] If the infant has a normal fellow eye, no surgical intervention of the abnormal eye may be warranted, irrespective of severity.

Rieger's Anomaly

Like the spectrum of abnormalities seen in the central corneal (i.e., posterior keratoconus, Peter's anomaly with or without lens corneal adhesion), a spectrum of abnormalities is found in peripheral cornea.[73] The most common abnormality, of no clinical significance and seen in 8% to 15% of normal eyes, is an anteriorly displaced and prominent Schwalbe's line.[65, 74, 75] If prominent iris processes insert into this ridge, the deformity is termed Axenfeld's anomaly; if glaucoma is present, it is Axenfeld's syndrome. If hypoplasia of the anterior iris stroma and peripheral corneal opacity is added to the aforementioned, the malformation is termed *Rieger's anomaly* (Fig 17–6). Rieger's anomaly is associated with nonocular abnormalities such as maxillary hypoplasia, microdontia, limb or spine malformations, and umbilical hernia; such associations are termed *Rieger syndrome*.[73, 76, 77] It has been proposed that the distinction between Axenfeld's and Rieger's anomalies is artificial and unnecessary and that

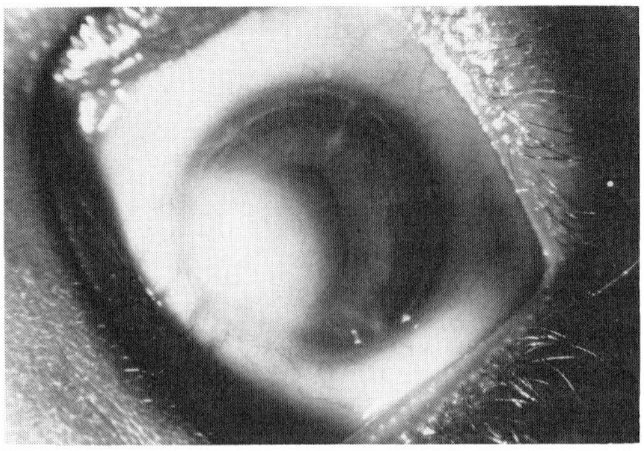

FIG 17–6.
Rieger's anomaly: iris and corneal anomalies, including opacity, prominent anteriorly displaced Schwalbe's line, and iris processes.

they should be referred to as the *A-R syndrome*.[76] Typically, A-R syndrome is bilateral in an infant with a positive family history (autosomal dominant inheritance).[65,78] Secondary glaucoma is common.[79]

Inborn Errors of Metabolism

Inborn errors of metabolism rarely yield congenital corneal opacities. More commonly metabolic products accumulate with time. A mild corneal haze may be present at birth in certain defects, particularly Hurler's, Maroteaux-Lamy, and Scheie's variants of the mucopolysaccharidoses.[80] These conditions, however, have characteristic facial and skeletal abnormalities that suggest the diagnosis. Other endocrine and metabolic derangements are manifested later in infancy and childhood.

CORNEAL DYSTROPHIES

Of many corneal dystrophies, only congenital hereditary endothelial dystrophy (CHED), posterior polymorphous dystrophy (PPMD), and congenital hereditary stromal dystrophy (CHSD) present at or shortly after birth. Dystrophies are usually bilateral, and a positive family history is common. The two most common, CHED and PPMD, may be difficult to differentiate.

Congenital Hereditary Endothelial Dystrophy

CHED is characterized by bilateral diffuse corneal edema not related to elevated intraocular pressure (Fig 17–7). As in all instances of congenital corneal clouding, glaucoma must be excluded. Inheritance of CHED has been reported as both autosomal recessive and autosomal dominant,[81–83] yet the cases thought to be autosomal dominant may represent PPMD. Symptoms are rare. Nystagmus is common when the condition is present at birth.[81] The degree of corneal clouding may vary from a mild haze to a severe opacification obscuring examination of the anterior segment.[84] Abnormalities in Descemet's membrane vary from abnormally thin to diffusely thickened.[74,75,82,83] Palliative therapy consists of medical methods to make the cornea less turgescent; definitive treatment requires keratoplasty.

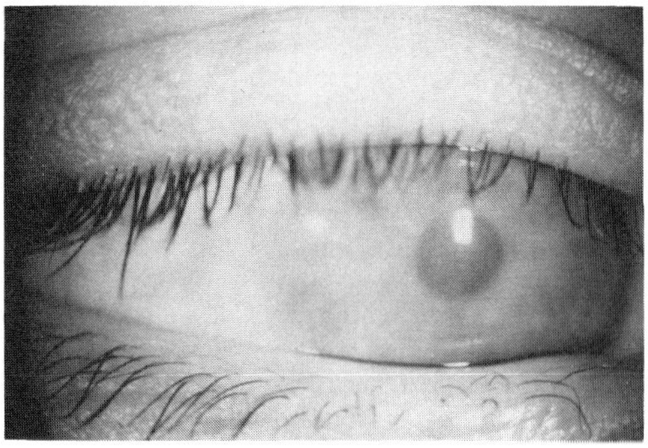

FIG 17–7.
CHED: ground-glass haze, the result of endothelial abnormality and corneal edema.

Posterior Polymorphous Dystrophy

The PPMD of Schlichting[85] is a bilateral, dominantly inherited abnormality of the corneal endothelium. Pedigrees consistent with autosomal recessive inheritance have been described.[86] Many cases are very mild; they are typically asymptomatic and observed as an incidental finding on routine examination in later life. Intrafamilial variability is common.[86,87] Areas of polymorphous opacities, often vesicular in character, are present at the level of Descemet's membrane (Fig 17–8). Severe cases may obscure visualization of Descemet's membrane[86] and thus may mimic CHED. Severe PPMD may be generally differentiated from CHED by normal stromal thickness; however, in some cases of PPMD the stroma is diffusely edematous.[86,88] Histopathologic examination reveals abnormal endothelial cells that resemble epithelium. PPMD has been associated with calcium deposition (band keratopathy), pupillary distortion (ectropion), peripheral anterior synechia, and glaucoma.[86,87]

Congenital Hereditary Stromal Dystrophy

Congenital hereditary stromal dystrophy (CHSD) is a very rare, unique entity characterized by dominantly inherited, nonprogressive, congenital corneal clouding (Fig 17–9). The epithelium is smooth and regular. Descemet's membrane and endothelium appear normal. The stroma, however, is characterized by diffuse feathery clouding, more prominent in central anterior stroma than peripheral deep stroma. Alternating esotropia and searching nystagmus are common. CHSD is differentiated clinically from CHED by normal stromal thickness.[88, 89] Pathological examination of corneal buttons have confirmed normal corneal thickness. Light microscopy has demonstrated a normal epithelium and Bowman's membrane with the usual population and distribution of keratocytes and a regular uninterrupted Descemet's membrane covered by a normal-appearing endothelium. Electron microscopy has confirmed the normal appearance of the epithelium, its basement membrane, Bowman's layer, and the endothelium. Descemet's membrane has failed to demonstrate the characteristic anterior banded portion but was otherwise unremarkable. The stroma, however, has demonstrated pathological changes of the lamellae. The normal arrangements of collagen fibrils are separated by abnormal layers made up of collagen filaments of smaller than normal diameter, abnormally arranged and loosely embedded in ground substance.[89]

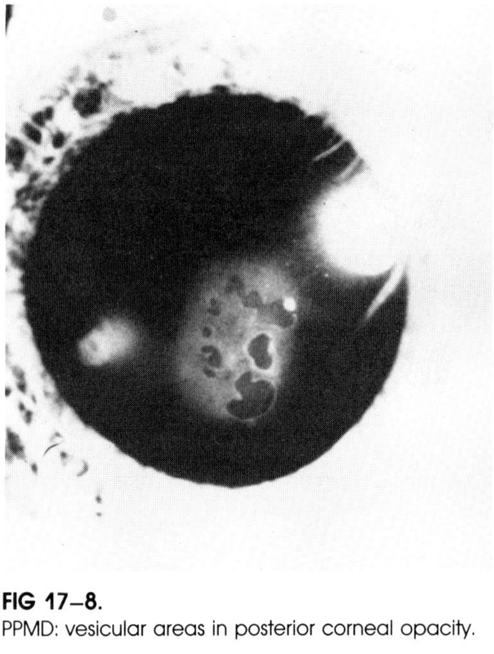

FIG 17–8.
PPMD: vesicular areas in posterior corneal opacity.

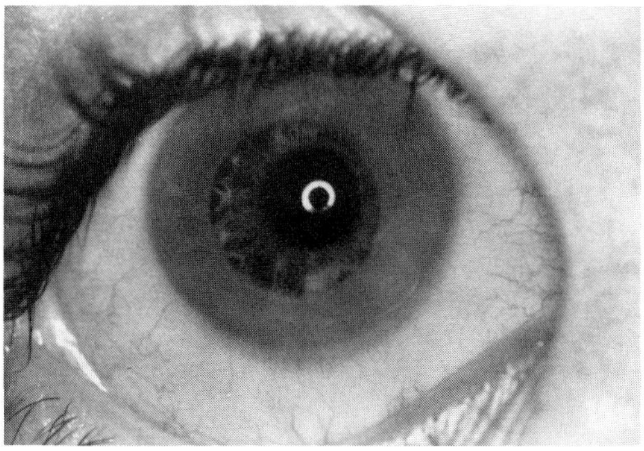

FIG 17–9.
CHSD: prominent corneal opacity without edema (note the clear central transplanted cornea).

CONGENITAL GLAUCOMA

Primary infantile (congenital) glaucoma may present at birth or within the first year of life. The condition is rare (approximately 1 in 20,000 births) but is a distinct and treatable entity. Early diagnosis facilitates optimal outcome. The signs and symptoms include photophobia, tearing, and blepharospasm. As the disease progresses, the cornea (indeed, the entire eye) enlarges rapidly. The rapid expansion causes dehiscences in corneal endothelium and Descemet's membrane, which permits aqueous humor to enter the corneal stroma. The resultant edema causes corneal clouding (Fig 17–10).[90] In time and with control of intraocular pressure, these posterior corneal defects heal and leave linear microscopic scars (Haab's striae) (Fig 17–11). The tearing associated with blockage of the nasolacrimal duct (NLD) system often may be differentiated by observing for nasal secretions. A wet eye and dry nose suggests NLD stenosis; excessive tearing from congenital glaucoma causes the nose to be wetter than normal. Treatment is surgical (goniotomy, trabeculotomy, trabeculectomy) and should be performed as soon after diagnosis as feasible.

EPIBULBAR TUMORS

Congenital epibulbar tumors generally are variable choristomatous malformations named by location and primary histopathologic tissue. Dermoids are differentiated from epidermoid structures by the presence of dermal elements. When lipid is predominant, they are termed lipodermoids; if mature bony elements are the primary tissue, they are osseous choristomas. If all three germ cell layers are present, the lesion is a teratoma.[91–93]

Dermoid

The most common epibulbar tumors in newborns are dermoids. Dermoids may be orbital (dermoid cysts) or epibulbar (dermoid tumors of conjunctiva, limbus, or cornea). They are generally lightly colored (yellow, tan, or pink), elevated, and solid (Fig 17–12).[93] Occurrence confined strictly to the cornea is extremely rare; nonetheless, the resultant visual deficit may be profound and necessitate intervention.[93–95] A limbal dermoid often requires observation only (depending on size). If it is particularly large, it may extend intraocularly or centrally and prevent normal visual development.[91, 93, 96–99] Small- to moderate-sized lesions may cause moderate to high astigmatism with refractive amblyopia (Fig 17–13).[100] The triad of auricular anomalies (appendages, pretragal fistulas), epibulbar dermoid, and vertebral anomalies constitutes oculoauriculovertebral dysplasia (Goldenhar syndrome).[101–104] Corneal dermoids occur sporadically, although isolated case reports suggest an autosomal recessive mode of inheritance.[105, 106] Dermoids threatening visual development may rarely require excision at an early age for normal visual development to occur. A lamellar keratectomy may suffice. However, the surgeon should be prepared for a localized penetrating keratoplasty or lamellar patch graft because the precise stromal depth of large tumors is difficult to determine

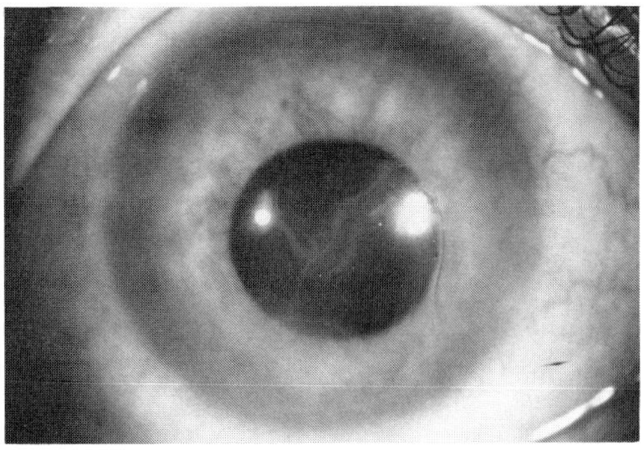

FIG 17–11.
Congenital glaucoma (resolved). Central posterior corneal linear opacities represent healed breaks in Descemet's membrane.

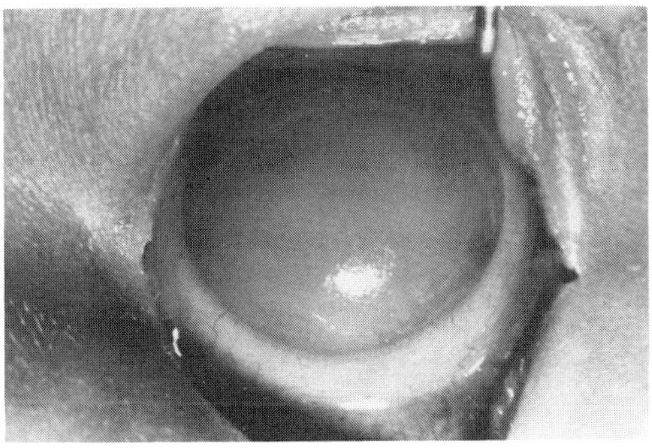

FIG 17–10.
Congenital glaucoma: enlarged edematous cornea with markedly elevated intraocular pressure.

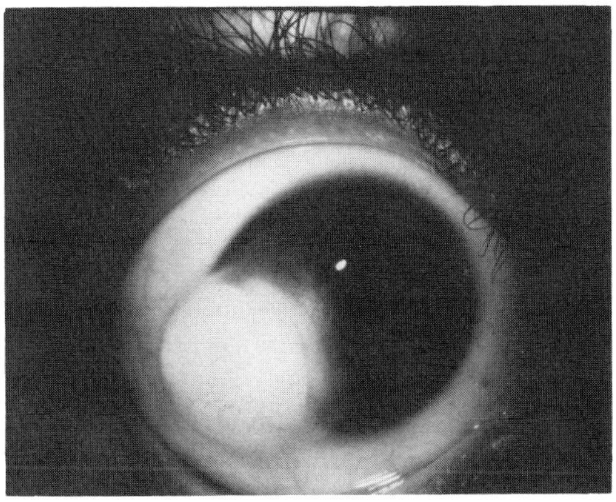

FIG 17–12.
Limbal dermoid, primarily lipodermal choristomatous tissue.

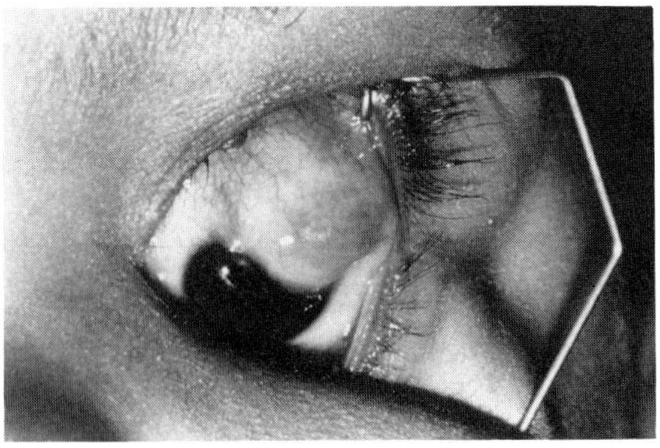

FIG 17–13.
Epibulbar choristoma. Tissues may include bone, cartilage, dermal elements, fat, and/or ectopic lacrimal gland.

preoperatively.[95] A two-stage approach to large corneal dermoids has been suggested—a large lamellar keratoplasty followed by a smaller penetrating keratoplasty.[98] Evaluation and monitoring of refractive error, visual acuity, and binocularity is advisable in all instances.

Osseous Choristomas

Osseous choristomas are very rare ocular lesions. These tumors involve the conjunctiva and episclera more frequently than cornea and may adhere to the muscle sheath.[107] They are composed of mature bone, and radiography aids diagnosis.[108, 109] Bony elements have been reported in only two dermoids: one, a congenitally deformed eye; the other, a mixed epibulbar osseous choristoma and dermoid.[107] Management is similar to that for dermoids.

BIRTH TRAUMA

Corneal forceps injuries may result in corneal edema and opacity. The improperly applied forcep may create a shearing force (typically vertically oriented) across the anterior globe and, tear posterior corneal layers (endothelium and Descemet's membrane). Aqueous humor from the anterior chamber enters the corneal stroma, and corneal edema ensues. In time, endothelial cells will migrate (perhaps replicate) to cover the defect, the edema will subside, and new Descemet's membrane is formed. The end result is often significant astigmatism, myopia, and amblyopia.[110] Should edema persist during the critical period of fixation reflex development, the amblyopia may be intractable. Treatment is directed to correction of refractive error and amblyopia. Keratoplasty may be warranted in severe cases, though such procedures performed for unilateral congenital corneal disease are controversial. (For further discussion, see Chapter 24.)

CORNEAL SURGERY IN INFANTS

Prior to 1965, there was a reluctance to perform penetrating keratoplasty in infants; surgical intervention for congenitally opaque corneas was generally restricted to optical iridectomies and lamellar keratoplasties.[111–113] Reports of successful penetrating keratoplasties in infants are balanced by reports of technical difficulties, complications, and admonitions for caution.[114–116] Modern surgical techniques combined with a better understanding of corneal physiology and mechanisms of graft rejection raise expectations for improved results.[117, 118] However, penetrating keratoplasty for a congenitally opaque cornea requires significant commitment from both the surgeon and the patient's family, and barriers to success are multiple.[116, 119]

Penetrating keratoplasty in infants is technically more challenging than in adults.[111, 114]

> The scleral rigidity is low. As a result, there tends to be anterior displacement of the lens iris diaphragm, rarely leading to spontaneous explusion of the lens. One response to this problem has been the use of a (support) ring. Fibrin exudation in the anterior chamber seems more profound in pediatric eyes, leading to an appearance that may mimic lens injury. In addition, the intense outpouring of fibrinoid material may lead to difficulty in dilating the pupil in the postoperative phase and perhaps contributes to the increased incidence of iris adherence to the wound that has been observed. Further, there are difficulties in handling pediatric corneal tissue. Wound ap-

position is difficult and occasionally donor buttons that are either 0.25 or 0.5 mm larger than recipient beds have been placed to facilitate wound closure. Dissection and suturing of pediatric corneal tissue is more demanding, relating to the nature of young corneal tissue. There seems to be a lack of "corneal rigidity," analogous to low scleral rigidity, in children.[115]

Complications are common, particularly related to flaccidity of recipient tissues. Postoperatively, examinations are difficult and suboptimal.[118] The infant cannot communicate typical warning signals. Glaucoma is relatively more common.[111, 114] Wound healing is rapid; corneal vascularization and graft rejection occur more rapidly and probably more frequently in infants. Loose sutures are common and a constant threat to the clarity of the graft; they may stimulate graft reaction, often requiring early and immediate removal.[116, 118] Postkeratoplasty eyes should be examined frequently, under general anesthesia if necessary. Parents must play an active role and inspect the eye for redness, graft clarity, and loose sutures (indicated by adherent mucous).[114, 117] If there is question of graft integrity, examination under anesthesia should be performed. Despite excellent immediate operative appearance and proper good postoperative care, graft failure may necessitate repeat grafting. Matching of donors and recipients by tissue typing holds promise. Intractable amblyopia remains a significant barrier requiring early occlusion therapy.[115] Given the aforementioned, transplantation of monocular congenitally opaque corneas remains controversial, and such procedures are not recommended by many corneal surgeons.[111, 116, 119]

In summary,

> Functional failure may occur in keratoplasty at any age. In adults causes may be categorized as operative complications, primary tissue failure, graft rejection, or recurrent disease. In infants and children all of the above may be present and would seem not only to be more common but possibly some more severe as well. In addition, amblyopia, noted and acknowledged by all observers who comment on pediatric keratoplasty, represents an additional major barrier to functional success in young children. Amblyogenesis preoperatively may ensue from occlusion or distortion. Postoperatively, even in the presence of a clear graft, amblyopia may result from a surgically induced astigmatism or from an induced spherical anisometropia.[115]

Given these barriers to functional success and the high risk of complications, the authors are reluctant to perform keratoplasty on any unilateral congenital corneal opacity. Keratoplasty in acquired corneal disease of infancy, where established fixation reflexes have been achieved, is demanding and occasionally rewarding, yet amblyopia, technical difficulties, and complications are omnipresent considerations.

REFERENCES

1. Jakobiec FA (ed): Ocular anatomy, embryology and teratology, in *Biomedical Foundations of Ophthalmology,* Vol 1. Philadelphia, JB Lippincott Co, 1982.
2. Johnston MC, Noden DM, Hazelton RD, et al: Origins of avian ocular and periocular tissues. *Exp Eye Res* 1979; 29:27.
3. Beauchamp GR, Knepper PA: Role of the neural crest in anterior segment development and disease. *J Pediatr Ophthalmol Strabismus* 1984; 21:209.
4. Bahn CF, Falls HF, Varley GA, et al: Classification of corneal endothelial disorders based on neural crest origin. *Ophthalmology* 1984; 91:558.
5. Wilmer HA, Seammon RE: Growth of the components of the human eyeball. *Arch Ophthalmol* 1950; 43:599.
6. Hirst LW: Congenital corneal problems. *Int Ophthalmol Clin* 1984; 24:55
7. Friedman MW, Wright ES: Hereditary microcornea and cataract in 5 generations. *Am J Ophthalmol* 1952; 35:1017.
8. Holmes LB, Walton DS: Hereditary microcornea, glaucoma, and absent frontal sinuses: A family study. *J Pediatr* 1969; 74:968.
9. Sommers IG: *Histology and Histopathology of the Eye.* New York, Grune & Stratton, 1949, p 635.

10. David R, MacBaeth L, Jenkins T: Aniridia associated with microcornea and subluxated lenses. *Br J Ophthalmol* 1978; 62:118.
11. Polomeno RC, Cummings C: Autosomal dominant cataracts and microcornea. *Can J Ophthalmol* 1979; 14:227.
12. Francois J: *Heredity in Ophthalmology*. St Louis, CV Mosby Co, 1961, p 291.
13. Francois J, Neetens A: Microcornee associee a une hydrophthalmie et a d'autres anomalies hereditaries. Acta Genet Med Gemel 1955; 4:217.
14. Durham DG: Cutis hyperelastic (Ehlers-Danlos syndrome) with blue scleras, microcornea, and glaucoma. *Arch Ophthalmol* 1953; 49:220.
15. Wood WJ, Green WR, Marr WG: Megalocornea: A clinicopathologic clinical case report. *Md State Med J* 1974; 23:57.
16. Hogan MJ, Zimmerman HE: *Ophthalmic Pathology: An Atlas and Textbook*, ed 2, Philadelphia, WB Saunders Co, 1962, p 289.
17. Skuta GL, Sugar J, Ericson ES: Corneal endothelial cell measurement in megalocornea. *Arch Ophthalmol* 1983; 101:51.
18. Vail DT: Adult hereditary anterior megalophthalmus sine glaucoma: A definite disease entity. *Arch Ophthalmol* 1931; 6:39.
19. Duke-Elder S (ed): Congenital deformities, in *System of Ophthalmology*, Vol 3. St Louis, CV Mosby Co, 1963, pp 498–502.
20. Howard RD, Abrahams IW: Sclerocornea. *Am J Ophthalmol* 1971; 71:1245.
21. Collier M: Progressive facial hemiatrophy with megalocornea, micropupil, and central nebulbar dystrophy of the cornea. *Acta Ophthalmol (Copenh)* 1971; 49:946.
22. Mansour AM, Traboulsi EI, Frangiah GT, et al: Unilateral megalocornea in lamellar icthyosis. *Ann Ophthalmol* 1985; 17:466.
23. Rogers GL, Polomeno RC: Autosomal-dominant inheritance of megalocornea associated with Down's syndrome. *Am J Ophthalmol* 1974; 78:526.
24. Biglan AW, Brown SI, Johnson BL: Keratoglobus and blue sclera. *Am J Ophthalmol* 1977; 83:225.
25. Hymas S, Dar H, Neumann E: Blue sclera and keratoglobus. Ocular signs of a systemic connective tissues disorder. *Br J Ophthalmol* 1969; 53:53.
26. Jacobs DS, Green WR, Maumenee AE: Acquired keratoglobus. *Am J Ophthalmol* 1974; 77:693.
27. Cavara V: Keratoglobus and keratoconus: A contribution to the nosological interpretation of keratoglobus. *Br J Ophthalmol* 1950; 34:621.
28. Arkin W: Blue sclera with keratoglobus. *Am J Ophthalmol* 1963; 58:678.
29. Gupta VF, Jain RK, Angra SK: Acute hydrops in keratoglobus with vernal keratoconjunctivitis. *Indian J Ophthalmol* 1985; 33:121.
30. Fishman AJ, Ackerman J, Kanarek I, et al: Cornea plana: A case report. *Ann Ophthalmol* 1982; 14:47.
31. Larsen V, Eriksen A: Cornea plana. *Acta Ophthalmol* 1949; 27:275–286.
32. May MA, Beauchamp GR: Collagen maturation defects in Ehlers-Danlos keratopathy. *J Pediatr Ophthalmol Strabismus* 1987; 24:78.
33. Duke-Elder S (ed): Congenital deformities, in *System of Ophthalmology*, vol 3. St Louis, CV Mosby Co, 1972, pp 505–508.
34. Elliott JH, Feman SS, O'Day DM, et al: Hereditary sclerocornea. *Arch Ophthalmol* 1985; 103:676.
35. Kanai A, Wood TC, Polak FM, et al: The fine structure of sclerocornea. *Invest Ophthalmol* 1971; 10:687.
36. Rodrigues MM, Calhoun J, Weinreb S: Sclerocornea with an unbalanced translocation (17p, 10q). *Am J Ophthalmol* 1974; 78:49.
37. Goldstein JE, Cogan DG: Sclerocornea and associated congenital anomalies. *Arch Ophthalmol* 1962; 67:199.
38. Howard RO, Abrahams IW: Sclerocornea. *Am J Ophthalmol* 1971; 71:1254.
39. Schanzlin DJ, Goldberg DB, Brown SI: Hallermann-Streiff syndrome associated with sclerocornea, aniridia, and a chromosomal abnormality. *Am J Ophthalmol* 1980; 90:411.
40. Harbin RL, Katz JI, Frias JL, et al: Sclerocornea associated with the Smith-Opitz syndrome. *Am J Ophthalmol* 1977; 84:72.
41. Waring GO, Rodrigues MM: Ultrastructure and successful keratoplasty of sclerocornea in Mieten's syndrome. *Am J Ophthalmol* 1980; 90:469.
42. Perry LD, Edwards WS, Bramson RT: Melnick-Needles syndrome. *J Pediatr Ophthalmol Strabismus* 1978; 15:226.
43. DeSuignes P, Pouliquen Y, Legras M, et al: Aspect conographique d'une cornea plana

dans une maladie de lobstein. *Arch Ophthalmol* 1967; 27:585.
44. March WE, Chalkley TH: Sclerocornea associated with Dandy-Walker cyst. *Am J Ophthalmol* 1974; 78:54.
45. Karlin DB, Wise GN: Keratoconus posticus. *Am J Ophthalmol* 1961; 52:119.
46. Jacobs MB: Traumatic keratoconus posticus. *Br J Ophthalmol* 1957; 41:40.
47. Ross JUM: Keratoconus posticus generalis. *Am J Ophthalmol* 1950; 33: 801.
48. Mukherjee G, Patnaik N, Mohan M: Acquired keratoconus posticus. *Indian J Ophthalmol* 1982; 30:357.
49. Young ID, Macrae WG, Hughes HE, et al: Keratoconus posticus circumscriptus, cleft lip and palate, genitourinary abnormalities, short stature, and mental retardation in sibs. *J Med Genet* 1982; 19:332.
50. Barry WE, Tredici TJ: Keratoconus in USAF flying personnel. *Aerospace Med* 1972; 43:1027.
51. Greene PB: Keratoconus posticus circumscriptus: Report of a case. *Arch Ophthalmol* 1945; 34:432.
52. Hagedoorn A, Velzeboer GMJ: Postnatal partial spontaneous correction of a severe congenital anomaly of the anterior segment of an eye. *Arch Ophthalmol* 1959; 62:685.
53. Streeten BW, Karpik AG, Spitzer KH: Posterior keratoconus associated with systemic abnormalities. *Arch Ophthalmol* 1983; 101:616.
54. Haney WR, Falls HF: The occurrence of congenital keratoconus posticus circumscriptus in two siblings presenting a previously unrecognized syndrome. *Am J Ophthalmol* 1961; 52:53.
55. Migeon BR: Short arm deletions in group E and chromosomal deletion syndrome. *J Pediatr* 1966; 69:432.
56. Linksz A: Physiology of the eye, in *Optics,* vol 1. New York, Grune & Stratton, 1950, p 281.
57. Peters A: Uber angeborene Defektildung der oescemetschen Membran. *Klin Monatsbl Augenheilkd* 1906; 44:27, 105.
58. Baqueiro A, Hein PA: Familial congenital leukoma. Case report and review of the literature. *Am J Ophthalmol* 1980; 50:810.
59. Bateman JB, Maumenee IH, Sparkes RS: Peters' anomaly associated with partial deletion of the long arm of chromosome 11. *Am J Ophthalmol* 1984; 97:11.
60. Townsend WM, Font RL, Zimmerman LE: Congenital corneal leukomas. 2. Histopathologic findings in 19 eyes with central defect in Descemet's membrane. *Am J Ophthalmol* 1974; 77:192.
61. Fineman RM, Ablow, RC, Howard RO, et al: Trisomy 8 mosaicism syndrome. *Pediatrics* 1975; 56:762.
62. Miller M, Epstein RJ, Sugar J, et al: Anterior segment anomalies associated with the fetal alcohol syndrome. *J Pediatr Ophthalmol Strabismus* 1984; 21:8.
63. Reese AB, Ellworth RM: The anterior chamber cleavage syndrome. *Arch Ophthalmol* 1966; 75:307.
64. Varley GA, Beauchamp GR, Meisler DM: Cornea. *Cornea* 1988; 7:63–66.
65. Alkemade PPH: *Dysgenesis Mesodermalis of the Iris and the Cornea.* Assen, The Netherlands, Royal van Gorcum, 1969, pp 83–98.
66. Townsend WM: Congenital corneal leukoma. I. Central defect in Descemet's membrane. *Am J Ophthalmol* 1974; 77:80.
67. Kenyon KR: Mesenchymal dysgenesis in Peters' anomaly, sclerocornea, and congenital endothelial dystrophy. *Sys Res* 1975; 21:125.
68. Bull MJ, Maum JL: Peters' anomaly with pulmonary hypoplasia. *Birth Defects* 1976; 12:181.
69. Ide CH, Matta C, Holt JE, et al: Dysgenesis mesodermalis of the cornea (Peters' anomaly) associated with cleft lip and palate. *Ann Ophthalmol* 1975; 7:841.
70. Townsend WM, Font RL, Zimmerman LE: Congenital corneal leukomas. 3. Histopathologic findings in 13 eyes with noncentral defect in Descemet's membrane. *Am J Ophthalmol* 1974; 70:400.
71. Collier M: La dysplasie marginale postericure de la cornee dans la cadre des anomalies squelettiques et ectodermiques. *Ann Oculist* 1961; 195:512.
72. Naumann GOH: Surgery for Peters' anomaly. *Dev Ophthalmol* 1985; 11:156.
73. Waring GO III, Rodrigues MM, Laibson PR: Anterior chamber cleavage syndrome: A stepladder classification. *Surv Ophthalmol* 1975; 20:3.
74. Burian HM, Braley AE, Allan L: External and gonioscopic visibility of the ring of

Schwalbe and the trabecular zone: An interpretation of the posterior corneal embryotoxon and the so called congenital hyaline membrane on the posterior corneal surface. *Trans Am Ophthalmol Soc* 1955; 51:389.

75. Axenfeld T: Embryotoxon corneae posterius. *Dtsch Ophthalmol Gasamte* 1920; 42:301.
76. Shields MB: Axenfeld-Reiger syndrome: A theory of mechanism and distinction from the iridocorneal endothelial syndrome. *Trans Am Ophthalmol Soc* 1983; 81:736.
77. Tabbara KF, Khouri FP, der Kaloustian VM: Rieger's syndrome with chromosomal anomaly (report of a case). *Can J Ophthalmol* 1973; 8:488.
78. Henkind P, Siegel IM, Carr RE: Mesodermal dysgenesis of the anterior segment: Rieger's anomaly. *Arch Ophthalmol* 1965; 73:810.
79. Sugar HS: Juvenile glaucoma with Axenfeld's syndrome: A histopathologic report. *Am J Ophthalmol* 1965; 59:1012.
80. Smith RE, Lee JS: The cornea in systemic disease, in Duane T (ed): *Clinical Ophthalmology*, vol 4. Philadelphia, Harper & Row, Publishers, Inc, 1986.
81. Judisch GF, Maumenee IH: Clinical differentiation of recessive congenital hereditary endothelial dystrophy and dominant hereditary endothelial dystrophy. *Am J Ophthalmol* 1978; 85:606.
82. Kenyon KR, Maumenee AE: The histological and ultrastructural pathology of congenital hereditary corneal dystrophy: A case report. *Invest Ophthalmol* 1968; 7:475.
83. Pearce WG, Tripathi RC, Morgan G: Congenital endothelial corneal dystrophy: Clinical, pathological and genetic study. *Br J Ophthamol* 1969; 53:577.
84. Maumenee AE: Congenital hereditary corneal dystrophy. *Am J Ophthalmol* 1960; 50:1114.
85. Schlichting H: Blasen und dellenformige Endotheldystrophe der Horenhaut. *Klin Monatsbl Augenheilkd* 1941; 107:425.
86. Cibis GW, Krachmer JA, Phelps CD, et al: The clinical spectrum of posterior polymorphous dystrophy. *Arch Ophthalmol* 1977; 95:1529.
87. Cibis GW, Krachmer JA, Phelps CD, et al: Iridocorneal adhesions in posterior polymorphous dystrophy. *Trans Am Acad Ophthalmol Otolaryngol* 1976; 81:770.
88. Rodrigues MM, Waring GO, Laibson PR, et al: Endothelial alterations in congenital corneal dystrophies. *Am J Ophthalmol* 1975; 80:678.
89. Witschel H, Fine BS, Grutzner P, et al: Congenital hereditary stromal dystrophy of the cornea. *Arch Ophthalmol* 1978; 96:1034.
90. Morin JD, Coughlin WR: Corneal changes in primary congenital glaucoma. *Trans Am Ophthalmol Soc* 1980; 78:123.
91. Boniuk M, Zimmerman LE: Epibulbar osteoma (episcleral osseous choristoma). *Am J Ophthalmol* 1962; 53:290.
92. Howard GM: Cystic tumors, in Jones IS, Jakobiec FA (eds): *Diseases of the Orbit*. Hagerstown, Md, Harper & Row, Publishers, Inc, 1979, p 135.
93. Dailey EG, Lubowitz RM: Dermoids of the limbus and cornea. *Am J Ophthalmol* 1962; 53:661.
94. Ash JE: Epibulbar tumors. *Am J Ophthalmol* 1950; 33:1203.
95. Shields JA, Laibson PR, Augsburger JJ, et al: Central corneal dermoid: A clinicopathologic correlation and review of the literature. *Can J Ophthalmol* 1986; 21:23.
96. Garner LL: Dermoid of the limbus involving the iris, angle, and lens. *Arch Ophthalmol* 1951; 46:69.
97. Schulze RR: Limbal dermoid tumor with intraocular extension. *Arch Ophthalmol* 1966; 75:803.
98. Zaidman GW, Johnson B, Brown SI: Corneal transplantation in an infant with corneal dermoid. *Am J Ophthalmol* 1982; 93:78.
99. Mann I: A rare congenital abnormality of the eye. *Br J Ophthalmol* 1930; 14:321.
100. Swann KC, Emmens TH, Christensen L: Experiences with tumors of the limbus. *Trans Am Acad Ophthalmol* 1947; 52:458.
101. Goldenmar M: Associations malformations de J'oeil et de l'oreille, en particulier le syndrome dermoide epibulbaire-appendices auricularies-fistula auris congenita ot ses relations avec la dysostose mandibulo-sociale. *J Genet Hum* 1952; 1:243.
102. O'Connor M, Johnson SS, Kidd MN, et al: Goldenhar's syndrome. Bull Soc Belge Ophthalmol 1984; 211:7.
103. Baum JL, Feingold M: Ocular aspects of Goldenhar's syndrome. *Am J Ophthalmol* 1973; 75:25.
104. Gorlin RJ, Jue KL, Jacobsen Y, et al: Oculoauriculovertebral dysplasia. *J Pediatr* 1963; 63:991.
105. Guizar-Vazquez I, Luengas-Munoz FJ, Antil-

lon F: Brief clinical report: Corneal dermoids and short stature in brother and sister—A new syndrome? *Am J Med Gen* 1981; 8:229.
106. Henkind P, Marinoff G, Manas A, et al: Bilateral corneal dermoids. *Am J Ophthalmol* 1973; 76:972.
107. Ferry A, Hein H: Epibulbar osseous choristoma within an epibulbar dermoid. *Am J Ophthalmol* 1970; 70:764.
108. Beckman H, Sugar HS: Episcleral osseous choristoma: A report of two cases. *Arch Ophthalmol* 1964; 71:377.
109. Dreizen NG, Schachat AP, Shields JA, et al: Epibulbar osseous choristoma. *J Pediatr Ophthalmol Strabismus* 1983; 20:247.
110. Angell LK, Robb RM, Berson FG: Visual prognosis in patients with ruptures in Descemet's membrane due to forceps injuries. *Arch Ophthalmol* 1981; 99:2137.
111. Thomas JWT: On advising a corneal graft. *Br Med J* 1956; 1:880.
112. Leigh AG: Corneal grafting. *Br J Clin Pract* 1958; 12:329.
113. Noble BA, Easty DL: Late corneal grafting in congenitally opaque corneas. *Dev. Ophthalmol* 1985; 11:75.
114. Schanzlin DJ, Goldberg DB, Brown SI: Transplantation of congenital opaque corneas. *Ophthalmology* 1980; 87:1253.
115. Beauchamp GR: Pediatric keratoplasty: Problems in management. *J Pediatr Ophthalmol Strabismus* 1979; 16:388.
116. Waring GO III, Laibson PR: Keratoplasty in infants and children. *Trans Am Acad Ophthalmol Otolaryngol* 1977; 83:283.
117. Stulting RD, Sumers KD, Cavanagh HD, et al: Penetrating keratoplasty in children. *Ophthalmology* 1984; 91:1222.
118. Brown SI: Corneal transplantation of the infant cornea. *Trans Am Acad Ophthalmol Otolaryngol* 1974; 78:461.
119. Waring GO III, Laibson PR: Keratoplasty in children, in Kwito ML (ed): *Surgery of the Infant Eye*. New York, Appleton-Century-Crofts, 1979, pp 197–215.

18 The Uveal Tract

Marilyn B. Mets, M.D.
Venkat Reddy, B.A.

The uveal tract is composed of the iris, the ciliary body, and the choroid and is considered to be the vascular coat of the eye. The iris is the anterior-most portion of the uveal tract. It forms the posterior wall of the anterior chamber except centrally where there is a sphincter-bordered aperture in the iris tissue known as the pupil. The contraction and dilation of the pupil is what controls the amount of light that is able to reach the posterior segment of the eye. The iris comprises four layers, the anterior limiting layer, the stroma, the dilator muscle, and the posterior epithelium.[1]

The ciliary body is the middle ground of the uveal tract. It is about 6 mm wide and extends from the base of the iris to the choroid. Its junction with the choroid occurs at the ora serrata. There are essentially two parts to it. The anterior portion is called the pars plicata and the posterior portion the pars plana. It has two major functions. Its muscular components are responsible for accommodation and relaxation of the pupil, and the nonpigmented ciliary epithelium of the pars plicata produces aqueous humor.

The choroid is the vascular coat of the posterior segment of the eye, and it contains the majority of the pigmentation in that segment. It extends from the ora serrata to the optic nerve. It provides the vascular supply to the retinal pigment epithelium and the outer layers of the retina. The congenital disorders of the uveal tract will be organized according to the aforementioned.

IRIS

Aniridia

In aniridia, much or most of the iris tissue is missing. Its prevalence in the general population is reported as 1 in 50,000 in Michigan[2] and 1 in 100,000 in Denmark.[3] Characteristically, there is a lack of iris tissue that may be associated with cataracts, foveal hypoplasia, nystagmus, glaucoma, corneal pannus, and vision in the range of 20/200. The typical presentation is a baby with apparent absence of the irides or with the appearance of fully dilated pupils (Fig 18–1,A and B), nystagmus, and photophobia. On examination, the associated cataracts and foveal hypoplasia can be found (see Fig 18–1,C). The cataracts are often anterior polar and have been observed to be associated with a persistent pupillary membrane (see Figure 18–1,B). The nystagmus is, most likely, a sensory type due to decreased vision from foveal hypoplasia and possibly cataracts if they are extensive. In the first and second decades of life, there is the associated development of glaucoma and corneal pannus. The glaucoma appears to be due to migration of the peripheral iris stroma up the angle wall until the iris essentially occludes the trabecular meshwork.[4] The corneal pannus is also not typically present in infancy, and in cases where there is some patchy iris tissue present, it forms where the iris is absent.[5]

There are two forms of aniridia, familial and sporadic, and both present with the afore-

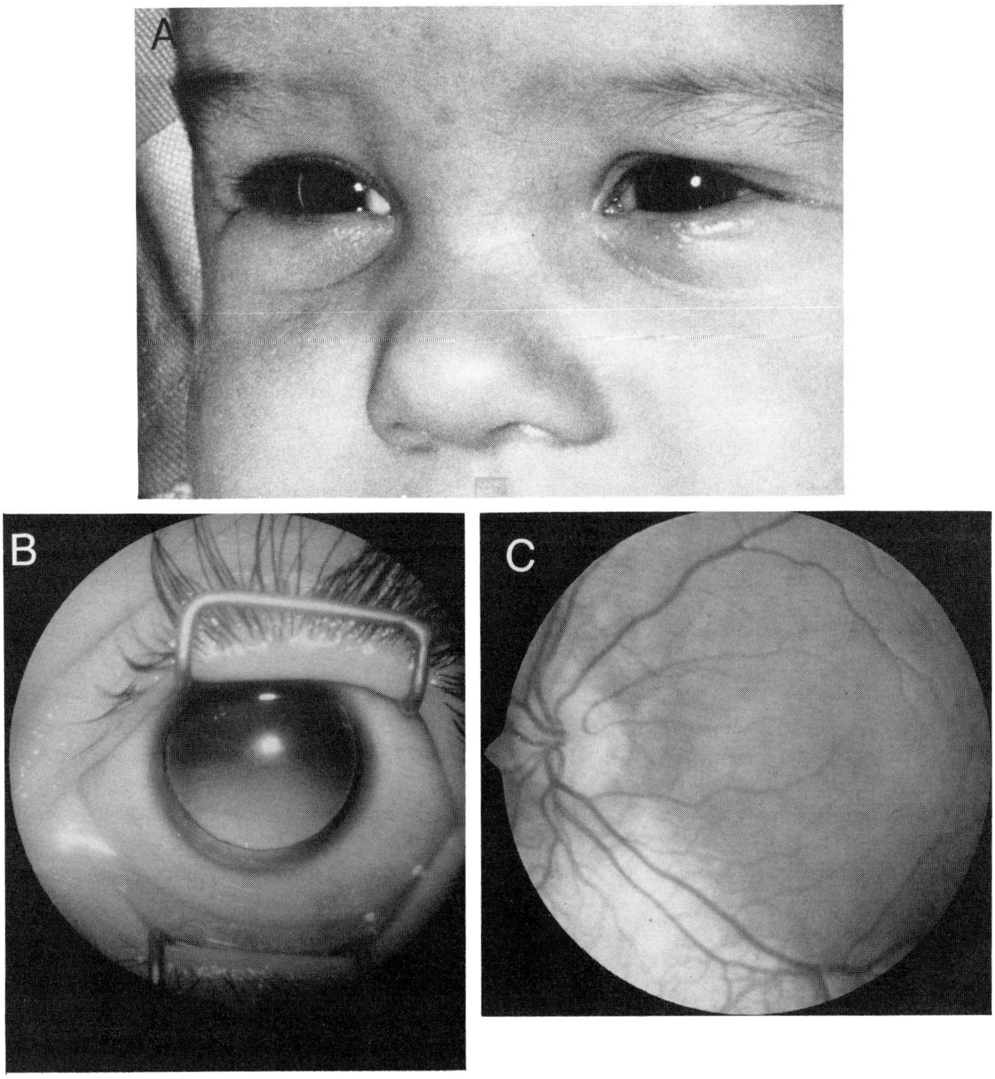

FIG 18–1.
A, 3-month-old child with sporadic aniridia. Note the equators of the lenses visible temporally on the left and nasally and temporally on the right. **B**, the same child's left eye at the age of 5 years which shows an apparent absence of the iris. The equator of the lens is visible everywhere except from the 10:00 to the 1:00 position. In addition, a persistent pupillary membrane and a central anterior polar cataract can be seen. **C**, the left fundus of the same child which shows vessels going right into the area of the macula and demonstrates the foveal hypoplasia found in aniridia.

mentioned clinical findings. The familial form is autosomal dominant with fairly complete penetrance and variable expressivity. Extensive family studies have been reported.[2,6,7] In addition, there have been several families reported in which there have been members with uncharacteristically good vision.[8,9]

The sporadic form was first identified by Miller and colleagues in a study of 440 patients with Wilms' tumor.[10] They noted aniridia in 6 of their cases, a prevalence of 1:74, which is much higher than the frequency reported in the general population. Subsequently, Fraumeni and Glass reported Wilms' tumor in 5 of 15 hospitalized patients with aniridia.[11] It is now known that there is a significant association between sporadic aniridia and Wilms' tumor, with the tumor developing in one third of aniridia patients.[12] Also, one case of Wilms' tumor has been reported in a child with familial aniridia.[11] (Most likely, this case represents a familial 11p13 deletion.) All children with sporadic aniridia should have repeated abdominal examinations supplemented by ultrasound or intravenous pyelography. Our protocol at the University of Chicago is to have the child be seen every 3 months until the age of 5, every 6 months until the age of 10, and once a year until the age of 16.

In addition, the sporadic form of aniridia is associated with other systemic abnormalities including mental retardation, craniofacial dysmorphism, ptosis, microcephaly, and other genitourinary anomalies.[10,11,13] Deletion analysis has been used by Riccardi and associates to assign the complex of aniridia, ambiguous genitalia, and mental retardation (AGR) to chromosome 11p.[14] They described three unrelated patients with 11p interstitial deletions. These deletions were all overlapping band 13. One of the three also had a Wilms' tumor. They concluded that a partial deletion of 11p 13 causes the characteristic syndrome of AGR and a nephroblastic diathesis, with a tumor developing in only a portion of cases.

Coloboma

Coloboma is defined as a "multiliation or defect" and is derived from the Greek *koloboma*.[15] The English term is used almost exclusively with reference to the eye. Coloboma of the uveal tract will be discussed as one topic. Iris colobomas may be typical or atypical depending on their location. Atypical colobomas are those found anywhere except the inferior nasal quadrant and are usually restricted to the iris. Typical colobomas are found in the inferior nasal quadrant and are due to an embryological arrest resulting in incomplete closure of the fetal fissure of the optic cup. Typical colobomas may involve the iris, ciliary body, choroid, retina, and optic nerve, isolated or in combination. Colobomas can be considered to be part of a continuum that extends to microphthalmia and anophthalmia because there have been several autosomal dominant families with members showing these variable manifestations.[16–18]

Characteristically, the child presents clinically with a keyhole appearance of one or both irides as seen in Figure 18–2. Nystagmus may be present if there is also a chorioretinal coloboma involving the fovea. On examination of the posterior segment, one may find an entirely normal posterior segment or chorioretinal and optic nerve coloboma occurring in association or individually (Fig 18–3). There has been a report of an associated peripheral corneal pannus, like that seen in aniridia, that presented in a family with autosomal dominant iris coloboma, but this is not a typical finding.[19]

Autosomal dominant forms of isolated uveal tract colobomas are well noted in the literature.[20–22] As mentioned before, some of these families show manifestations ranging from coloboma to microphthalmia and anophthalmia.[16,17] Autosomal recessive forms of coloboma have been suggested, but there is some question about older reports published before the use of the indirect ophthalmoscope.[23]

There is a nonspecific association between uveal tract coloboma and almost any chromosomal abnormality. In addition, there are several chromosomal anomalies that are more characteristically associated with ocular colobomas[24–33]:

- Trisomy 13
- Triploidy
- Cat-eye syndrome
- 4p−
- 11q−
- 13q−
- 18q
- 18r
- 13r
- Trisomy 18
- Klinefelter syndrome
- Turner syndrome

Trisomy 13, or Patau syndrome, is per-

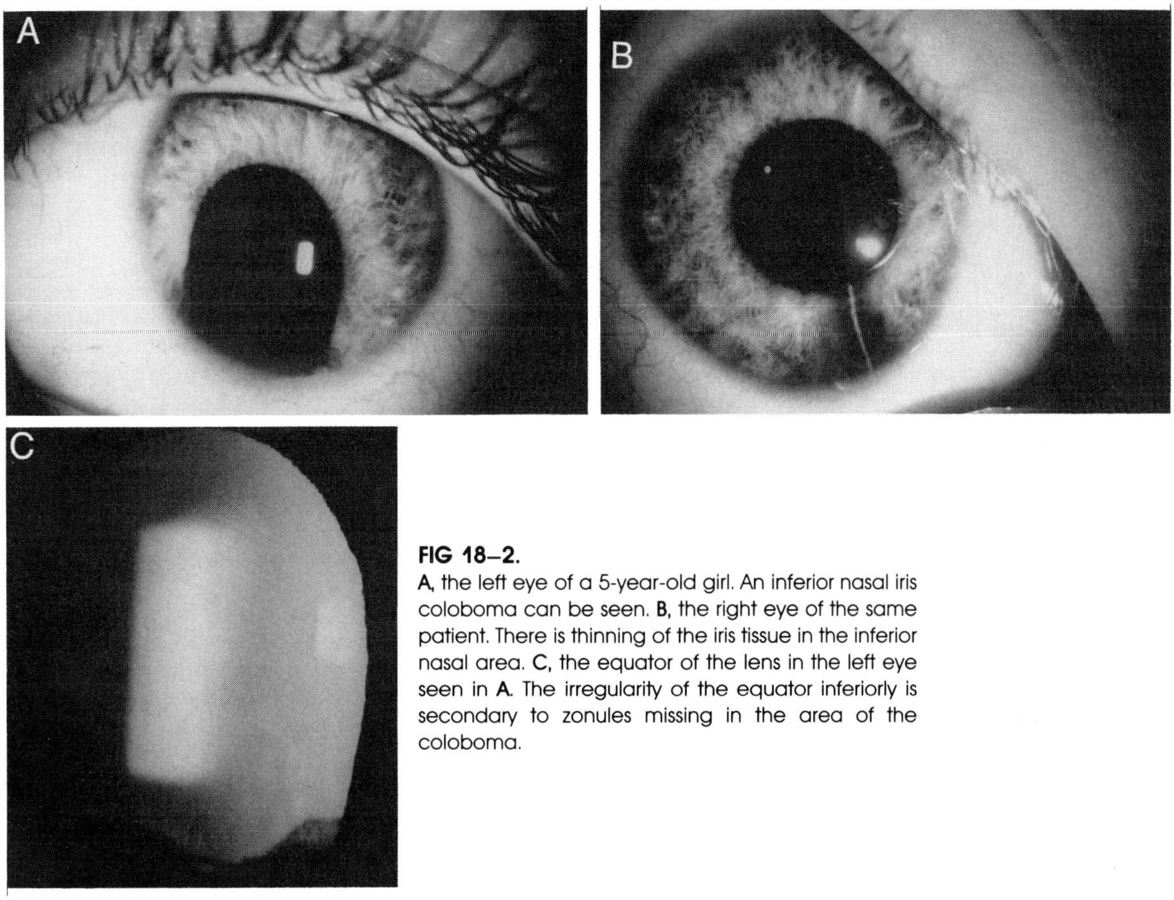

FIG 18–2.
A, the left eye of a 5-year-old girl. An inferior nasal iris coloboma can be seen. **B**, the right eye of the same patient. There is thinning of the iris tissue in the inferior nasal area. **C**, the equator of the lens in the left eye seen in **A**. The irregularity of the equator inferiorly is secondary to zonules missing in the area of the coloboma.

haps the most frequent and well known of these associations.

Several known syndromes have uveal tract colobomas associated with them[34–49]:

- Aicardi syndrome
- CHARGE syndrome
- Basal cell nevus syndrome
- Goldenhar syndrome
- Goltz focal dermal hypoplasia
- Lentz microphthalmos syndrome
- Linear sebaceous nevus syndrome
- Meckel syndrome
- Median facial cleft syndrome
- Rubenstein-Taybi syndrome
- Warburg syndrome

Of these, the CHARGE syndrome (*C*oloboma, *H*eart disease, *A*tresia choanae, *R*etarded growth and retarded development and/or central nervous system [CNS] anomalies, *G*enital hypoplasia, and *E*ar anomalies, and/or deafness) is the most common. A syndrome of coloboma and multiple congenital anomalies was first reported in 1961 by Edwards and associates and Angelman.[50, 51] Then, in 1979, Hall described 17 unrelated patients with choanal atresia and associated abnormalities.[52] Following this, in 1981 Pagon and associates synthesized previous reports and described 21 patients with the CHARGE association.[53] In this paper, the features were considered an association rather than a syndrome to allow for comparison of a larger number of probands to better deliniate the heterogeneity of the possible etiologies. Pagon et al. refer to at least two forms of inheritance, autosomal dominant and autosomal recessive. Subsequently, Mitchell and colleagues have reported an autosomal dominant family.[54] Pagon et al. also cite the possibility of teratogens and mentions thalidomide, al-

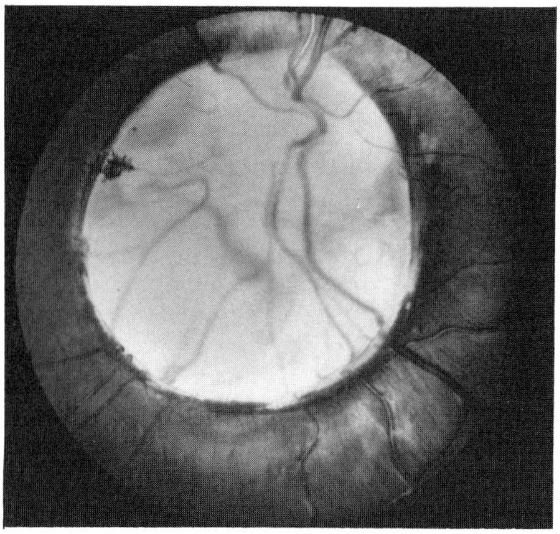

FIG 18–3.
The left eye of a 5-year-old girl with a chorioretinal coloboma that also involves the optic nerve.

though most of these patients have normal intelligence. In 1986, Davenport and colleagues reported nine sporadic and six familial cases and suggest that CHARGE be considered a syndrome rather than an association.[55]

The eye findings in the CHARGE syndrome range from typical iris coloboma with no visual impairment to clinical anophthalmos and include the full spectrum of chorioretinal and optic nerve colobomas and microphthalmos as described earlier.

There is a known association between uveal tract colobomas and known teratogens such as thalidomide.[56, 57] Thalidomide cases in particular are seen in association with limb malformations and are caused by damage around the 40th to 42nd day of gestation.

Uveal tract colobomas are fairly common eye anomalies that may be due to many etiologies as we have discussed. Pagon suggests that affected individual should be evaluated by having (1) a complete ophthalmologic examination; (2) a medical evaluation to determine whether the eye findings are isolated or part of a multisystem disorder, (3) a careful pregnancy history to look for teratogens, (4) a family history to look for other members with colobomatous defects, and (5) an ophthalmologic examination of parents and siblings.[23] In addition, the patient should be followed for anisometropia and a possible associated amblyopia. Also, choroidal colobomas predispose to retinal detachment, and this should be monitored.[58]

Primary Iris Cyst

A primary iris cyst may be defined as an epithelium-lined space that is found in some part of the iris and has no known etiology.[59] There are pigmented and unpigmented types[60] and they may be located at the pupillary margin, in the posterior epithelial layer of the iris, or as free floating cysts in the aqueous or vitreous. Their pathogenesis remains a puzzle. It was thought that they grew over time and resulted in secondary glaucoma and loss of vision.[61] However, a more recent study of 82 patients by Shields shows that the vast majority of primary iris cysts are stationary, do not progress, and do not cause visual complications.[59]

Persistent Pupillary Membrane

Significant persistent pupillary membrane presents clinically as strands of pigmented anterior iris stroma crossing the pupil from the lesser arterial circle (or collarette). These may be very minimal or very extensive. The pathogenesis is the result of an arrest in the normal process of atrophy of the vessels and intervening connective tissue that form the pupillary membrane prenatally.[60] Persistence of part of the membrane is very common. Mann quotes Waardenburg as saying that 80% of dark eyes and 35% of light eyes show minimal persistences of fine threads attached to the lesser circle.[60] The majority are sporadic, but there have been some autosomal dominant families reported.[62, 63] Merin and colleagues report that members of one family have surprisingly good vision (20/30 to 20/80) in view of the appearance of their membranes.[63] They suggest that the condition should not be treated surgically except in very young children before amblyopia develops.

Brushfield's Spots

Spots on the anterior surface of the iris in normal individuals were initially described by Wolfflin in 1902 and Kruckmann in 1907.[64, 65] Then in 1924, Thomas Brushfield reported spots on the iris surface in Down syndrome and considered them to be characteristic of the disease[66] (Fig 18–4). In a large controlled study of iris spots, Donaldson found Brushfield's spots in 85% of mongoloids and the somewhat similar Kruckmann-Wolfflin spots in 24% of irides of normal individuals.[67] Both types of spots are seen in both blue and brown irides although they appear somewhat more distinct in blue irides. Brushfield's spots differ from those seen in normal individuals (Kruckmann-Wolfflin) because they tend to be more centrally located, more numerous, and more distinct. The characteristic distinctness is probably due to the contrast of these spots against a background of iris hypoplasia, which is also seen in Down syndrome. Brushfield's spots may be a useful clinical sign when considering the diagnosis of Down syndrome in an infant, but as discussed, 24% of normal individuals have similar anterior iris spots.

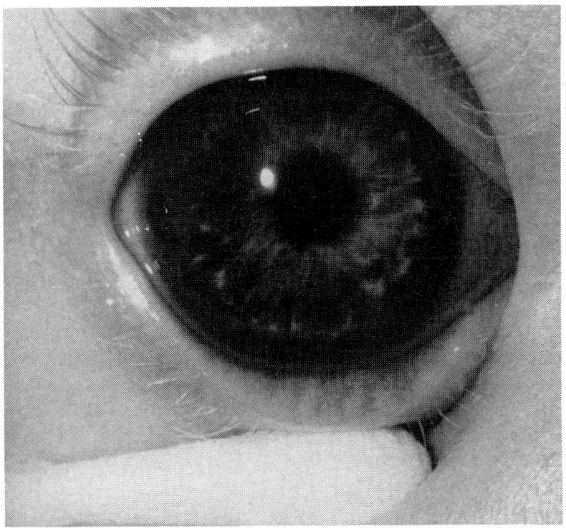

FIG 18–4.
The right eye of a 12-month-old boy with Down syndrome that shows Brushfield's spots. Note that this child also has congenital glaucoma causing a fine haziness in the cornea.

CILIARY BODY

Medulloepithelioma

Medulloepithelioma, also known as diktyoma, is a tumor of the ciliary body or iris that appears in infancy or early childhood. It may occur in either benign or malignant forms but rarely metastasizes. The usual presentation is an iris or ciliary body mass that covers much of the affected structure. The tumor may erode anteriorly and block the trabecular meshwork, thereby resulting in glaucoma and buphthalmos. Extension posteriorly can result in a white pupillary reflex and reduced visual acuity.[68]

Medulloepitheliomas are unilateral tumors that arise from the anterior portion of the inner neuroectoderm. Tumors containing only neuroectodermal elements are termed *nonteratoid*. If neuroectodermal and heteroptic elements such as cartilage, striated muscle, and brain tissue are present in the tumor, it is termed a *teratoid medulloepithelioma*.[69] Since the potential for spread is low, local excision or cryotherapy have been advocated for anteriorly placed localized tumors.[70] Unless diagnosis is made at an early stage, enucleation is the recommended form of therapy for two reasons: (1) medulloepitheliomas are radio insensitive, and (2) Broughton and Zimmerman reported 4 tumor deaths occurring in 10 patients with extraorbital tumor extension in a study of 37 malignant medulloepitheliomas.[68, 69]

CHOROID

Hemangioma

Hemangioma of the choroid occurs in two specific forms. First, a circumscribed hemangioma without associated systemic manifestations occurs more often in adulthood. The second type of choroidal hemangioma appears diffusely red (tomato-catsup fundus) and is detected in 40% of infants with Sturge-Weber syndrome.[71] The Sturge-Weber syndrome consists of the following: (1) a facial angioma (nevus flammeus or port-wine stain), usually

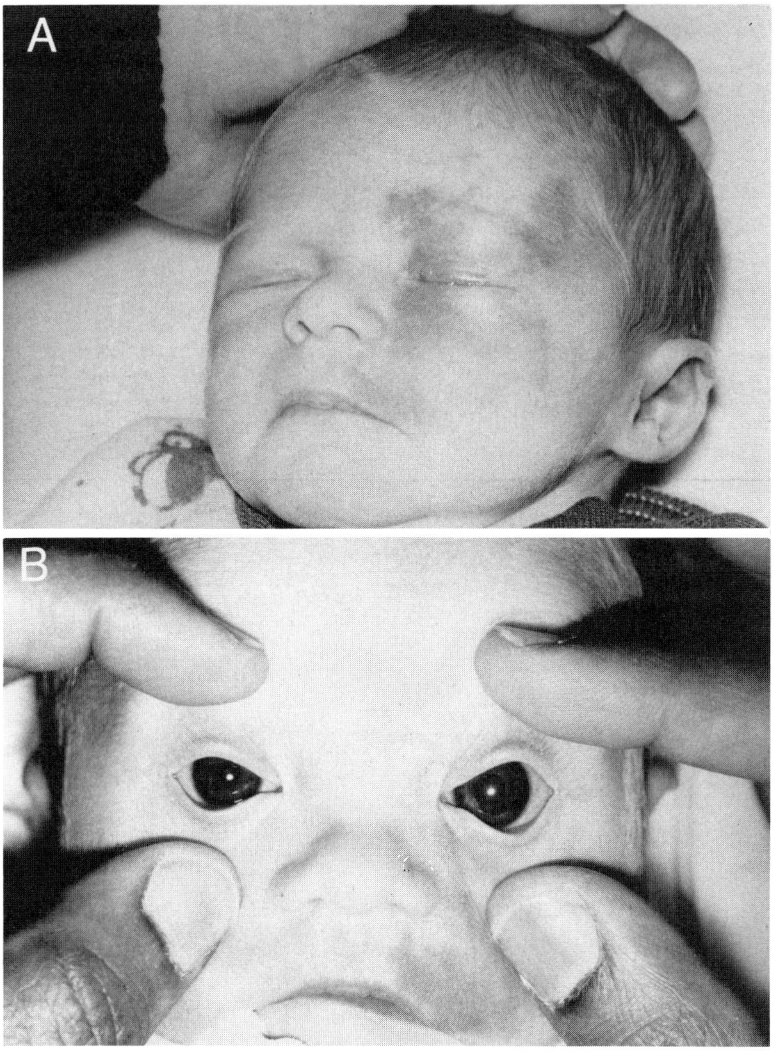

FIG 18–5.
A, a 5-day-old baby girl with a left-sided facial hemangioma. **B,** the same child showing the slightly enlarged and cloudy cornea on the left side secondary to associated glaucoma.

unilateral and distributed along the trigeminal nerve; (2) choroidal hemangioma; (3) unilateral glaucoma and buphthalmos on the same side as the facial hemangioma; and (4) various CNS abnormalities including leptomeningeal angiomas, cerebral calcifications, seizure disorder, mental retardation, and hemiparesis[72] (Fig 18–5,A and B).

In Sturge-Weber syndrome, the hemangioma occurs temporal to the optic disc and grows very slowly. The retina proximal to the tumor may degenerate, first becoming edematous and later cystic and atrophic. Serous retinal detachment is a frequent complication. The glaucoma occurs on the side of the facial angioma and may be congenital or develop later in childhood. The congenital form usually occurs when the facial angioma involves the eyelids or conjunctiva.[73] Several mechanisms have been proposed for the glaucoma. Congenital malformation of the anterior chamber angle with anterior insertion of the ciliary muscle may cause increased resistance to aqueous outflow.[72] Another proposed mechanism is that episcleral vascular malformations elevate the episcleral venous pressure, thus impeding aqueous outflow.[67]

The diagnosis of choroidal hemangioma within the Sturge-Weber syndrome is made with relative ease on fundus examination. However, some lesions may be subtle and necessitate the use of fluorescein angiography and A-scan ultrasonography. If the hemangioma is asymptomatic, no treatment is indicated; as it grows larger and threatens vision, photocoagulation and cryotherapy may be used to destroy the tumor.[74, 75] Serous retinal detachments are treated by photocoagulating the tumor surface to prevent further fluid accumulation.[76] Treatment of glaucoma is usually difficult. It may be best approached with trabeculotomy ab externo, goniotomy, or trabeculectomy followed by medical treatment as needed to maintain normal intraocular pressure.[73]

Isolated hemangiomas of the iris and ciliary body are extremely rare. The diagnosis is very difficult and often incorrect. One must be certain to rule out malignant melanoma, juvenile xanthogranuloma, and neovascularization secondary to an underlying process before diagnosing an anterior uveal hemangioma.[77]

Choroideremia

Choroideremia is a bilateral, progressive atrophy of the choroid and its vessels, with secondary atrophy of the retinal pigment epithelium (RPE) and outer part of the retina.[78] It is inherited as an X-linked recessive trait with complete manifestation in males and partial manifestation in females, a feature allowing for clinical detection of carriers. By using restriction fragment-length polymorphisms, Lewis and associates have localized the mutation for choroideremia to the region of Xq13-q24.[79]

In choroideremia, bilateral fundus changes are present from birth, and night blindness becomes evident within the first 2 decades. Visual field constriction and central visual losses are noted by the age of 40 when the atrophy finally extends into the macula.[80] The fundus in the male infant is diffusely granular with pigment epithelial stippling and thinning of the choroid. This progresses to atrophy and disappearance of RPE and choroidal vessels, a process starting from the midperiphery and spreading to the disc and fovea (Fig 18–6). At this stage, the fundus appears white due to exposed sclera. Aggregates of pigment may be seen to course along remaining choroidal vessels, and not retinal vessels as seen in retinitis pigmentosa. The retina and optic disc are uninvolved until very late in the process.[80] Visual diagnostic tests show a reduced or extinguished scotopic phase on the electroretinogram,[81] elevated dark adaptation thresholds,[78] and a loss of choriocapillaris when using fluorescein angiography.[82]

Visual function is typically normal in the female carrier who presents with abnormal fundus exam findings. The fundus changes are very similar to those of the male infant, with mottling of pigment epithelium in the periphery and paramacular area. These changes are evident at birth and do not progress.[78] There are, however, rare cases of female car-

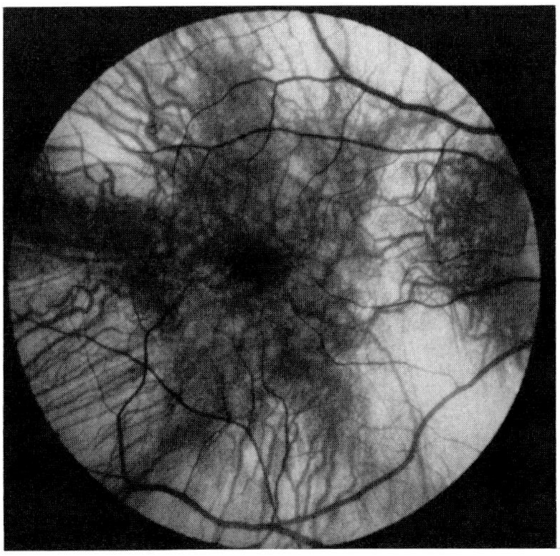

FIG 18–6.
The right fundus of a teenaged child with X-linked choroideremia. The photograph was taken with a red-free filter to demonstrate the choroidal vessels and the atrophy of the retinal pigment epithelial. The retinal pigment epithelium remains in the star-shaped pattern around the macula.

riers displaying a progressive disorder similar to the affected male, a finding explained as an extreme case of X-chromosome inactivation on the basis of the Lyon hypothesis.[83, 84]

Choroideremia may be associated with other ocular anomalies including heterchromia iridis, conjunctival melanosis,[85] and posterior subcapsular cataracts.[86] Systemic associations have been reported twice. Van den Bosch described males in an isolated Dutch family with choroideremia, mental retardation, acrokeratosis verruciformis, anhidrosis, and skeletal deformity.[87] More recently, Ayazi reported a syndrome of choroideremia, congenital deafness, and obesity that was compatible with X-linked inheritance in which carrier females had only ophthalmic findings.[88]

REFERENCES

1. Green WR: The uveal tract, in Spencer WH (ed): *Ophthalmic Pathology: An Atlas and Textbook,* vol 3. Philadelphia, WB Saunders Co, 1986.
2. Shaw MW, Falls HF, Neel JF: Congenital aniridia. *Am J Genet* 1960; 12:389.
3. Mollenbach CJ: Congenital defects in the internal membrane of the eye: *Opera Ex Domo Biologia Heriditariae Humane Universitatis Hafniensis,* vol 15. Copenhagen, Ejner, Munksgaard, 1947.
4. Grant WM, Walton DS: Progressive changes in the angle in congenital aniridia with development of glaucoma. *Am J Ophthalmol* 1974; 78:842.
5. Mackman G, Brightbell FS, Opitz JM: Corneal changes in aniridia. *Am J Ophthalmol* 1979; 87:497.
6. Grove JH, Shaw, MW, Borque G: A family study of aniridia. *Arch Ophthalmol* 1961; 65:81.
7. Shaffer RN, Cohen JS: Visual reduction in aniridia. *J Pediatr Ophthalmol* 1975; 12:220.
8. Elsas FJ, Maumenee IH, Kenyon KR, et al: Familial aniridia with preserved ocular function. *Am J Ophthalmol* 1977; 83:718.
9. Hittner HM, Riccardi VM, Ferrell RE, et al: Variable expressivity in autosomal dominant aniridia by clinical electrophysiologic, and angiographic criteria. *Am J Ophthalmol* 1980; 89:531.
10. Miller RW, Fraumeni JF, Manning MD: Association of Wilms' tumor with aniridia, hemi-hypertrophy and other congenital malformations. *N Engl J Med* 1964; 270:922.
11. Fraumeni JF, Glass AG: Wilms' tumor and congenital aniridia. *JAMA* 1968; 206:825.
12. Cotlier E, Rose M, and Moel SA: Aniridia, cataracts, and Wilms' tumor in monozygous twins. *Am J Ophthalmol* 1978; 86:129.
13. DiGeorge AM, Harley, RD: The association of aniridia, Wilms' tumor and genital abnormalities. *Arch Ophthalmol* 1966; 75:796.
14. Riccardi VM, Sujansky E, Smith AC, et al: Chromosomal imbalance in the aniridia-Wilms' tumor association: 11p interstitial deletion. *Pediatrics* 1978; 61:604.
15. *Dorland's Illustrated Medical Dictionary,* 24th ed. Philadelphia, WB Saunders Co, 1965, p 325.
16. Waardenburg PJ, Franceschetti A, Klein D: Colobomas and microphthalmia seen from a neurological angle, in *Genetics and Ophthalmology,* vol. 2. Springfield, Ill, Charles C Thomas, Publishers, 1963, pp 1197–1200.
17. Warburg M: Genetic eye disease: Retinitis pigmentosa and other inherited eye disorders. *Birth Defects* 1982; 18:31–50.
18. Fraser GR: Severe visual handicap in childhood, in Goldberg MF (ed): *Genetic and Metabolic Eye Disease:* Little, Brown, & Co, Boston, 1974, pp 30–31.
19. Soong HK, Raizman MB: Corneal changes in a familial iris coloboma. *Ophthalmology* 1986; 93:335.
20. Cross HE: Ocular colobomas, in Bergsma D (ed): *Birth Defects Compendium.* New York, Alan R. Liss, Inc, 1979, p 791.
21. McKusick VA: *Medelian Inheritance in Man.* Baltimore, Johns Hopkins University Press, 1978.
22. Francois J: Colobomatous malformations of the ocular globe. *Int Ophthalmol Clin* 1968; 8:797.
23. Pagon RA: Ocular coloboma. *Surv Ophthalmol* 1981; 25:223.
24. Cogan DG: Congenital anomalies of the retina. *Birth Defects.* 1971; 7:41.
25. Fulton AB, Howard RD, Albert DM, et al: Ocular findings in triploidy. *Am J Ophthalmol* 1977; 84:859.
26. Zellweger H, Ionasecu V, Simpson J, et al: The problems of trisomy 22. *Clin Pediatr* 1976; 12:601.

27. Jay M: The eye in chromosome duplications and deficiencies. *Ophthalmic Sem* 1977; 22.
28. Schnizel A, Auf de Maur P, Moser H: Partial deletion of the long arm of chromosome 11 del (11) (q 23): Jacobsen syndrome. *J Med Genet* 1977; 14:438.
29. Butler LG, Snodgrass JAL, France NE, et al: E (16–18) trisomy syndrome: Analysis of 13 cases. *Arch Dis Child* 1965; 40:600.
30. François J, Matton van Leuven MT, Gombautt P: Uveal colobomas and true Klinefelter syndrome. *J Med Genet* 1970; 7:213.
31. Hashmi MS, Karseras AG: Uveal colobomata and Klinefelter syndrome. *Br J Ophthalmol* 1976; 60:661.
32. Epstein RJ, Mets MB, Wong PW, et al: Uveal colobomas and the Klinefelter syndrome. *Am J Ophthalmol* 1984; 98:241.
33. Mullaney J: Curious colobomata. *Trans Ophthalmol Soc UK* 1977; 97:517.
34. Aicardi J, LeFebvre J, Lerique A: Spasms in flexion, callosal agenesis, ocular abnormalities: A new syndrome. *Electroencephalogr Clin Neurophysiol* 1965; 19:609.
35. Del Pero RA, Mets MB, Tripathi RC, et al: Anomalies of retinal architecture in Aicardi syndrome. *Arch Ophthalmol* 1986; 104:1659.
36. Hall BD: Choanal atresia and associated multiple anomalies. *J Pediatr* 1979; 95:395.
37. Hittner HM, Hirsch NJ, Kreh GM, et al: Colobomatous microphthalmia, heart disease, hearing loss, and mental retardation—A syndrome. *J Pediatr Ophthalmol Strabismus* 1979; 16:122.
38. Gorlin RJ, Goltz, RW: Multiple nevoid basal cell epithelioma, jaw cysts and bifid rib. *N Engl J Med* 1960; 262:908.
39. Gorlin RJ, Pindborg JJ, Cohen MM Jr: *Syndromes of the Head and Neck.* New York, McGraw-Hill International Book Co, 1976.
40. Limaye SR: Coloboma of the iris and choroid and retinal detachment in oculoauricular dysplasia (Goldenhar syndrome). *Eye, Ear, Nose, Throat Monogr* 1972; 51:28.
41. Warburg M: Focal dermal hypoplasia: Ocular and general manifestations with a survey of the literature. *Acta Ophthalmol (Copenh)* 1970; 48:525.
42. François J: A new syndrome, dyscephalia with birdface and dental anomalies, nanism, hypotrichosis, cutaneous atrophy, microphthalmia and congenital cataract. *Arch Ophthalmol* 1958; 60:842.
43. Herrmann J, Opitz JM: The Lenz microphthalmia syndrome. *Birth Defects* 1969; 5:138.
44. Feurerstein RC, Mims LC: Linear sebaceous nevus with convulsions and mental retardation. *Am J Dis Child* 1962; 104:675.
45. Marden PM, Venters HD: A new neurocutaneous syndrome. *Am J Dis Child* 1966; 112:79.
46. MacRae DW, Howard RO, Albert DM, et al: Ocular manifestations of the Meckel syndrome. *Arch Ophthalmol* 1972; 88:106.
47. François J, Eggermont E, Evens L, et al: Agenesis of the corpus callosum in the medial facial cleft syndrome and associated ocular malformations. *Am J Ophthalmol* 1973; 76:241.
48. Roy FH, Summitt RL, Hiatt RL, et al: Ocular manifestations of the Rubinstein-Taybi syndrome. *Arch Ophthalmol* 1968; 79:272.
49. Warburg M: The heterogeneity of microphthalmia in the mentally retarded. *Birth Defects* 1971; 7:136.
50. Edwards JG, Young DB, Finlay HVL: Coloboma with multiple anomalies. *Br Med J* 1961; 2:586.
51. Angelman H: Syndrome of coloboma with multiple congenital abnormalities in infancy. *Br Med J* 1961; 1:1212.
52. Hall BD: Choanal atresia and associated multiple anomalies. *J. Pediatr* 1979; 95:395.
53. Pagon RA, Graham JM, Zonana J, et al: Coloboma, congenital heart disease, and choanal atresia with multiple anomalies: CHARGE association. *J Pediatr* 1981; 99:223.
54. Mitchell JA, Giangiacoma J, Hefner MA et al: Dominant CHARGE association. *Ophthalmic Paediatr Genet* 1985; 1:271.
55. Davenport SLH, Hefner MA, Mitchell JA: The spectrum of clinical features in CHARGE syndrome. *Clin Genet* 1986; 29:298.
56. Cullen JF: Ocular defects in thalidomide babies. *Br J Ophthalmol* 1964, 48:151.
57. Cullen JF: Ocular muscle anomalies in thalidomide children. *Br Orthopt J* 1967; 24:2.
58. Jesberg DO, Schepens CL: Retinal detachment associated with coloboma of the choroid. *Arch Ophthalmol* 1961; 65:163.
59. Shields JA: Primary cysts of the iris. *Trans Am Ophthalmol Soc* 1981; 79:771
60. Mann I: *Developmental Abnormalities of the Eye.* Philadelphia, JB Lippincott Co, 1957.
61. Duke-Elder S: *System of Ophthalmology.* St Louis, CV Mosby Co, 1974, p 9.

62. Levy WJ: Congenital iris lesion. *Br J Ophthalmol* 1957; 4:120.
63. Merin S, Crawford MD, Cardarelli J: Hyperplastic persistent pupillary membrane. *Am J Ophthalmol* 1970; 72:717.
64. Wolfflin E: Ein klinischer Beitrag zur Kentniss der Structur der Iris. *Arch F Augenh* 1902; 45:1.
65. Kruckmann E: In von Graefe A, Saemish T (eds): *Die Erkrankugen des Uveal Tractus und des Glaskopers Regenbogenhaut,* ed 2. Leipzig, E Englemann, 1907, pp 1–11.
66. Brushfield T: Mongolism. *Br J Child Dis* 1924; 21:241.
67. Donaldson DD: The significance of spotting of the iris in mongoloids. *Arch Ophthalmol* 1961; 4:50.
68. Broughton WL, Zimmerman LE: A clinicopathologic study of 56 cases of intraocular medulloepitheliomas. *Am J Ophthalmol* 1971; 7:23.
69. Zimmerman LE: Verhoeff's "Terato-Neuroma." A clinical reappraisal in light of new observations and current concepts of embryonic tumors. *Am J Ophthalmol* 1971; 72:1039.
70. Jakobiec FA, Howard GM, Ellsworth RM, et al: Electron microscopic diagnosis of medulloepitheliomas. *Am J Ophthalmol* 1975; 79:321.
71. Witschel H, Font RL: Hemangioma of the choroid: A clinicopathologic study of 71 cases and a review of the literature. *Surv Ophthalmol* 1976; 20:415.
72. Font RL, Ferry AP: Phakomatoses. *Int Ophthalmol Clin* 1972; 12:1.
73. Phelps CD: Glaucoma in Sturge-Weber syndrome. *Ophthalmology* 1978; 85:276.
74. L'Esperance FA: *Ocular Photocoagulation: A Stereoscopic Atlas.* St Louis, CV Mosby Co, 1975, pp 169–173.
75. Humphrey WT: Chorodial hemangioma: Response to cryotherapy. *Ann Ophthalmol* 1979; 11:100.
76. Sanborn GE, Augsburger JJ, Shields JA: Treatment of circumscribed choroidal hemangiomas. *Ophthalmology* 1982; 89:1374.
77. Ferry AP: Hemangiomas of the iris and ciliary body. Do they exist? A search for a histologically proved case. *Int Ophthalmol Clin* 1972; 12:177.
78. François J: Heredity of the choroidal dystrophies. *Adv Ophthalmol* 1978; 35:1.
79. Lewis RA, Nussbaum RL, Ferrell R: Mapping X-linked ophthalmic diseases. Provisional assignment of the locus for choroideremia to Xq13-q24. *Ophthalmology* 1985; 92:800.
80. McCulloch C: Choroideremia: A clinical and pathologic review. *Trans Am Ophthalmol Clin* 1969; 67:142.
81. Sieving PA, Niffenegger JH, Berson EL: Electroretinographic findings in selected pedigrees with choroideremia. *Am J Ophthalmol* 1986; 101:361.
82. Noble KG, Carr RE, Siegel IM: Fluorescein angiography of the hereditary choroidal dystrophies. *Br J Ophthalmol* 1977; 61:43.
83. Jay B: X-linked retinal disorders and Lyon hypothesis. *Trans Ophthalmol Soc UK* 1985; 104:836.
84. Harris GS, Miller JR; Choroidermia. Visual defects in a heterozygote. *Arch Ophthalmol* 1968; 80:423.
85. François J: Choroideremia. *Int Ophthalmol Clin* 1968; 8:949.
86. Heckenlively J: The frequency of posterior subcapsular cataract in the hereditary retinal degenerations. *Am J Ophthalmol* 1982; 93:733.
87. van den Bosch J: A new syndrome in three generations of a Dutch family. *Ophthalmologica* 1959; 137:422.
88. Ayazi S: Choroideremia, obesity and congenital deafness. *Am J Ophthalmol* 1981; 92:63.

19 Developmental Glaucoma

Christopher J. Dickens, M.D.
H. Dunbar Hoskins, Jr., M.D.

The developmental glaucomas are a group of disorders characterized by improper development of the eye's aqueous outflow system. Glaucoma in the newborn is an uncommon disease and is estimated to affect less than 0.05% of all ophthalmology patients. However, the impact on a child's visual development can be extreme. Early recognition and appropriate therapy for the glaucoma can significantly improve a child's visual future.

The congenital glaucomas are divided into two major categories. The first is primary congenital glaucoma in which the developmental anomaly is restricted to a maldevelopment of the trabecular meshwork. The second major category is glaucoma associated with other ocular or systemic congenital anomalies. Most cases of glaucoma seen in infants are primary congenital glaucoma. A third category of glaucomas that occur in infancy is caused by other ocular diseases such as inflammation, trauma or neoplasms. These are acquired, not congenital disorders, and thus will not be covered in this chapter.

TERMINOLOGY

The terminology of the glaucomas that can affect infants has been somewhat inconsistent and, at times, confusing. More precise terminology has become possible and should be used whenever possible.

Developmental glaucoma refers to glaucoma that is associated with developmental anomalies of the eye that are present at birth. This includes both primary congenital glaucoma and glaucoma associated with other developmental anomalies, either in the eye or systemically.

Congenital glaucoma is a synonymous term for developmental glaucoma, being distinguished from glaucomas that are secondary to other ocular diseases such as inflammation, trauma, or tumors.

Primary congenital glaucoma is a specific term referring to a specific type of glaucoma. These eyes have an isolated maldevelopment of the trabecular meshwork not associated with other developmental anomalies, and there are no other ocular diseases present that can raise the intraocular pressure.

Infantile glaucoma is a term that has been used in a variety of contexts. Some have used this term synonymously with primary congenital glaucoma while others have referred to it to mean any glaucoma occurring during the first several years of life. Its meaning should thus be specified or its use avoided.

Juvenile glaucoma is a nonspecific term referring to any type of glaucoma occurring in later childhood or the teenage years of life.

Buphthalmos and *hydrophthalmos* are both descriptive terms that should not be used diagnostically. *Buphthalmos* literally means "ox eye" and refers to the marked enlargement that can occur as a result of any type of glaucoma present in infancy. *Hydrophthalmos* refers to these enlarged aqueous-filled eyes.

TABLE 19–1
Shaffer-Weiss Classification of Congenital Glaucoma Patients

I. Primary congenital glaucoma
II. Glaucoma associated with congenital anomalies
  A. Late-developing infantile glaucoma (late-developing primary congenital glaucoma)
  B. Aniridia
  C. Sturge-Weber
  D. Neurofibromatosis
  E. Marfan's syndrome
  F. Pierre Robin syndrome
  G. Homocystinuria
  H. Goniodysgenesis (iridocorneal mesodermal dysgenesis: Rieger's anomaly and syndrome, Axenfeld's anomaly, Peter's anomaly)
  I. Lowe's syndrome
  J. Microcornea
  K. Microspherophakia
  L. Rubella
  M. Chromosome abnormalities
  N. Broad-thumb syndrome
  O. Persistent hyperplastic primary vitreous
III. Secondary glaucoma in infants
  A. Retrolental fibroplasia
  B. Tumors
    1. Retinoblastoma
    2. Juvenile xanthogranuloma
  C. Inflammation
  D. Trauma

CLASSIFICATION OF DEVELOPMENTAL GLAUCOMA

A variety of classifications of the developmental glaucomas has been used. In this chapter we will use the Shaffer-Weiss classification (Table 19–1) of congenital glaucoma patients, which divides patients into those having primary congenital glaucoma and those with glaucoma associated with other congenital ocular or systemic anomalies.[1,2] A third category of glaucoma in infants is that of the secondary glaucomas. This is included in the Shaffer-Weiss classification but will not be discussed in this chapter because these are acquired rather than developmental glaucomas.

An anatomic classification of the developmental glaucomas has also recently been developed.[3,4] Anatomic defects of the eye that are apparent on examination of the child form the basis for this classification (Table 19–2).

Maldevelopment of the anterior segment is present in all forms of developmental glaucoma. This maldevelopment may involve the trabecular meshwork alone or the trabecular meshwork in combination with either the iris and/or cornea. Identification of the type of anatomic defect can be helpful in determining therapy and prognosis for the infant.

Isolated Trabeculodysgenesis

In over 50% of infants presenting with glaucoma, isolated trabeculodysgenesis is the only congenital anomaly of the eye. There are no developmental anomalies of the iris or cornea present, although abnormalities secondary to the intraocular pressure elevation and its effects on these structures may be evident.

This maldevelopment of the trabecular meshwork presents in one of two forms. In the most common form, the iris inserts flatly into the trabecular meshwork either at or anterior to the scleral spur (Figs 19–1 and 19–

TABLE 19–2
Hoskins' Anatomic Classification of the Developmental Glaucomas

I. Isolated trabeculodysgenesis.—Malformation of trabecular meshwork in the absence of iris or corneal anomalies
  A. Flat iris insertion
    1. Anterior insertion
    2. Posterior insertion
    3. Mixed insertion
  B. Concave (wraparound) iris insertion
  C. Unclassified
II. Iridotrabeculodysgenesis.—Trabeculodysgenesis with iris anomalies
  A. Anterior stromal defects of the iris
    1. Hypoplasia
    2. Hyperplasia
  B. Anomalous iris vessels
    1. Persistence of tunica vasculosa lentis
    2. Anomalous superficial vessels
  C. Structural anomalies of the iris
    1. Holes
    2. Colobomas
    3. Aniridia
III. Corneotrabeculodysgenesis.—Usually has associated iris anomalies
  A. Peripheral
  B. Midperipheral
  C. Central
  D. Corneal size

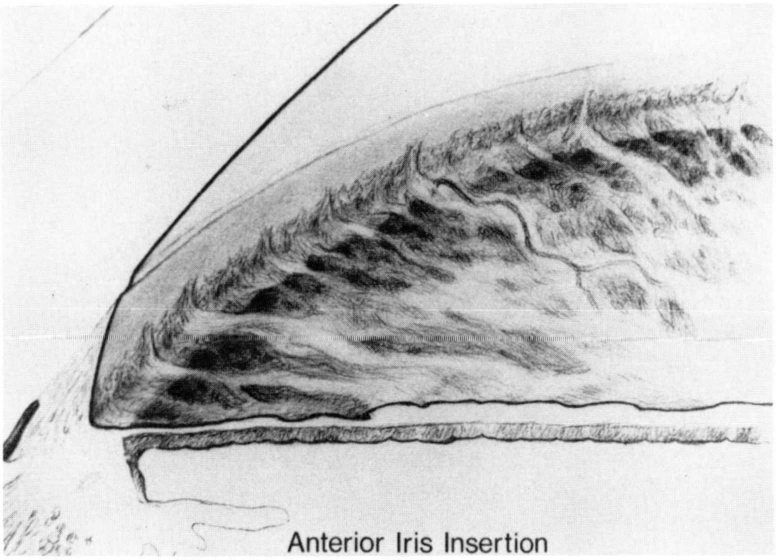

FIG 19–1.
Isolated trabeculodysgenesis with flat anterior iris insertion. The iris inserts flatly and abruptly into trabecular meshwork. (From Hoskins HD Jr, Shaffer RN, Hetherington J: Anatomical classification of the developmental glaucomas. *Arch Ophthalmol* 1984; 102:1333. Used with permission.)

2). The ciliary body is usually obscured by this insertion, although the anterior ciliary body may be seen through a thick trabecular meshwork if one views the angle obliquely. The iris insertion may vary in its level along the chamber angle, with some portions of the iris inserting anterior to the scleral spur while other areas insert at the spur or even posterior to the spur. The surface of the trabecular meshwork may have a stippled, orange-peel appearance, and the peripheral iris stroma may appear thinned due to the stretching effects resulting from enlargement of the eye.

The second form of isolated trabeculodysgenesis is one in which the iris has a concave insertion into the surface of the trabecular meshwork (Fig 19–3). The plane of the iris is posterior to the scleral spur, but the anterior stroma sweeps upward over the trabecular meshwork, obscures the scleral spur, and inserts into the upper portion of the trabecular meshwork just posterior to Schwalbe's line.

Isolated trabeculodysgenesis must be differentiated from the normal gonioscopic appearance of the anterior chamber angle in a normal newborn eye. In a normal newborn the insertion of the iris is usually into the ciliary body, posterior to the scleral spur. The ciliary body is seen as a distant band anterior to the iris insertion. The iris insertion into the angle wall is flat because the angle recess does not form until the first 6 to 12 months of life. The adult angle configuration in which the iris turns posteriorly before inserting into the ciliary body is thus not normally evident at birth.

Iridotrabeculodysgenesis

Congenital anomalies of the iris associated with maldevelopment of the trabecular meshwork may involve the anterior stroma, the iris vessels, or the full thickness of the iris. In these disorders, the appearance of the trabecular meshwork is similar to that found in isolated trabeculodysgenesis.

Anterior Stromal Defects

Hypoplasia of the anterior iris stroma is the most common iris defect one sees associated with congenital glaucoma. In this disorder, there is malformation of the iris collarette with a reduction or complete absence of the crypt layer. The pupillary sphincter may appear to be quite prominent.

In hyperplasia of the anterior iris stroma, the stroma has a thickened, pebbled appearance. This is uncommon, and we have seen it only in association with Sturge-Weber syndrome.

Anomalous Iris Vessels

Developmental anomalies of the iris vasculature can occur in the form of persistence of the tunica vasculosa lentis or in the form of irregularly wandering superficial iris vessels. With persistence of the tunica vasculosa lentis, there is a regular arrangement of vessels seen looping into the pupillary axis either in front of or behind the lens.

With superficial anomalous iris vessels, one sees the vessels wandering irregularly over the iris surface with a distorted pupil. The iris surface usually has a whorled appearance.

These vessels are not associated with any particular syndrome. It is unclear at this time whether they represent an earlier onset of primary congenital glaucoma or an entirely different syndrome. They do indicate a grave prognosis, and all cases we have observed have required multiple surgeries.

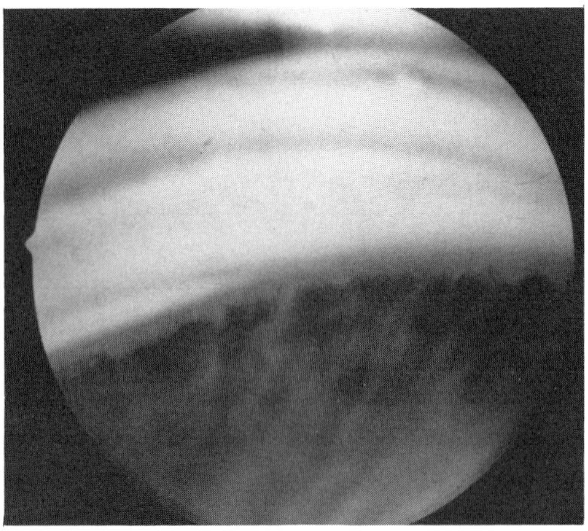

FIG 19–2.
Clinical appearance of flat anterior iris insertion *(at right)*. The goniotomy incision is present to the left. (From Hoskins HD Jr, Shaffer RN, Hetherington J: Anatomical classification of the developmental glaucomas. *Arch Ophthalmol* 1984; 102:1333. Used with permission.)

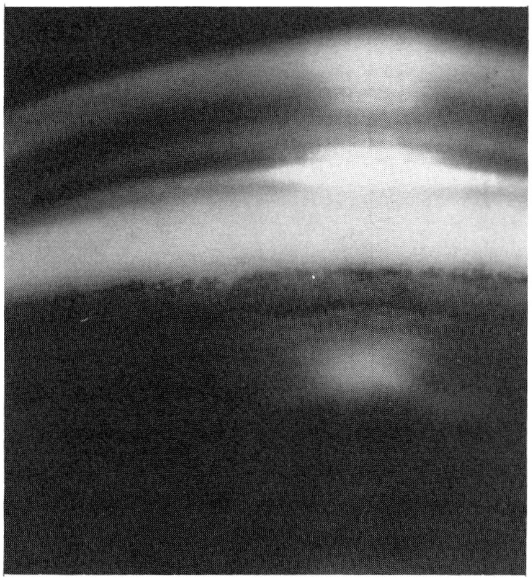

FIG 19–3.
Concave iris insertion. (From Hoskins HD Jr, Shaffer RN, Hetherington J: Anatomical classification of the developmental glaucomas. *Arch Ophthalmol* 1984; 102:1334. Used with permission.)

Structural Iris Defects

Structural iris defects may present with a full-thickness hole through the iris with no involvement of the sphincter muscle. There may be a full-thickness coloboma involving the sphincter, or aniridia may be present in which the majority of the iris is absent.

Corneotrabeculodysgenesis

One should keep in mind that the corneal stretching and clouding that occur secondarily to the elevated intraocular pressure are not congenital defects. True congenital corneal defects may involve the peripheral, midperipheral, or central portions of the cornea or may present as abnormalities of corneal size. In the vast majority of cases, associated iris anomalies are also found.

The most common peripheral corneal abnormality is a prominent cordlike Schwalbe's line to which iris adhesions are seen. This so-called posterior embryotoxon is characteristic of Axenfeld's anomaly and extends no more than 2.0 mm into the clear cornea. Peripheral iridocorneal adhesions may rarely be seen in the absence of a posterior embryotoxon.

With midperipheral lesions, the iris is attached to the cornea in broad areas of apposition that extend toward the center of the cornea. Pupillary anomalies and holes of the iris are commonly associated. The cornea is frequently opacified in the areas of the iris adhesions.

Central corneal anomalies usually have adhesions between the collarette of the iris and the posterior aspect of the central cornea. The cornea is usually opacified centrally and may be thinned. Usually there is an area of clear cornea between the central defect and the corneoscleral limbus. This is typically seen in Peter's anomaly.

Abnormalities of corneal size may present with both small and large corneas. Microcornea may be seen in a variety of congenital anomalies including microphthalmos, nanophthalmos, Rieger's anomaly, and persistent hyperplastic primary vitreous. Macrocornea must be distinguished from the corneal stretching that occurs because of an elevated intraocular pressure. It may be seen in patients with Axenfeld's syndrome or as an X-linked recessive megalocornea.

PATHOPHYSIOLOGY OF INTRAOCULAR PRESSURE ELEVATION

The aqueous humor is a clear fluid that fills the anterior and posterior chambers of the eye. It is produced by the ciliary epithelium and provides nutrition to the anterior portion of the eye, particularly the avascular lens and cornea. The aqueous humor is also responsible for maintaining an intraocular pressure that is consistent with the normal functioning of the eye.

After being produced by the ciliary epithelium, the aqueous humor passes through the pupil and enters the anterior chamber from which it leaves by two main outflow pathways. Approximately 25% passes into the iris and the ciliary body and then leaves the eye through the venous drainage system within the uveal tissue. The majority of the aqueous humor leaves the eye via the trabecular meshwork, which is located at the anterior chamber angle formed by the junction of the iris and cornea. Once through the trabecular meshwork, the aqueous humor enters the canal of Schlemm, passes into collector channels, and eventually reaches the episcleral venous circulation. Resistance to this directional flow of aqueous humor at any point along this pathway may result in an elevation of the intraocular pressure and glaucoma.

The two main subdivisions of the mechanistic types of glaucoma are open-angle glaucoma and closed-angle glaucoma. In *open-angle glaucoma,* the block to aqueous outflow occurs at the level of the trabecular meshwork or beyond. This may result from maldevelopment as seen in the congenital glaucomas or a malfunctioning of the trabecular meshwork area as in open-angle glaucoma of the elderly. The trabecular meshwork may also be obstructed by particulate matter such as inflammatory cells, tumor particles, red blood cells, edema, fibrovascular membranes, or scarring. These processes occur in the acquired secondary types of glaucoma.

The second main type of glaucoma is termed *closed-angle glaucoma.* In this type of glaucoma the obstruction to the aqueous outflow results from the iris covering the trabecular meshwork area. The iris may be pushed against the trabecular meshwork by pressure posterior to the plane of the iris as in a pupillary block, or it may be pulled into the trabeculum.

A pupillary block occurs when there is a relative or total blockage at the pupil that prevents the aqueous humor from passing from the posterior chamber to the anterior chamber. As a result, the aqueous humor is trapped behind the iris and pushes it forward into the trabecular meshwork. This process may cause a rapid rise in intraocular pressure. In children, a pupillary block is most commonly seen when there is an abnormally shaped spherical lens such as in spherophakia or a dislocation of the lens as in Marfan's syndrome or homocystinuria. A pupillary block may also occur from adhesions forming between the iris and the lens as a result of inflammation. Tumors, cysts, or fibrovascular tissue posterior to the iris may also push the iris up against the trabecular meshwork. Inflammatory membranes or fibrovascular tissue may also pull the iris into the trabecular meshwork and cause the formation of peripheral anterior synechiae (adhesions) and a blockage of aqueous outflow.

EFFECTS OF ELEVATED INTRAOCULAR PRESSURE ON THE INFANT EYE

Within the first 3 years of life the collagen fibers of the eye are softer and more elastic than those in older children or adults. Elevation of intraocular pressure can thus cause an enlargement of the globe that is apparent as a progressive enlargement of the cornea. As the cornea and limbal area enlarge, the corneal endothelium and Descemet's membrane are stretched. This can lead to stromal and epithelial edema of the cornea as well as actual ruptures of Descemet's membrane.

With enlargement of the eye, the iris may also be stretched and the stroma thinned. The scleral ring through which the optic nerve passes is also enlarged, which can lead to rapid cupping of the optic nerve head. A reversal of this cup size enlargement can also occur rapidly following normalization of the intraocular pressure. This is not seen in adults and is probably related to the increased elasticity of the connective tissues of the optic nerve head that allows an elastic response to changes in intraocular pressure.[5,6]

Infant eyes with advanced disease are enlarged in all dimensions. The iris root and trabecular meshwork area are found to be thin and degenerated, and Schlemm's canal may not be evident. The ciliary body, retina, and choroid are atrophic, and the zonules may be degenerated with displacement of the lens. Scarring of the cornea due to long-standing edema and tears in Descemet's membrane is evident. The optic nerve shows complete cupping.

CLINICAL PRESENTATION

The infant with glaucoma will present with unique signs and symptoms when compared with older children and adults. These are present regardless of the cause of the glaucoma and are due to the fact that the infant eye is elastic and stretches under the influence of the elevated intraocular pressure. Epiphora, photophobia, and blepharospasm are the cardinal symptoms present, being secondary to corneal irritation that results from corneal epithelial edema. A hazy appearance and enlargement of the cornea may be noted by the parents.

The large eyes are often not a concern to the parents because they are believed to enhance the beauty of their child, but they must be considered a warning sign to the ophthalmologist or pediatrician. With further stretching of the cornea there may be ruptures of Descemet's membrane with a sudden influx of aqueous humor into the cornea, which exacerbates the signs and symptoms. The child may become irritable and so photophobic that he will bury his head in a pillow to avoid light.

EXAMINATION

A reasonably good office examination can sometimes be performed on infants younger than 3 months when using the infant diagnostic lens of Richardson and Shaffer. The lens is well tolerated when placed onto the eye following application of topical anesthesia and enables a good examination of the anterior part of the eye and the optic nerve head.

Pacifying the infant with a bottle is helpful for obtaining intraocular pressure measurements with either a Schiotz' or hand-held electronic tonometer. The pneumotonometer and hand-held applanation instruments can also be useful.

However, general anesthesia is usually required for a thorough examination of these infants. In a healthy child with anesthesia administered by an anesthesiologist experienced in dealing with these small children, there is little risk involved. Usually delivery of anesthesia by mask with an oral airway is adequate and safe for short examinations. If prolonged examination or surgery is required, endotracheal intubation should be performed.

One should check the intraocular pressure as soon as it is safely possible because most general anesthetics will lower the intraocular pressure by variable amounts and at variable times after administration. Tonometry can be performed either with a Schiotz' or hand-held applanation tonometer. Either one is usually adequate, although if uncertainty exists, both can be used. Applanation tonometry is definitely helpful in cases with microcornea. A useful upper limit of intraocular pressure is 21 mm Hg but is not absolute, and one must also rely on signs such as increased corneal diameter, corneal haze, increased cup-to-disc ratio, or evidence of trabecular malformation to confirm a diagnosis of glaucoma.

The normal neonatal horizontal corneal diameter is 10.0 to 10.5 mm in term newborns (or smaller in preterm neonates) and increases to 11.0 to 12.0 mm by 1 year of life. An effective measurement of the corneal diameter can be obtained by using calipers to measure the horizontal diameter from the first appearance of the white scleral fibers on one side to the same point on the other side. It is important to have a good baseline measurement both for initial diagnosis and for detection of subsequent corneal enlargement.

When examining the cornea, one must also look for corneal haziness and tears in Descemet's membrane. Developmental anomalies of the iris and cornea must also be searched for because they may alter one's diagnosis and treatment.

Gonioscopy is performed by using a smooth-domed Koeppe 14- to 16-mm lens with a Barkan light and hand-held binocular microscope. If marked corneal clouding is evident, the view may be improved by removing the epithelium with a blade or 70% alcohol solution and a cotton applicator.

The Koeppe lens can also aid in visualizing the crystalline lens, vitreous, and fundus. The lens neutralizes irregular corneal reflexes and also improves the view through a small pupil, thus allowing one to see the entire optic nerve head in one field.

Cupping of the optic nerve is an early sign of increased pressure and occurs much more quickly and at lower pressures in infants than in older children and adults. These changes can occur within hours to days. Cup-to-disc ratios greater than 0.3 are rare in normal infants and must be considered indicative of glaucoma.[7] Inequality of cupping between the optic nerves is also suggestive of glaucoma. It is uncommon for a normal individual to have a cup/disc ratio difference between the two eyes of greater than 0.2, and therefore, asymmetry of this magnitude or greater must be considered pathognomonic of glaucoma. In infants, the glaucomatous cup can be oval in configuration but is more often round and central, with circumferential enlargement of the cup noted (Fig 19–4).

With successful control of the intraocular pressure, the cup will either remain stable or decrease in size. Such a reduction in cup size is most commonly seen in the first year of life. An increasing cup size is indicative of uncon-

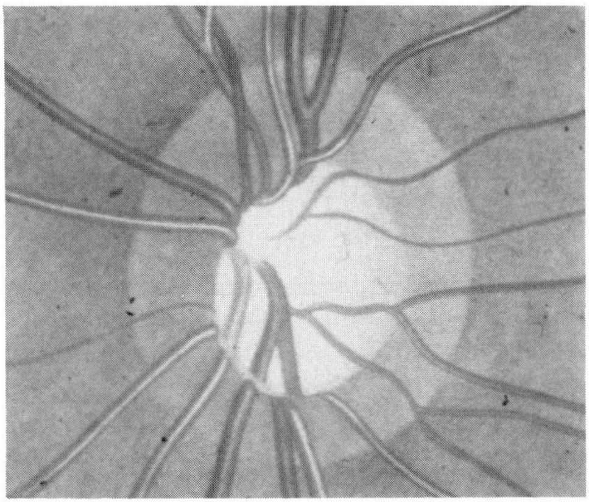

FIG 19–4.
Disc of glaucomatous infant with deep, central cupping.

trolled glaucoma, and one must make careful drawings or take photographs for future comparison.

A thorough systemic evaluation is also indicated in these infants both to check for any signs of syndromes that may be associated with glaucoma and to ensure the safety of general anesthesia.

Cycloplegic refraction must be performed to correct significant differences in refractive errors between the two eyes and help prevent the development of anisometropic amblyopia, especially in cases of unilateral glaucoma. Greater myopia or less hyperopia in one eye may be an early sign of glaucoma.

The specific types of developmental glaucomas will be presented by using the Shaffer-Weiss classification.

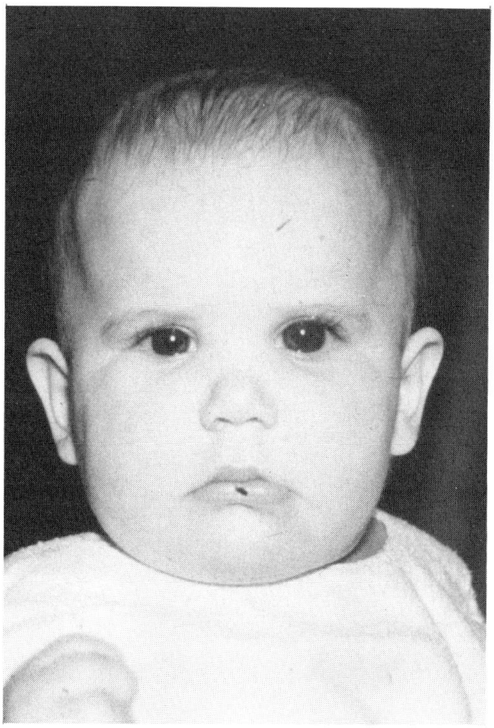

FIG 19–5.
Primary congenital glaucoma: enlarged and mildly hazy left cornea.

PRIMARY CONGENITAL GLAUCOMA

Primary congenital glaucoma is the most common glaucoma of infancy (Figs 19–5 and 19–6). It is characterized by the specific angle anomaly of isolated trabeculodysgenesis. There are no associated ocular or systemic developmental anomalies or other ocular diseases present that can raise the intraocular pressure.

Although it is the most common glaucoma seen in infancy, it is still an uncommon disease, and a general ophthalmologist is unlikely to see more than one new case in several years. When it does occur, it is bilaterally present in approximately 75% of cases, and males account for 65% of cases. More than 80% of cases of primary congenital glaucoma is evident within the first year of life.

The majority of cases are sporadic in occurrence and do not exhibit a hereditary pattern. In the approximately 10% that do show a hereditary pattern, it is either autosomal recessive or polygenic.[8,9] The important point is that one must examine other children in the family if one child does have this disease.

Clinically, these patients present with symptoms of epiphora, photophobia, and blepharospasm. Examination reveals an increase in the cup-to-disc ratio, an increased corneal diameter, possible corneal haziness, and tears in Descemet's membrane. Gonioscopy shows isolated trabeculodysgenesis, and the intraocular pressure will be over 21 mm Hg in most cases.

In the differential diagnosis, one should consider other causes of these signs. Such corneal abnormalities include megalocornea, metabolic diseases such as the mucopolysaccharidoses, congenital hereditary endothelial dystrophy, posterior polymorphous dystrophy, obstetric trauma, and keratitis. Other causes of epiphora or photophobia include an obstructed nasolacrimal duct, conjunctivitis as caused by silver nitrate prophylaxis, corneal abrasions, Meesman's corneal dystrophy and Reis-Buckler's corneal dystrophy. Other causes of optic nerve abnormalities include congenital malformations such as pits, colobomas, and hypoplasia. Large physiological cupping should also be kept in mind but is usually not a problem in the differential diagnosis in infants with their presenting symptoms and signs of glaucoma. This is a more difficult diagnosis to make in older children where other signs are not present.

Once the diagnosis of primary congenital glaucoma is made, surgery is indicated. Surgery is preferred in these patients because there is a poor response of infants to medications and there are significant problems with compliance and concerns over systemic effects. Most importantly, there is a high success rate and a low complication rate with current surgical procedures.

In these infants under 1 year of age, a goniotomy is the recommended initial procedure.[10, 11] One or two goniotomies will control the intraocular pressure in the majority of cases. A trabeculotomy is a reasonable alternative to goniotomy as the procedure of choice.[12] If severe corneal clouding is evident so that one cannot visualize the anterior chamber angle, a trabeculotomy should be performed. Preoperative medications can help clear corneal clouding, as can scraping of the corneal epithelium at the time of surgery. These methods can significantly improve the surgeon's view for a goniotomy.

GLAUCOMA ASSOCIATED WITH CONGENITAL ANOMALIES

Late-Developing Infantile Glaucoma (Late-Developing Primary Congenital Glaucoma)

Late-developing primary congenital glaucoma occurs in children whose intraocular pressure has been insufficiently high to cause marked corneal enlargement or significant symptoms but has caused damage to the optic nerve. The angle may have the appearance of an isolated trabeculodysgenesis or partial development of the angle recess. This disorder manifests itself after infancy and may be difficult to distinguish from early developing, primary open-angle glaucoma.

Aniridia

Aniridia is a bilateral congenital anomaly in which there is marked hypoplasia of the iris, frequently associated with keratopathy, foveal hypoplasia, cataract, ectopia lentis, and optic nerve hypoplasia (Fig 19–7). A retardation in psychomotor development may also be evident.

Aniridia is most commonly a hereditary disorder transmitted in an autosomal dominant fashion. It can also occur with no evident hereditary pattern. In these sporadic cases, approximately 20% of patients have been found to have Wilms' tumor.[13]

Although the defective iris is readily apparent at birth, in most cases glaucoma does not develop until later childhood or early adulthood. Glaucoma does not develop in all cases.[14] When the onset of the glaucoma does occur in the first year of life, the globe will stretch with similar signs and symptoms as in primary congenital glaucoma. The glaucoma may be due to trabeculodysgenesis or may be due to a progressive pulling up of the residual iris stump that occludes the trabecular meshwork with synechia formation.

The iris is never completely absent. It may vary from being fairly well developed in areas to only a rudimentary stump in other areas. During early life, the iris stump may progressively adhere to the trabecular meshwork and

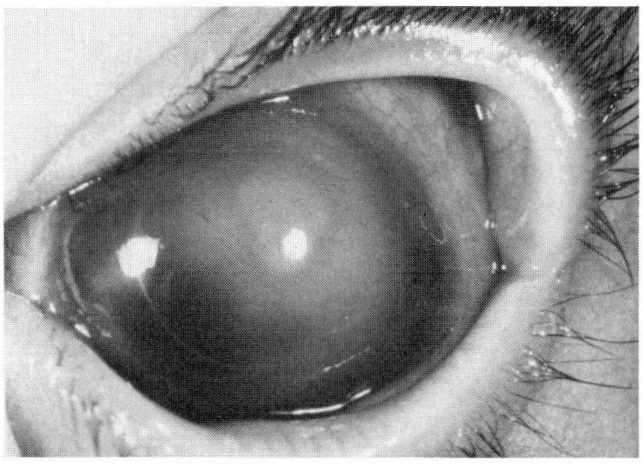

FIG 19–6.
Primary congenital glaucoma: increased corneal diameter and marked corneal clouding.

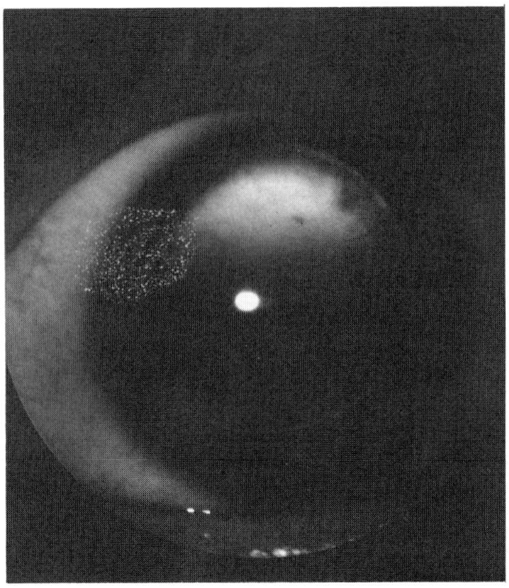

FIG 19–7.
Aniridia: periphery of lens is visible due to marked iris hypoplasia.

cause further obstruction to aqueous outflow with the development or worsening of glaucoma.

A corneal dystrophy is seen in the majority of cases. This is initially evident as a circumferential and peripheral opacification of the epithelial and subepithelial layers, with vessels advancing into these areas from the limbus. This pannus can extend centrally over many years and rarely can completely opacify the cornea. Cataracts develop in most aniridic patients, and the lens may be displaced with a segmental absence of zonules evident. Foveal hypoplasia is present in most instances and limits vision to no better than 20/200 with accompanying pendular nystagmus. Hypoplasia of the optic nerve is found occasionally.

If glaucoma does present in infancy, a goniotomy or trabeculotomy is indicated. Medical therapy may also be required. Walton has suggested that an early goniotomy to prevent the progressive adherence of the peripheral iris to the trabecular meshwork may be helpful.[15]

In older children, medical therapy should be tried prior to any surgical procedure.

Sturge-Weber Syndrome

Sturge-Weber syndrome, also known as encephalofacial angiomatosis, presents with a flat facial hemangioma that follows the distribution of the fifth cranial nerve (Fig 19–8). The facial hemangioma is usually unilateral but may occasionally be bilateral. In addition, a meningeal hemangioma that can produce a seizure disorder in the child may be present. The meningeal hemangioma may be associated with calcification that can be seen on x-ray examination after the age of 1 year. Choroidal hemangiomas and episcleral hemangiomas are also commonly seen, and leakage from the choroidal hemangioma may cause retinal edema. The genetic transmission of this disease is unclear.

Glaucoma associated with Sturge-Weber syndrome often occurs in infancy but also may not develop until later childhood or early adulthood. The glaucoma usually occurs when the facial hemangioma involves the lid or con-

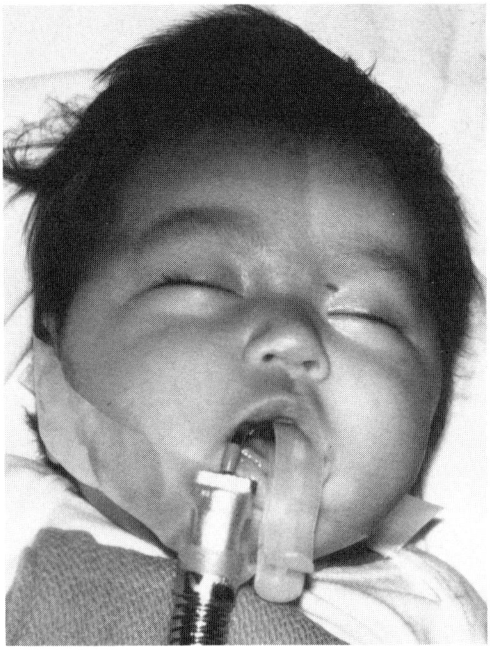

FIG 19–8.
Sturge-Weber syndrome: unilateral facial hemangioma.

junctiva on the same side as the facial disorder.

The glaucoma in infancy presents with an isolated trabeculodysgenesis type of angle anomaly. As the child ages, the elevated intraocular pressure seems to be due to elevation of episcleral venous pressure, which results from arteriovenous shunts through the episcleral hemangiomas.[16]

When the glaucoma presents in infancy, goniotomy can be successful and should be performed as the initial procedure of choice. In older children, medical therapy is indicated initially. If medical therapy is not successful, then a trabeculotomy or trabeculectomy should be considered.

Filtering surgery may result in a rapid expansion of the choroidal hemangioma with a possible effusion of fluid into the surrounding tissues. The anterior chamber flattens and may be impossible to reform through the surgical or paracentesis site. Posterior sclerotomy should be performed in an attempt to drain fluid from the suprachoroidal space and followed by anterior chamber reformation. If no fluid is obtained and the anterior chamber does not reform, one should close the trabeculectomy site. The expansion will then gradually subside. Filtering surgery can be reconsidered later because the choroidal hemangioma may scar, thereby enabling one to successfully perform the procedure without a recurrence of the expansion or effusion.

Klippel-Trenaunay-Weber syndrome is similar and may be a form of Sturge-Weber syndrome. It is similar to Sturge-Weber syndrome except that the hemangioma involves the body and limbs and has associated hypertrophy of one or more of the limbs on the affected side.

Neurofibromatosis (von Recklinghausen Disease)

Neurofibromatosis is characterized by multiple café au lait spots and neurofibromas of the skin, skeletal defects that can include congenital absence of a portion of the sphenoid bone, neurofibromatous lesions of the viscera, and neurofibromas of the peripheral and central nervous system (Fig 19–9). An autosomal dominant transmission pattern is typically seen, although sporadic cases can occur.

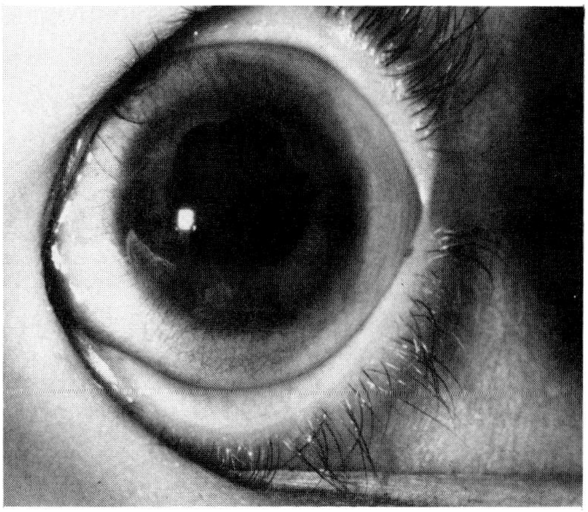

FIG 19–9.
Neurofibromatosis: ectropian uvea.

Ocular involvement includes neurofibromatous nodules on the iris, ectropion uvea, optic nerve gliomas, retinal astrocytic hamartomas, proptosis that may be evident as a pulsating exophthalmos secondary to sphenoid bone maldevelopment, herniation of brain tissue into the orbit, proptosis secondary to optic nerve glioma, and enlargement of the globe aside from that caused by glaucoma.

Glaucoma should be suspected when the neurofibromas involve the upper eyelid or the eye itself. The anterior chamber angle may take on several appearances. Isolated trabeculodysgenesia may be evident. There may be synechial closure due to neurofibromatous tissue posterior to the iris, or there may be neurofibromatous infiltration of the angle itself, that is accompanied by synechial closure. A sheet of avascular, opaque, dense tissue may arise from the periphery of the iris and extend anteriorly into the angle.

The treatment of choice in infants is usually goniotomy, with trabeculotomy recommended if iris adhesions are prominent.

Marfan Syndrome

Marfan syndrome is characterized by arachnodactyly, congenital weakness of the aorta, aortic and mitral valve disease, congenital weakness of the joints, hypotonia, scoliosis, and ocular abnormalities. The transmission is usually autosomal dominant, with approximately 15% being sporadic.

Ocular abnormalities include ectopia lentis, microphakia, myopia, megalocornea, keratoconus, hypoplasia of the iris stroma and dilator muscle, and retinal detachment in addition to glaucoma.[17,18]

One form of glaucoma may result from a pupillary block secondary to malposition of the lens. The lens is usually subluxed upward, being held by zonules that are attenuated and often broken. However, the lens can become dislocated into the pupil or anterior chamber, thus resulting in pupillary block glaucoma. This is initially managed by dilation of the pupil. A peripheral iridectomy or lens extraction may be indicated.

Open-angle glaucoma can also develop in these patients. It frequently develops in childhood or the juvenile years of life and is associated with congenital abnormalities of the anterior chamber angle. Iris processes, often dense in appearance, can bridge the angle recess and insert well anterior to the scleral spur. A concave configuration of this iris tissue may be evident.[19]

Although rare, if open-angle glaucoma were to appear during the first year of life, a goniotomy or trabeculotomy would be the preferred procedure. When the glaucoma occurs in older childhood, medical therapy should be attempted for initial control of the intraocular pressure.

Pierre Robin Syndrome

Pierre Robin syndrome is characterized by micrognathia, glossoptosis, cleft palate, and cardiac and ocular anomalies. Ocular disorders include cataracts, high myopia, retinal detachments, microphthalmos, and developmental glaucoma.[20]

The type or types of glaucoma are not yet fully described. Isolated trabeculodysgenesis may be present and would indicate goniotomy as the initial procedure.

Homocystinuria

Homocystinuria is an autosomal, recessively inherited metabolic abnormality with a defect in the enzyme cystathionine synthetase. Arachnodactyly may be present, although less commonly than in Marfan's syndrome. Osteoporosis, mental retardation, and seizures may also be present. The patients are often lightly pigmented with blond hair and blue eyes. A hazard of general anesthesia in these patients is that thromboembolism can be precipitated.

Ocular abnormalities include retinal detachment and ectopia lentis. Anomalies of the anterior chamber angle have not been described. The lens is usually subluxed inferiorly but may move anteriorly as well, which results in pupillary-block glaucoma.

Treatment of the glaucoma consists of dilation of the pupil, peripheral iridectomy to break the pupillary block, and lens extraction when the lens has dislocated into the anterior chamber. General anesthesia should be avoided because of the risk of the thromboembolic phenomena that occur in these patients.

Goniodysgenesis (Iridocorneal Mesodermal Dysgenesis: Axenfeld's Anomaly, Rieger's Anomaly and Syndrome, Peter's Anomaly)

Axenfeld's anomaly and Rieger's syndrome involve corneotrabeculodysgenesis of the peripheral (Axenfeld's) and midperipheral (Rieger's) portions of the cornea and iris. These disorders represent variations of a similar disease process. Central corneotrabeculodysgenesis is present in Peter's anomaly.

Axenfeld's Anomaly

Axenfeld's anomaly (Fig 19–10) is characterized by a prominent anteriorly displaced Schwalbe's line termed *posterior embryotoxon*. Posterior embryotoxon can be found in normal eyes. However, when bands of iris tissue extend across the anterior chamber angle and attach to the posterior embryotoxon, this is termed *Axenfeld's anomaly*. Approximately 50% of these patients will develop glaucoma. In some patients there is hypoplasia of the anterior iris stroma, but more severe defects of the iris are not present. The disease is usually present bilaterally, and the inheritance pattern is autosomal dominant.

The glaucoma may occur in infancy and can respond to goniotomy or trabeculotomy. If it occurs in later childhood, medical therapy should initially be tried, with trabeculotomy or trabeculectomy considered as surgical procedures.

Rieger's Anomaly and Syndrome

Reiger's anomaly (Fig 19–11) may or may not have posterior embryotoxon with adherent iris strands as in Axenfeld's anomaly, but

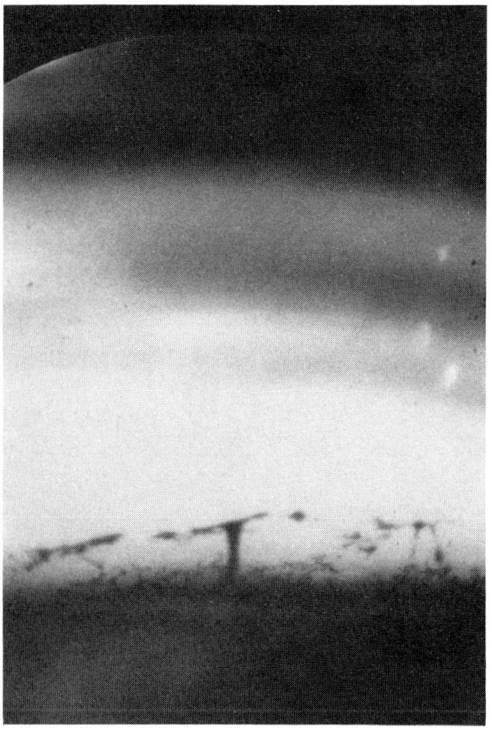

FIG 19–10.
Axenfeld's anomaly: iris strands attached to Schwalbe's line.

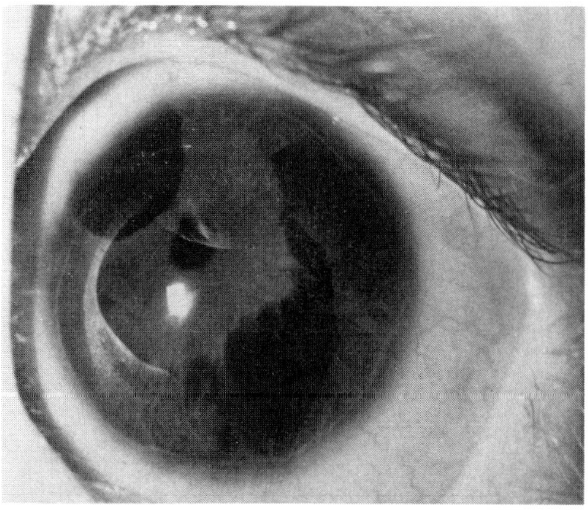

FIG 19–11.
Rieger's anomaly: hypoplastic iris with a distorted, corectopic pupil.

in addition, midperipheral iris adhesions to the cornea may be present as well as significant iris abnormalities that can include marked hypoplasia of the anterior iris stroma as well as pupillary abnormalities such as distortion of the pupil, polycoria, and corectopia. Microcornea or macrocornea may also be evident.

When the ocular abnormalities are associated with dental and facial abnormalities, the term *Rieger syndrome* is applied. The dental and facial anomalies include hypodentia, microdentia, and occasional anodentia as well as malar hypoplasia (Fig 19–12). The ocular abnormalities are usually present bilaterally, and autosomal dominant transmission is the inheritance pattern.

Glaucoma occurs in approximately 50% of affected individuals.[21, 22] The glaucoma may occur in infancy but is usually delayed until later in life. In infants, a goniotomy if the angle is visible or trabeculotomy is the indicated procedure, with filtering surgery subsequently required in many cases. In older children, medical therapy should be tried prior to any surgical procedures.

Peter's Anomaly

Peter's anomaly is manifested by central corneal opacification with adhesions of the central part of the iris and possibly lens to the posterior surface of the cornea. Frequently, these iris attachments arise from the collarette with an absence of Descemet's membrane and thinning of the posterior corneal stroma.

Glaucoma occurs in approximately 50% of cases and may be present even when the anterior chamber angle appears grossly normal, although peripheral corneotrabeculodysgenesis may also be found. The glaucoma may present in infancy or later in life. When glaucoma exists in infants, goniotomy, trabeculotomy, and trabeculectomy have all been used, with the choice of procedure individualized to each patient. Medical therapy becomes important in older children.

Penetrating keratoplasty and cataract extraction may be required to provide a clear visual axis. More advanced forms of this disorder may demonstrate varying degrees of corneal thinning, with severe cases showing actual full-thickness holes through the cornea with flat anterior chambers and adherence of the lens to the posterior cornea.

Lowe Syndrome (Oculocerebrorenal Syndrome)

Lowe syndrome is characterized by aminoaciduria and mental retardation in male infants. The inheritance pattern is sex linked recessive. Glaucoma and cataracts are the most significant ocular abnormalities present.[23] The glaucomatous angle can have an isolated trabeculodysgenesis appearance and respond to goniotomy or trabeculotomy, although filtering surgery may be required. One case of severe hemorrhage following goniotomy has been reported.

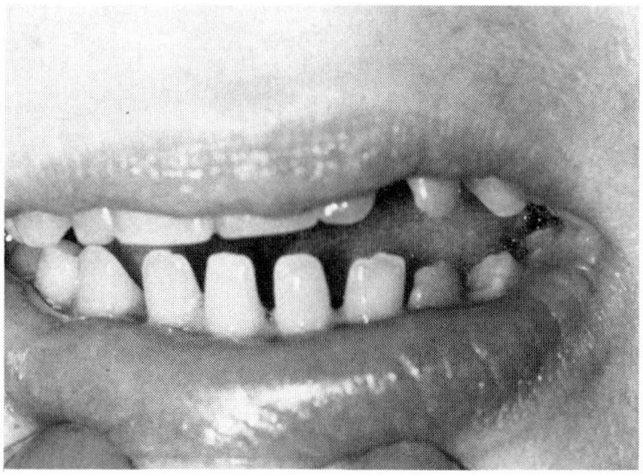

FIG 19–12.
Rieger syndrome: dental anomalies.

Microcornea

Microcornea is not a specific diagnosis but may be found in patients with rubella syndrome, persistent hyperplastic primary vitreous, Rieger's anomaly, nanophthalmos, and microphthalmos. The term generally refers to patients with microphthalmos in which the eye is hyperopic and has a corneal horizontal diameter less than 10 mm. Shallow anterior chambers and narrow angles may contribute to an attack of acute angle-closure glaucoma. Treatment is directed toward the angle-closure glaucoma.

Microspherophakia

Microspherophakia may occur as an isolated ocular anomaly or in association with the systemic anomalies of Marchesani's syndrome, which include brachydactyly, a short pyknic build, brachycephaly, and mental retardation. An autosomal dominant or recessive inheritance pattern may be evident. The most prominent ocular abnormality is a small spherical lens. The edges of the lens can often be seen through a mid-dilated pupil. High degrees of myopia are usually present.

The lens may assume an abnormal position in the posterior chamber or may move anteriorly and result in pupillary-block glaucoma, which is worsened by treatment with miotics. The angle-closure glaucoma may occur in an acute form that can be treated by mydriasis, iridectomy, or lens extraction or in a chronic form causing progressive formation of peripheral anterior synechiae. The glaucoma usually occurs later in childhood or early adulthood.

Rubella

Rubella in the newborn can produce glaucoma, cataract, microcornea, keratitis, uveitis, and a pigmented retinopathy. Cardiac, auditory, and central nervous system involvement may also be present.

The glaucoma may present in infancy and have the appearance of isolated trabeculodysgenesis. This form is best managed by goniotomy.

The rubella virus with its accompanying inflammation may affect a normally developed trabecular meshwork and produce an elevation in intraocular pressure. If there is evidence of inflammation, this mechanism must be suspected. These patients would respond poorly to goniotomy and should be treated with aqueous suppressants during the acute phase.

Chromosome Abnormalities

Several types of chromosomal defects have been associated with congenital glaucoma. These include trisomy 21, trisomy 13–15, trisomy 17–18, Turner syndrome, and trisomy 20. Multiple ocular and systemic defects may be evident, with a large variation in their presentations. The necessity for surgical or medical management must be individualized to each patient. If isolated trabeculodysgenesis is evident on examination, a goniotomy would be the initial procedure of choice.

Broad-Thumb Syndrome (Rubenstein-Taybi Syndrome)

Broad thumbs and great toes are the most evident abnormalities in this syndrome.[24] They may occur in association with mental and motor retardation, lid colobomas, and cataract as well as congential glaucoma. Large physiological optic disc cupping without glaucoma can also be seen in these patients. Goniotomy can be successful in controlling the glaucoma.

Persistent Hyperplastic Primary Vitreous

Persistent hyperplastic primary vitreous typically occurs unilaterally in a microphthalmic eye. It results from failure of atrophy of the primary vitreous and its vascular structures. A retrolental fibrovascular membrane can attach to the posterior aspect of the lens as well as to the ciliary processes and draw the processes into the pupillary space. The membrane can be seen as a whitish mass in the pupil and is thus in the differential diagnosis for leukocoria.

Angle-closure glaucoma may be produced by progressive opacification and swelling of the lens or contraction of the retrolental membrane which pushes the lens forward. Hemorrhages into the eye may also result in glaucoma. Removal of the lens and the membrane may prevent closure of the angle.

Familial Hypoplasia of the Iris With Glaucoma

Familial hypoplasia of the iris with glaucoma is characterized by hypoplasia of the anterior iris stroma, a prominent pupillary sphincter, trabeculodysgenesis, and glaucoma. Its hereditary pattern is autosomal dominant. The anterior stroma of the iris is markedly hypoplastic, and the pupillary sphincter is obvious as a tan, distinct ring around the pupil. Glaucoma may occur at any time from birth until late adulthood but eventually develops in almost 100% of cases.[25–28] Childhood cases can respond to goniotomy or trabeculotomy. Cases with later onset have been successfully managed with medical therapy, argon laser trabeculoplasty, trabeculotomy, or trabeculectomy.

GENERAL GUIDELINES FOR THE TREATMENT OF GLAUCOMA

Treatment consists of lowering the intraocular pressure. Surgical therapy is preferred in infants with primary congenital glaucoma and in many of the glaucomas associated with congenital anomalies as well. In such cases, medications may be used to control any damage that might occur prior to surgery. Medications are also used in the long-term management of difficult cases that have not responded well to surgical intervention.

Medical Therapy

There are four basic types of medical therapy for glaucoma: cholinergic agents, β-adrenergic blocking agents, adrenergic agents, and carbonic anhydrase inhibitors.

Cholinergic Agents

The cholinergic drugs act to increase the outflow of aqueous humor from the eye with a resultant lowering of the intraocular pressure. They come in two forms, one being the direct-acting cholinergic agents such as pilocarpine and carbachol. The second group comprises the anticholinesterase drugs, which inhibit the enzyme cholinesterase and allow acetylcholine to build up at the nerve endings. Drugs in this category are echothiophate iodide (Phospholine Iodide) and demecarium bromide (Humorsol).

Stimulation of the parasympathetic system causes a contraction of the ciliary and pupillary sphincter muscles, which causes an increased outflow of aqueous humor, miosis, an increase in myopia, and in most cases, a widening of the anterior chamber angle.

In children, the most troublesome side effect of these agents is increased myopia, which can be visually disabling. Other side effects include allergic or toxic conjunctivitis, dimness of vision, ocular pain or browache, iritis, and retinal tears with possible detachment. In narrow-angle eyes, the anterior chamber angle may actually narrow rather than widen, and gonioscopy must be performed to ensure that a narrow angle has not closed in these individuals.

The longer-acting anticholinesterase agents produce a more constant degree of myopia that can be better corrected with glasses. However, these drugs can also produce cataracts as well as systemic toxicity. They can reduce the circulating cholinesterase levels in the blood to 1/10 of normal, and a sensitive patient may develop weakness, diarrhea, salivation, bradycardia, and other evidence of parasympathetic stimulation. Children using anticholinesterase agents who require general anesthesia must not receive succinylcholine because this may cause prolonged apnea. Also, a child in an area sprayed with anticholinesterase insecticide may develop a further reduction in his cholinesterase levels.

Alternative forms of cholinergic therapy include a pilocarpin system (Ocusert) and pilocarpine gel (Pilopine H.S. Gel). Ocusert is a plastic membrane delivery system that is placed in the conjunctival sac once weekly to provide a gradual release of pilocarpine over this period of time. When it is retained and is comfortable, it can be very helpful by providing a more constant therapeutic level of the medication, although occasional "bursts" of excess pilocarpine may cause intermittent side effects. The pilocarpine gel is applied only at bedtime and may be better tolerated by some children because the increase in myopia primarily occurs during sleep. The development of subtle subepithelial opacifications has been noted in some individuals using the pilocarpine gel.

β-Adrenergic Blocking Agents

The nonselective β-adrenergic blocking agents such as timolol (Timoptic) and levobunolol (Betagan) and the selective β_1-adrenergic blocking agent betaxolol (Betoptic) can lower intraocular pressure by inhibiting the production of aqueous fluid. The ocular side effects are much less troublesome than those seen with the cholinergic agents, and in general, these agents are better tolerated by children. They do not change the size of the pupil or the refractive error. Ocular side effects include conjunctival hyperemia, superficial punctate keratitis, corneal anesthesia, allergic conjunctivitis, and burning on instillation.

The greatest concern in the use of β-adrenergic blocking agents is the potential for serious systemic side effects including asthmatic attacks, bradycardia, light-headedness, dizziness, drowsiness, hyperactivity, and dissociated behavior.[28–30] Precipitation of acute asthmatic attacks can occur when timolol is administered to a patient with a history of asthma, and thus it must be used very cautiously if at all in these patients. The selective

β_1-adrenergic blocking agents have less effect on the airways and thus are safer for use in patients with a history of asthma or other lung disease such as cystic fibrosis. Infants with cardiac disease must also be evaluated very carefully prior to administering any β-adrenergic blocking agents because they may exacerbate congestive heart failure and bradycardia. Central nervous system side effects are uncommon and may be overlooked if not checked for carefully. Parents thus must observe carefully for a child's change in behavioral patterns. In infants this may be impossible to recognize. Betaxolol may have fewer pulmonary and possibly even cardiac side effects. However, this remains to be evaluated in infants.

Timolol is available in both a 0.25% and 0.5% solution. Levobunolol and betaxolol are available only as 0.5% solutions. If one is using timolol as the medication of choice, one should initiate therapy with the 0.25% solution in most cases and increase to 0.5% only if the intraocular pressure–lowering effect is not adequate. One should then re-evaluate to be certain that better control has been obtained when using the stronger dose.

The Food and Drug Administration has not ruled on the safety or efficacy of these drugs in children, and parents should be made aware of this fact. Parents should also be warned of any potential side effects that can occur with these medications so that treatment with the drug can be discontinued if side effects develop.

Adrenergic Agents

The adrenergic agents, which are epinephrine derivatives, are a third type of topical medication available for glaucoma patients. They do not affect the refractive error or vision and thus may be better tolerated than are the cholinergic agents. They can dilate the pupil and should be avoided in patients with narrow angles.

Allergic reactions are common after the prolonged use of adrenergic agents. A rebound hyperemia of the conjunctiva frequently occurs several hours after instillation of the drops. This is usually a harmless side effect but can be troubling to the parents who see the redness of the eyes. Parents may be tempted to place the drop more frequently due to the initial constriction of the blood vessels that whitens the eye.

Burning and an aching periorbital pain may also occur from the instillation of these agents. Melanin-like adrenochrome deposits, usually noted in the conjunctiva and rarely on the cornea, can also develop after prolonged use. Cystoid macular edema may occur in patients who have had cataract extraction. Systemic side effects include an increase in blood pressure, tachycardia, palpitations, and behavioral changes. These side effects are the result of stimulation of the sympathetic nervous system in predisposed individuals. These drugs lower intraocular pressure by decreasing aqueous production and increasing aqueous outflow.

Antiglaucomatous epinephrine agents include the hydrochloride, bitartrate, and borate compounds. The agents are all about equally effective, although the epinephrine borate is more comfortable on instillation.

The epinephrine pro-drug, dipivefrin, is the most commonly used adrenergic agent. It is many times more lipophilic than is epinephrine, which enhances its ocular penetration and allows a much lower concentration of the drug to be applied externally to achieve therapeutic intraocular levels. This enhances the drug's effectiveness and reduces systemic side effects. The 0.1% concentration of this drug is as effective as 1% epinephrine hydrochloride.

Carbonic Anhydrase Inhibitors

The carbonic anhydrase inhibitors are oral agents that reduce intraocular pressure by decreasing the formation of aqueous humor. Acetazolamide is the agent most commonly used because it has been the most extensively studied. In infants, it is administered in a dosage of 5 to 10 mg/kg of body weight. Other agents such as methazolamide and dichlorphenamide are also available but are used less commonly in infants.

The main value of the carbonic anhydrase inhibitors is the short-term lowering of intraocular pressure preoperatively or in self-limited secondary forms of glaucoma. They must be administered cautiously due to their many systemic side effects including a rapid and severe acidosis. Consultation with the pediatrician is important if their use is to be prolonged, and long-term use should be avoided whenever possible. Other systemic side effects include paresthesias, changes in behavior, and gastrointestinal symptoms including anorexia, nausea, and diarrhea. As with other sulfonamides, there is also a risk of aplastic anemia or exfoliative dermatitis. Genitourinary symptoms may include frequency of urination, which usually diminishes after several weeks of use, but ureteral calculi may be seen with prolonged use of these agents. The most common ocular side effect from the carbonic anhydrase inhibitors is that of a transient myopia.

Surgical Therapy

Surgical procedures available for the treatment of the developmental glaucomas include operations to increase aqueous outflow, decrease aqueous production, and correct pupillary block.

A key point in the surgical management of infants is that if *isolated trabeculodysgenesis* is present on examination, a *goniotomy* is the indicated procedure.

Surgery to Increase Aqueous Outflow

Goniotomy.—Goniotomy involves a direct incision of the superficial layers of the trabecular meshwork (Fig 19–13). This is performed by entering the anterior chamber through the cornea slightly inside the limbus and then passing the goniotomy knife across the anterior chamber where a direct incision is made into the trabecular meshwork. Accurate visualization is obtained by using the operating microscope and a goniotomy contact lens. Goniotomy is particularly successful in those types of glaucoma where the block

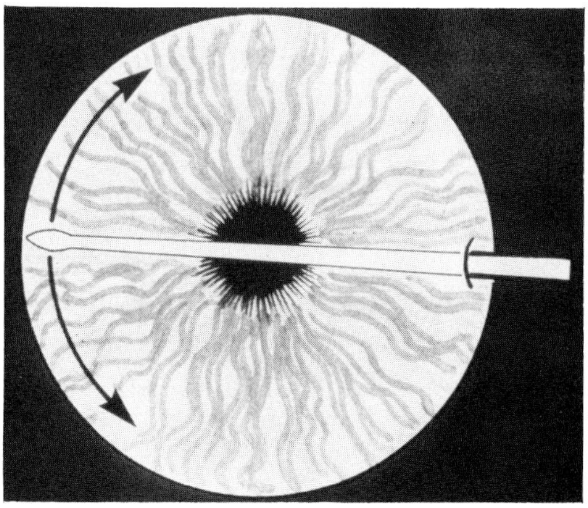

FIG 19–13.
Goniotomy. A goniotomy knife is passed across the anterior chamber to incise the trabecular meshwork.

to aqueous flow lies in the superficial layers of the trabecular meshwork.

Trabeculotomy.—Trabeculotomy is performed by creating a scleral flap to locate the canal of Schlemm, which is opened by using a surgical blade (Fig 19–14). A trabeculotome is then inserted along the course of the canal and rotated into the anterior chamber, thus breaking through the trabecular meshwork. The goal of this procedure is to remove the trabecular meshwork as a blockade to the flow of the aqueous into Schlemm's canal.

Trabeculectomy.—In the performance of a trabeculectomy, a conjunctival flap is dissected and a partial-thickness scleral flap is created that is hinged anteriorly at the cornea (Fig 19–15). The anterior chamber is entered, and a block of tissue including the trabecular meshwork and Schlemm's canal is removed and a peripheral iridectomy performed. This procedure provides a direct outflow of aqueous humor through the surgical opening into the subconjunctival tissues. Trabeculectomies have fewer complications such as flat anterior chambers, cataract formation, bleb complications, and staphyloma formation than do full-thickness filtering procedures. For this reason, a trabeculectomy is usually performed prior to performing full-thickness surgery. If trabeculectomy fails, a full-thickness filtering operation is then considered.

Full-Thickness Filtering Procedures.—Full-thickness filtering procedures are operations that create a hole through the sclera beneath a conjunctival flap at the corneoscleral limbus. No scleral flap is created as is done with the trabeculectomy. This opening provides a direct pathway for the flow of aqueous humor out of the anterior chamber and into the subconjunctival space. The opening may be created with cautery (thermal sclerostomy), a scleral punch (posterior or anterior lip sclerectomy), or a trephine (Elliot's trephination). A peripheral iridectomy is also performed with this procedure.

Cyclodialysis.—Cyclodialysis creates a communication between the anterior chamber and the suprachoroidal space by disinserting the ciliary body from the scleral spur via a scleral incision posterior to the limbus. The decrease in intraocular pressure is probably due to a combined decrease in aqueous humor production as well as an increase in aqueous flow into the suprachoroidal space and out of the eye. This procedure is seldomly effective in infants and is rarely used.

Adjuncts to Filtering Surgery.—Trabeculectomy and full-thickness filtering surgery may fail due to scar formation. Inhibitors of scar formation such as the antimetabolite 5-fluorouracil and the long-acting steroid triamcinolone acetonide may be injected subconjunctivally to help prevent this fibrosis from occurring.[31, 32]

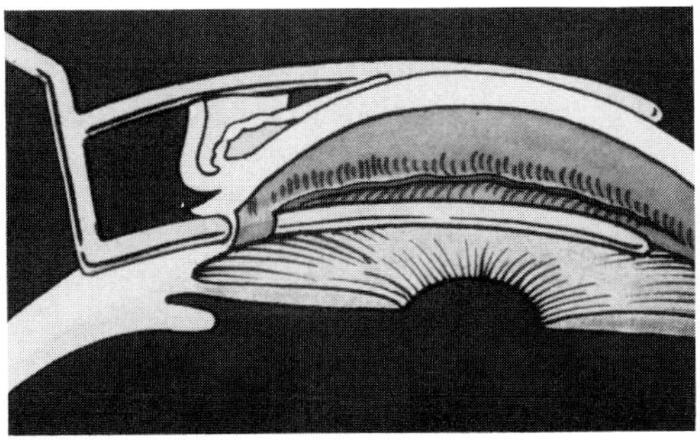

FIG 19–14.
Trabeculotomy. The trabeculotome is being rotated from its position within Schlemm's canal through the trabecular meshwork into the anterior chamber.

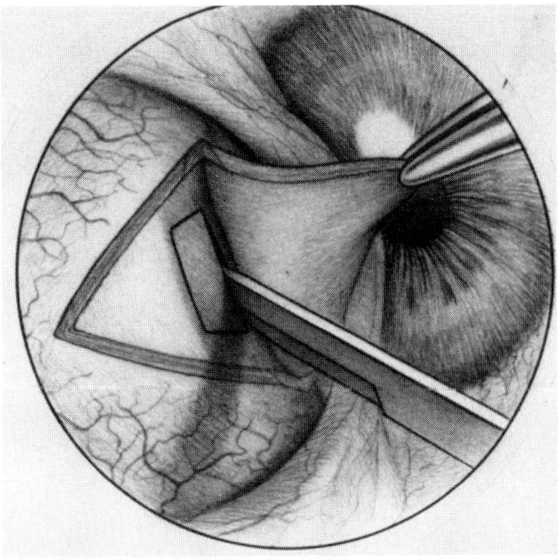

FIG 19–15.
Trabeculectomy. A block of tissue including the trabecular meshwork and Schlemm's canal is removed.

Synthetic Drainage Devices.—Synthetic drainage devices may be inserted subconjunctivally to provide an opening between the anterior chamber and the subconjunctival space. Many types of synthetic drainage devices have been used through the years with generally poor results. Recently, the implant of Molteno and colleagues has shown more promising results than have previous devices and should be considered in patients where filtering surgery has failed.[33] Investigations of these synthetic drainage devices are ongoing and will, it is hoped, lead to improvements.

Surgery to Decrease Aqueous Humor Production

Cyclocryotherapy.—Cryoapplication to the sclera overlying the aqueous-producing portion of the ciliary body can damage the ciliary epithelium and decrease aqueous secretion. This can result in a variable lowering of the intraocular pressure. It often causes severe pain in children and frequently must be repeated. It is usually used when repeated surgery to improve aqueous outflow has failed.

Ultrasound.—The therapeutic use of ultrasound is being investigated as a treatment for patients with refractory glaucoma. The results in children have been disappointing.[34]

Surgery for Pupillary-Block Glaucoma

Iridectomy.—In cases of pupillary-block glaucoma, a passage is created between the posterior and anterior chambers by surgically making an opening in the iris (Fig 19–16). This allows aqueous humor to flow through this surgical opening, which relieves the pupillary block. The procedure is performed through an incision into the anterior chamber at the corneoscleral limbus. In adults, an iridectomy may be created by using an argon or Nd-YAG laser. However, at the present time, these lasers require the cooperation of the patient and are thus not applicable for infants.

Treatment of Amblyopia

An important feature in managing patients with developmental glaucoma is the treatment of amblyopia, which can result from tears in Descemet's membrane that involve the visual axis and from anisometropia. A significant amount of myopia with or without irregular astigmatism can be present. A cycloplegic refraction must be performed as soon as possible and the proper lens correction given. Occlusion therapy must also be considered, especially in monocular cases, and may need to be continued for years.

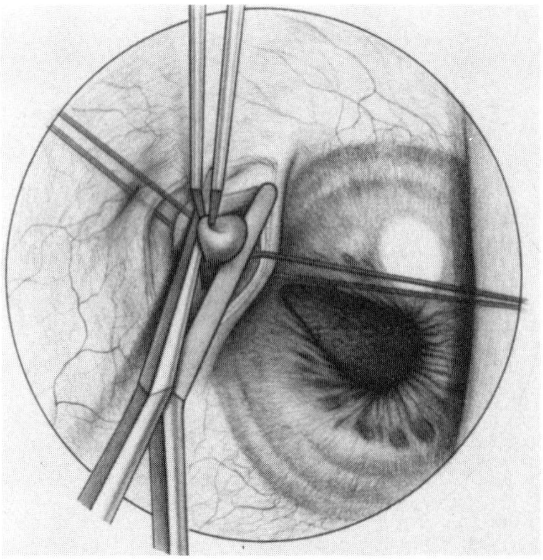

FIG 19–16.
Iridectomy. An opening in the iris is created.

REFERENCES

1. Shaffer RN, Weiss DI: *Congenital and Pediatric Glaucomas.* St Louis, CV Mosby Co, 1970.
2. Becker B, Shaffer RN: *The Diagnosis and Therapy of Glaucomas.* St Louis, CV Mosby Co, 1983.
3. Hoskins HD Jr, Shaffer RN, Hetherington J: Anatomical classification of the developmental glaucomas. *Arch Ophthalmol* 1984; 102:1331.
4. Hoskins HD Jr, Hetherington J, Shaffer RN, et al: Developmental glaucoma: Diagnosis and classification, in *Proceedings of the New Orleans Academy of Ophthalmologic Glaucoma Symposium.* St Louis, CV Mosby Co, 1981.
5. Shaffer RN, Hetherington J: The glaucomatous disc in infants—A suggested hypothesis for disc cupping. *Trans Am Acad Ophthalmol* 1969; 73:923.
6. Quigley HA: Childhood glaucoma—Results with trabeculotomy and study of reversible cupping. *Ophthalmology* 1982; 89:219.
7. Richardson KT, Shaffer RN: Optic nerve cupping in congenital glaucoma. *Am J Ophthalmol* 1966; 62:507.
8. Jay MR, Phil M, Rice NSC: Genetic implications of congenital glaucoma. *Metabolic Ophthalmol* 1978; 2:257–258.
9. Merin S, Morin D: Heredity of congenital glaucoma. *Br J Ophthalmol* 1972; 56:414.
10. Shaffer RN: Prognosis of goniotomy in primary infantile glaucoma (trabeculodysgenesis). *Trans Am Ophthalmol Soc* 1982; 80:321.
11. Hoskins HD Jr, Shaffer RN, Hetherington J: Goniotomy vs. trabeculotomy. *J Pediatr Ophthalmol Strabismus* 1984; 21:153.
12. Anderson DR: Trabeculotomy compared to goniotomy for glaucoma in children. *Ophthalmology* 1983; 90:805.

13. Fraumeni JH: The aniridia Wilms' tumor syndrome. *Birth Defects* 1969; 5:198.
14. Nelson LB, Spaeth GL, Nowinski TS, et al: Aniridia—A review. *Surv Ophthalmol* 1984; 28:621.
15. Walton DS: Aniridic glaucoma—The results of goniosurgery to prevent and treat this problem. *Trans Am Ophthalmol Soc* 1986; 84:59.
16. Phelps CD: The pathogenesis of glaucoma in Sturge-Weber syndrome. *Ophthalmology* 1978; 85:276.
17. Cross HE, Jensen AD: Ocular manifestations in Marfan's syndrome and homocystinuria. *Am J Ophthalmol* 1973; 75:405.
18. Allen RA, Straatsma DR, Apt L, et al: Ocular manifestations of the Marfan's syndrome. *Trans Am Acad Ophthalmol Otolaryngol* 1973; 76:18.
19. Burian HM, Allen L: Histologic study of the chamber angle in patients with Marfan's syndrome. *Arch Ophthalmol* 1961; 65:323.
20. Smith JL, Stowe FR: The Pierre Robin syndrome (glossoptosis, micrognathia, cleft palate)—A review of 39 cases with emphasis on associated ocular lesions. *J Pediatr* 1961; 27:128.
21. Alkemade PPH: *Dysgenesis Mesodermalis of the Iris and Cornea.* Assen, The Netherlands, Charles C Thomas, 1969.
22. Waring GO III, Rodrigues MM, Laibson PR: Anterior chamber cleavage syndrome—A stepladder classification. *Surv Ophthalmol* 1975; 29:3.
23. Lowe CU, Terrey M, MacLachlan EA: Organic aciduria, decreased renal ammonia production, hydrophthalmus, and mental retardation—A clinical entity. *Am J Dis Child* 1952; 83:164.
24. Rubenstein JH, Taybi H: Broad thumbs and toes and facial abnormalities. *Am J Dis Child* 1963; 105:588.
25. Weatherhill JR, Hart CT: Familial hypoplasia of the iris stroma associated with glaucoma. *Br J Ophthalmol* 1969; 53:433.
26. Jerndal T: Dominant goniodysgenesis with late congenital glaucoma. *Am J Ophthalmol* 1972; 74:28.
27. Martin JP, Zorab EC: Familial glaucoma. *Br J Ophthalmol* 1974; 58:536.
28. Hoskins HD Jr, Hetherington J, Magee SD, et al: Clinical experience with timolol in childhood glaucoma. *Arch Ophthalmol* 1985; 103:1163.
29. Boger WP: Timolol in childhood glaucoma. *Surv Ophthalmol* 1983; 28:259.
30. Zimmerman TJ, Kooner KS, Morgan KS: Safety and efficacy of timolol in pediatric glaucoma. *Surv Ophthalmol* 1983; 28:262.
31. Heuer DK, Parish RK II, Gressel MG, et al: 5-Fluorouracil and glaucoma filtering surgery—A pilot study. *Ophthalmology* 1984; 91:384.
32. Giangiacomo J, Dueker DK, Adelstein E: The effect of preoperative subconjunctival triamcinolone administration on glaucoma filtration. *Arch Ophthalmol* 1986; 104:838.
33. Molteno ACB, Ancker E, VanBiljon G: Surgical technique for advanced juvenile glaucoma. *Arch Ophthalmol* 1984; 102:51.
34. Burgess SEP, Silverman RH, Coleman DJ, et al: Treatment of glaucoma with high intensity focus ultrasound. *Ophthalmology* 1986; 93:831.

20A Disorders of the Lens

David A. Hiles, M.D.
Robert W. Hered, M.D.

Disorders of the lens in the human infant's eye constitute a major deterent to the development of visual function. Lens abnormalities occur as defects in shape, position, or clarity and project blurred or distorted images onto the retina of the developing infant. Distortions occurring in children prior to visual maturation (between 6 to 8 years of age) frequently lead to severe and often irreversible deprivation amblyopia.

The management of these patients has been profoundly altered by the research of Wiesel and Hubel[1–4] and von Noorden and his associates on the effect of visual deprivation in animals.[5,6] A "sensitive" period exists in which a reversal of amblyopia may occur, but its exact duration in the human remains unknown. Complete reversal of deprivation amblyopia in infants with complete congenital cataracts, theoretically, may be possible up to 2 to 3 months of age. This is followed by a period of decreasing visual recovery potential throughout a 6- to 10-year age range.[7,8] Therefore, infants and young children with lens abnormalities require very early diagnosis, surgical treatment when required, and vigorous aphakic rehabilitation to achieve maximum visual success. Children developing cataracts after the ages of 8 to 10 years do not lose visual acuity or develop amblyopia even following prolonged occlusion of their visual axes.

CLASSIFICATION

Disorders of the lens may be classified according to morphology or etiology.[9–26] Not all of the following diseases or syndromes have lens abnormalities present at birth or occurring in early infancy. The following guide is presented to aid the reader in diagnosis, and the references in this section point to other sources with greater detail.

Morphology

Congenital Aphakia

Congenital aphakia is a rare syndrome consisting of the total absence of the crystalline lens due to developmental failure or degeneration and reabsorption of the lens fibers.

Microspherophakia

Microspherophakia, a rarely isolated anomaly, is often associated with other ocular or systemic syndromes as Marfan, homocystinuria, and Weill-Marchesani and produces small, bilateral, spherical-shaped displaced lenses.

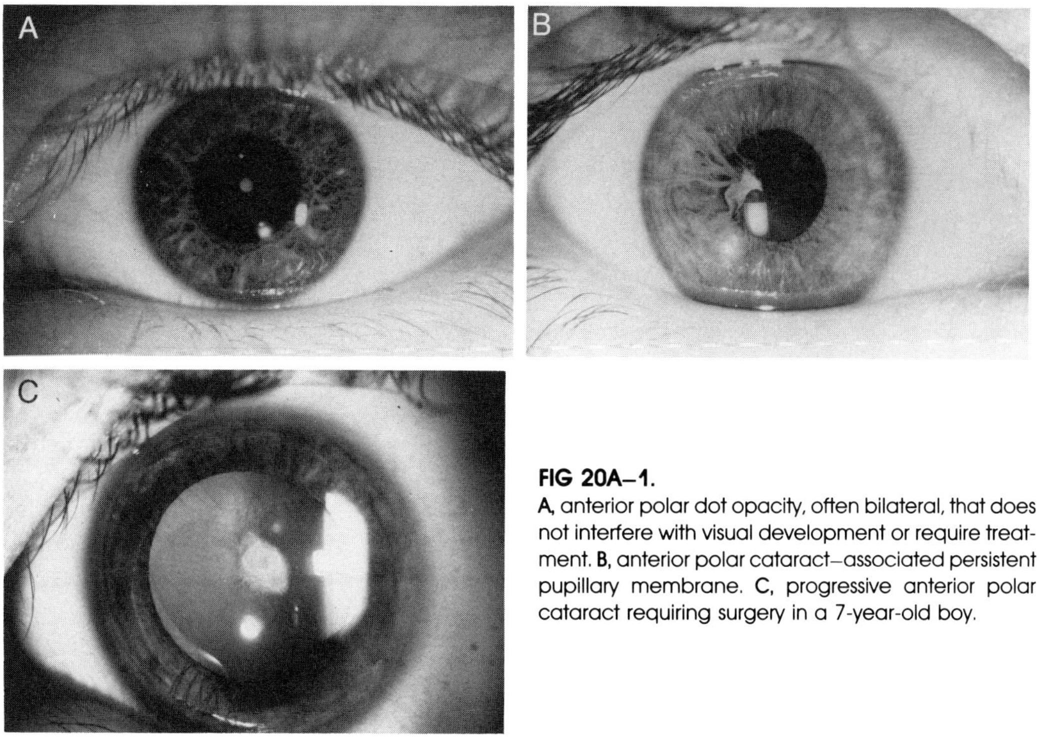

FIG 20A–1.
A, anterior polar dot opacity, often bilateral, that does not interfere with visual development or require treatment. **B**, anterior polar cataract–associated persistent pupillary membrane. **C**, progressive anterior polar cataract requiring surgery in a 7-year-old boy.

Coloboma

Colobomas of the lens are produced by segmental deficiencies of the zonular fibers or their attachment to the lens. These absent or weakened fibers produce an indentation or notching in the equatorial region of the lens.

Cataracts

Cataracts are opacifications of the crystalline lens. Some are nonprogressive without visual distortion or loss while others are "cataracts" in the clinical sense of inducing visual loss requiring observation or medical and surgical treatment.

Zones of discontinuity within the infant lens are formed as early lens fibers are laid down to create the bulk of the lens. The clear embryonic nucleus constitutes the center of the lens and is formed within the first few weeks of gestation. The secondary fetal nuclear fibers overlie the embryonic nucleus and are laid down between the third and eighth month of gestation. These fibers join to form the anterior upright Y and posterior inverted-Y sutures and are fully formed by the end of the third month of gestation. Additional fibers forming the infantile nucleus are laid down from the last weeks of gestation through puberty when the adult nucleus is formed. Superficial, soft cortex lies between the nucleus and anterior capsular epithelial cells and lens capsule.

Lens opacities in children frequently occur in identifiable zones of the lens, with clear lens fibers deposited over the opacified ones. This stratification is useful in distinguishing the occurrence of a prenatal toxic lens insult from a more superficial insult occurring in the postnatal period.

Polar Cataracts.—*Congenital anterior polar cataracts.*—Many anterior polar cataracts are bilateral, symmetrical, stationary, dot opacities less than 1 mm in diameter, and the visual acuity is usually not affected (Fig 20A–1,A). The defect is often familial. The familial variety, an autosomal dominant trait, is divided into three groups: one associated with lamellar lens opacities, a second associated with microphthalmos and aniridia, and a third associated with hyperplastic pupillary membranes that themselves may partially or totally occlude the pupil or attach to the lens to produce an anterior polar opacity (Fig 20A–1,B). This latter defect may be associated with lamellar, anterior lenticonus, or pyramidal cataracts.

Jaafar and Robb and Nelson et al. have recently reported patients with progressive, larger anterior polar cataracts that eventually lead to surgical removal of the lens. The occurrence of amblyopia, strabismus, and anisometropia in these patients mandates frequent ophthalmologic examination and eventual surgery in some[27,28] (Fig 20A–1,C).

Congenital posterior polar cataracts.— Posterior polar cataracts, usually stable, may progress with increasing density and size. The diameter of the opacity is usually larger than anterior polar cataracts and, therefore, interferes more with visual development. They may be familial or sporadic in inheritance; the familial type is usually autosomal dominant. The sporadic type is often unilateral and is associated with posterior lenticonus or remnants of the hyaloid artery system.

Posterior Lenticonus and Lentiglobus.— Posterior lenticonus is a common, unilateral, circumscribed round or oval posterior bulge (lentiglobus) of the posterior lens capsule[29,30] (Fig 20A–2). The lenticonus slowly increases in size over the first several years of life and is frequently associated with an adjacent posterior cortical cataract. Frequent amblyopia monitoring is essential. Following cataract surgery, aphakic visual acuity is often markedly improved in these eyes due to the slow preoperative progression of the visual loss over prolonged periods of visual development before surgery is required.

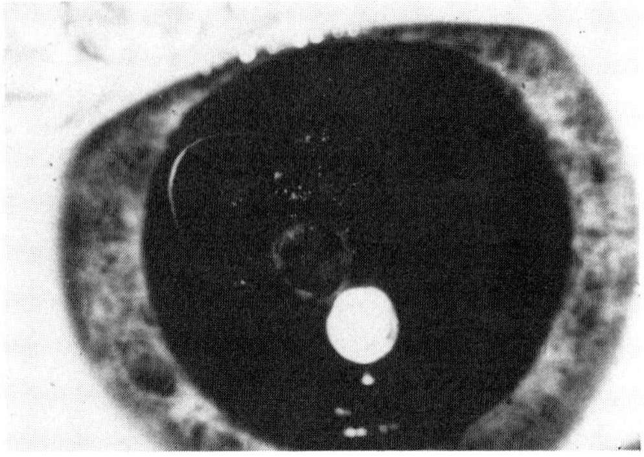

FIG 20A–2.
Posterior lenticonus with surrounding posterior cortical powdery opacites inducing slowly progressive visual loss in later childhood (*above,* white light reflex).

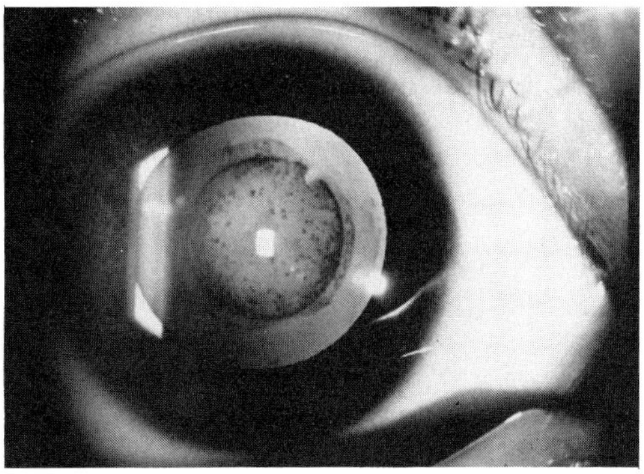

FIG 20A–3.
Hereditary lamellar cataract: clear nucleus surrounded by a cataract that is surrounded by clear cortex.

Zonular or Lamellar Cataracts.—Zonular cataracts are confined to specific zones of the developing lens. They may be nuclear with or without surrounding riders, cortical, sutural, stellate, floriform, coralliform, spear shaped, etc. The opacity may progress to involve other areas of the lens also.

Lamellar cataracts are the most common type of zonular cataract and consist of a zone or layer of opacification surrounding a clear zone of lens that in turn is surrounded by a clear zone of cortex (Fig 20A–3). Secondary subcapsular cortical opacities may develop in the presence of lamellar opacities. Lamellar cataracts are the result of a transient insult to the lens during its development, and the earlier the lens insult, the deeper and smaller is the lens opacity. Lamellar cataracts may occur simultaneously with other forms of zonular cataracts such as nuclear or sutural cataracts. The visual acuity of eyes with lamellar cataracts varies according to the density of the opacification. If an axial opacity is 3 mm in diameter or greater, amblyopia is more prone to develop, and surgery is indicated at an earlier age.[31]

Nuclear Cataracts.—Nuclear cataract, a form of zonular cataract, is common in infancy and is always congenital. They may involve the embryonic nucleus alone or the embryonic and fetal nuclei. These opacities are usually bilateral and vary in size, and the visual acuity may be affected earlier and more severely (Fig 20A–4).

Total or Complete Cataracts.—Total or complete cataracts are those in which no view of the retina by direct or indirect ophthalmoscopy is possible (Fig 20A–5). Complete cataracts often progress from incomplete cataracts, and this process may be slow or rapid depending upon the insult that produced the opacification. Long-term, early-onset, total cataracts develop more severe deprivation amblyopia.

Membranous Cataracts.—Membranous cataracts are thin, dense, and sometimes fibrotic lens opacities that may be congenital. More commonly, they develop from the absorption of lens cortex and nuclear material of mature cataracts, which allows the lens capsule and capsular cells to form dense plaques.

Infections and Tumors

Infections of the lens may occur intrinsically or extrinsically following penetrating injuries of the globe and are usually accompanied by an associated endophthalmitis.

Tumors of the lens in children are unknown in this author's experience.

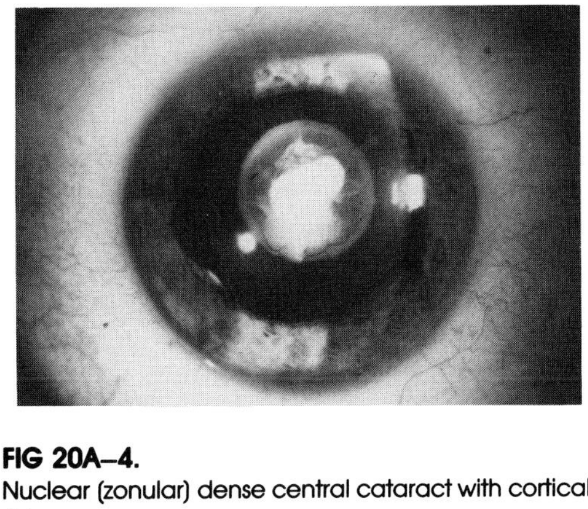

FIG 20A–4.
Nuclear (zonular) dense central cataract with cortical riders.

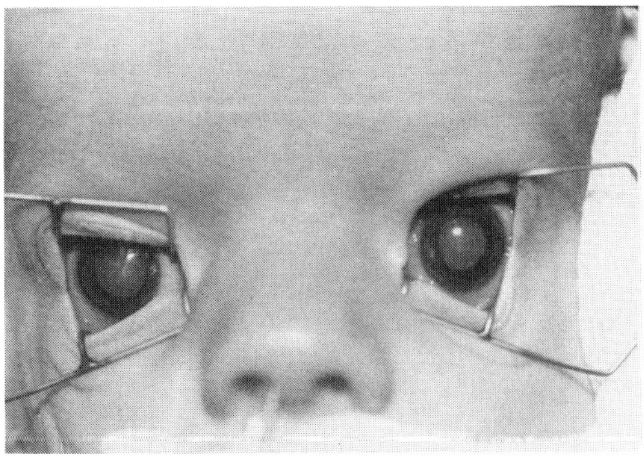

FIG 20A–5.
Bilateral, symmetrical, complete congenital cataracts in a newborn with autosomal dominant familial inheritance.

Etiologies of Cataracts

The etiology of cataracts and lens dislocations is determined from the genetic evaluation, medical history, physical examination, the age of onset, morphological characteristics of the cataract, and laboratory and radiological investigations (Table 20A–1). Lens defects may occur as isolated findings in otherwise normal patients or as part of a constellation of findings related to a syndrome, systemic abnormality, or other ocular abnormalities.

Sporadic Cataracts

Sporadic cataracts constitute approximately one third of pediatric cataracts. They arise de novo and are not associated with other ocular or systemic diseases. Merin and Crawford have estimated that as many as one fourth of these patients have a new autosomal dominant mutation.[19] They also suggest that some of these defects may be related to systemic diseases with symptoms too mild to be recognized.

Hereditary Cataracts

Hereditary cataracts may be isolated or

TABLE 20A–1.
Evaluation of Infantile Cataract Patients

- I. Ophthalmologic history
  - A. Birth weight
    - 1. Low
      - a. Hypoglycemia
  - B. Family history
    - 1. Inherited disease
      - a. Retinitis pigmentosa
      - b. Optic atrophy
      - c. Cataracts
      - d. Glaucoma
  - C. Ocular history
    - 1. Trauma
    - 2. Uveitis
    - 3. Retinal detachment
    - 4. Drug ingestion
      - a. Corticosteroids
      - b. Vitamin D
      - c. Thorazine
    - 5. Maternal drug ingestion
    - 6. Ionizing radiation
  - D. Onset of cataracts
- II. Ophthalmologic examination
  - A. Corneal abnormalities
    - 1. Megalocornea
    - 2. Wilson disease
    - 3. Cerebro-ocular-facial-skeletal syndrome
    - 4. Trisomy 18
    - 5. Turner syndrome
    - 6. Lowe syndrome
    - 7. Fabry disease
    - 8. Down syndrome
  - B. Iris
    - 1. Aniridia
      - a. Marinesco-Sjögren syndrome
    - 2. Coloboma
      - a. Trisomy 13–15
  - C. Slit lamp
    - 1. Vacuoles
      - a. Diabetes
      - b. Hyperalimentation
    - 2. Spoke opacities
      - a. Congenital cataract
      - b. Fabry disease
      - c. Mannosidosis
    - 3. Multicolored flecks
      - a. Hypoparathyroidism
      - b. Pseudohypoparathyroidism
      - c. Myotonic dystrophy
    - 4. Green sunflower
      - a. Wilson disease
    - 5. Lamellar
      - a. Hypoglycemia
      - b. Galactosemia
      - c. Congenital cataract
    - 6. Discoid lens
      - a. Lowe syndrome
    - 7. Spoke opacities
      - a. Homocystinuria
      - b. Rubella
  - D. Retina
    - 1. Retinal pigmentation
      - a. Rubella
      - b. Laurence-Moon-Biedl syndrome
      - c. Hallgren syndrome
    - 2. Fundus albipunctatus
      - a. Alport syndrome
    - 3. Retinal depigmentation
      - a. Turner syndrome
    - 4. Atrophy
      - a. Cockayne syndrome
    - 5. Dysplasia
      - a. Trisomy 13–15
  - E. Optic nerve
    - 1. Atrophy
      - a. Trisomy 18
      - b. Cockayne syndrome
      - c. Hallgren syndrome
      - d. Trisomy 13–15
      - e. Homocystinuria
      - f. Laurence-Moon-Biedl syndrome
    - 2. Drusen
      - a. Alport syndrome
  - F. Glaucoma
    - a. Lowe syndrome
    - b. Trisomy 18
    - c. Rubella
- III. Laboratory Evaluation
  - A. Complete blood count
    - 1. Anemia
  - B. Blood
    - 1. Glucose (repeated examination)
      - a. Diabetes
      - b. Hypoglycemia
    - 2. Blood urea nitrogen
      - a. Renal disease
      - b. Lowe syndrome
    - 3. SMA-12-18 (protein, calcium, phosphorus, glucose)
      - a. Hypoparathyroidism
    - 4. Galactose enzymes (red blood cell) [RBC] galactose-1-phosphate uridyl transferase activity)
      - a. Galactosemia
    - 5. Rubella titer
      - a. Rubella
    - 6. Serological test for syphilis
      - a. Syphilis
    - 7. Virus cultures
      - a. Rubella
      - b. Herpes
    - 8. Platelet count (thromocytopenia)
      - a. Rubella
    - 9. Galactosidase A activity—plasma (also tears and fibroblasts)

(Continued)

TABLE 20A – 1 (cont.).

10. Liver function copper levels
    a. Wilson syndrome
11. Cholesterol
    a. Cerebral cholesterinosis

C. Urine
1. Urinalysis (following milk and meat meal)
   a. Renal disease (hematuria-proteinuria)
2. Sediment (Maltese cross figures under Polaroid light)
   a. Alport syndrome

D. Nitroprusside
1. Ketone excretion
   a. Homocystinuria
2. Benedict's test
   a. Diabetes
   b. Galactokinase deficiency

E. Amino acid
1. Chromatography
   a. Lowe syndrome

F. Ferric chloride
1. Phenylketonuria

G. Toluidine blue
1. Mucopolysaccharides
   a. Hurler disease

IV. X-ray evaluation

A. Skull
1. Bony facial abnormalities
   a. Hallermann-Streiff syndrome
   b. Pierre Robin syndrome
   c. Treacher Collins syndrome
2. Craniofacial stenosis
   a. Crouzon disease
   b. Apert syndrome
3. Calcified basal ganglia
   a. Hypoparathyroidism
   b. Pseudohypoparathyroidism
4. Calcifications
   a. Toxoplasmosis
   b. Cytomegalic inclusion disease
   c. Albers-Schönberg disease

B. Chest
1. Heart disease
   a. Rubella
   b. Conradi's disease
   c. Trisomy 18
   d. Ellis–van Creveld syndrome
   e. Down syndrome
   f. Zellweger syndrome
   g. Cerebro-oculo-facial-skeletal syndrome
   h. Laurence-Moon-Biedl syndrome
   i. Oto-oculo-musculo-skeletal syndrome
2. Dwarfism
   a. Hallermann-Streiff syndrome
   b. Rothmund-Thomson
   c. Progeria
   d. Mannosidosis
   e. Chondrodysplasia punctata
   f. Crome syndrome
   g. Weill-Marchesani syndrome
   h. Laurence-Moon-Biedl syndrome
   i. Kwiest syndrome
3. Stippled epiphyses
   a. Chondrodysplasia punctata
   b. Conradi syndrome
4. Joint abnormalities
   a. Kwiest syndrome
   b. Hallermann-Streiff syndrome

V. Audiological and intellectual evaluation

A. Deafness
1. Rubella
2. Turner syndrome
3. Alport syndrome
4. Laurence-Moon-Biedl syndrome
5. Cockayne syndrome
6. Hallgren syndrome
7. Oto-oculo-musclo-skeletal syndrome
8. Marshall disease
9. Trisomy 13–15

B. Vestibular defects
1. Alport syndrome
2. Hallgren syndrome

C. Mental retardation
1. Rubella
2. Lowe syndrome
3. Cockayne syndrome
4. Down syndrome
5. Hallermann-Streiff syndrome
6. Homocystinuria
7. Laurence-Moon-Biedl syndrome
8. Marinesco-Sjögren syndrome
9. Trisomy 13–15
10. Turner syndrome
11. Galactosemia
12. Megalocornea
13. Hypoglycemia
14. Mannosidosis
15. Cerebral cholesterinosis
16. Crome syndrome
17. Rubinstein-Taybi syndrome

associated with other systemic abnormalities. Eight percent to 23% of congenital cataracts are familial. The most frequent mode of inheritance is autosomal dominant with almost complete penetrance, and transmission is regular throughout the generations. These defects occur as total cataracts, anterior and posterior polar cataracts, lamellar cataracts, or nuclear opacities. Autosomal recessive cataracts are less frequent and occur in consanguineous unions. X-linked heredity is rare, and the affected males have dense, nuclear cataracts that may remain stationary or progress to maturity. Microcorneas are associated defects. Female carriers exhibit sutural cataracts that do not affect visual acuity; the corneas are normal to only slightly reduced in diameter.[32]

Cataracts Associated With Syndromes and Systemic Diseases

Many cataracts are associated with syndromes and other systemic diseases. These syndromes with their systemic and ocular findings and modes of inheritance are listed in Table 20A–2, and representative syndromes are presented in Figures 20A–6 to 20A–10.

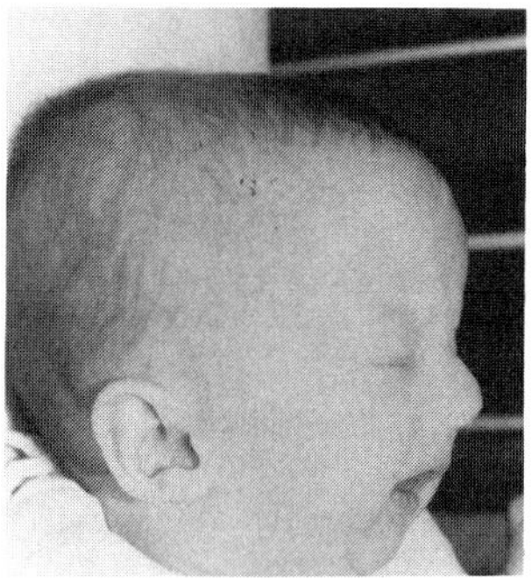

FIG 20A–6.
Hallermann-Streiff-François syndrome with bilateral complete congenital cataracts, bird facies, thin beaked nose, and micrognathia.

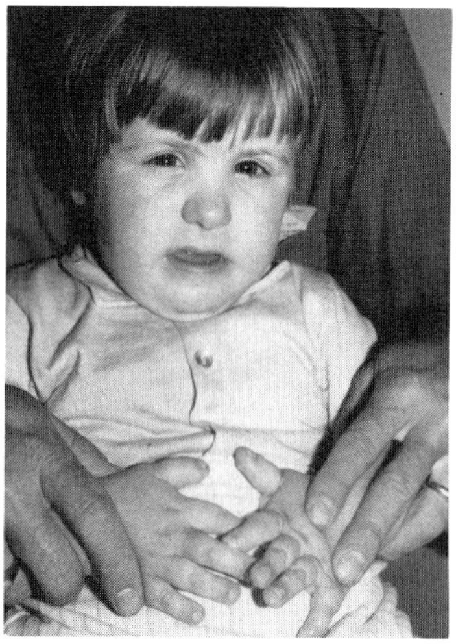

FIG 20A–7.
Mentally retarded child with Rubinstein-Tabyi syndrome. Note the broad thumbs, microcephaly, prominent forehead, and wide nasal bridge.

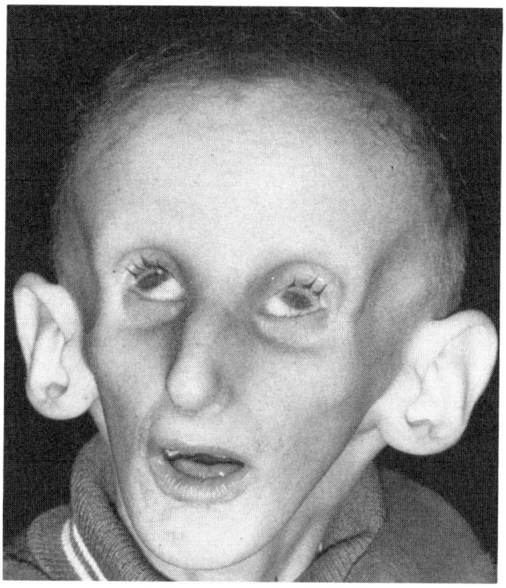

FIG 20A–8.
Teenage child with Cockayne syndrome. Bilateral aphakia, band keratopathy, absent dentition, deafness, cachetic dwarfism, and premature aging are noted.

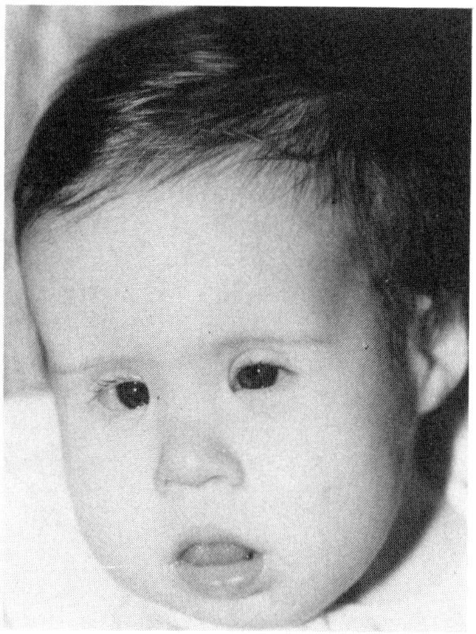

FIG 20A–9.
Down syndrome infant with typical facies, bilateral cataracts leading to aphakia, and bilateral epikeratophakia grafts.

TABLE 20A–2.
Syndromes Associated With Infantile Cataracts

Disorder	Inheritance	Systemic Findings	Ocular Findings	Lens
Craniofacial syndromes				
Crouzon disease (craniofacial dysostosis)	AD	Multiple synostoses, midface hypoplasia, prognathism	Shallow Orbits, exophthalmos V-pattern exotropia, late optic atrophy, microcornea, iris and choroidal colobomas, pupillary irregularities, retinal detachment	Occasional cataract
Apert syndrome (acrocephalosyndactyly)	Often AR	Oxycephaly (tower skull), midface hypoplasia, symmetrical syndactyly	Hypertelorism, strabismus, blepharoptosis	Rare cataract (usually zonular or lamellar), occasional, ectopia lentis
Engelmann disease	Variable, can be AD	Osteoclastic bone dystrophy with overgrowth of skull and skeleton, limb pain, muscular weakness, hypocalcemia	Exophthalmos, papilledema, optic atrophy, abducens palsy, blepharoptosis	Cortical dot cataracts, progressive, secondary to hypocalcemia
Lanzieri syndrome		Dwarfism, dyscephaly, congenital dental, and skin anomalies	Microphthalmos, anophthalmia, colobomas of iris, choroid, retina, and optic disc	Congenital cataract
Oxycephaly	AD	Tower skull, seizure disorder, mental retardation	Exophthalmos, optic atrophy	Occasional cataract
Rubinstein-Taybi syndrome		See apical syndromes		
Conradi syndrome		See skeletal syndromes		
Mandibulofacial syndromes				
Hallerman-Streiff syndrome (François syndrome) (mandibular oculofacial dyscephaly) (Fig 20A–6)	Sporadic, possibly AR	Birdlike facies, micrognathia, maldeveloped temporomandibular joint, teeth erupted at birth with early caries, small stature, sparse hair, low-set ears, joint hyperextensibility, pulmonary insufficiency	Relative nanophthalmos, high hypermetropic strabismus, nystagmus, peripapillary atrophy, coloboma of iris, retina, choroid, optic disc	Bilateral dense congenital cataracts, lens may spontaneously resorb

(Continued)

TABLE 20A–2 (cont.).

Disorder	Inheritance	Systemic Findings	Ocular Findings	Lens
Pierre Robin syndrome	Sporadic	Mandibular hypoplasia, glossoptosis, cleft palate, 1/3 have Stickler's syndrome (see skeletal syndromes)	Esotropia, microphthalmos, high myopia, glaucoma, retinal detachment	Rare congenital cataract
Treacher Collins syndrome (mandibulofacial dysostosis) (Franceschetti syndrome)	AD	Malar and mandibular hypoplasia, external ear defects, deafness	Antimongoloid slant of palpebral fissures, coloboma of lateral third of lower eyelid Microphthalmos	Rare cataract, rare ectopia lentis
Aberfeld-Schwartz-Jampel syndrome	Possibly AR	Dwarfism, myotonia, hypokalemia, muscle atrophy, hypoplastic facial bones	Blepharophimosis, strabismus, myopia, microcornea, posterior synechiae	Congenital cataract
Smith-Lemli-Opitz syndrome (cerebrohepatorenal syndrome)	AR	Mental retardation, microcephaly, hypotonia, low-set ears, high-arched palate, congenital pyloric stenosis, hepatomegaly, intrahepatic biliary dysgenesis, renal cysts, genital anomalies, congenital heart disease, syndactyly, death in early infancy	Synophrys, blepharoptosis, epicanthal folds, strabismus, nystagmus, optic nerve demyelination	Congenital cataract
Marshall syndrome		See dermatologic syndromes		
Skeletal syndromes				
Conradi syndrome (congenital stippled epiphyses)	AD AR	Abnormal calcium deposition, short limbs, joint stiffness, syndactyly, Micrognathia, Club foot, Dislocated hips, Craniosynostosis, early death (recessive form), from calcium deposition, in cardiac valves	Heterochromia iridis, optic atrophy, prominent Schwalbe's line, iridocorneal synechiae, iris hypoplasia	Early-onset, complete cataracts (recessive form), cataract less common in dominant form

Marfan syndrome	AD	Tall stature, arachnodactyly, joint hyperextensibility, congenital heart disease, dissecting aortic aneurysms	High refractive errors, strabismus, amblyopia, retinal detachment	Ectopia lentis, rare cataract
Albers-Schönberg disease (osteopetrosis, marble bone disease)	AD AR	Osteoclastic bone dystrophy, with dense sclerosis of long bones and base of skull, fatal when congenital and AR	Cranial nerve compression, strabismus, optic atrophy	Rare congenital cataract
Van der Hoeve syndrome (osteogenesis imperfecta)	AD, rarely AR	Brittle bones, deafness, dental anomalies	Blue sclera, glaucoma	Cataract
Weill-Marchesani syndrome	AR	Short stature, stubby hands and feet, brachycephaly	Lenticular myopia, pupillary-block glaucoma	Frequent ectopia lentis and microspherophakia, occasional cataract
Stickler syndrome (hereditary progressive arthro-ophthalmopathy)	AD	Joint anomalies with hyperextensibility and pain, long limbs, midfacial hypoplasia, micrognathia, cleft palate	High axial myopia, high astigmatism, vitreal degeneration, retinal pigment epithelial atrophy, lattice retinal degeneration, retinal detachments, giant retinal tears, keratopathy, strabismus	Complicated cataract, occasional cataract, prior to retinal detachment
Kwiest syndrome (achondrodystrophy)	AD	Disproportionate dwarfism, moon facies, saddle nose, short arms and legs, joint swelling, motor retardation, hearing deficit, muscular weakness, cleft palate, normal intelligence	High myopia, vitreoretinal degeneration, giant retinal tear following cataract extraction	Rare cataract
Sprangler rhizomelic dwarfism, (Sprangler-Wiedemann syndrome)		Connective tissue disorder involving spine and epiphyses of long bones and pelvis, cleft palate, deafness	Progressive high myopia, lattice retinal degeneration, strabismus, iritis with posterior synechiae, retinal detachment, glaucoma	Secondary cataract in adolescence

(Continued)

TABLE 20A–2 (cont.).

Disorder	Inheritance	Systemic Findings	Ocular Findings	Lens
Albright hereditary osteodystrophy, (pseudohypoparathyroidism syndrome)	AD	Short stature, mental retardation, intracranial calcifications, two forms of disease (pseudohypoparathyroid and pseudopseudohypoparathyroidism)	Strabismus, blue sclera, papilledema, hypertelorism, keratitis, scleral calcification	Punctate cataract common with pseudohypoparathyroidism but rare with pseudopseudohypoparathyroidism
Chondrodysplasia punctata	AD or AR	Bony dysplasia, commonly death in first year of life		Cataract uncommon in AD, frequent in AR form
Robert syndrome	AR	Cleft lip, cleft palate, phocomelia, prominent phallus	Hypertelorism	Congenital cataract
Pena-Shokeir II syndrome (COFS syndrome) (Cerebro-oculofacioskeletal syndrome)	AR	Large ear pinnae, hypotonia, microcephaly, osteoporosis, early death, kyphosis, scoliosis	Microphthalmos, blepharophimosis, nystagmus	Cataract
Apical syndromes				
Laurence-Moon-Bardet-Biedl syndrome (Retinitis pigmentosa–polydactyly–adiposogenital syndrome)	Usually AR, may be AD or XR	Mental retardation, obesity, hypogenitalism, polydactyly, congenital heart disease	Retinitis, nystagmus, strabismus	Lamellar cataract
Meyer-Schwickerath syndrome (oculodentodigital dysplasia)	Probably AR	Syndactyly, camptodactyly of 4th and 5th finger, hypoplastic nasal alae, dental enamel hypoplasia	Microphthalmos, iris anomalies	Occasional cataract
Rubinstein-Taybi syndrome (Fig 20A–7)	Polygenetic or possibly AR	Mental retardation, motor retardation, recurrent respiratory infections, broad thumbs, broad great toes, high-arched palate, short stature, obesity, joint hyperextensibility, microcephaly, prominent forehead, broad nasal bridge, beaked nose	Long cilia, antimongoloid slant of palpebral fissures, epicanthal folds, strabismus, blepharoptosis, glaucoma, dacryostenosis, optic atrophy	Frequent congenital cataract

Ellis–van Creveld syndrome (chondroectodermal dysplasia)	AR	Polydactyly, dysplastic nails and teeth, dwarfism, epiphyseal dysplasia, congenital heart defects, may be mentally retarded, dental anomalies, mental retardation	Strabismus, coloboma of iris	Rare congenital cataract
Meckel-Gruber syndrome (dysencephalia splanchnocystica syndrome)	AR	Sloping forehead, posterior encephalocele, short neck, polysyndactyly, polycystic kidneys, cryptorchidism, cleft lip, cleft palate, death in early infancy	Cryptophthalmos, clinical anophthalmia, microphthalmos, mongoloid slant of palpebral fissures, sclerocornea, microcornea, aniridia, retinal dysplasia, posterior staphyloma optic nerve hypoplasia	Congenital cataract
Central nervous system syndromes				
Sjögren syndrome (Sjögren-Larsson syndrome)	AR	Mental retardation, congenital ichthyosis	Hypertelorism, atypical retinitis pigmentosa	Congenital cataract (usually zonular, can be polar or total)
Marinesco-Sjögren syndrome (congenital spinocerebellar ataxia–congenital cataract oligophrenia syndrome)	AR	Mental retardation, cerebellar ataxia	Epicanthal folds, nystagmus, esotropia	Zonular congenital cataract
Zellweger syndrome (oculocerebrohepatorenal syndrome)		Hypotony, hepatomegaly, albuminuria, lethal syndrome	Corneal opacity, microphthalmos, retinal hole, glaucoma, optic disc anomalies	Cataract
Krause syndrome (congenital encephalo-ophthalmic dysplasia)	Sporadic	Congenital cerebral dysplasia, hydrocephalus, microcephaly	Microphthalmos, blepharoptosis, strabismus, secondary glaucoma, iris atrophy, scleral atrophy, retinal and choroidal dysplasia, coloboma, intraocular hemorrhages	Congenital cataract

(Continued)

TABLE 20A–2 (cont.).

Disorder	Inheritance	Systemic Findings	Ocular Findings	Lens
Hallgren syndrome (retinitis pigmentosa–deafness–ataxia syndrome)	AR	Mental retardation, deafness, ataxia	Retinitis pigmentosa, nystagmus	Cataract
Meckel-Gruber syndrome		See apical syndromes		
Muscular diseases				
Myotonic dystrophy	AD	Myotonia, muscular wasting, hypogonadism, cardiomyopathy	Pigmentary retinopathy	Anterior and posterior subcapsular cataract in 1st decade of life (punctate and flake opacities)
Walker-Warburg syndrome (Cerebro-ocular dysplasia–muscular dystrophy [COD-MD] syndrome)	AR	Hydrocephaly, congenital muscular dystrophy	Microphthalmos, retinal dysplasia	Cataract, posterior lenticonus
Dermatologic syndromes				
Congenital anhidrotic ectodermal dysplasia	XR	Anhidrosis, hypotrichosis, dental anomalies	Microphthalmos corneal degeneration	Cataract
Rothmund-Thomson syndrome (infantile poikiloderma)	AR	Skin atrophy, telangiectasis, sparse hair, absent dentition, hypogonadism	Hypertelorism, madarosis, retinal hyperpigmentation	Congenital lamellar or complete cataract or cataract at age 2 to 7 yr
Marshall syndrome (oculoauditory ectodermal dysplasia)	AD	Saddle nose, midfacial hypoplasia, frontal bossing, acquired hearing defect	High myopia, secondary glaucoma	Congenital cortical or posterior polar cataract or juvenile posterior subcapsular cataract, spontaneous absorption of cataract
Shafer syndrome (congenital dyskeratosis)	Probably XR	Palmar and plantar keratosis hyperhidrosis, alopecia, thickened nails, microcephaly, hypogenitalism	Corneal lesions	Congenital cataract
Congenital ichthyosis	Various modes, AD (ichthyosis vulgaris), AR (ichthyosiform erythroderma)	Hyperkeratosis, scaling	Punctate keratitis, corneal opacities	Congenital cataract

Siemens syndrome (hereditary ectodermal dysplasia)	AR, males > females	Alopecia, mental retardation, anhidrosis, hypotrichosis	Madarosis, dry eye, ectropion, corneal erosions	Congenital cataract
Bloch-Sulzberger syndrome (incontinentia pigmenti)	XD, seen only in females	Bullous skin eruptions changing to areas of hyperpigmentation, dental anomalies, skeletal anomalies, mental retardation	Strabismus, optic atrophy, nystagmus, retrolental pseudoglioma	Cataract
Cockayne syndrome (Fig 20A–8)	AR	Photosensitive dermatitis, short stature, hyperostosis of skull, intracranial calcifications, deafness, precocious puberty, mental retardation, precocious senile appearance	Enophthalmos, retinal pigmentary degeneration, strabismus, optic atrophy	Unilateral or bilateral cataract
Hutchinson-Gilford syndrome (progeria)	Unknown	Short stature, atrophy of skin and subcutaneous adipose tissue, oligodentia, premature arteriosclerosis	Microphthalmos	Cataract
Gorlin-Goltz syndrome (basal cell nevus syndrome)	AD	Multiple basal cell nevi, rib anomalies, kyphoscoliosis	Hypertelorism, glaucoma, corneal leukomas	Cataract
Bonnevie-Ullrich syndrome (pterygolymphangiectasia)	Female preponderance	Hyperplastic skin, hypertrichosis, facial paralysis	Epicanthal folds, blepharoptosis, ocular palsy	Congenital cataract
Curtius syndrome (ectodermal dysplasia with ocular malformations)		Hypodontia, ichthyosis, acrofacial syndactylic dysostosis	Hypertelorism, nystagmus, tapetoretinal degeneration, coloboma	Congenital cataract
Ward syndrome (epitheliomatous phakomatosis)	AD	Basal cell nevi, epithelioima adenoides cysticum	Hypertelorism, eyelid nevi, congenital corneal opacity, colobomas	Congenital cataract
Renal diseases				
Lowe syndrome (oculocerebrorenal syndrome)	XR	Mental retardation, growth retardation, hypotonia, renal rickets,	Glaucoma, anterior chamber cleavage defects	Congenital cataract (usually complete in a small, poorly differen-

(Continued)

TABLE 20A–2 (cont.).

Disorder	Inheritance	Systemic Findings	Ocular Findings	Lens
		renal tubular acidosis, aminoaciduria		tiated lens), female carriers have central or cortical cataracts that do not impair vision
Alport syndrome (hereditary familial congenital hemorrhagic nephritis)	AD, possibly XR	Hemorrhagic nephritis, sensorineural hearing loss	Retinal pigment, epitheliopathy	Progresive anterior lenticonus, subcapsular cataract
Potter syndrome (renal agenesis syndrome)	May be form of trisomy 18	Flat nasal bridge, low-set ears, micrognathia, cystic renal dysplasia or renal agenesis, spina bifida	Hypertelorism, epicanthal folds, antimongoloid slant of palpebral fissure	Cataract
Zellweger syndrome	Chromosomal anomaly	See central nervous system disorders		
Miscellaneous syndromes				
Norrie disease	XR	Mental retardation, hearing defects	Bilateral retrolental mass of detached retina, elongated ciliary process, phthisis bulbi	Complete cataract in early childhood
Congenital hemolytic icterus	AD with variable penetrance	Icterus, splenomegalic anemia, abnormal erythrocyte fragility	Microphthalmos	Bilateral cataracts
Pseudo-Turner syndrome (Noonan syndrome)	Sporadic	Mental retardation, short stature, pulmonic stenosis, Turner's syndrome phenotype	Blepharoptosis, hypertelorism, myopia, keratoconus, strabismus	
Prematurity	Sporadic	Bronchopulmonary dysplasia, intraventricular hemorrhages	Retinopathy of prematurity, myopia, strabismus	Usually transient bilateral, symmetrical, vacuolar cataracts anterior to the posterior lens capsule
Metabolic and endocrine diseases				
Hypocalcemia (hypoparathyroidism, pseudohypoparathyroidism, idiopathic hypocalcemia of infancy,				Morphology of cataract related to time of hypocalcemia; intrauterine: embryonal or fetal nu-

and steatorrhea) (Fig 20A–10)				clear opacity; infancy: zonular opacities; older child: discrete white cortical opacities
Hypoglycemia		Neonatal hypoglycemia: low birth weight, complicated pregnancy		Zonular cataracts
Galactosemia galactose-1-phosphate uridyl transferase deficiency	AR	Hepatosplenomegaly, mental retardation		"Oil droplet" cataracts from diffusion of galactose into lens and converting into dulcitol; cataract forms in first weeks of life, progressing to a mature cataract
Galactokinase deficiency	AR			Early-onset bilateral cataracts, heterozygote forms cataracts later in life
Diabetes mellitus (infant of diabetic mother)		Large for gestational age		Children of diabetic mothers have a higher incidence of congenital cataracts
Thyroid disease (infant of dysthyroid mother)				Children of dysthyroid mothers have a higher incidence of congenital cataracts
Fabry disease (ceramide trihexosidase deficiency)	XR	Proteinuria, hematuria, keratinized angiomatous skin lesions, painful paresthesias	Whorl-like corneal opacities	Feathery, spokelike cataract of posterior sutures, posterior subcapsular cataract, inferior wedge-shaped anterior subcapsular cataract
Refsum disease (phytanic acid hydroxylase deficiency)	AR	Cerebellar ataxia, peripheral polyneuropathy, tremors, pes cavus	Retinal pigmentary degeneration, nystagmus, corneal epithelial degeneration, glaucoma	Posterior subcapsular cataract

(Continued)

TABLE 20A–2 (cont.).

Disorder	Inheritance	Systemic Findings	Ocular Findings	Lens
Mannosidosis (α-mannosidase deficiency)	AR	Psychomotor retardation, coarse facies, hepatosplenomegaly, gibbous deformity, (resembles Hurler syndrome phenotypically)	Strabismus, optic disc pallor	Occasional cataract (spokelike petaloid cataract
Lowe syndrome	XR	See renal diseases		
Alport syndrome	AD, possibly XR	See renal diseases		
Chromosomal disorders				
Down syndrome (Fig 20A–9)	Trisomy 21	Characteristic facies, microcephaly, mental retardation, skeletal anomalies, palmar simian creases, cardiac anomalies	Mongoloid slant of palpebral fissures, epicanthus, esotropia, myopia, Brushfield's spots, peripheral iris hypoplasia, keratoconus	Congenital cataract or arcuate, sutural, or flake-shaped acquired cataracts
Turner syndrome	XO or XO/XX	Webbed neck, mental retardation, cardiac anomalies, renal anomalies	Epicanthal folds, blepharoptosis, strabismus, blue sclera, pigmentation of eyelids, eccentric pupils	Cataracts
Patau syndrome	Trisomy 13–15	Deafness, cleft lip, cleft palate, capillary hemangioma, renal abnormalities, fatal infancy	Microphthalmos coloboma of uvea, persistent hyperplastic primary vitreous, intraocular cartilage, retinal dysplasia, optic nerve hypoplasia, cyclopia	Congenital cataract
Edwards syndrome	Trisomy 18	Low-set ears, micrognathia, high-arched palate, cardiac anomalies, cryptorchidism, mental retardation	Epicanthal fold, blepharoptosis, hypertelorism, corneal opacity, microphthalmos, congenital glaucoma, coloboma of uvea	Congenital cataract
Cat-eye syndrome (Schmid-Fraccaro syndrome) partial G trisomy	Trisomy 13–15 or 21–22	Anal atresia, preauricular fistula, cardiac anomalies	Coloboma of iris, choroid, or retina, microphthalmos	Cataract

*Abbreviations: AD = autosomal dominant; AR = autosomal recessive; XR = X-linked recessive.

Cataracts Associated with Embryopathies

An embryopathy is a nongenetic disease affecting the fetus.

Rubella Syndrome.—The rubella syndrome results from a maternal infection occurring during the first trimester of pregnancy. It is the single most common cause of embryopathic congenital cataracts. The cataracts characteristically are almost complete, with a small portion of clear peripheral lens remaining. The cataracts are the result of the invasion of the lens by rubella virus. Microphthalmos and characteristic retinal pigmentary changes are common (Fig 20A–11).

In addition to the ocular anomalies, cardiac defects, deafness, mental retardation, and hematologic and skeletal defects occur.

Other Infections Causing Cataracts.—Cataracts have also been attributed to rubeola, chickenpox, smallpox, herpes simplex and zoster, poliomyelitis, influenza, hepatitis, infectious mononucleosis, and cytomegalic inclusion disease.

Syphilis is a rare cause of congenital cataracts; cases have been reported in which a congenital cataract involved the embryonic nucleus in association with interstitial keratitis and syphilitic choroiditis.

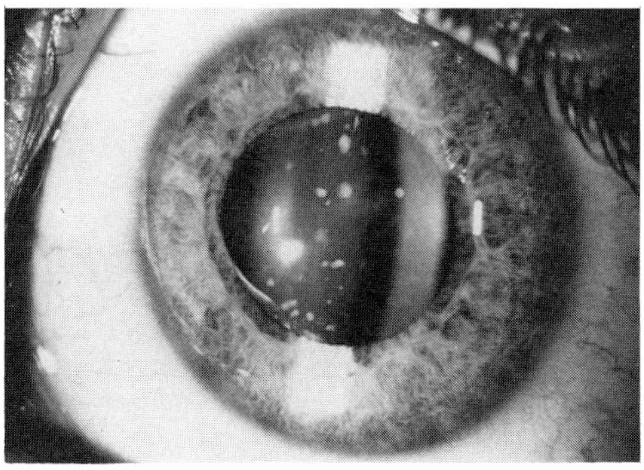

FIG 20A–10.
Discrete white cortical opacities suggesting Down syndrome, diabetes mellitus, myotonic dystrophy, or hypocalcemia.

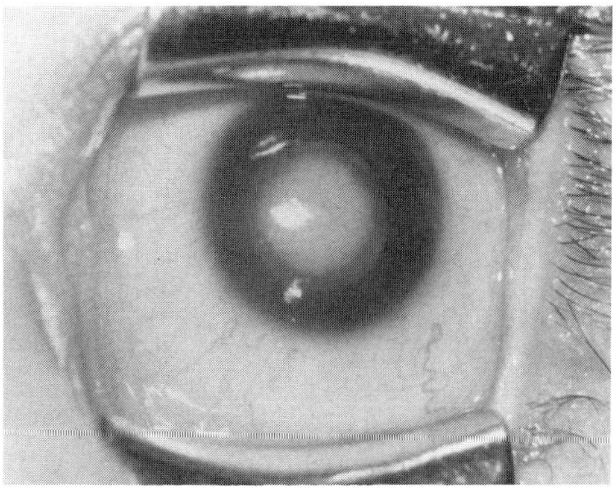

FIG 20A–11.
Rubella syndrome cataract with typical nuclear opacity and liquefied cortex in a microphthalmic eye.

Infantile cataract is rarely seen with congenital toxoplasmosis, but it may occur secondarily to uveitis.

Infestation of the eye with *Toxocara canis* may produce secondary lens opacities.

Toxic Cataracts

Corticosteroids.—Prolonged topical and systemic corticosteroids may lead to irreversible posterior subcapsular cataracts. They occur in patients who have received corticosteroid therapy for longer than 1 year in systemic dosages greater than 15 mg/day.

The cataracts appear as irregular iridescent reflections in the posterior subcapsular area beginning in front of the posterior pole and spreading forward into the cortex and along the surface of the posterior capsule.

Hypoxia.—Intrauterine hypoxia may lead to multiple developmental defects including congenital cataract formation.

Other Toxic Medications.—Other known cataractogenic agents in humans include triparanol, dinitrophenol, dinitro-*o*-cresol, bis(phenylisopropyl)-piperazine, busulfan, chlorpromazine, and sodium cyanate.

Cataracts Secondary to Ionizing Radiation

Ionizing radiation, including x-rays and gamma rays, penetrate the cornea and disrupt the lens epithelial cells and cortical fibers. The immature lens is more radiosensitive. Intrauterine radiation–induced cataracts are possible but have not been documented.

Low doses of radiation (250 to 800 R) cause the germinal pre-equatorial cells to cease mitotic division; later they resume mitosis at an accelerated rate and form abortive cells that migrate to the posterior pole where they accumulate as dust like opacities in the posterior subcapsular region. Radiation in excess of 1,000 R accentuates this process, but the epithelial cells cease forming new fibers. The youngest fibers fail to dehydrate and gradually become opaque.

Cataracts Secondary to Ocular Disease or Anomalies

Cataracts in children may be produced secondarily to ocular diseases. These consist of:

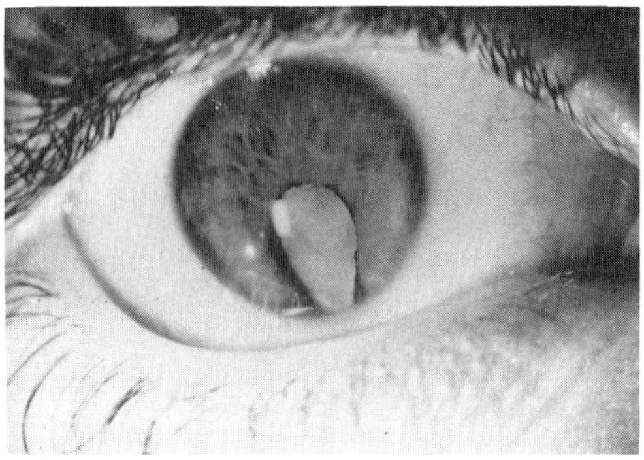

FIG 20A–12.
Microphthalmos: typical iris coloboma and mature cataract.

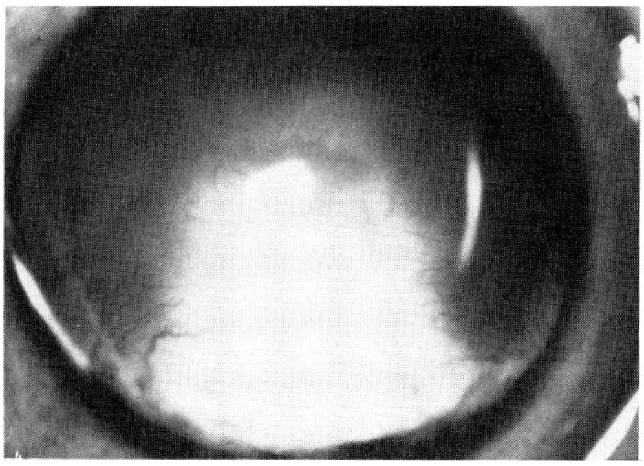

FIG 20A–13.
Persistent hyperplastic primary vitreous with dense fibrovascular plaque, a clear microspherophakic lens, and elongated ciliary processes.

- Trauma
- Retrolental fibroplasia
- Congenital glaucoma
- Retinoblastoma
- Uveitis
- Retinal detachment
- Retinitis pigmentosa

Ocular anomalies also associated with a variety of infantile cataracts include:

- Microphthalmos (Fig 20A–12)
- Keratoconus
- Sclerocornea
- Anterior chamber cleavage syndrome (mesodermal dysgenesis)
- Coloboma
- Aniridia
- Heterochromia
- Persistent pupillary membrane
- Ectopia lentis
- Retinal dysplasia
- Megalocornea
- Persistent hyperplastic primary vitreous (Fig 20A–13)
- Posterior lenticonus and lentiglobus

ECTOPIA LENTIS

A clear or cataractous lens may be displaced, subluxated, or dislocated from the visual axis, thereby inducing refractive errors, astigmatism, decreased visual acuity with amblyopia, photophobia, unilateral diplopia, or bilateral quadropia. These usually bilateral defects are frequently associated with systemic diseases and are asymetrical in position. Unilateral dislocations most frequently follow trauma.

The supporting zonular lens fibers may be absent or weakened and stretched in localized segments thus producing colobomas, or are generalized weaknesses leading to spherophakia. The lens may also dislocate into the anterior chamber or vitreous.

Syndromes associated with ectopia lentis are described in Table 20A–3[33] and Figures 20A–14 and 20A–15.

CATARACT SURGERY

Any discussion of pediatric cataract surgery must be prefaced by outlining the indications for cataract surgery. The following are my current recommendations.

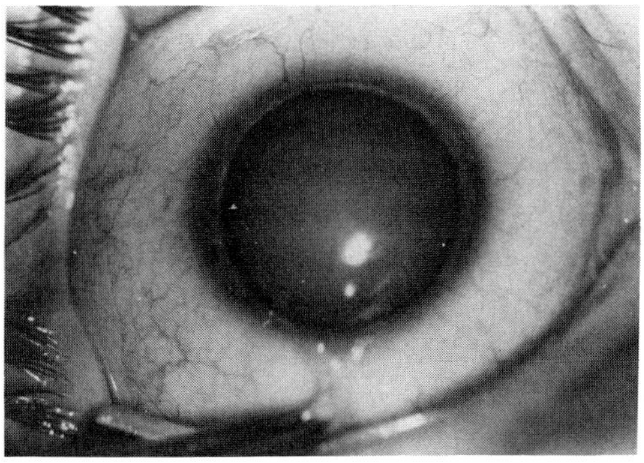

FIG 20A–14.
Spherophakia, an isolated finding, but more commonly associated with systemic syndromes.

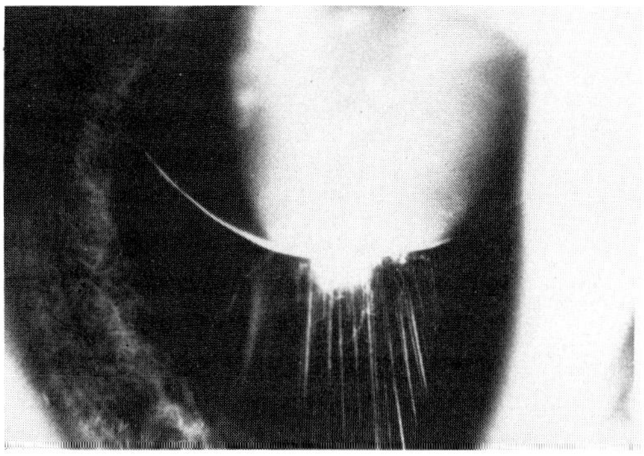

FIG 20A–15.
Upward displacement of the lens, with stretched and broken zonules in a child with Marfan syndrome.

Conservative Cataract Management

Some children have cataracts compatible with good and prolonged visual development.[31] Frequent re-evaluation of the visual reflexes or acuity is required to ascertain the progression of visual development, however. Atropine dilation with refractive error correction and +2.50 bifocals in tinted glasses is recommended. Occlusion of the fellow eye prevents amblyopia in patients with unilateral or asymmetrical bilateral cataracts. Surgery is deferred until fixation is lost, vision decreases, strabismus occurs, or school performance lags behind the child's learning capability.

Surgical Indications

Bilateral Cataracts

Infants with bilateral complete cataracts are often diagnosed early in life with leukokoria (white pupil), a lack of visual attention, or the onset of nystagmus or strabismus.[34, 35] Cataract surgery and optical rehabilitation must be accomplished before the onset of nystagmus, which occurs between 2 to 3 months of age, to secure central visual fixation (Fig 20A–16).

TABLE 20A–3.
Disorders Associated With Ectopia Lentis

Disorder	Inheritance	Systemic Findings	Ocular Findings	Lens
Ocular disorders				
Simple congenital ectopia lentis	AD, occasionally AR		Lenticular myopia, glaucoma, retinal detachment	Upward subluxation, microspherophakia, complicated cataract
Ectopia lentis et pupillae	AR		Oval or slit-shaped pupil	Ectopia lentis
Spherophakia (Fig 20A–14)	Unknown		Colobomas of uvea, pupillary membrane, cornea plana, glaucoma, microphthalmos	Spherophakia, ectopia lentis
Concussive ocular trauma			Hyphema, glaucoma, choroidal rupture, retinal detachment, optic nerve injury	Subluxation, luxation, cataract
Aniridia	AD or sporadic	Wilms' tumor in sporadic cases	Rudimentary iris, macular hypoplasia, nystagmus, glaucoma, corneal opacity	Ectopia lentis, anterior polar cataract
Anterior megalophthalmos	XR		Megalocornea, iris and angle abnormalities, ectopic pupil	Ectopia lentis, cataract
Systemic disorders				
Marfan syndrome (Figure 20A–15)	AD	Tall stature, arachnodactyly, joint laxity, congenital heart disease, dissecting aortic aneurysm	High refractive errors, strabismus, amblyopia, retinal detachment	Usually upward subluxation, rarely cataract
Homocystinuria (cystathionine B synthetase deficiency)	AR	Mental retardation, osteoporosis, tall stature, arachnodactyly, thromboembolism	Secondary glaucoma, retinal detachment, thickened zonules	Inferior or inferonasal subluxation, luxation into vitreous or anterior chamber
Weill-Marchesani syndrome	AR	Short stature, stubby hands and feet, brachycephaly	Myopia, secondary glaucoma	Microspherophakia, ectopia lentis

Crouzon disease (craniofacial dysostosis)	AD	Multiple synostoses, midface hypoplasia, prognathism	Shallow orbits, exophthalmos, V-pattern exotropia, late optic atrophy, microcornea, iris and choroidal colobomas, pupillary irregularities, retinal detachment	Occasional cataract, ectopia lentis
Apert syndrome (acrocephalosyndactyly)	Often AR	Oxycephaly (tower skull), midface hypoplasia, symmetrical syndactyly	Hypertelorism, strabismus, blepharoptosis	Rarely cataract (usually zonular or lamellar), occasional ectopia lentis
Treacher Collins syndrome (mandibulofacial dysostosis; Franceschetti syndrome)	AD	Malar and mandibular hypoplasia, external ear defects, deafness	Antimongoloid slant of palpebral fissures, coloboma of lateral third of lower eyelid, microphthalmos	Rarely cataract, rarely ectopia lentis
Ehlers-Danlos syndrome	AD with low penetrance	Thin hyperelastic atrophic skin, excessive articular laxity, dissecting aortic aneurysm	Angioid streaks, blue sclera, keratoconus, choroidal hemorrhages	Ectopia lentis following minor trauma
Sulfite oxidase deficiency	AR	Progressive muscular rigidity, decerebrate behavior, death in early childhood		Ectopia lentis
Rieger syndrome	AD	Hypodontia, hypoplastic maxilla, umbilical hernia	Microphthalmos, congenital glaucoma, iris hypoplasia, acentric pupil, posterior embryotoxon	Ectopia lentis
Hyperlysinemia	AR	Hypotonia, mental retardation, seizure disorder, joint hyperextensibility	Strabismus	Ectopia lentis, spherophakia
Congenital syphilis		Mental retardation, deafness, anemia, hepatosplenomegaly, mucocutaneous lesions, periostitis, dental deformities, depressed nasal bridge, frontal bossing	Dacryocystitis, optic atrophy, gumma of conjunctiva, eyelid, and orbit, uveitis, glaucoma, interstitial keratitis, retinitis, choroiditis	Ectopia lentis

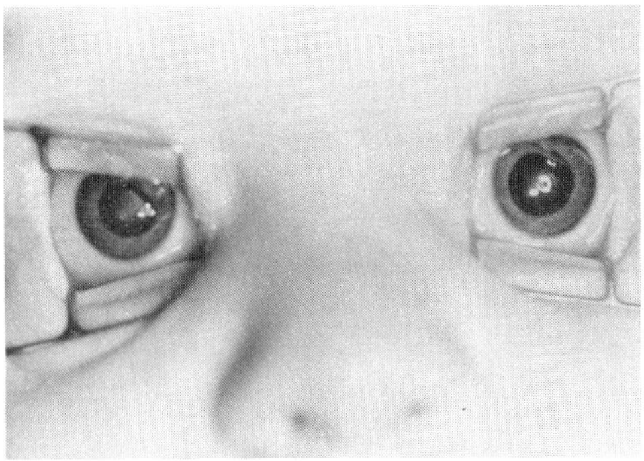

FIG 20A–16.
Bilateral incomplete asymmetrical cataracts in an infant that are significant enough for surgical intervention.

Infants with symmetrical, dense, axial, or complete bilateral infantile cataracts require surgery of one eye within the first week of life.[36] The second eye is operated on 1 to 2 weeks later, depending upon the residual surgical inflammation remaining in the first eye. This schedule permits surgery and optical rehabilitation of the second eye to occur within the sensitive period, yet after the possible onset of uveitis, endophthalmitis, or pupillary-block or angle-closure glaucoma in the first eye.

Children with asymmetrical bilateral cataracts may develop amblyopia secondary to occlusion of the visual axis by the cataract or after surgical aphakia.[37] Aphakic optical correction and amblyopia occlusion therapy for the phakic eye is recommended to achieve equal vision in each eye.

Patients with bilateral, incomplete progressive cataracts may exhibit increasing behavioral abnormalities associated with visual loss as the cataracts become more opaque.[37] However, this slow progression of lens opacification permits early visual development with an enhanced aphakic visual result. In older children, cataract surgery is indicated when the corrected visual acuity falls below 20/70 with pupillary dilation and full optical correction. Glare testers may be used to detect reduced visual efficiency in the home or school situations. Often the visual acuity noted in a clinical environment is better than that achieved casually by the child in his own environment, which suggests that these patients may require cataract surgery earlier because of reduced acuity induced by glare.

Unilateral Cataracts

Children with large, dense, axial, unilateral cataracts discovered in the neonatal period suffer severe deprivation amblyopia and almost uniformly achieve poor aphakic visual results.[37–41] Frequently other ocular defects such as microphthalmos and strabismus coexist, which further reduces visual potential.

Surgery for complete cataracts or those with 3 mm or larger axial opacities should be accomplished within the first week of life or as soon after discovery of the cataract as possible. Patients over the age of 8 to 9 years with unoperated congenital cataracts retain severe, irreversible deprivation amblyopia following cataract surgery and optical rehabilitation. However, cosmetic cataract surgery may be indicated to create a black pupil. Other older children, particularly those with posterior lenticonus, may develop enhanced aphakic vision if they have had an opportunity to develop form vision prior to the formation of dense axial lens opacities.

Traumatic Cataracts

Traumatic cataracts are most often unilateral and very rare in infants. Their onset may be either acute or delayed.[37] Acute cataracts are associated with perforating injuries and ruptured lens capsules. Child abuse should be suspected in infants with ocular trauma. Cataract surgery is performed at the time of the repair of the penetrating wound, but through a separate cataract incision following repair of the initial wound. Cataracts following contusion injuries, ionizing radiation, or traumatic lens dislocation develop increasingly dense lens opacities more slowly, and surgery is performed when the corrected visual acuity decreases to the 20/70 to 20/100 range or when the visual fixation reflex of preverbal children is poorly maintained. Intraocular pressures altered by trauma should be within the normal range prior to surgery.

Children under 6 years of age with traumatic cataracts respond in a similar manner to the cataract's presence and therapy as do patients with unilateral congenital or infantile cataracts. The visual result depends upon the age of the child at the time of the occlusion of the visual axis, the time elapsed before cataract surgery is performed, plus the time lapsed before the placement of the optical correction. The result is also compromised by the effects of the trauma to other ocular structures.

Acquired Cataracts

Surgery of acquired, developmental, or metabolic cataracts is indicated when the visual acuity falls below 20/70 to 20/100 or the fixation reflexes are not well maintained.[35] In patients with chronic intraocular inflammation, the most minimal preoperative anterior chamber reaction of flare and cells is preferred; however, surgery may be performed at any time during the inflammatory cycle. Oral and topical preoperative corticosteroids are used to suppress the inflammation both before and after surgery. Surgery is complicated by the presence of a pupillary membrane, posterior and peripheral anterior synechiae, and smoldering uveitis, which frequently leads to intractable glaucoma and ultimate loss of vision.

The Child's Eye

The child's eye differs markedly from the adult eye in its operative and postoperative responses to surgery. The scleral sac has increased pliancy with decreased rigidity so that when the child's eye is opened there is pressure upon the intraocular contents from scleral collapse, which predisposes to vitreous loss. This loss may be exaggerated by variations of intraocular pressure during various levels of general anesthesia.[42] The anesthesiologist should be informed that the eye is open and, therefore, maintain a steady, deep anesthesia.

Children's eyes exhibit very active inflammatory reactions to injury, with early fibrin excretion and later fibrotic healing processes. These processes may become excessive and lead to peripheral anterior synechiae, pupillary occlusion, cyclitic membranes, vitreous membranes, retinal detachment, glaucoma, or phthisis bulbi. The stimuli to fibrotic overgrowth are trauma and the presence of blood, lens cortex, epithelial cells, uveal elements, and vitreous occurring in abnormal positions within the eye.

Cataract Surgery Techniques

Aspiration-Irrigation

Scheie's small limbal incision aspiration-irrigation procedure originally consisted of a discission of the anterior capsule followed by a separate lens aspiration operation a few days later.[43] With modifications by others, this procedure was soon accomplished as a single operation.[44–46] Anterior chamber depth is maintained through irrigating systems by using secondary corneal ports. The aspirating and irrigating needles can be shifted in these ports to facilitate lens aspiration at the superior pole.

The complications of needle aspiration-irrigation are repeated anterior chamber collapse, lens elements' regurgitation during aspiration, fluid and lens particle turbulence within the anterior chamber with loss of corneal endothelial cells, and posterior capsular rupture with vitreous loss. Vitreous loss requires repeated wound sweeping with cellulose sponges followed by scissors and vitreous excision. Frequently, vitreous remains attached to the wound and distorts the pupil and iris surface. This situation obstructs the pupil and places tension on the peripheral and posterior portions of the retina, which leads to late retinal detachments. Dense, calcified nuclei and cortical material as well as capsular placques have to be extracted with forceps. Intact posterior capsules often opacify and require several secondary discissions.[42, 46, 47]

Automated Aspiration-Irrigation Machines

The Kelman phacoemulsifier disrupts lens elements with a rapidly moving, longitudinally oscillating titanium cylinder driven by a low-frequency ultrasonic transducer.[48] The irrigation fluid, which enters the eye via a silicon sleeve around the titanium needle, maintains the anterior chamber depth and prevents chamber collapse. Aspiration of the disrupted, emulsified lens elements occurs through the titanium needle's bore. The machine's console incorporates a valve system to prevent anterior chamber collapse and lens element regurgitation. The posterior capsule remains intact at the conclusion of the operation because the device cannot emulsify lens capsule or formed vitreous. Operative complications of phacoemulsification are accidental rupture of the posterior capsule leading to vitreous loss and iris trauma leading to synechiae formation.[49]

Other inventors developed machines with small-diameter intraocular tips of concentric tubes or needles.[47] An integrated infusion system or an infusion system through a second corneal port is needed to maintain anterior chamber depth and intraocular pressure during lens aspiration. The cutting mechanism is either adjacent to a port at the tip or is located on the side of the outer needle. A rotating, guillotine or oscillating cutting action is developed by the inner needle. Suction draws the lens elements toward the aspiration port where the cutting mechanism engages and reduces them to small particles that are aspirated from the eye through the bore of the inner needle. These machines also have a control console to allow adjustment of the suction and infusion pressures and to activate the cutting mechanism and its speed. The major drawback of these devices is the prolonged aspiration time required to fragment a hard lens. Fortunately, hard lenses are unusual in infants. They often are not capable of engaging and fragmenting fibrous tissue, plaques, or a thickened hypertrophied lens capsule. Their advantage is the ability, with a single device, to engage and fragment a thin lens capsule, lens cortex, and vitreous and remove them from the eye. This creates a permanent, large, tissue-free visual axis in a single operation (Fig 20A–17).

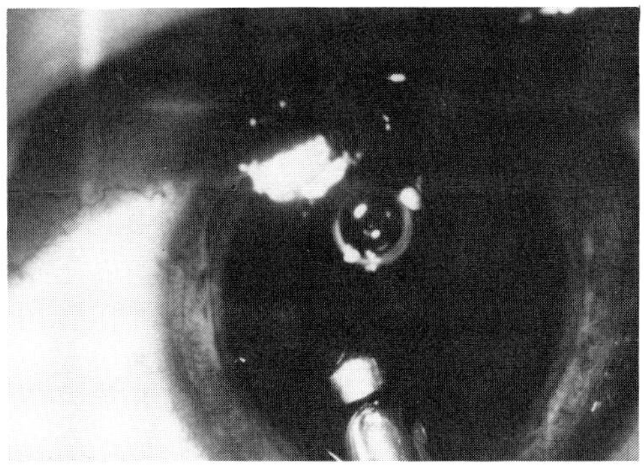

FIG 20A–17.
Clear visual axis after a lensectomy-vitrectomy procedure with a mechanical aspirating-irrigating vitrectomy device.

Limbal Incisions

Either a peritomy or a limbus-based flap is prepared at the 12-o'clock position, and a 3-mm corneoscleral incision is made through the surgical limbus.[47] A wide anterior capsulectomy is performed to remove as many anterior capsular epithelial cells as possible. Aspiration and irrigation of the cortex and nucleus is then accomplished.[42] Pupillary dilatation is maintained by the addition of 1 to 3 ampules of 1:1,000 epinephrine solution without preservative per liter of irrigating solution. The lens cortex at the superior pole is gently teased into the pupillary space by the pull of the suction apparatus or is removed by shifting the aspirating needle to an inferior corneal port.

Pars Plana Incisions

An incision is made through the pars plana. The cutting-aspiration instrument is passed through the incision into the pupillary space, and under direct observation, the posterior capsule, lens cortex, nucleus, and anterior capsule as well as the anterior and central vitreous body are removed.[50, 51]

The Posterior Capsule

The management of the posterior capsule has evolved rapidly with the advent of vitreous suction-cutting devices. Originally the posterior capsule was allowed to remain intact, and a secondary discission was performed 3 to 6 weeks or more after the cataract was aspirated.

In the early 1980s, sodium hyaluronate (Healon) became a readily available viscoelastic agent used for anterior segment surgery. A primary posterior capsulotomy was performed with a discission knife or hook, after the administration of Healon, through the cataract incision and after the eye had been sutured closed. Healon maintained the anterior chamber depth and prevented vitreous displacement.[47]

The more recent approach is to perform a primary posterior capsulotomy with a vitreous suction-cutting instrument and remove a large central section of the posterior capsule as well as the anterior vitreous body.[52–57] This procedure eliminates opaque secondary membranes, occluded pupils, and the hazards of a second anesthesia needed for a discission. The elapsed time to visual recovery is reduced because both optical and amblyopia therapy may be started in the early postoperative period.

Postoperative Complications

Postoperative complications of infantile cataract surgery are secondary membrane formation, peripheral anterior or posterior synechiae, corneal endothelial cell loss with corneal edema and opacification, glaucoma, retinal detachment, and cystoid macular edema (CME).

Secondary membranes arise from the proliferation and metaplastic changes of anterior capsular epithelial cells. Wide anterior capsulotomies remove much of the anterior capsular epithelium, and this reduces the sources of fibrous tissue proliferation.[47, 58–60] In addition, a posterior capsulotomy and anterior vitrectomy remove the posterior capsular and anterior vitreous face matrix necessary for the proliferation of secondary membranes.

The preservation of the corneal endothelial cells remains important because these cells are essential for maintaining corneal transparency.[61] The corneal endothelium has a healing reserve to compensate for some cell loss following injury. The remaining cells enlarge, become pleomorphic, and slide to cover the traumatized corneal endothelium surface. When the population of the corneal endothelial cells is reduced to a critical level, corneal edema with bullous keratopathy ensues, which results in further visual loss.

Aphakic glaucoma is related to surgical trauma, retained lens cortex, secondary surgeries, prolonged postoperative inflammation, posterior and peripheral anterior synechiae, angle closure, and inadequate iridectomies.[62, 63] Prolonged use of corticosteroids may induce glaucoma in steroid responders. Chronic open-angle glaucoma develops slowly and may not become apparent for many years after cataract surgery. Thus continued follow-up of these children into adulthood is mandatory.

The incidence of retinal detachment following aspiration-irrigation cataract extraction techniques has been markedly reduced since we have abandoned multiple discissions, linear extractions, and operations with the retention of the posterior part of the capsule. The surgical correction of pediatric aphakic retinal detachment achieves the same surgical success for reattachment as does the adult aphakic eye.[62, 64, 65]

The occurrence, severity, duration, and effect on vision of CME has not been well documented in infants and children. One series following aspiration-irrigation showed no CME 5 weeks to 4 years after surgery, even if the vitreous face had been disturbed.[66] A second study of Hoyt and Nickel indicated that infant eyes undergoing lensectomy-vitrectomy procedures develop a high percentage of CME. Modifications of technique reduced this complication to a rare occurrence.[67] A third series using oral fluorescein angioscopy in 11 eyes of 7 children following lensectomy-vitrectomy procedures reported no evidence of CME. [68] A fourth study indicated that pars plana lensectomy-vitrectomy may even protect the child's eye against CME formation.[69]

APHAKIC OPTICAL CORRECTION

The optical rehabilitation of the pediatric aphakic eye is one of the most important aspects of the management of children with cataracts. Without the use of a correcting lens, the aphakic image on the retina remains defocused, blurred, and amblyopiogenic.[70]

No Optical Correction

While all children theoretically require aphakic optical correction, some unfortunate ones will not receive such aids.[70] Patients who are severely mentally retarded, combative, or destructive may not tolerate optical devices and may destroy them. Clearing of the visual axis alone may be enough for these children to navigate, dress and feed themselves, and enjoy a greater awareness in their custodial environment.

Children with severe anterior segment disorganization, retinal detachments, optic atrophy, phthisis bulbi, or blind eyes will not benefit from optical correction. Spectacles, cosmetic shells, or contact lenses may be prescribed to minimize unsightly and strabismic blind eyes.

Aphakic Spectacles

Aphakic spectacles with +2.50 bifocal additions remain the primary rehabilitation mode for children 1 to 2 years of age and older with bilateral aphakia. However, children 6 months of age and less have worn spectacles successfully[70] (Fig 20A–18). Low-vision aids using telescopes for distance or magnifiers for near may be incorporated into especially designed aphakic spectacles. Young children often do not wear glasses as well as older children because of the excessive weight of the high-plus lens powers. To reduce this weight, a 20-D Fresnel power prism is applied to a carrier spectacle lens in which the residual sphere, cylinder, and bifocal are incorporated. Plastic aspheric lenses also reduce the weight, but these lenses do not absorb ultraviolet and infrared light rays as well as glass.

Spectacle advantages are no contact with the eye, no ocular discomfort, easy adjustments, and a low loss rate. They also offer another aphakic optical modality following the failure of other modes of aphakic optical correction.

Glasses for correction of unilateral aphakia are almost always unsuccessful because of their high degree of anisometropia and aniseikonia

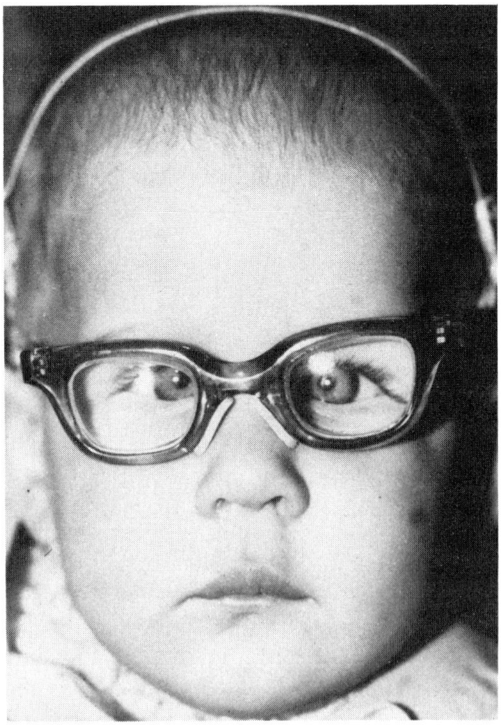

FIG 20A–18.
Infant aphakic spectacles for bilateral aphakia. A headband supports the frames.

that results in diplopia and leads to further suppression and amblyopia. The unilateral aphakic lens is also heavy and cosmetically unsightly. The normal fellow eye should be occluded in children up to 8 years of age to treat the coexistent amblyopia.

One disadvantage of aphakic spectacles is their high magnification that induces spatial disorientation with false projection and depth.[71, 72] Peripheral magnification induces the pincushion effect and concave contraction. Swim, induced by prismatic effects, is a psychological phenomenon caused by rotation of the eyes or head while viewing through the aphakic glasses. Aberrations occurring at the periphery of the aphakic spectacles induce radial astigmatism and curvature of the image plane. A restricted visual field is due to the small sizes of the lenticular glasses, the presence of ring and frame scotomas, and the unrefracted field outside of the spectacle glass. Errors in refraction with the addition of meridional magnification due to astigmatic correction may also be magnified in the aphakic glass. A poor spectacle fit, therefore, contributes to continued amblyopia. Most pediatric wearers of glasses do not complain of the aforementioned aberations, but some children wish to discontinue use of their glasses because of excessive scratches, weight, and poor cosmesis.

Contact Lens

Contact lenses offer increased optical zones, decreased glare and dazzle, and improved cosmetic appearance to the aphakic child. The quality of aphakic vision and the depth and size of the visual field are also enhanced over correction by glasses. Contact lens rehabilitation may be instituted immediately following surgery, which aids in the reduction of amblyopia. Hard contact lens are prescribed for infants because of their ease of insertion into the small interpalpebral spaces. The contact lens are worn with greatest success by patients with acquired unilateral or bilateral cataracts, but patients with infantile cataracts also achieve significant visual successes with their use.[70]

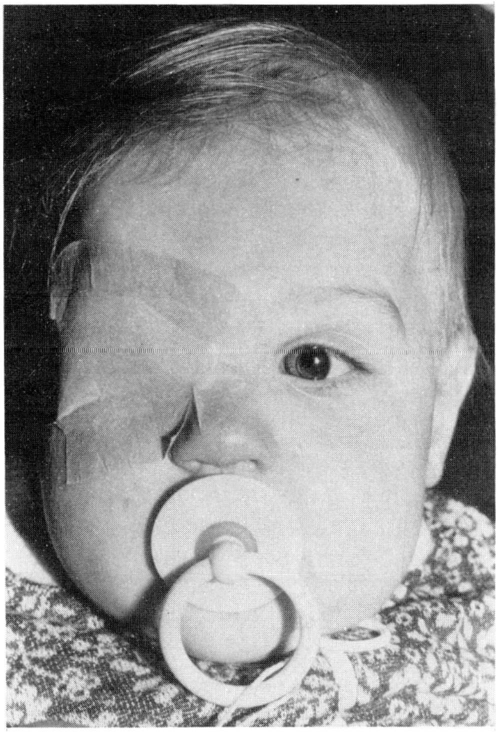

FIG 20A–19.
Aphakic infant with unilateral cataract, hard contact lens, and amblyopia occlusion of the dominant eye.

At the present time, the treatment of choice for infants with cataracts is to remove the lens as early as possible and fit them with hard contact lenses. If contact lens failure occurs, other modalities such as spectacles, secondary intraocular lens (IOL) implants, and epikeratophakia are applied (Fig 20A–19).

Improvements in polymer chemistry have created soft and extended-wear contact lens composed of high–water content hydrogel and silicone polymers. These lens have the advantages of greater comfort, expanded optical zones, and less glare and may be fitted at an earlier postoperative time. Keratometer readings are not necessary, and no corneal abnormalities are induced. However, not all children are able to wear them comfortably. The lenses require frequent maintenance to keep them clean and free of debris. Corneal erosions or abrasions may become contaminated by bacteria residing in the lens and result in severe visual loss. Corneal vascularization, allergy, mucous coating, and precipitates on the lens surface contribute to decreased comfort or cessation of wear. Other disadvantages of soft lenses are their higher replacement rate due to breakage or tearing, greater difficulties of insertion into infant's eyes, and a reduced ability to correct high cylinders in addition to their higher cost per lens.

Contact lens wear reduces retinal image size disparity in unilateral aphakia. However, a residual aniseikonia of 7% to 9% remains.[73] Contact lenses may re-establish single binocular vision in children who possessed it before the onset of the cataract. Other children achieve peripheral fusion because central fusion cannot exist with aniseikonia of 5% to 6% or more.[74, 75] If single binocular vision or peripheral fusion is reduced or absent, motivation for contact lens wear is often poor. Strabismic angles, in the presence of poor visual acuity, may be reduced with contact lens wear, for the lens encourages the redevelopment of peripheral fusion, which helps to maintain a normal ocular alignment. Nystagmus has also been reduced by the application of contact lenses.[70]

The complications of contact lens wear are corneal abrasions, red or irritated eyes, corneal vascularization, and infection. Most complications result from overwear, a poor lens fit, or poor lens hygiene.

Failure to wear a contact lens for prolonged time periods is frequent among children. The reasons for these failures consist of parental disinterest, lens wear difficulties, hostilities toward the lens, difficulties of insertion and removal in active or squirming children, refusal by the child to wear the lens, or the occurrence of intervening ocular pathology. Contact lens failures are greatest within the first 10 years of life and within the first 3 years after the lens has been prescribed.[70] The parents must be willing to withstand the greater cost, care, and frequency of contact lens follow-up visits. The greater weight of the aphakic lenticular contact lens may induce vertical phorias, which lead to additional suppression and amblyopia. If the visual acuity is not adequate or binocularity is absent, children will often lose interest in contact lens wear. The loss rate is higher in patients with hard contact lenses than with the larger, more comfortable soft lenses.

Intraocular Lenses

IOL, continue to play an important role for optical correction of aphakia in children. While the use of IOLs in adults is widespread, the IOL is not as frequently considered for aphakic rehabilitation for children because of the risk of an intraocular device being in a child's eye for many years. However, if the lens is well fixed in the proper position in the eye and the visual axis is clear of iris and lens remnants, vision is developed to the same extent as for other optical devices and remains constant over prolonged periods of time. In addition, as surgeons become more familiar with the technique and as new lens designs are developed, the use of IOLs will continue to increase because the optics are constantly in place and because of high resolution.

Indications for IOL Implantation

Patients are selected for IOL implantation if the parent or the child refuses the concept of contact lens wear, the ophthalmologist deems that contact lens wear would not be successful due to patient or parent noncompliance, or because other social or economic factors preclude adequate contact lens follow-up.[70] The IOL offers the advantage of a full-time optical device, and amblyopia-prone children require only amblyopia occlusion. Over-glasses, if necessary, are well tolerated and accepted by most children. Patients with bilateral cataracts may receive a primary IOL in one eye if that cataract requires surgery while the fellow eye retains useful vision. A secondary IOL may be implanted in an eye that has had cataract surgery and subsequently becomes contact lens noncompliant, especially when the fellow eye's cataract does not require surgery in the near future. These children function as though they had unilateral cataracts.

Contraindications to IOL Implantation

Lens implantations are reserved for children who are contact lens noncompliant. IOL implantation in children should be reserved for patients with unilateral cataracts. Bilateral implantations are generally not indicated because of the lack of sufficient, very long term data relative to the safety and efficacy of pediatric IOL implantation.

Patients with microphthalmic eyes (corneas less than 10 mm in diameter) do not receive implants because the anterior chamber lacks sufficient space to ensure that corneal endothelial touch during or following implantation will not occur. Eyes with congenital, familial, or acquired aniridia following trauma may not provide enough support by the iris root for anterior chamber lenses. If the capsular bag and zonules are intact at the conclusion of the cataract surgery, secure capsular fixation alone may occur with a posterior-chamber "in-the-bag" lens. Eyes with syndrome-related dislocated lenses are not selected for implantation because of their high incidence of retinal detachment and/or secondary glaucoma. Infantile glaucoma eyes also are rejected, for they may redevelop glaucoma that is extremely difficult to control medically or surgically. No IOLs are implanted into eyes with chronic intraocular inflammation, including the rubella syndrome. Late exacerbations of these inflammations that are accompanied by synechiae formation and secondary glaucoma may occur. Eyes with known retinal detachments, macular lesions, optic nerve defects or atrophy, or diabetes with progressive proliferative retinopathy are not IOL candidates.

Intraocular Lens Power

The IOL powers are either selected empirically or are calculated from keratometric readings, A-scan axial lengths, anterior chamber depths, and refractive errors. Calculations of lens powers in young children with changing refractive errors may induce power errors of increasing magnitude, particularly in those receiving implants during the first year of life. An IOL of a power suitable for an adult eye is therefore selected that allows the child's eye to grow toward emmetropia. If the postoperative IOL power is not plano, suitable spectacles with residual sphere, cylinder, and bifocals are prescribed. If the child is older than 10 to 12 years of age, accurate power calculations are determined, and that IOL is implanted. The average power for anterior chamber lenses is 19 D and that for posterior chamber lenses is 20 D.[70, 76]

If an IOL power error is large and the eye has not become severely and irreversibly amblyopic, an IOL exchange may be considered. Removing an IOL from the eye of a child is surgically difficult because of marked synechiae formation that may lead to disruption of the anterior vitreous face, with vitreous loss, the possibility of inducing chronic CME, and corneal endothelial cell loss.

Intraocular Lens Selection

It was originally theorized that an IOL could be implanted into the eyes of babies and that further optical rehabilitation would only require amblyopia occlusion therapy. This concept did not take into consideration the rapid myopic shift that occurs during the first years of life or the prolific production of secondary membranes following cataract surgery.

The iris suture lens offered the advantage of lightweight Prolene loops fixed by iridocapsular adhesions plus the additional fixation supplied by the 10/0 nylon iris suture. This lens was small and did not encroach upon the anterior chamber angle or permit the haptic to become enmeshed within the capsular sac. Complications arose with this lens, and it has been abandoned.

Anterior-Chamber Intraocular Lenses.— As the lensectomy-vitrectomy cataract operation gained increasing popularity among pediatric ophthalmologists, the anterior chamber IOL offered the only possibility of secondary IOL aphakic rehabilitation for these patients. Four-point flexible, open-looped, single-piece polymethylmethacrylate (PMMA) IOLs were selected because of the possibility of slowly decreasing loop compression with resulting expansion of the loops as the child's eye grew (Fig 20A–20). Anterior-chamber IOLs also afford the surgeon the opportunity to implant a primary IOL in those patients in whom the posterior part of the capsule was inadvertently ruptured and vitreous lost during the cataract aspiration.

This style of IOL is recommended for all contact lens–noncompliant children between 3 and 6 years of age as well as for all children over 3 years of age who require secondary lens implantation. If a membrane occurs, a surgical discission under the lens is performed without dislocating the IOL, or Nd-YAG laser capsulotomy may be performed in children older than 6 years of age.

Posterior-Chamber IOLs.—The posterior-chamber lens is implanted in all children 6 years of age and older with otherwise normal anterior segments who are undergoing primary IOL implantation at the time of cataract surgery. Posterior-chamber lenses are selected for primary implantation when the posterior part of the capsule remains intact or has a small central posterior capsulotomy without vitreous presentation following cataract aspiration.[70] The posterior-chamber lens selected is the Sinskey C loop design with 10-degree forward anterior angulation of the haptic Prolene loops[77] (Fig 20A–21).

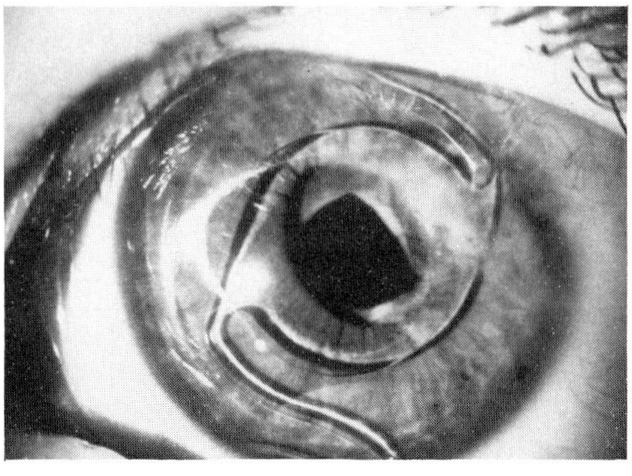

FIG 20A–20.
Secondary, anterior-chamber, single-piece, flexible, 4-point–fixation PMMA IOL. A secondary membrane with a square central opening is seen behind the IOL.

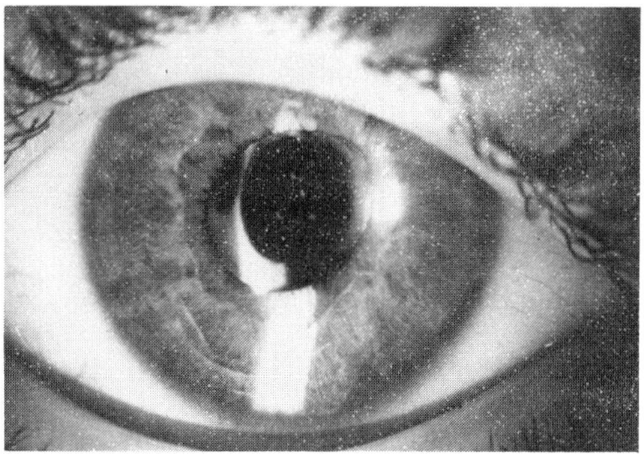

FIG 20A–21.
A primary posterior-chamber IOL with white lens remnants on the anterior surface of the IOL.

Posterior-chamber lens implantation is contraindicated as a secondary procedure unless an intact posterior capsule or adequate peripheral capsule is present to support the lens. In addition, sufficient iris and capsular synechiae formation to the haptics is required to prevent lens malposition, and these synechiae are frequently not forthcoming secondarily, with resultant IOL dislocation.

Nd-YAG laser posterior capsulotomies may be accomplished in children over 6 years of age. This technique induces less trauma to the eye than does an operative discission, does not require general anesthesia, and may be repeated if additional capsular opacification occurs. Patients less than 6 years of age are poor candidates for Nd-YAG laser capsulotomy because they are frightened by the machinery and contact lens application and do not remain sufficiently quiet for accurate focusing of the laser beam. Additionally, the capsulotomy must be performed under general endotracheal anesthesia, with the child placed in an upright position at the laser, which is often located outside of the operating room environment.

EPIKERATOPHAKIA

Epikeratophakia corneal onlay refractive grafts are the latest alternative to aphakic glasses, contact lenses, and IOLs.

Epikeratophakia consists of the applica-

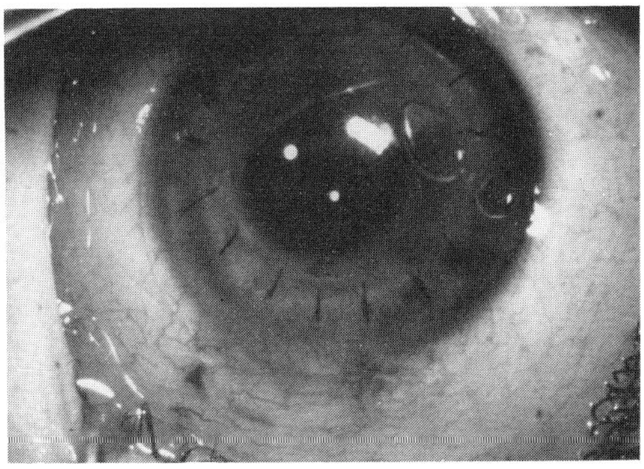

FIG 20A–22.
Clear epikeratophakia graft with sutures in place and covered with a bandage contact lens.

tion of human donor corneal tissue that has been microcryolathed to an appropriate power based upon the recipient eye's refraction at the corneal plane, keratometric readings, and A-scan axial lengths (Fig 20A–22). The commercially prepared graft or lenticule is lyophilized and is supplied to the surgeon in a dry, nonsterilized state. The graft is rehydrated in a gentamicin-balanced salt solution for 20 minutes prior to application.[78]

Epikeratophakia Indications

Epikeratophakia is indicated for optical correction of cataract lens-intolerant or –noncompliant children with traumatic, congenital, or acquired unilateral and bilateral cataracts. The graft may be applied primarily at the time of cataract aspiration or, more commonly, secondarily for contact lens–noncompliant aphakic children. Bilateral aphakic individuals receive epikeratophakia grafts on each eye, at separate operations, when they become spectacle or contact lens intolerant (Fig 20A–23).

Epigrafts are indicated for those patients in whom traumatic or congenital anterior segment disorganization would not support an IOL or an IOL would induce continued corneal endothelial cell loss or CME. Epigrafts may be applied to eyes following penetrating keratoplasty or with traumatic corneal scars with or without vascularization.[79] Epigrafts are also indicated for patients who have distorted intraocular anterior segments, decreased endothelial cell counts, acquired or congenital maculopathies, nystagmus, controlled glaucoma, and postaphakic retinal detachments. Epigrafts may be applied on the aphakic eyes of Down's syndrome or other retarded, nonself-abusive infants and children.

Timing of Epikeratophakia Application

The timing of aphakic graft application has been altered recently by the findings of Arffa and colleagues who noted significant undercorrections in children 6 months of age and younger.[80] Children over the age of 1 year achieved refraction results closer to emmetropia. Arffa et al. recommend grafts for children over 1 year of age to prevent a significant residual hyperopic refractive error and to avoid the rapid myopic shift with loss of graft power. The cataracts should be removed as early as discovered and a contact lens fitted. If contact lens wear is successful, it remains the method of aphakic optical correction. If contact lens wear fails, a secondary epigraft may be applied.

Epikeratophakia Contraindications

Microphthalmic eyes with corneas less than 9 mm in diameter are rejected for epikeratophakia, for the 7-mm lenticule allows less than 1.5 mm of peripheral cornea for suturing, and vessels are attracted into the host cornea toward the graft.[78] Eyes with poor an-

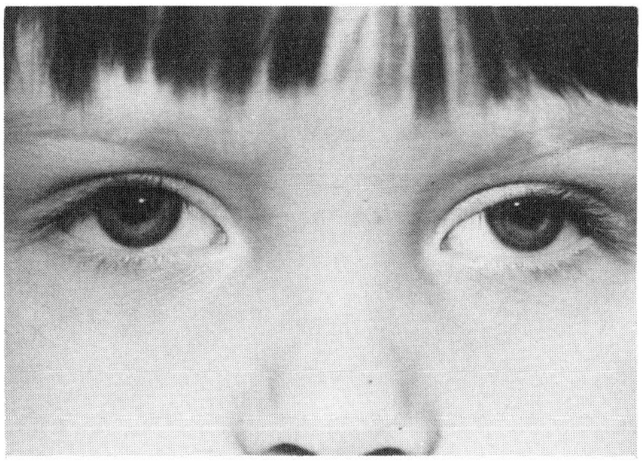

FIG 20A–23.
Secondary bilateral epikeratophakia grafts in 3-year-old child with bilateral aphakia.

ticipated vision secondary to corneal, vitreal, uveal, retinal, or optic nerve pathology are also excluded, as are patients with poor acuity in the fellow eye. Unreliable patients or parents are not candidates, for frequent re-evaluations are necessary for graft success. Debilitated children do not heal as well or as rapidly following epikeratophakia surgery and should not become graft candidates.

Epikeratophakia Advantages

There are many advantages to epikeratophakia. The lenticule, originally devoid of cells, becomes a living human optical device populated by the patient's keratocytes and covered with his own epithelium. Over the central area of the cornea, the posterior lenticule's stroma and host's Bowman's membrane are continuously opposed along the interface but do not become adherent.

The graft provides constant surface optics with stable long-term corneal curvature by keratometric determinations after the third postoperative month. The graft and the axial length of the eye increase normally as the child grows. The grafts do not induce astigmatism but reduce it by as much as 1.75 D. Epigrafts also reduce irregular astigmatism, for the graft covers the patient's irregular corneal surface and presents a regular surface to the incoming image source.[80,81]

Corneal endothelial cell counts are not decreased following surgical application of epigrafts.[82,83] The intraocular pressure may be accurately measured by applanation or Schiotz's tonometry.[84] Corneal sensitivity is decreased in the region of the donor lenticule for the first 2 postoperative years, but the patient retains a normal blink reflex.[85] The epigraft moves with the eye and does not create optical distortions as occurs with glasses. Patients with unilateral aphakia accept and tolerate amblyopia occlusion therapy with less resistance when only one therapeutic parameter is applied to the child at a time.[86] Epikeratophakia grafts may be applied to bilateral aphakic children. Secondary surgery such as strabismus operations, discission of secondary membranes, pupilloplasties, capsulectomies, vitrectomies, retinal detachment, and glaucoma operations may be performed without disturbing the graft.[87]

Cataract surgery may be combined with epigrafting. However, it is my practice following cataract aspiration without epigrafting to treat the child with atropine and antibiotic-corticosteroid topical medications. These eyes exhibit less inflammatory reaction than eyes not receiving these medications. The epigraft is nonviable tissue when applied to the eye. Corticosteroids inhibit re-epithelialization, which may promote infection of the graft, and are therefore avoided in the early postoperative period. The measurements for the epigraft power are recorded at the time of the cataract surgery, and 2 to 3 weeks later, the secondary epigraft is applied.

If graft failure occurs or the power of the graft is not accurate, the graft may be surgically removed and replaced. The optical zone of the host cornea remains intact except for removal of the epithelium and the keratectomy defect in the peripheral Bowman's membrane and stroma.[88] Refraction and keratometry determinations return to the pre-epigraft state after graft removal.[80]

Epikeratophakia Disadvantages

The application of the epigraft requires a tedious surgical procedure. A bandage contact lens is applied to children at the conclusion of the grafting procedure and is left in place for the first 2 postoperative weeks.[89] A hazy graft and lid edema may further occlude the visual axis during the recovery period. The child must be returned to the operating room under general insufflation anesthesia 2 weeks later for suture removal. Some patients experience a delay in graft clearing or persistent epithelial defects that lead to persistent graft stromal haze or clouding. All of the aforementioned complications that occlude the visual axis may enhance amblyopia and delay amblyopia therapy.

Systemic antibiotic therapy is used for 28 postoperative days even with the complications of diarrhea, medication sensitivity, or allergy. Treatment with topical antibiotics and atropine and wearing an eye shield are continued during this same period. These medications are essential to prevent infection of the epigraft and control operative keratouveitis.

The epikeratophakia graft powers may not be as precise as those obtained with contact lens, spectacles, or IOLs, and over-and undercorrections occur.[86] The large graft powers frequently necessary for young children are difficult to manufacture. However, the post-graft refractive errors have been approximately emmetropic in the majority of eyes of older patients.

VISUAL RESULTS

The visual results following cataract surgery in the eyes of children remain approximately the same with glasses, contact lens, IOLs, and epikeratophakia grafts. Each parameter is an optical device and is not, in itself, an amblyopia-reducing agent. It is stressed to all parents of children in the amblyopia-forming age group of 8 years and less that their child must receive an aphakic optical correction and amblyopia occlusion therapy to achieve a satisfactory visual result.

REFERENCES

1. Wiesel TN, Hubel DH: Effects of visual deprivation on morphology and physiology of cells in the cats lateral geniculate body. *J Neurophysiol* 1963; 26:978.
2. Wiesel TN, Hubel DH: Single-cell responses in striate cortex of kittens deprived of vision in one eye. *J Neurophysiol* 1963; 26:1003.
3. Wiesel TN, Hubel DH: Comparison of the effects of unilateral and bilateral eye closure on cortical unit responses in kittens. *J Neurophysiol* 1965; 28:1029.
4. Wiesel TN, Hubel DH: Extent of recovery from the effects of visual deprivation in kittens. *J Neurophysiol* 1965; 28:1060.
5. von Noorden GK: Experimental amblyopia in monkeys. Further observation and clinical correlations. *Invest Ophthalmol* 1973; 12:721.
6. Baker FH, Grigg P, von Noorden GK: Effects of visual deprivation and strabismus on the responses of neurons in the visual cortex of the monkey, including studies on the striate and pre-striate cortex in the normal animal. *Brain Res* 1974; 66:185.
7. Awaya S: Stimulus vision deprivation amblyopia in humans, in Reinecke RD (ed): *Strabismus: Proceedings of the Third Meeting of the International Strabismological Association*. New York, Grune & Stratton, 1978, p 31.
8. Vaegan TD: Critical period for deprivation amblyopia in children. *Trans Ophthalmol Soc UK* 1979; 99:432.
9. Bellows JG: *Cataract and Abnormalities of the Lens*. New York, Grune & Stratton, 1975.
10. Cordes FC: Cataract types, *American Academy of Ophthalmology and Otolaryngology Manual,* 1961.
11. Duke-Elder S: *Normal and Abnormal Development: System of Ophthalmology,* vol 3. St Louis, CV Mosby Co, 1963.
12. Duke-Elder S: Diseases of the lens, vitreous, glaucoma and hypotony, in *System of Ophthalmology*, vol 11. St Louis, CV Mosby Co, 1969.
13. Duke-Elder S, MacFaul PA: *Injuries. System of Ophthalmology,* vol 14. St Louis, CV Mosby Co, 1972.
14. François J: Syndromes with congenital cataract. *Am J Ophthalmol* 1961; 52:207.
15. Kohn BA: The differential diagnosis of cataracts in infancy and childhood. *Am J Dis Child* 1976; 130:184.
16. Mausolf FA (ed): *The Eye and Systemic Disease*. St Louis, CV Mosby Co, 1975.
17. McDonald PR: Disorders of the lens, in Harley RD (ed): *Pediatric Ophthalmology*. Philadelphia, WB Saunders Co, 1975.
18. Merin S: Congenital cataracts, in Goldberg MF (ed): *Genetic and Metabolic Eye Disease*. Boston, Little, Brown & Co, 1974.
19. Merin S, Crawford JS: The etiology of congenital cataracts. A survey of 386 cases. *Can J Ophthalmol* 1971; 6:178.
20. Hiles DA, Carter ET: Classification of cataracts in children. *Int Ophthalmol Clin* 1977; 17:15.
21. McKusick VA: *Mendelian Inheritance in Man,* ed 5. Baltimore, Johns Hopkins University Press, 1978.
22. Wybar K, Taylor D: *Pediatric Ophthalmology. Current Aspects*. New York, Marcel Dekker, Inc, 1983.

23. Harley RD: *Pediatric Ophthalmology,* ed 2. Philadelphia, WB Saunders Co, 1983.
24. Franfelder FT, Roy FH: *Current Ocular Therapy 2.* Philadelphia, WB Saunders Co, 1985.
25. Roy FH: *Ocular Syndromes and Systemic Diseases.* Orlando, Fla, Grune & Stratton, 1985.
26. Regenbogen LS, Coscas GJ: *Oculo-Auditory Syndromes.* New York, Masson Publishers USA, Inc, 1985.
27. Jaafar MS, Robb, RM: Congenital anterior polar cataract: A review of 63 cases. *Ophthalmology* 1984; 91:249.
28. Nelson LB, Calhoun JH, Simon JW, et al: Progression of congenital anterior polar cataracts in childhood. *Arch Ophthalmol* 1985; 103: 1842.
29. Crouch ER, Parks MM: Management of posterior lenticonus complicated by unilateral cataracts. *Am J Ophthalmol* 1978; 85:503.
30. Khalil M, Saheb W: Posterior lenticonus. *Ophthalmology* 1984; 91:1429.
31. Crawford JS: Conservative management of cataracts. *Int Ophthalmol Clin* 1977; 17:31.
32. O'Neill JF, Bateman JB: The lens and pediatric cataracts, in Metz HS, Rosenbaum AL (eds): *Pediatric Ophthalmology.* Garden City, NY, Medical Examination Publishing Co, 1982, p 235.
33. Fielder AR: Dislocated lenses, in Wybar K, Taylor D (eds): *Pediatric Ophthalmology.* New York, Marcel Dekker, Inc, p 165.
34. Hiles DA, Biglan AW: Indications for infantile cataract surgery. *Int Ophthalmol Clin* 1977; 17:39.
35. Taylor D, Rice NSC: Congenital cataract, a cause of preventable child blindness. *Arch Dis Child* 1982; 57:165.
36. Rogers GL, Tishler CL, Tsou BH, et al: Visual acuities in infants with congenital cataracts operated on prior to six months of age. *Arch Ophthalmol* 1981; 99:999.
37. Hiles DA: Cataract surgical indications in children. *Int J Cataract Surg* 1984; 1:8.
38. Helveston EM, Saunders RA, Ellis FD: Unilateral cataracts in children. *Ophthalmic Surg* 1980; 11:102.
39. Pratt-Johnson JA, Tillson G: Visual results after removal of congenital cataracts before the age of one year. *Can J Ophthalmol* 1981; 16:19.
40. Ryan SJ, Maumanee AE: Unilateral congenital cataracts and their management. *Ophthalmic Surg* 1977; 8:35.
41. Beller R, Hoyt CS, Marg E, et al: Good visual function after neonatal surgery for congenital monocular cataracts. *Am J Ophthalmol* 1981; 91:559.
42. Hiles DA: Phacoemulsification of infantile cataracts. *Int Ophtholmol Clin* 1977; 17:83.
43. Scheie HG: Aspiration of congenital or soft cataracts: A new technique. *Am J Ophthalmol* 1960; 50:1048.
44. Ryan SJ, Blanton FM, von Noorden GK: Surgery of congenital cataracts. *Am J Ophthalmol* 1965; 60:583.
45. Scheie HG, Rubenstein RA, Kent RB: Aspiration of congenital or soft cataracts: Further experience. *Am J Ophthalmol* 1967; 63:3.
46. Parks MM, Hiles DA: Management of infantile cataracts. *Am J Ophthalmol* 1967; 63:10.
47. Hiles DA: Infantile cataracts—Cataract surgery in children. Part II. *Int J Cataract Surg* 1984; 1:7.
48. Kelman CD: Phacoemulsification and aspiration. *Am J Ophthalmol* 1967; 64:23.
49. Hiles DA, Wallar PH: Phacoemulsification versus aspiration in infantile cataract surgery. *Ophthalmic Surg* 1974; 5:13.
50. Peyman GA, Rachand M, Goldberg M: Surgery of congenital and juvenile cataracts: A pars plicata approach with the vitrophage. *Br J Ophthalmol* 1978; 62:780.
51. Peyman GM, Raickand M, Oesterle C, et al: Pars plicata lensectomy and vitrectomy in the management of congenital cataracts. *Ophthalmology* 1981; 88:437.
52. Calhoun JH, Harley RD: The roto-extractor in pediatric ophthalmology. *Trans Am Ophthalmol Soc* 1975; 73:292.
53. Parks MM: Posterior lens capsulectomy during primary cataract surgery in children. *Ophthalmology* 1983; 90:344.
54. Calhoun JH: Cutting-aspiration instruments. *Int Ophthalmol Clin* 1977; 17:103.
55. Price RL, Crawford JR, Yeh H, et al: Medical and surgical management of children with cataracts. *Perspect Ophthalmol* 1978; 2:49.
56. Douvas NG: Phakectomy with shallow anterior vitrectomy in congenital and juvenile cataracts. *Dev Ophthalmol* 1981; 2:163.
57. Calhoun JH: Cutting-aspiration instruments. *Int Ophthalmol Clin* 1977; 17:103.
58. Hiles DA: Phacoemulsification of infantile cataracts. *Int Ophthalmol Clin* 1977; 17:83.
59. Hiles DA, Johnson BL: The role of the crystalline lens epithelium in post-pseudophakos

membrane formation. *Am Intraocular Implant Soc J* 1980; 6:141.
60. McConnell PJ, Zarbin MA, Green WR: Posterior capsule opacification in pseudophakic eyes. *Ophthalmology* 1983; 90:1548.
61. Hiles DA, Biglan AW, Fetherolf EC: Central corneal endothelial cell counts in children. *Am Intraocular Implant Soc J* 1979; 5:292.
62. Chrousos GA, Parks MM, O'Neill JF: Incidence of chronic glaucoma, retinal detachment and secondary membrane surgery in pediatric aphakic patients. *Ophthalmology* 1984; 91:1238.
63. Phelps CD, Arafat NI: Open-angle glaucoma following surgery for congenital cataracts. *Arch Ophthalmol* 1977; 95:1985.
64. Toyofuku M, Hirose T, Schepens CL: Retinal detachment following congenital cataract surgery. *Arch Ophthalmol* 1980; 98:669.
65. Everett WG, Sorr, EM: Retinal detachment following congenital cataract surgery. *Int Ophthalmol Clin* 1977; 17:187.
66. Poer DV, Helveston EM, Ellis FD: Aphakic cystoid macular edema in children. *Arch Ophthalmol* 1981; 99:249.
67. Hoyt CS, Nickel B: Aphakic cystoid macular edema. *Arch Ophthalmol* 1982; 100:746.
68. Morgan K, Franklin RM: Oral fluorescein angioscopy in aphakic children. *J Pediatr Ophthalmol Strabismus* 1984; 21:33.
69. Gilbard SM, Peyman GA, Goldberg MF: Evaluation for cystoid maculopathy after pars plicata lensectomy-vitrectomy for congenital cataracts. *Ophthalmology* 1983; 90:1201.
70. Hiles DA: Infantile cataracts—Aphakic optical correction. Part III. *Int J Cataract Surg* 1984; 1:20.
71. Dabezies O: Defects of vision through aphakic spectacles. *Ophthalmology* 1979; 86:352.
72. Milder B: Spectacles in children, in Engelstein JM (ed): *Cataract Surgery—Current Options and Problems.* New York, Grune & Stratton, 1984, p 11.
73. Spaeth PG, O'Neill OT: Functional results with contact lens in unilateral congenital cataract, high myopia and traumatic cataracts. *Am J Ophthalmol* 1960; 49:548.
74. Ogle KN, Burian HM, Bannon RE: On the correction of unilateral aphakia with contact lenses. *Arch Ophthalmol* 1958; 59:639.
75. Blaxter PL: The use of contact lens on infants. *Trans Ophthalmol Soc UK* 1963; 83:41.
76. Hoffer KJ: Selection of lens power for implantation in infants and children. *Am Intraocular Implant Soc J* 1975; 1:49.
77. Sinskey RM, Patel J: Posterior chamber intraocular lens implantation in children: Report of a series. *Am Intraocular Implant Soc J* 1983; 9:157.
78. Hiles DA: Epikeratophakia—An alternative to glasses, contact lenses and intraocular lenses for optical correction of aphakia in children. *Trans Pa Acad Ophthalmol Otolaryngol* 1985; 38:279.
79. Morgan KS, Stephenson GS: Epikeratophakia in children with corneal lacerations. *J Pediatr Ophthalmol Strabismus* 1985; 22:105.
80. Arffa RC, Maravelli TL, Morgan KS: Keratometric and refractive results of pediatric epikeratophakia. *Arch Ophthalmol* 1985; 103:1656.
81. Morgan KS, Stephenson GS, McDonald MB, et al: Epikeratophakia in children. *Ophthalmology* 1984; 91:780.
82. Guss RB, Asbell PA, Berkowitz RA, et al: Endothelial cell counts after epikeratophakia surgery. *Ann Ophthalmol* 1983; 15:408.
83. Singh G, Bohnke M, VonDomarus D, et al: Endothelial cell densities in corneal donor material. *Ann Ophthalmol* 1983; 90:1213.
84. Olson PF, McDonald MB, Werblin TP, et al: The measurement of intraocular pressure after epikeratophakia. *Arch Ophthalmol* 1983; 101:1111.
85. Koenig SB, Berkowitz RA, Beuerman RW, et al: Corneal sensitivity after epikeratophakia. *Ophthalmology* 1983; 90:1213.
86. Morgan KS, Asbell PA, May JG, et al: Surgical and visual results of pediatric epikeratophakia. *Metab Pediatr Syst Ophthalmol* 1983; 7:45.
87. Asbell PA, Werblin TP, Loupe DN, et al: Secondary surgical procedures after epikeratophakia. *Ophthalmic Surg* 1982; 13:555.
88. Morgan KS, Asbell PA, McDonald MB, et al: Preliminary visual results of pediatric epikeratophakia. *Arch Ophthalmol* 1983; 101:1540.
89. Morgan KS, Werblin TP, Friedlander MH, et al: Epikeratophakia in the pediatric patient: A case report. *Ocular Ther Surg* 1982; 1:198.

20B Contact Lens Application After Infantile Cataract Surgery

Barry A. Weissman, O.D., Ph.D.
Paul B. Donzis, M.D.

The optical correction of pediatric aphakia presents numerous challanges to both the ophthalmic professional and the involved family. Spectacles may theoretically be used, especially in bilateral cases. But there are several sources of problems with spectacles including

1. Optical distortion and magnification
2. Difficulty in obtaining adequate frames
3. Problems maintaining the lenses properly situated on the infant's face during times of normal activity
4. Aniseikonia (dissimilar retinal image sizes between the two eyes) in instances of unilateral aphakia

Because of these problems and the generally poor visual results, especially in instances of unilateral aphakia, newer methods of optical correction have been advocated including contact lenses,[1] intraocular lenses,[2] and epikeratophakia.[3] Intraocular lenses can theoretically give the least optical distortion and magnification,[4] but normal ocular growth quickly makes any static power correction obsolete. Thus, some form of overcorrection or secondary invasive surgery would be required as the eye grows. Furthermore, there is concern about the potential for long-term adverse effects inasmuch as clinical experience with intraocular lenses is less than the 70 or so years expected for these lenses to reside in the patients' eyes.

Epikeratophakia offers some advantages in that it is a less invasive procedure and the lenticle can more easily be removed and replaced if necessary. The main advantage of epikeratophakia is its potential ease of compliance. Although there have been some problems in children under 1 year of age undergoing this procedure such as less accurate original lenticule power and difficulties in responding to power requirement changes associated with development, epikeratophakia has shown excellent results in children over 1 year of age who are contact lens intolerant.[5]

CONTACT LENSES

Contact lens correction has advantages and some disadvantages of its own. The clear advantage of contact lens wear is that the practitioner can visually obtain adequate optical correction of refractive error that is easily changed in response to ocular growth. Furthermore, contact lenses minimize the optical distortion and magnification inherent with the use of spectacles, and no surgery other than the cataract extraction is required. These qualities make contact lenses an ideal mode of aphakic optical correction for children under 1 year of age. Contact lenses may be rigid (either polymethylmethacrylate [PMMA] or gas-permeable material), flexible (silicone), or soft (hydrogel). Depending on the lens type, they may be used on daily-wear or extended-wear schedules. Difficulties include lens care, maintenance, and handling. Naturally, any contact lens care for neonates must be undertaken by the parents or guardians, and some are reluctant to devote the necessary time and energy. Other parents may have a psychological reluctance to using contact lenses. Lens loss or breakage may also become a disadvantage by causing interruptions in visual therapy, possibly complicating amblyopia management, and frequent lens replacement can be quite costly.

Rigid contact lenses have been used for many years with relative success.[1,6–8] Advantages of this modality are relative inexpense, good optical performance (in most cases neutralizing astigmatic as well as spherical components of refractive error), and ease of handling. Disadvantages include occasional lens loss and some initial discomfort for the child but, more importantly, some anticipation by the parents of this discomfort for the child. Clinically, physiological results have usually been good with daily wear of rigid PMMA lenses, and improvements can be anticipated with the use of recently introduced and expanding rigid oxygen-permeable materials. Potential extended-wear versions of these materials will soon be available as well.

Many aphakic infants are currently fitted with extended-wear flexible silicone lenses.[9–12] Disadvantages of this technique include the expense of the lenses, inability to obtain complete correction (these lenses may only be available in 3-D steps over +20 D), and the risks associated with extended wear of contact lenses.[13,14] For example, Matsumoto and Murphree[12] report success with this modality, yet document that 16% of their patients had epithelial abrasions. Silicone rubber lenses often soil quickly, can transmit water vapor and deplete the tear film under the lens,[15] and may generate negative pressures[16] as well; all these factors may contribute to the occurrence of abrasion. The primary advantages of this modality are that extended wear is convenient for both the doctor and parents and lens loss is less than that reported for hydrogel lenses.[10,12] A reduction in lens loss and the use of lenses for all open-eye experience (i.e., extended-wear, full-time use) may facilitate antiamblyopia therapy. Hydrogel lenses have also been used for infant extended-wear use.[7,10] The use of hydrogel contact lenses on an extended-wear basis in adults, however, has been associated with an increased risk of infection, vascularization, soiling of lenses, and giant papillary conjunctivitis (GPC). Because of these problems extended-wear use of hydrogel lenses should probably be avoided.

Hydrogel lens use for daily-wear correction of infantile aphakia has been used almost from the inception of this modality.[6,17–19] The availability of custom lenses from several manufacturers allows practical application to the pediatric population. Disadvantages include frequent and rapid lens loss in some cases, poor correction of residual refractive astigmatism, and difficulty in insertion. Physiological complications with daily-wear use of hydrogel lenses in the pediatric population, however, are rare in our experience.

The use of contact lenses on a daily-wear basis initially demands a substantial investment in time and patience from both the doctor and parents. During the first several weeks of care, the process of lens handling and care must be taught to and then mastered by the parents—but after that period, in most instances, the procedure becomes familiar and convenient.

UCLA EXPERIENCE

At UCLA, we have primarily used hydrogel

daily-wear lenses for many aphakic infants over the past 7 years. Several laboratories (i.e., American Hydron, Flexlens, Optech, Kontur) have supplied custom lenticular construction hydrogel contact lenses with powers in excess of + 20 D (+ 54 D has been the highest power thus far used) and various base curve/diameter combinations (base curve ranges from 7.00 to 8.75 mm and diameter ranges from 12.5 to 15.5 mm) to enable proper fitting of these infants. When corneal distortion or astigmatism is such that optically the child would benefit from a rigid lens as opposed to a hydrogel lens (which has happened in rare instances) or if a child becomes adept at hydrogel lens removal and loses several lenses in rapid succession,[18] rigid lenses have been applied in management. In these cases, PMMA lenses were used to determine lens design, and then rigid gas-permeable materials (either CAB [cellulose acetate butyrate] or silicone acrylates) were used as the final lens material. Two children have been managed with flexible silicone lenses because of several factors. Except for the latter two patients and two other children where extended wear was attempted but later abandoned due to minor complications (e.g., neovascularization and rapid lens soilage or loss), all our pediatric patients are using lenses on a daily-wear basis.

FITTING TECHNIQUE

Most children are initially examined under anesthesia (EUA), either immediately preceding cataract extraction or soon thereafter. If the child is to undergo cataract extraction on the same date, only quantification of corneal curvature is made (see the next paragraph) and the initial diameter and power of the contact lens is selected by either knowledge of age norms or from keratometry measurements and axial length measurements made at the time of surgery.

Corneal curvature may be assessed by using a keratometer,[12] but for contact lens fitting we have found it easier to use a set of trial hard contact lenses[17] (all 10.0-mm in diameter) with base curves varying from 7.2 to 8.2 mm in 0.1-mm steps. Fluorescein evaluation with these "template" lenses in situ allows an experienced observer to determine the lens that best aligns with the underlying cornea; a "steep" lens produces distinct central pooling of fluorescient tears, a "flat" lens produces an absence of fluorescence centrally, and a lens in alignment with corneal curvature produces a uniform distribution of dye. If the child is sufficiently cooperative, this can often be done in the office with or without mild sedation. At times, however, an EUA is required for accurate initial measurements.

The hydrogel lens base curve is usually selected to be about 1 mm flatter than the corneal curvature as measured by the hard lens templates. With flexible silicone lenses we begin diagnostic fitting with a trial lens about 0.2 mm flatter than the corneal curvature and attempt to obtain *minimal* apical touch as observed by fluorescein evaluation. Rigid lenses are initially selected with base curve in alignment with the flatter (i.e., longer) corneal curvature to maximize mass distribution and optimize tear exchange in situ while maintaining adequate lens centering and movement (as observed during fluorescein diagnostic evaluation).

For the neonate, we usually order a hydrogel lens diameter between 12.5 and 14.0 mm to fit within the small palpebral aperture. If the child is 2 months old or older, the usual diameter selected is 15.0 mm so that the lens is used as a semiscleral design that minimizes lens loss (Fig 20B–1). Flexible silicone lenses are used almost exclusively in the 11.3-mm diameter with the Silsoft design and slightly smaller with the Danker Sila-Rx design. Rigid lenses are fitted as most other aphakic rigid contact lenses: effort is made to use a lens with a light apical touch, as discussed earlier with diameter selected to achieve good centering and movement—usually of about 9.4 to 9.6 mm in diameter and of lenticular design. Occasionally, "single-cut" (i.e., nonlenticular) designs have been used as well in both relatively large and relatively small (i.e., Opticap) formats. Oxygen-permeable materials

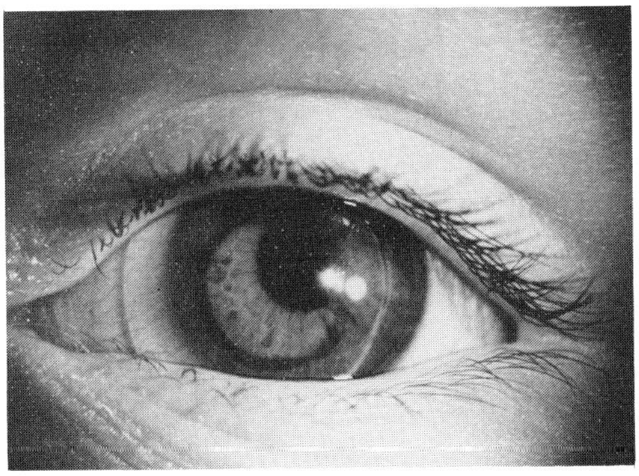

FIG 20B–1.
A daily-wear custom hydrogel contact lens in place on one pediatric patient's eye. Note the large diameter (15.0 mm) and semiscleral fit.

are usually suggested for a "final" prescription, although some trial lens work may be made with PMMA.

CONTACT LENS POWER DETERMINATION

If the child is examined postoperatively, power is first determined with retinoscopy, often during the EUA, and then confirmed with a diagnostic high-plus–power hydrogel or silicone elastomer contact lens in situ. It is important to correct for vertex distance or use a trial contact lens because of the large effect of vertex distance on power determination in these small eyes. Power determination can also be estimated at the time of surgery by obtaining the axial length and keratometry measurement. We have found that using a theoretical intraocular lens power formula with an anterior chamber depth of 0 gives an accurate estimate of the power (F) in diopters required at the contact lens plane:

F = (1,336/axial length in mm) − corneal curvature in diopters

The younger the child, the higher the anticipated power (usually between +25 and +30 D in neonates). If the eye is microphthalmic, as in persistent hyperplastic primary vitreous [PHPV], the anticipated power may be even higher (+35 to +50 D). When lenses are ordered, power is deliberately ordered with somewhat more plus power than measured to allow for the young child to be in best focus at about arms' length, which is the anticipated visual focal point.[18]

DISPENSING VISIT

Effort is made at the dispensing visit to first become acquainted with the parents and then examine the child and the aphakic eye. The initial lens is then placed on the eye with the parents assisting and observing the dispenser's technique. The child is placed prone on a soft table and then gently restrained while the lens is removed from its shipping container, rinsed, inspected, and then slipped under the upper lid of the patient. Some effort is usually needed to hold the child during this maneuver. It is important at this point to inspect the eye and observe that the lens is in proper position; the parents should be instructed to also observe the lens and monitor its position. We tell the parents what to observe in terms of a steep lens (nonmoving, which may induce a sectoral or complete compression "ring" indentation in the sclera if hydrogel) or loose lens (which produces some edge lift, increased lens excursions, and poor centering). We also tell the parents that the child should quiet quickly with the lens in place and that if the child continues to cry more than about 5 minutes the lens may be torn, chipped, cracked, inside-out or there may be a foreign body underneath. If the child continues to be uncomfortable the lens should be removed and inspected. If the lens is found to be undamaged, it should be carefully rinsed prior to reinsertion. If it continues to cause discomfort, lens wear is to be discontinued and the situation professionally reassessed immediately.

After the lens has been allowed to settle 15 to 30 minutes, retinoscopy is performed to check the lens power, and a hand-held biomicroscope is used to examine the lens for proper centering and movement. Rigid and silicone elastomer lenses are evaluated as well with the aid of fluorescein to assess alignment with the corneal surface. If the lens fit is felt to be improper, further diagnostic lens evaluations may be necessary. Often, however, a second lens may be ordered from observation of the initial lens and the initial lens still dispensed if only a small change (e.g., 1 D of power or less) is needed. The parents are instructed in proper methods for lens care, removal, and handling under the guidance of the clinician or delegated technician.

For lens disinfection, we primarily use normal thermal disinfection for low–water content hydrogel contact lenses and chemical disinfection for other lens types. Initial lenses are dispensed as quickly as possible (as long as the parents are felt to be competent in lens handling and care), even if not precise, to improve amblyopia management and improved lens designs ordered on a "rush" basis from the laboratory. When the clinician is convinced the parents can adequately care for the lens, they can be given a wearing schedule (usually 6 hr/day for the first week) and a return appointment (for 1 week). The parents may be told to let the child sleep with the lens on for short naps only over the first week or so and then not to leave the lens on at all during sleep after that.

SUBSEQUENT PROGRESS EVALUATIONS

The child should return several times over the first month of lens wear as physiological adaptation occurs and the parents become familiar with lens care. Wearing time is rapidly increased to all waking hours if no particular problems are encountered, but any sleeping or napping with the lens in place is discouraged after the first several weeks. Parents should be certain that the lens is always adequately cleaned and disinfected prior to reinsertion. Monthly progress evaluations should occur over the first year or so, and then the child should be seen about four times a year. A history should always be obtained including normal wearing time and wearing time on the day of examination. Questions should be directed at any difficulties handling the lens, any lens loss, any irritation of the eye(s), and behavioral visual progress.

During the first year of life the eye grows rapidly, from an axial length of approximately 16.8 mm at birth to almost 20 mm by 1 year of age.[20] As the eye grows, the aphakic power requirements will decrease. An assessment of retinoscopy in these young children has shown a decrease of approximately 10 D over the first year of life[21] (Fig 20B–2). The most rapid ocular growth phase is during the first 6 months of life. Also during the first 6 months of life, the cornea rapidly changes by both increasing its overall diameter and decreasing the radius of curvature.[22] Thus the importance of frequent early visits cannot be overemphasized. Lens changes should be made if retinoscopy indicates a power change of 1 D or more. When the child is about a year in age, power should be corrected properly for distance fixation, and an additional near-"reading" correction supplied in a spectacle form.

A hand-held biomicroscope helps to determine whether both contact lens fit (base curve/diameter or ocular topography relationship) and physiological response is adequate. Hydrogel lenses often appear to loosen in the *immediate* postoperative period, and the child often appears to demonstrate a need for a larger and steeper fit. This may be related to decreasing inflammation of the adnexal and lid tissues after surgery. As the cornea later flattens, the lens base curve should be lengthened (i.e., made flatter) and the diameter increased. Rarely does a young child need a smaller-diameter lens, although when the child reaches the age of 5 or 6 years, the power usually drops below +20 D which permits a refit with an "adult"-series hydrogel lens from any major manufacturer with the lens diameter decreased to about 14.0 mm.

As the child matures, he slowly assumes certain responsibilities associated with lens care. Lens removal seems to be the first task learned, and often younger children are able to tell their parents when a lens has come out on its own or remove their lenses for their parents at the proper time. One should always be careful to teach rules of good lens hygiene to the child (like washing hands prior to lens manipulation) and let the child perform tasks that are appropriate for his level of maturity.

CONCLUSIONS

Cataracts occur in the pediatric group with low frequency. Often cataracts are dense enough to preclude the possibility of visual development, either unilaterally or bilaterally. These cataracts may be associated with trauma, or intrauterine infection (i.e., rubella), other sporadic events (i.e., PHPV), or genetic. Overall experience suggests that best management is early cataract removal and aggressive contact lens therapy for any unilateral and most bilateral patients whose potential visual development may be compromised by the lenticular opacity. For patients unable to tolerate contact lenses, surgical procedures, epikeratophakia in particular, have given encouraging results in children over 1 year of age. For many children with congenital or traumatic cataracts in the first year of life, conscientious professional and family care may produce visual improvement far in excess of that expected if no intervention had occurred. However, both parents and clinicians must recognize from the outset of such care that it is both expensive

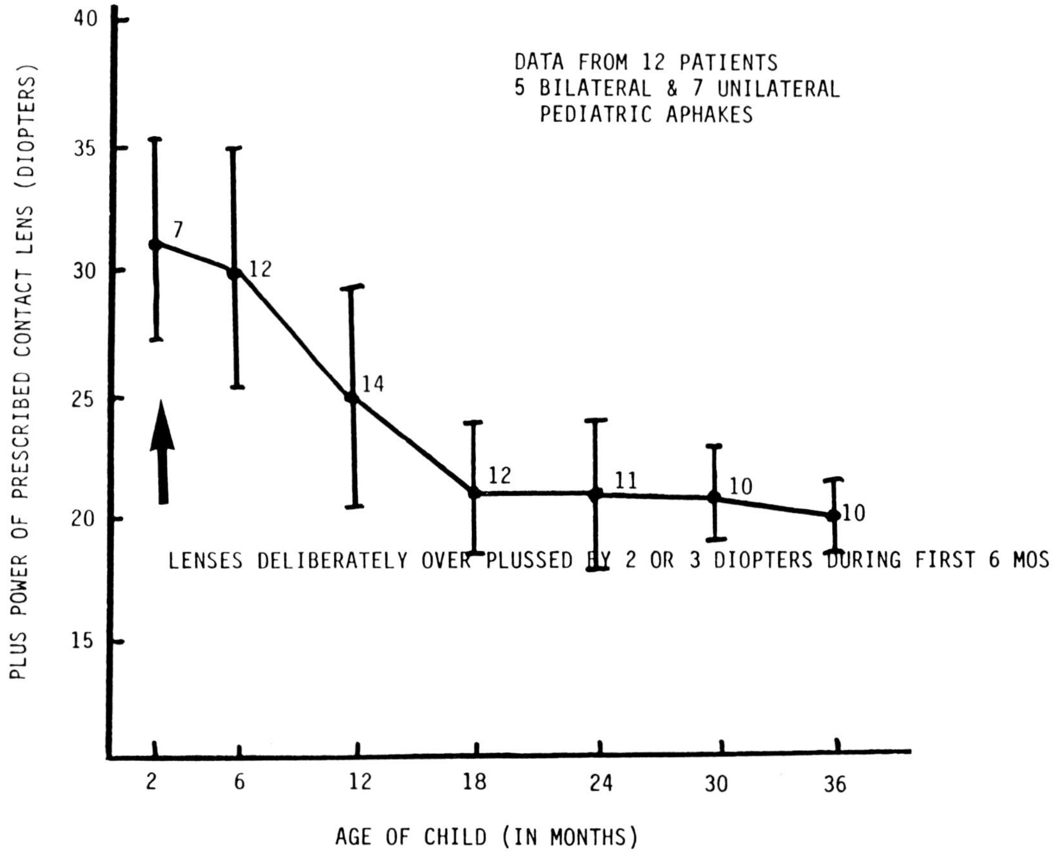

FIG 20B–2.
Decrease in required hydrogel contact lens power over time for 12 aphakic patients from the UCLA study group (5 bilateral and 7 unilateral aphakic patients). Power is determined by retinoscopy by one experienced clinician (BAW) over dispensed hydrogel lenses. Note that all children began with lenses deliberately overcorrected by 2 to 3 D. The number of children participating at each point is just above the respective data point, which represents the mean value, while brackets represent 1 SD.

and labor intensive and not always successful.

Clinicians must use their best professional judgment in caring for these young patients and use all skills to maximize the development of visual potential.

REFERENCES

1. Parks MM, Hiles DA: Management of infantile cataracts. *Am J Ophthalmol* 1967; 63:10–15.
2. Hiles DA: The need for intraocular lens implantation in children. *Ophthalmic Surg* 1977; 8:162–169.
3. Morgan KS, Arffa RC, Marvelli TL, et al: Five year follow-up of epikeratophakia in children. *Ophthalmology* 1986; 93:423–432.
4. Ogle K, Burian H, Bannon R: On correction of unilateral aphakia with contact lenses. *Arch Ophthalmol* 1958; 59:639–657.
5. Arffa RC, Marvelli TL, Morgan KS: Keratometric and refractive results of pediatric aphakia. *Arch Ophthalmol* 1986; 104:662–667.
6. Levinson A: Comparative study of the fitting of hard and Soflens contact lenses on infants and children. *Optician* 1976; 171:10–14.
7. Saunders RA, Ellis FD: Empirical fitting of hard contact lenses in infants and young children. *Ophthalmology* 1981; 88:127–130.
8. Pratt-Johnson JA, Tillson G: Hard contact lenses in the management of congenital cataracts. *J Pediatr Ophthalmol Strabismus* 1985; 22:94–96.
9. Harris M: Correction of pediatric aphakia with silicone contact lenses. *CLAO J* 1985; 11:343–347.
10. Cutler SI, Nelson LB, Calhoun JH: Extended wear contact lenses in pediatric aphakia. *J Pediatr Ophthalmol Strabismus* 1985; 22:86–91.
11. Nelson LB, Cutler SI, Calhoun JH, et al: Silsoft extended wear contact lenses in pediatric aphakia. *Ophthalmology* 1985; 92:1529–1531.
12. Matsumoto E, Murphree AL: The use of silicone elastomer lenses in aphakic pediatric patients. *Int Eyecare* 1986; 2:214–217.
13. Weissman BA, Mondino BJ, Hofbauer JD, et al: Corneal ulcers associated with extended-wear soft contact lenses. *Am J Ophthalmol* 1984; 97:476–481.
14. Mondino BJ, Weissman BA, Farb MD, et al: Corneal ulcers associated with daily-wear and extended-wear contact lenses. *Am J Ophthalmol* 1986; 102:58–65.
15. Refojo MF, Leong F-L: Water pervaporation through silicone rubber contact lenses: A possible cause of complications. *CLAO J* 1981; 7:226–233.
16. Fatt I: Negative pressure under silicone rubber contact lenses. *Contacto* 1979; 23:6–8.
17. Enoch JM: Fitting parameters which need to be considered when designing soft contact lenses for the neonate. *CLAO J* 1979; 5:31–317.
18. Parks MM: Visual results in aphakic children. *Am J Ophthalmol* 1982; 94:441–449.
19. Weissman BA: Fitting aphakic children with contact lenses. *J Am Optom Assoc* 1983; 54:235–237.
20. Gordon RA, Donzis PB: Refractive development of the human eye. *Arch Ophthalmol* 1985; 103:785–789.
21. Beller R, Hoyt CS, Marg E, et al: Good visual function after neonatal surgery for congenital monocular cataracts. *Am J Ophthalmol* 1981; 91:559–565.
22. Donzis PB, Insler MS, Gordon RA: Corneal curvatures in premature infants. *Am J Ophthalmol* 1985; 99:213–215.

21 Optic Nerve and Cortical Blindness

Creig S. Hoyt, M.D.

OPTIC NERVE

Embryology of the Optic Nerve

The optic nerve develops in the substance of the optic stalk. This stalk becomes apparent at the 4-mm human embryo stage. At the 17-mm stage, nerve fibers begin to grow from ganglion cells of the retina, and the embryonic cleft begins to close. As this occurs, the inner retinal wall of the optic cup at its proximal portion, having folded around the hyaloid artery, is initially in direct contact with the rest of the retina. As the first axons of the ganglion cells reach this point on their journey toward the brain, they turn at right angles and traverse the retinal layer to reach the optic stalk. Some retinal cells surrounding the stalk are believed to become sequestered or cut off at this point as a small clump of glial cells in the center of the presumptive optic disc. This cone-shaped mass of cells is known as the primitive epithelial papillae of Bergmeister. Many mild optic nerve anomalies are related to this important embryological event.[1] At the 25-mm stage the whole stalk is occupied with nerve fibers.

As development proceeds from the 25-mm stage, the cavity of the optic vesicle no longer communicates with that of the forebrain. Only the optic recess in the floor of the third ventricle is left to mark the cerebral end of the original wide connection between the optic vesicle and the forebrain. From the surrounding mesoderm, blood vessels invade the periphery of the nerve, beginning proximally and extending distally. These blood vessels bring with them mesodermal elements, primarily elastic tissue, and these elements together with the mesoderm associated with the hyaloid vessels eventually complete the septal system.

The optic nerve rapidly grows in both diameter and length. The most rapid growth occurs during the fifth month when the dural sheath consolidates, at which time the nerve length increases from 3 to 7 or 8 mm. At birth, the diameter of the optic nerve is approximately 2 mm, and its length is 24 mm. Largely owing to the increase in thickness of the myelin sheathes, the nerve diameter increases to 2.4 mm during the third month after birth. Around the sixth month after birth, the nerve begins to lengthen considerably to accommodate the growth of the orbit and brain until at puberty its diameter is 3 to 4 mm and its length averages 40 mm.

An important embryological event in understanding congenital anomalies of the optic nerve is the massive degeneration of supernumerary axons during the normal development of the visual pathways. Rhesus monkeys and chicks have been noted to have a 40%

loss of optic nerve axons during embryonic development and even a further loss postnatally. Similarly, Provis and coworkers found a peak of 3.7 million axons in human fetuses at 16 to 17 weeks of gestation with a rapid decline to 1.1 million axons by the 31st gestational week.[2] This process may be carried to an extreme in some instances and give rise to optic nerve hypoplasia. The selective elimination of supernumerary axons may serve as a mechanism whereby the topography of the visual pathways is established. Hoff and Peterson provided support for this argument by demonstrating that axonal projections during embryonic development are initially randomly distributed and only later assume a laminar arrangement.[3]

Optic Nerve Aplasia

Optic nerve aplasia implies a total absence of the optic disc, ganglion cells, nerve fiber layer, and retinal vessels as well as an absence of the pupillary response to direct light. This is an extremely rare anomaly, and most cases of optic nerve aplasia have been, in fact, extreme cases of optic hypoplasia. Optic nerve aplasia may be associated with the absence or gross maldevelopment of the globe, although normal-appearing eyes may also be present.[4]

Optic Nerve Hypoplasia

Optic nerve hypoplasia is a nonprogressive developmental anomaly associated with a diminished number of axons in the involved optic nerve (Figs 21–1 to 21–3).[5–7] It was once considered to be a rare and isolated congenital defect, but recent reports have emphasized both its more frequent occurrence and wide spectrum of functional deficits.[5–8] Over the past decade, it has become apparent that it is a major cause of visual loss in children. In addition, several clinically important endocrine and central nervous system abnormalities are now recognized as frequently associated conditions.[8–10]

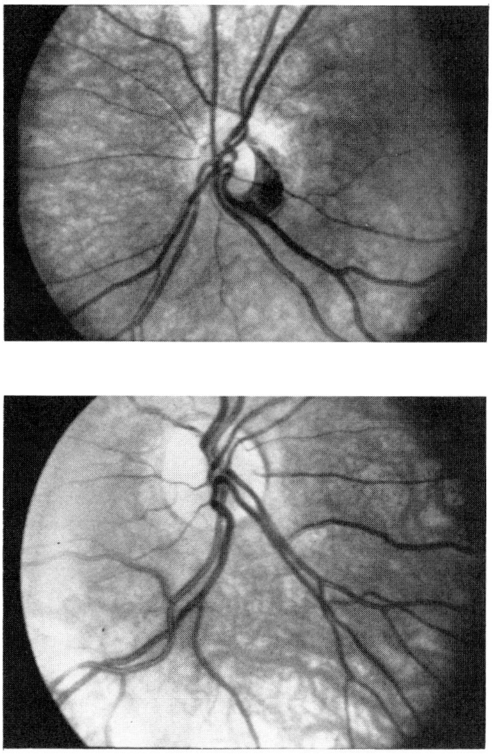

FIG 21–1.
Normal-sized right optic nerve is shown in the top section. At the bottom is the left optic nerve, which is less than 50% of the size of the right. Note the oval-shaped pigmentation on the nasal side of the left optic nerve.

Hypoplasia of the optic nerve has a wide spectrum of variation and ranges from severely reduced optic nerves to subtle segmental changes.[5] In its most florid presentation, it is characterized by a small nerve, usually one-third to one-half normal size, surrounded by a pigment ring and a yellowish mottled peripapillary halo that has been referred to as the double-ring sign. However, it may be as subtle as a slight incongruity of one border of the optic nerve with thinning of the adjacent nerve fiber. Visual acuity may range from severe visual loss compatible with the diagnosis of legal blindness to normal central visual acuity and only subtle peripheral field loss.[5]

A number of objective means of evaluating optic nerves for hypoplasia have been proposed. They include the use of red-free photography, slit-lamp examination with a posterior fundus contact lens, and careful measurement of the ratio of the disc diameter to the distance from the disc to macula. Unfortunately, all these tests require greater cooperation than is usually possible in infants. Subnormal diameters of the optic foramina and optic nerves may also be demonstrated radiographically but are not present consistently enough to provide a reliable means of corroborating the diagnosis. Furthermore, while Acers noted that the orbital portion of hypoplastic nerves is frequently subnormal in diameter when imaged by electrode sonography, he was unable to establish a correlation between the diameter of the optic nerves and visual function.[6] Despite the fact that direct ophthalmoscopy may be difficult in infants and magnification and minification errors may exist in eyes with high refractive errors, direct ophthalmoscopy remains the most reliable means of establishing the diagnosis in most cases in infancy. Indirect ophthalmoscopy does not provide magnification sufficient enough to examine subtle details of the optic disc. Bilateral cases, which are much more prevalent than unilateral cases, are often diagnosed early in infancy as part of an evaluation for poor visual development and coexisting nystagmus. Less severely affected bilateral cases may not be discovered until adulthood as an incidental finding in evaluating peripheral field defects.[11] Unilateral cases are frequently noted first because of secondary strabismus in the affected eye that usually commences after the first year of life.

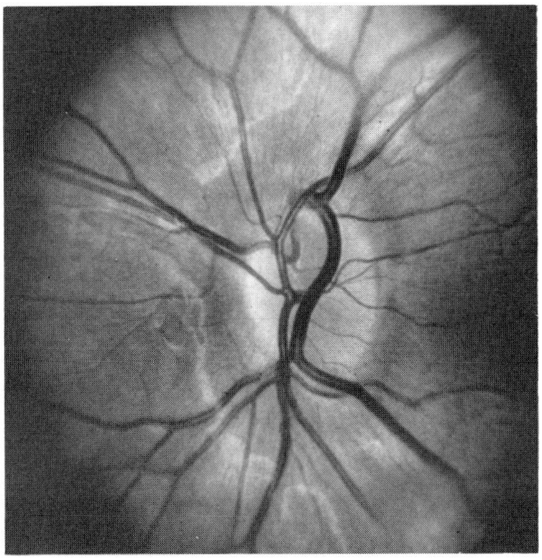

FIG 21–2.
Mild optic nerve hypoplasia that is segmentally affecting the nasal side of the optic disc. Note the prominent anomaly of retinal veins.

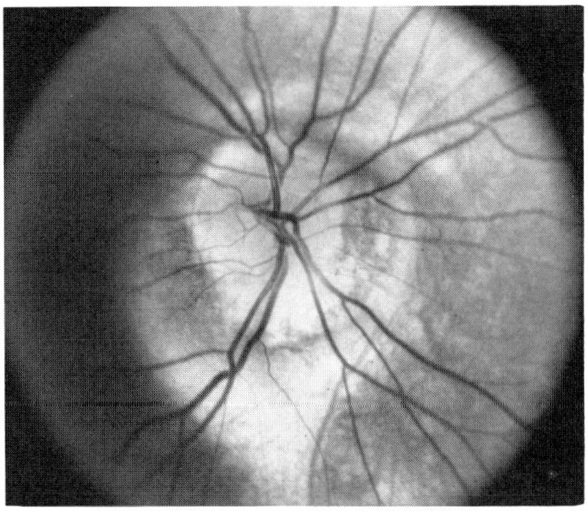

FIG 21–3.
Segmental hypoplasia involving the inferior portion of the optic disc is seen in association with a geographic loss of retinal pigment epithelium and choroidal pigmentation. This is the right eye of the patient seen in Figure 21–4.

Conditions Associated With Optic Nerve Hypoplasia Including Septo-optic Dysplasia

Septo-optic dysplasia is a syndrome named by DeMorsier in 1956,[9] but was first recognized by Reeves in 1941 in a blind 7-month-old infant lacking a septum pellucidum.[12] DeMorsier, a neuropathologist, noted that midline abnormalities of the brain including absence of the septum pellucidum, partial or complete agenesis of the corpus callosum, and dysplasia of the third ventricles were frequently associated with optic nerve hypoplasia.[9] In his series, 25% of patients with agenesis of the septum pellucidum had optic nerve hypoplasia. This syndrome has subsequently been noted to be frequently associated with endocrinologic abnormalities, especially pituitary dwarfism.[6,8] Deficiencies or hypersecretion of most of the topic hormones have since been shown to be associated with this syndrome. These include hypothyroidism, sexual infantilism or precocity, neonatal hypoglycemia, hypoadrenalism, diabetes insipidus, and hyperprolactinemia.

While a deficiency of growth hormone is the most prevalent endocrine abnormality with septo-optic dysplasia, multiple tropic hormone abnormalities may also be present. Optic nerve hypoplasia is often first noted in children during an endocrinologic evaluation where, in one series, 15% of all children with growth hormone deficiency had septo-optic dysplasia.[13] Variable levels of visual function may be associated with this syndrome, ranging from normal acuity to no light perception, depending upon the degree of optic nerve underdevelopment. In addition to neonatal jaundice, seizures, feeding problems, and lethargy are frequently noted in affected infants. Growth is usually normal in the first 2 to 3 years of life, presumably because of normal or elevated levels of prolactin.

Optic nerve hypoplasia has also been reported to occur with a number of other disorders affecting the central nervous system. These include anencephaly, porencephalia, cerebral atrophy, hydranencephaly, colpocephaly, and encephaloceles (Fig 21–4).[8] Taylor has emphasized the importance of performing computerized tomographic (CT) studies on children with optic nerve hypoplasia and bitemporal field changes since craniopharyngiomas and pilocytic astrocytomas may be associated with these findings.[14] A large prospective study by Skarf and Hoyt[8] noted neuroradiographic abnormalities in 39% of children with bilateral optic nerve hypoplasia presenting as poor vision with nystagmus. In contrast, unilateral cases are associated with intracranial pathology in less than 10% of cases. Miller has recommended that all infants presenting with bilateral optic nerve hypoplasia and poor visual function undergo a thorough neuroradiographic and endocrinological evaluation.[15]

Several other ocular disorders have been shown to be associated with optic nerve hypoplasia including albinism, aniridia, optic disc

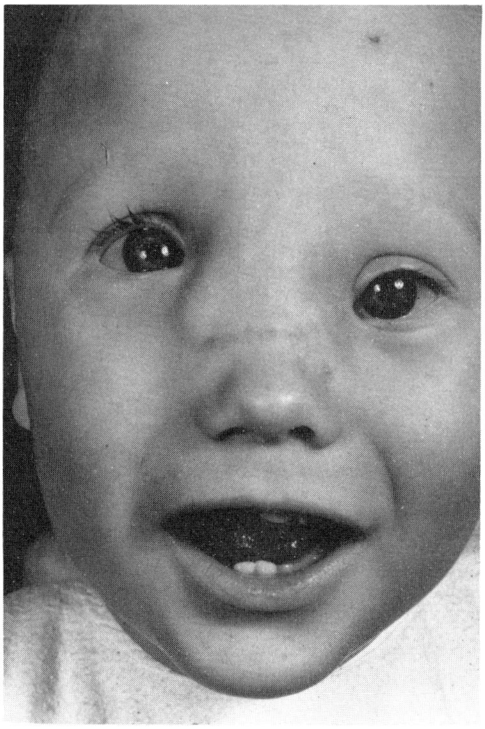

FIG 21–4.
A patient with a transethmoidal encephalocele is seen. Segmental optic nerve hypoplasia is a commonly associated finding in this disorder.

and chorioretinal colobomas, high myopia, and retinal vascular tortuosity. Several other congenital anomalies and syndromes have also been associated with optic nerve hypoplasia including Duane retraction syndrome, median cleft face syndrome, Klippel-Trenaunay-Weber syndrome, Goldenhar-Gorland syndrome, chondrodysplasia punctata, Meckel syndrome, orbital apex syndrome, hypertelorism, hemifacial atrophy, and blepharophimosis. However, the majority of infants with optic nerve hypoplasia, particularly if it is unilateral or segmental, will have no accompanying disorders.

Optic nerve hypoplasia is usually idiopathic, but in certain instances evidence suggestive of an etiology may be present. Isolated reports have noted that optic nerve hypoplasia may be inherited as an autosomal recessive or dominant trait. In addition, case reports have noted that optic nerve hypoplasia may infrequently occur in conditions resulting from chromosomal aberrations such as trisomy 18 and 19. An infectious etiology has also occasionally been invoked, and optic nerve hypoplasia has been reported to occur after intrauterine cytomegalovirus and hepatitis infections. However, since both of these infections are fairly common, the significance of this association is unclear.

A toxic agent may be responsible for some cases of optic nerve hypoplasia. The maternal use of phenytoin (Dilantin), quinine, lysergic acid diethylamide (LSD), and alcohol during pregnancy have all been associated with the occurrence of optic nerve hypoplasia in the offspring.[16, 17] Stromland reported the occurrence of optic nerve hypoplasia in 48% of infants with the fetal alcohol syndrome.[17] Two large studies have reported as 10% and 12% incidence of substance abuse among the mothers of children affected with optic nerve hypoplasia.[18] A number of reports have also emphasized that optic nerve hypoplasia occurs more commonly in firstborn children who are the offspring of young mothers.[10, 19] It is unclear whether the etiology stems from maternal age or a higher prevalence of substance abuse among these young mothers. The offspring of diabetic mothers appear to be at an increased risk for developing segmental optic nerve hypoplasia. These cases are rarely detected in infancy and often go undetected until adulthood.

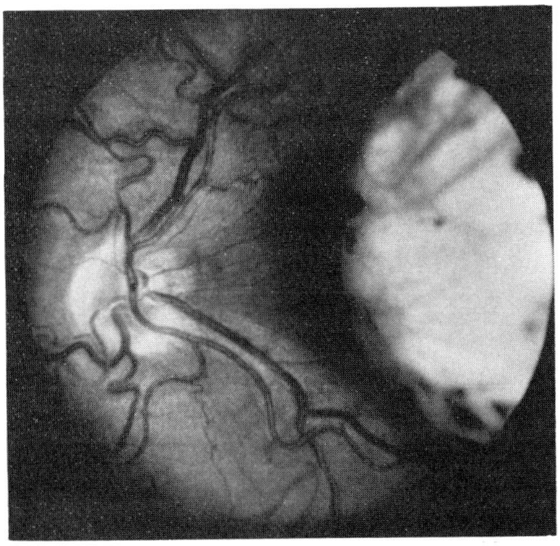

FIG 21–5.
Segmental optic nerve hypoplasia involving primarily the papillomacular bundle is seen in association with a large macular "coloboma." Visual acuity was markedly reduced in this eye.

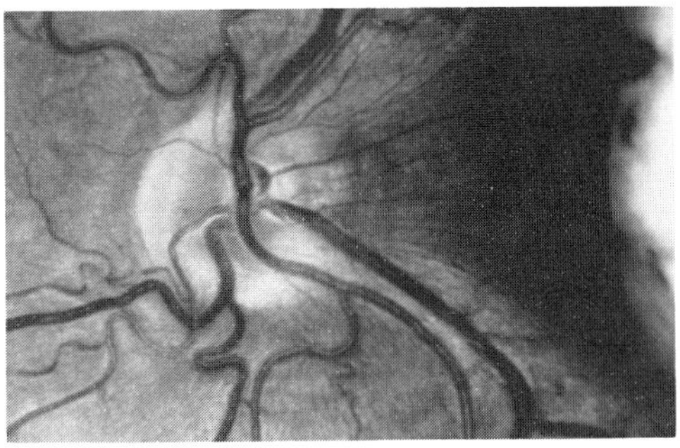

FIG 21–6.
Higher magnification of the optic disc seen in Figure 21–5. Note the loss of normal nerve fiber detail (seen as the gray and white striations radiating from the disc) in the papillomacular bundle.

Coloboma

Optic nerve coloboma is an anomaly that occurs due to defective closure of the fetal cleft of the optic cup in its extreme posterior segment (Figs 21–5 to 21–9). Associated with this anomaly is an abnormal development of the surrounding mesoblastic precursors, choroid and sclera, with ectasia of the resulting tissues. The clinical appearance of colobomatous defects varies considerably. There may be deep colobomatous cupping of the disc with ectasia of the tissue adjacent to the disc or merely an irregularity or pit at the disc margin. Visual function may be severely affected or merely confined to peripheral superior visual field loss. Severe bilateral optic nerve colobomas will present with poor visual function and nystagmus early in infancy.

Most cases of optic disc coloboma occur in isolation with no other associated neurological or systemic findings. They may be unilateral or bilateral. Although the majority of cases are sporadic, familial cases may occur. Autosomal dominant inheritance is the most common inheritance pattern. Colobomas of

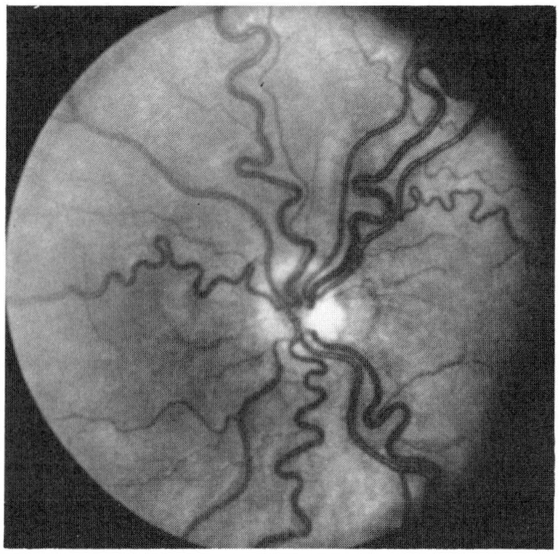

FIG 21–7.
A very tiny central optic disc is seen with anomalous tortuosity of the retinal veins. Note the so-called double pigment ring on the temporal side of the disc.

the optic disc may be associated with other colobomas involving the iris, lens, and/or choroid as well as with other ocular and systemic anomalies. The most important systemic anomalies associated with optic nerve colobomas include basal encephaloceles, Aicardi syndrome, the CHARGE association, and Warburg syndrome.[20] Patients with Aicardi syndrome may have optic disc colobomas associated with lacunar choroidal defects, vertebral anomalies, absence of the corpus callosum, infantile spasms, and mental retardation. Aicardi syndrome appears to be X-linked dominant, lethal to males since, with a rare exception, only affected females have been reported. Warburg syndrome has been suggested as the name for autosomal recessively inherited eye and brain anomalies first described by Warburg in 1971. This syndrome includes corneal leukomas, retinal dysplasia

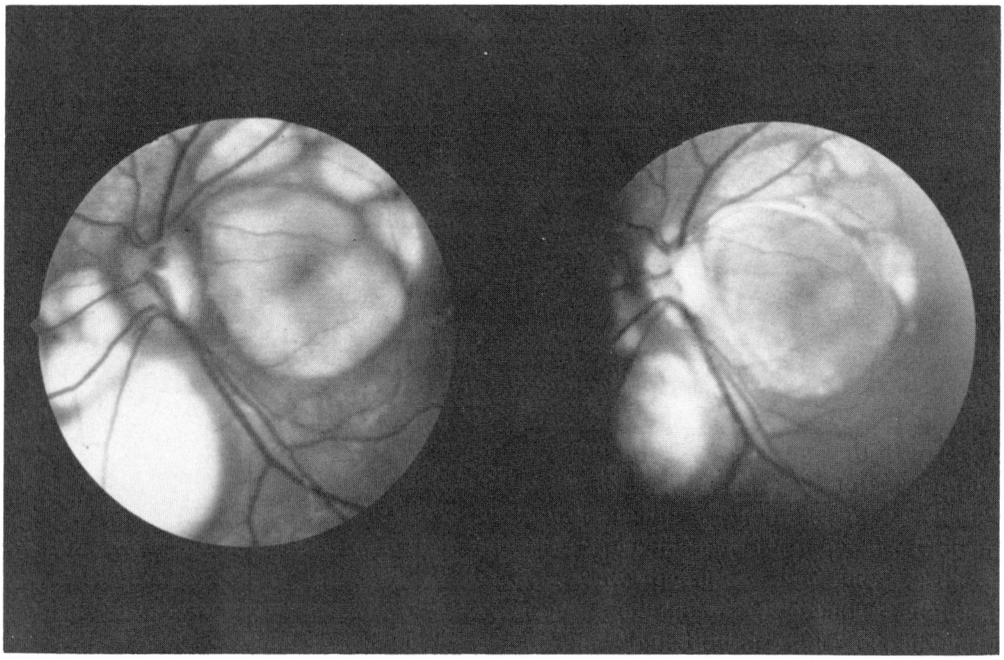

FIG 21–8.
Typical lesions involving the choroid and retina of a patient with Aicardi syndrome are associated with segmental optic nerve hypoplasia (seen as narrow, long oval discs). Colobomas of the optic nerve may also be seen in this syndrome.

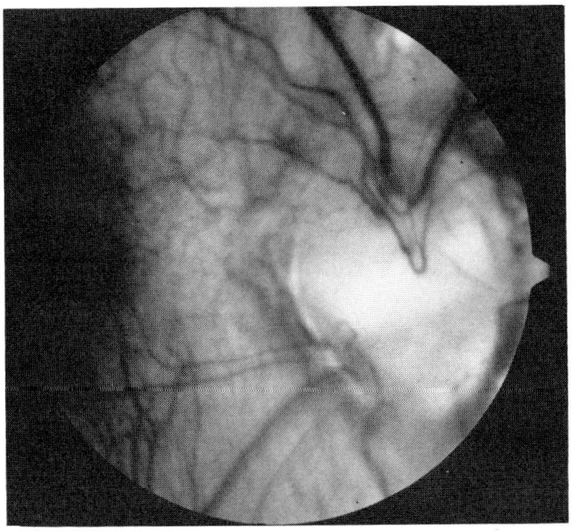

FIG 21–9.
A coloboma of the optic nerve involving the entire lower half of the disc is associated with very poor vision in this eye.

with or without coloboma, and congenital nonattachment of the retina without dysplasia. The brain anomalies include either servere hydrocephalus or dilated ventricles with microcephaly, absent cerebral gyri (agyria or lissencephaly), polymicrogyria, absent laminar structure of the cortex, and occasionally encephalocele. Recently the association of choanal atresia, congential heart disease, deafness, mental retardation, growth failure, and hypogonadism with ocular coloboma has been reported, and the mnemonic CHARGE association has been suggested.

Although optic nerve colobomas may exist in microphthalmic eyes, extreme degrees of myopia may be associated with this defect, and optical correction may be important in the rehabilitation of affected infants.

Optic Pits

Optic pits were first described almost 100 years ago as black depressions within the optic disc substance (Fig 21–10). The frequency of optic pits has been estimated at approximately 1:11,000, with equal male and female involvement. The majority of optic pits are situated on the temporal side of the disc inasmuch as nasal and inferior locations are extremely rare. Pits are usually described as round or oval, ranging in size from 0.1 to 0.7 D. The majority of pits appear to be predominantly gray in color, often with an olive tint or occasionally even black.

Most infants presenting with optic pits will have no visual symptoms unless there is an associated serous detachment of the macula. Although visual field defects have been documented in some patients with isolated optic pits, they are unlikely to be detected in early infancy. The association of congenital optic pits and serous detachment of the retina and macula is well established. However, this does not usually occur in early infancy. Nevertheless, parents should be advised of the potential for this complication to occur at a later date and of the need for routine ophthalmic examination of affected children.

Optic pits are almost always found as isolated phenomena, although they have occasionally been associated with ipsilateral retinochoroidal colobomas, unilateral pigmentary retinopathy, and most importantly, occasionally with basal encephaloceles. No inheritance pattern has been described.

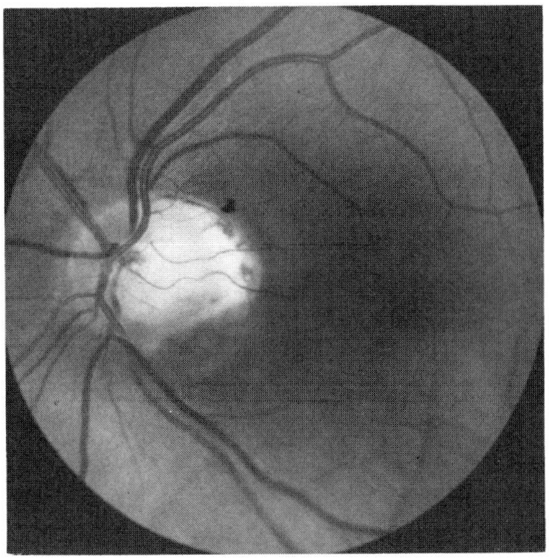

FIG 21–10.
An optic nerve pit is seen as a gray oval area of the inferior temporal portion of the optic disc. This may be associated with serious retinal detachment.

Optic Atrophy in Infancy

When irreparable damage to optic nerve fibers occurs, no matter what the nature of the initial insult, optic atrophy becomes manifested. It is usual to evaluate the presence or absence of optic atrophy by examining the color of the optic discs with a direct ophthalmoscope. This type of evaluation may be extremely difficult in some infants. This is because the ordinary appearance of the optic nerve in the first few weeks of life is oftentimes pale with little of the normal pinkish hue of the more adultlike optic nerve appearance. Moreover, in infants ophthalmoscopic examinations are made with difficulty, and efforts to keep the eyelids separated may produce inadvertent pressure on the eye. As a result, perfusion of the optic nerve may be inadvertently occluded, and pallor of the optic nerve may be entirely iatrogenic in nature. Therefore, evaluation of the peripapillary nerve fiber layer and its thickness may oftentimes give valuable information in estimating whether or not a pale optic nerve really represents an atrophic nerve in early infancy. Many infants who were once diagnosed as having optic atrophy were, in fact, examples of optic nerve hypoplasia. Congenital disc anomalies are a much more frequent source of optic nerve pathology in the first year of life than is optic atrophy.[10] However, optic atrophy may occur in association with certain problems, especially hydrocephalus.[21]

Most forms of inherited optic atrophy are not apparent in the first year of life. Only rarely is dominant optic atrophy manifested in this early period.[22] Occasionally cases of autosomal recessive optic atrophy have been reported. These are characterized by bilateral severe visual loss and nystagmus. Many of these cases probably represent panretinal degeneration (Leber's amaurosis) with associated optic atrophy. Before a diagnosis of autosomal recessive optic atrophy can be made, a complete retinal evaluation including electroretinography must be undertaken.

Compressive lesions of the anterior visual pathway may precipitate optic atrophy in the first year of life.[23] Optic atrophy may occur in association with hydrocephalus as the result of several different mechanisms. It may occur secondary to long-standing papilledema, as a consequence of compression of the chiasm by a dilated third ventricle, or by stretching of the chiasm and its blood supply as a result of intracranial displacement of the brain stem in an effort to accommodate increasing cerebral volume. It may also represent cortical damage with transsynaptic degeneration through the lateral geniculate body in infants. This last proposal for postnatal transsynaptic degeneration remains a controversial topic, and at the moment most authorities agree that transsynaptic degeneration implies prenatal insult.

Optic nerve gliomas may be associated with optic atrophy or, occasionally and much more rarely, optic nerve hypoplasia.[14] These tumors may present as an orbital lesion with axial proptosis and unilateral visual loss or as a chiasmal lesion with strabismus and/or nystagmus and visual loss. The chiasmal lesion may involve diencephalic structures or lead to obstructive hydrocephalus. Optic atrophy may occur in both forms of tumor. Treatment of this problem is controversial, and surgical treatment is probably not indicated unless the proptosis is disfiguring.[24] Whether or not radiation therapy is efficacious in this situation remains a highly controversial issue.

Craniopharyngioma is the most common intracranial tumor of nonglial origin in childhood.[23] It arises from displaced squamous cells of the embryonic hypophysis. The tumor may be primarily intrasellar and suprasellar in location. Visual loss is one of the cardinal signs of craniopharyngioma due to its compression of the chiasm or optic nerves. Papilledema is frequently evident and indicates elevated intracranial pressure. Interference with pituitary function often leads to dwarfism in children with these tumors. Calcification within the tumor is easily seen on plain skull films or on CT scanning. Meningiomas and pituitary adenomas are very rare in childhood and even more rare in infancy. Optic atrophy may be associated with these tumors, however. Children at any age presenting with nystagmus of any type and optic atrophy should be evaluated by complete neurological investigation including CT or magnetic resonance imaging (MRI) scanning in order to rule out the aforementioned associated conditions. Patients who appear to have the syndrome of spasmus nutans but exhibit optic atrophy will almost certainly harbor an optic nerve glioma.

Most metabolic causes of optic atrophy interfere with the normal metabolism of glucose (the only energy source for the brain and optic nerve). Thus, hypoxia, hypoglycemia, and deficiencies in the coenzymes (particularly the water-soluble vitamins) required for glucose metabolism may precipitate optic atrophy. However, the extent to which the optic nerve appears to be resistant to these metabolic insults is noteworthy. Despite the frequency with which hypoxia and hypoglycemia occur in the perinatal period, optic atrophy is not a common sequela of these metabolic disturbances, no matter how severe. Less than 15% of all infants who experience significant hypoxic encephalopathy develop optic atrophy.[25] In the presence of normal neurological examination findings and a normal CT scan, optic atrophy cannot be attributed to hypoxia.

Disc Edema or Swelling

The most common cause of disc swelling in infancy is papilledema. Papilledema should be a term restricted to imply disc swelling associated with increased intracranial pressure. One should recall that because of the open fontanelle, many infants with raised intracranial pressure will not develop papilledema. In contrast, those disorders that promote early suture closure and obliteration of the fontanelle may be associated with a high risk of occult hydrocephalus and papilledema, for example, Crouzon's or Apert's syndrome. In its complete expression, papilledema is characterized by edema of the optic nerve head, blurred margins of the disc, obliteration of the optic cup, hyperemia of the disc, engorgement of the veins, loss of venous pulsations, hemorrhages of the superficial retinal layers, and peripapillary soft exudates. In its incomplete forms, it may require repeated careful ophthalmic examinations to determine whether the changes in the nerve are diagnostic of papilledema. Characteristically, the visual function remains unaffected until late in the course of long-standing papilledema, and in early infancy only careful examination of the optic nerve head with direct ophthalmoscopy is likely to detect this problem. Although there are certain congenital anomalies of the optic nerve head that may mimic papilledema, they rarely do so in the first year of life. For example, the presence of optic nerve head drusen, a relatively common anomaly of the optic nerve head, is rarely confused with papilledema until later in life. This is because the hyaloid bodies that constitute this abnormality are buried and cause no apparent confusion on ophthalmoscopic inspection of the optic disc in early infancy.

Associated ocular abnormalities may be seen in association with papilledema in infancy. These include sixth-nerve palsies, poor upgaze, lid retraction, and concomitant esotropia. Any of these ocular motor disturbances should be carefully investigated, including meticulous examination of the optic nerve head in order to rule out the presence of papilledema.

Congenital Pigmentation of the Optic Disc

Pigmentation of the optic discs may occur in several forms, exclusive of the choroidal pigmentation that is frequently seen at the margins of the disc. These forms include occasional flecks lying on the optic disc or in the lamina cribosa, dense plaques lying on the disc or extending out from it, linear stripes of pigmentation, and a slate gray color of the entire disc. The last category of pigmentation is particularly important in the evaluation of the infant's optic nerve. This abnormality may be observed in early infancy or in adulthood. Beauvieux studied three infants who were felt to be blind.[26] Two of the infants had other abnormalities including buphthalmos, myopia, epicanthus, and posterior polar cataracts, and all three showed a lack of pupillary responses to direct light at the time of initial examination. All had incoordination of eye movements with a tendency to conjugate deviations and manifest nystagmus. All three infants showed a peculiar gray discoloration of the optic discs that was associated with normal-appearing vessels. Although the infants appeared blind initially, subsequent examination several months later revealed normal pupillary responses, normal ocular motility, and normal coloration of the discs. The three infants were all female, and there was no evidence of any systemic or neurological hereditary disease. Beauvieux implicated delayed myelinization as the etiology for this transient disc discoloration. Subsequent similar cases have been reported. Whether these cases represent forms of delayed visual maturation in infancy or a specific syndrome is not clear. However, the estimation of visual function in an infant presenting with abnormal pigmentation of the disc should be made carefully and cautiously after repeated examinations.

Morning Glory Anomaly

The "morning glory syndrome" optic disc presents a dramatic picture of radial traction folds of the entire retina inasmuch as it appears to be drawn into the interior and center of the optic papillae with glial tissue in the central part and no well defined cup. A peripapillary retinal pigment proliferation is seen adjacent to the peripheral scleral rim. This is usually associated with significant visual loss, and high refractive errors may be reported. The appearance of the optic nerve may superficially mimic an extreme example of glaucoma with optic nerve cupping. The morning glory syndrome is not an inherited disorder, although it may be associated with basal encephaloceles and other variants of congenital forebrain anomalies.

CORTICAL BLINDNESS

Cortical blindness refers to a loss of vision secondary to injuries to the geniculostriate pathways. Clinically it is manifested as the absence of vision and optokinetic nystagmus in the presence of normal ocular examination findings and intact pupillary light responses.[27] No manifest nystagmus accompanies this disorder.[28] Thus, it may be easily distinguished from those causes of blindness with associated ocular conditions and nystagmus.

It most commonly occurs in infants following hypoxic insults but may also arise as a sequela of meningitis, encephalitis, head trauma, hydrocephalus, or metabolic derangement.[28] While the recovery of vision may be rapid and complete, more often it is protracted and only partial. Since these children almost always regain some vision, Witting and coworkers have proposed that their visual loss be referred to as cortical visual impairment rather than cortical blindness.[29] Several theories have been proposed for the recovery of vision in cortically insulted children including the use of extrageniculostriate visual pathways, the recruitment of adjacent neurons, and the restoration of normal excitability to surviving neurons. Studies in humans that purport to demonstrate vision mediated by the extrageniculostriate pathways have largely been done, however, in the blind hemianopic fields of adults. These studies lack pathological proof that residual vision is not a consequence of incomplete destruction of the striate cortex mediating these visual fields.[30,31] Even in primates after bilateral occipital lobectomies, residual vision may reflect subtotal resection of the anterior striate cortex.[32] Others have suggested that the residual vision in these hemianopic fields may be an artifact of poor fixation or light scattering.[30] Most infants with recovery from visual cortical insults are cognizant of their visual function, which makes it unlikely that subcortical mechanisms are involved.[29]

More likely, children recover vision after

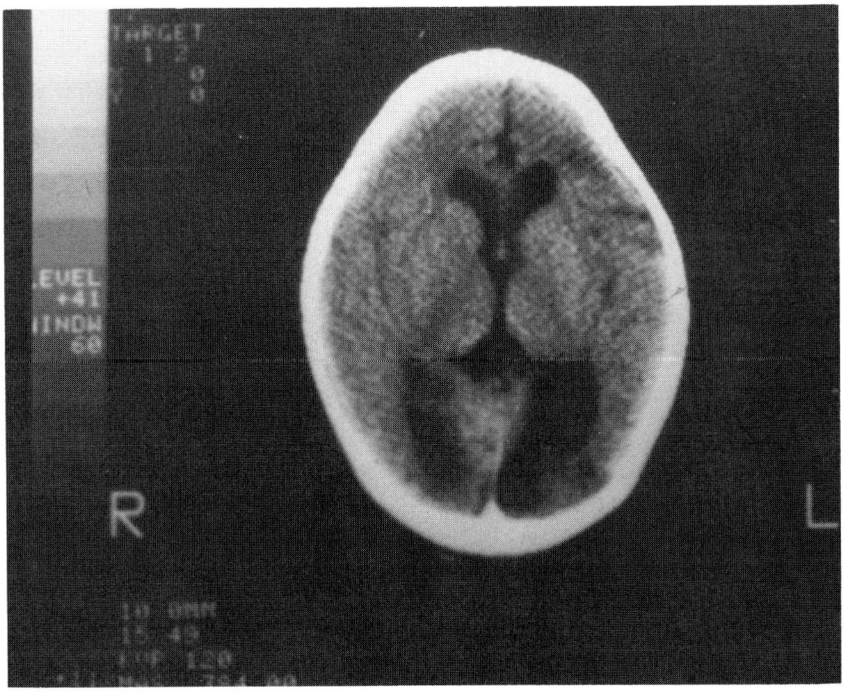

FIG 21–11.
A CT scan of a child who suffered severe perinatal hypoxia reveals "watershed infarction" of the visual cortex. This is seen as translucent areas contiguous with the ventricular systems. Mild damage to the motor cortex is also seen.

hypoxic or other insults to the primary visual cortex by a rewiring or neuronal connections in the visual cortex or neurochemical adaptations by the surviving neurons. Injuries to the immature central nervous system are compensated for by either collateral axonal sprouting, the expansion of dendritic surface areas, or the replacement of lost neurons by supernumerary neurons.[33] Supernumerary neurons are known to be present along the visual pathways during neural development.[2] Supernumerary neurons may be retained in the visual cortex of children with cortical visual insults. In addition to the morphological changes occurring after injury, recent studies have emphasized neurochemical adaptations that occur in surviving synapses such as denervation supersensitivity, which may help mediate a functional recovery. The gradual nature of the visual recovery of infants extends over months or years, and it would be consistent with such a regenerative process.[29] The degraded quality of visual recovery may stem from aberrant rewiring or a paucity of residual neurons in the surviving visual cortex.

Occasionally one sees infants who appear to be cortically blind but have no known cause for a cortical insult.[34] These children present in the first few months of life without any significant perinatal history and appear to have no visual function, no nystagmus, and no fixation responses. Over the course of 6 to 12 months, most develop normal visual function, although later they may develop other neurological abnormalities. It has been reported that these infants are frequently small for their gestational age or premature with associated delays in their general motor development.[35] Others have suggested that this delayed visual maturation may really just represent a mild form of cortical visual impairment with structural and functional abnormalities. However, it would appear that the long-term visual prognosis of these children is dramatically better than that of those with known cortical insults and that this fact alone justifies separation of these patients into a distinct clinical group.

A variety of tests have been used to diagnose and predict the visual outcome in cortically blind children including visual evoked potentials (VEP), electroencephalograms, and CT (Fig 21–11).[36, 37] Early reports emphasized the absence of marked attenuation of VEP occipital responses in patients with acute cortical blindness, with recovery of the responses as vision improved gradually over time.[38] It was initially noted that a correlation existed between short-latency VEP responses and visual recovery in children with cortical blindness. However, in large comparative studies, Frank and Torres have been unable to detect a significant difference between the VEP responses of children with cortical blindness and neurologically handicapped children without visual difficulties.[39] Others have even noted entirely intact VEPs in obviously cortically blind infants.[36] Similar difficulties have been encountered when trying to correlate EEGs of cortically blind children with their visual outcome. The most effective evaluation of these infants is with CT scanning or MRI with evaluation of the visual cortex and optic radiation. The most severe long-term visual problems occur in children with scans that reveal periventricular leukomalacia.[40]

REFERENCES

1. Harcourt B: Developmental abnormalities of the optic nerve. *Trans Ophthalmol Soc UK* 1973; 96:395.
2. Provis JN, Vandriel D, Billson FA: Human fetal optic nerve: Overproduction and elimination of retinal axons during development. *J Comp Neurol* 1985; 232:92.
3. Hoff JD, Peterson HRH: Craniopharyngiomas in children and adults. *J Neurosurg* 1972; 36:299.
4. Hotchkiss ML, Green WR: Optic nerve aplasia and hypoplasia. *J Pediatr Ophthalmol Strabismus* 1979; 16:225.
5. Friesen L, Holmegaard B: Spectrum of optic nerve hypoplasia. *Br J Ophthalmol* 1968; 62:7.
6. Acers TE: Optic nerve hypoplasia: Septo-optic pituitary dysplasia syndrome. *Trans Am Ophthalmol Soc* 1981; 79:425.
7. Hoyt CS: Optic nerve hypoplasia: A changing perspective, in *Transactions of New Orleans Academy of Ophthalmology*. New York, Raven Press, 1986, p 257.
8. Skarf B, Hoyt CS: Optic nerve hypoplasia in children. *Arch Ophthalmol* 1984; 102:62.
9. DeMorsier G: Agenesis du septum lucidum avec malformation du tractus optique. *Schweiz Arch Neurol Neurochir Psychiatr* 1956; 77:267.
10. Jan JE, Robinson GC, Tinnis C, et al: Blindness due to optic nerve atrophy and hypoplasia in children: An epidemiology study (1944–1974). *Dev Med Child Neurol* 1977; 19:353.
11. Graham MV, Wakefield GJ: Bitemporal visual field defects associated with anomalies of the optic disc. *Br J Ophthalmol* 1973; 57:307.
12. Reeves DL: Congenital absence of the septum pellucidum. *Bull Johns Hopkins Hosp* 1941; 69:61.
13. Margalith D, Tse WJ, Jan JE: Congenital optic nerve hypoplasia with hypothalamic-pituitary dysplasia. A review of 16 cases. *Am J Dis Child* 1985; 139:361.
14. Taylor DR: Congenital tumors of the anterior visual system with dysplasia of the optic discs. *Br J Ophthalmol* 1982; 66:455.
15. Miller NR: The disc that really isn't. *Surv Ophthalmol* 1985; 29:351.
16. Hoyt CS: Optic disc abnormalities in maternal congestion of LSD. *J Pediatr Ophthalmol* 1978; 15:286.
17. Stromland K: Ocular abnormalities in the fetal alcohol syndrome. *Acta Ophthalmol [Suppl] (Copenh)* 1985; suppl 1.
18. Margalith D, Jan JE, McCormick AQ, et al: Clinical spectrum of optic nerve hypoplasia. Review of 51 patients. *Dev Med Child Neurol* 1984; 26:311.
19. Lippe B, Kaplan FA, Lefranke F: Septo-optic dysplasia and maternal age. *Lancet* 1979; 2:92.
20. Pagan RA: Ocular coloboma. *Surv Ophthalmol* 1981; 25:223.
21. Costenbader FD, O'Rourk TR: Optic atrophy in childhood. *J Pediatr Ophthalmol* 1968; 5:77.
22. Kjer P: Infantile optic atrophy with dominant mode of inheritance. *Acta Ophthalmol (Copenh)* 1959; 54:1.
23. Rakic P: Prenatal genesis of connections serving ocular dominance in rhesus monkey. *Nature* 1976; 261:467.

24. Hoyt WF, Baghdassarian SA: Optic glioma of childhood: Natural history and rationale for conservative management. *Br J Ophthalmol* 1969; 53:793.
25. Good W, Hoyt CS: Optic atrophy and hypoxic encephalopathy. *Arch Ophthalmol*, in press.
26. Beauvieux J: La pseudo-atrophie optique de nouveaunes. *Ann Oculist* 1926; 163:881.
27. Barnett AB, Manson JI, Wilner E: Acute cerebral blindness in children. *Neurology* (NY) 1970; 20:1147.
28. Hoyt CS: Cortical blindness in infancy. Pediatric Ophthalmology and Strabismus, in *Transactions of the New Orleans Academy of Ophthalmology*. New York, Raven Press, 1986, p 235.
29. Witting S, Jan JE, Wong PKH: Permanent cortical visual impairment in children. *Dev Med Child Neurol* 1985; 27:730.
30. Campion J, Latto R, Smith YN: Is blind sight an effect of scattered light, spared cortex and near-threshhold vision? *Behav Brain Sci* 1983; 6:423.
31. Bridgeman B, Stagos B: Plasticity in human blind sight. *Vision Res* 1982; 22:1129.
32. Denny-Brown D, Chambers RA: Physiologic aspects of visual perception. *Arch Neurol* 1976; 33:219.
33. Marshall JF: Brain function: Neural adaptations and recovery from injury. *Annu Rev Psychol* 1984; 35:277.
34. Hoyt CS, Jastrzebski G, Marg E: Delayed visual maturation in infancy. *Br J Ophthalmol* 1983; 67:127.
35. Cole GF, Hungerford J, Jones RB: Delayed visual maturation. *Arch Vis Child* 1984; 59:107.
36. Ronen S, Nawratski I, Yanko L: Cortical blindness in infancy: A followup study. *Ophthalmologica* 1983; 187:217.
37. Weinberger HA, Van der Woude R: Prognosis for cortical blindness following cardiac arrest in children. *JAMA* 1962; 179:134.
38. Bodis-Wollner, I, Atkin A, Raab E: Visual association cortex and vision in man. Pattern evoked potentials in a blind boy. *Science* 1977; 198:629.
39. Frank Y, Torres F: Visual evoked potentials in the evaluation of "cortical blindness" in children. *Ann Neurol* 1979; 6:126.
40. Lambert SR, Hoyt CS, Jan JE, et al: Visual recovery from hypoxic cortical blindness during childhood: CT and MRI predictors. *Arch Ophthalmol* 1987; 105:1371.

22 Vitreous and Retina

Graham Quinn, M.D.

A chapter dealing with the subject of retinal and vitreous disorders that are first noted in the nursery and then through the first year of life cannot be comprehensive and must encourage the reader to place findings in general broad categories from which specific diagnostic groupings are apparent. Toward that end, this chapter is divided into development of the retina and vitreous, "inflammatory-type" retinal diseases, tumors, and abnormalities associated with systemic diseases (Table 22–1). Congenital and acquired retinal infections (Chapter 25), retinopathy of prematurity (ROP), (Chapter 26), chromosomal abnormalities (Chapter 11), and trauma (Chapter 24) are covered elsewhere in this volume.

RETINAL DEVELOPMENT

Leber's Congenital Amaurosis

Leber first described "amaurosis congenita" in 1869[1] to designate a type of blindness seen early in life that had no associated, readily apparent abnormalities of the eye. Since then, this entity has masqueraded in a variety of guises, e.g., retinal aplasia, dysgenesis neuroepithelialis retinae, and congenital tapetoretinal dysplasia. Alstrom and Olson[2] found that some 10% of children in schools for the blind could be assigned to this type of congenital blindness.

Infants with Leber's congenital amaurosis (LCA) are noted to be blind or at least have reduced vision soon after birth. The child will also have searching nystagmus, reflecting his poor vision, and may likely have sluggish or absent pupillary light reflexes. Photophobia and the oculodigital reflex (eye rubbing that produces phosgenes in the retina) are also frequently seen. Fundus examination findings in the infant with LCA are usually strikingly normal in view of the extent of the infant's visual compromise (Fig 22–1). During the first years of life, a normal pigmentary pattern or a mild pigmentary retinopathy is noted.[3] There is, however, the eventual appearance of a pigmentary retinopathy with bony spicules and irregular pigmentation, attenuated arterioles, and optic atrophy. Schroeder and colleagues[3] recently reported a nummular pigmentary pattern in two patients with LCA, one of whom was 8 months old. Optic pallor or edema have also been reported.

Leber's congenital amaurosis is frequently associated with systemic abnormalities, which prompted Foxman and coworkers[4] to suggest dividing children with LCA into two groups: uncomplicated and complicated. The uncomplicated form is defined as LCA in the "absence of known nonocular abnormalities." However, some children with this form of LCA may have macular colobomas. In general, these patients have extreme hyperopia (>5 D and, on the basis of A-scan ultrasound evidence,[5] are likely to have shorter-than-normal axial lengths.

Complicated LCA is defined as having nonocular abnormalities and may be associated with cerebrohepatorenal syndrome (Zellweger syndrome), nephronophthisis with epiphyseal abnormalities (Saldino-Mainzer

TABLE 22–1.
Retina and Vitreous Abnormalities in Early Life

I. Retinal development
  A. Leber's congenital amaurosis
  B. Retinal dysplasia
  C. Albinism
  D. Typical rod monochromatism
  E. Coloboma of the choroid
  F. Retinoschisis
  G. Myelinated nerve fibers
II. Vitreous development
  A. Hyaloid vasculature
  B. Persistent hyperplastic primary vitreous
  C. Coloboma of lens
III. "Inflammatory-like" disease
  A. Familial exudative vitreoretinopathy
  B. Coats disease
IV. Tumors
  A. Retinoblastoma
  B. Phakomatosis
V. Conditions seen early in life in systemic disease
  A. Cherry-red spot
  B. Norrie disease
  C. Stickler syndrome
  D. Spondyloepiphyseal dysplasia congenita
  E. Incontinentia pigmenti
  F. Lens dislocation

syndrome),[6] renal anomalies,[7] and congenital neurological abnormalities such as hyperreflexia and developmental motor and mental delay.[8] No extreme hyperopia is seen in this group of infants with LCA.

Regardless of refractive error or associated abnormalities, the suspicion of LCA should be confirmed with an electroretinogram ERG. The response to light stimulation in both light- and dark-adapted conditions will be extinguished regardless of age at testing. Such testing should be undertaken as soon as reasonable for accurate diagnosis and appropriate counseling for educational planning and the likelihood of recurrence in the child's subsequent siblings.

Autosomal recessive inheritance is the most common mode of transmission for LCA. In Noble and Carr's study of 33 patients,[9] 30% of the cases were likely to have been autosomal recessive. When there are associated systemic abnormalities, the inheritance pattern tends to be less clearly defined.

Children with LCA have very poor visual acuities, with a range from bare light perception to a relatively good 20/80.[9] An interesting subset of children with LCA was described in 1984 by Moore and Taylor.[7] These children exhibited not only the characteristic changes of LCA but also vertical and horizontal saccade palsies with relatively good acuities in the 20/60 to 20/80 range. In the three cases described with LCA and a type of oculomotor apraxia, the visions were felt to "improve" during the second year of life in spite of the absence of change in the ERG.

Retinal Dysplasia

Abnormal differentiation of the retina that produces folds, gliosis, and disorganization is termed *retinal dysplasia.* This description of congenital retinal proliferation is observed in a wide variety of clinical situations and, when bilateral, is often associated with systemic abnormalities.

The causes of retinal maldevelopment appear to be divided into environmental and genetic.[10] Radiation,[11] prenatal trauma,[12] prenatal virus,[13, 14] and Agent Orange[15] exposure have been associated with unilateral retinal dysplasia. Bilateral retinal dysplasia is usually seen with associated systemic abnormalities such as 13–15 trisomy,[16] Norrie's disease,[17]

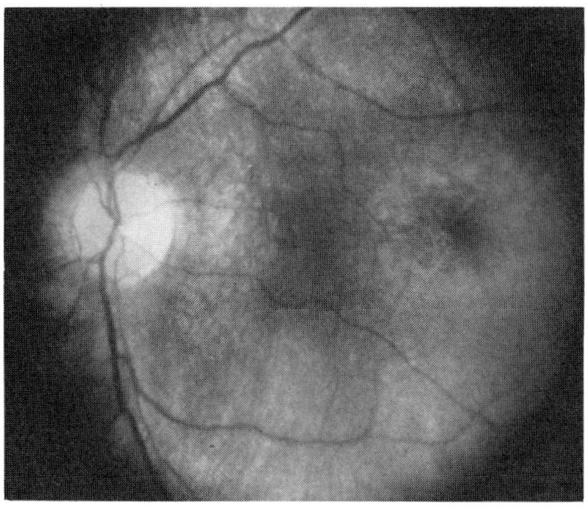

FIG 22–1.
LCA. The optic nerve and vessels appear normal in this patient with LCA, although there is a mild pigmentary disturbance in the macular area. (Courtesy of Gary Brown, M.D., and William Tasman, M.D.)

and Meckel syndrome.[18] The inheritance pattern of Norrie disease is X-linked recessive; Meckel syndrome is autosomal recessive. A primary vitreoretinal dysplasia transmitted in autosomal recessive pattern has also been described by Ohba et al.[10] with bilateral involvement without known systemic anomalies.

The child with bilateral retinal dysplasia is usually born at term after an uncomplicated delivery. "White pupils" are seen in the first weeks of life, and no fixation behavior is noted early in life. Ocular examination reveals searching nystagmus and severely impaired vision. The eyes are generally smaller than normal. The anterior chamber is often shallow, and the lens is usually clear at birth. Localized lenticular opacities may be noted in areas where retinal folds are attached to the posterior capsule. A mass of vascularized grayish white tissus is present in the retrolental space, with total retinal detachment in the most severe form. Systemic findings are those associated with the syndrome such as hearing loss, mental retardation, and dementia in Norrie disease[17] and microcephaly, encephalocele, polycystic kidneys, and syndactyly in Meckel syndrome.[18]

Unilateral cases with retinal dysplasia present as sighted children with the abnormality confined to one eye. Nystagmus should not be expected in unilateral disease. No detectable vision or pupillary response is likely to be elicited from an affected eye, which is clinically indistinguishable from that seen in bilateral cases. Preslan and colleagues[15] reported a case of unilateral retinal dysplasia and congenital glaucoma that presented with buphthalmos, increased intraocular pressure, and leukokoria. In this case, an association with Agent Orange exposure was suspected.

No visual rehabilitation is possible in these severely disorganized eyes, and counseling the parents about educational handicaps, systemic associations, and inheritance patterns is a vital part of the care of these children.

Albinism

Congenital hypopigmentation of the pigment epithelium of the eye is manifested by various types of albinism including oculocutaneous and ocular forms. The former is relatively easy to recognize because skin, hair, and eyes are all hypopigmented. There are four subtypes in oculocutaneous albinism: tyrosinase-positive, tyrosinase-negative, a yellow-mutant variety, and a tyrosinase-positive type associated with platelet dysfunction (Hermansky-Pudlak syndrome).[19] All are autosomal recessive, with the tyrosinase-positive form being most common. The subtypes are generally divided on the basis of electron microscopy of the skin and hair or hair bulb incubation with L-tyrosine or L-dopa.[20] Tyrosinase is an essential enzyme in melanin formation and is present in tyrosinase-positive albinism but lacking in the tyrosinase-negative form.

Nystagmus is noted early in life in children with albinism, and subnormal visual acuity should be expected (range, 20/100 to 20/400) as will be discussed. Photophobia, astigmatism, ametropia, and strabismus are also common early in life (Table 22–2). Ocular examination reveals iris transillumination due to hypopigmentation of the iris epithelium (Fig 22–2). The entire globe will often transilluminate diffusely. Hypoplasia of the macula is a constant finding with the absence of the foveal reflex, absence of normal hyperpigmentation of the foveal area, and absence of macula lutea pigment (Fig 22–3). Color vision testing results are usually normal, and the ERG may even be supernormal.[21]

The etiology of the visual impairment in albinism is multifactorial. Macular "hypoplasia" implies abnormal maturation of the foveal

TABLE 22–2.
Ocular Findings in Albinism

Macular hypoplasia
Absence of foveal reflex
Absence of normal foveal hyperpigmentation
Absence of macula lutea pigment
Iris transillumination
Nystagmus
Photophobia frequent
Strabismus common

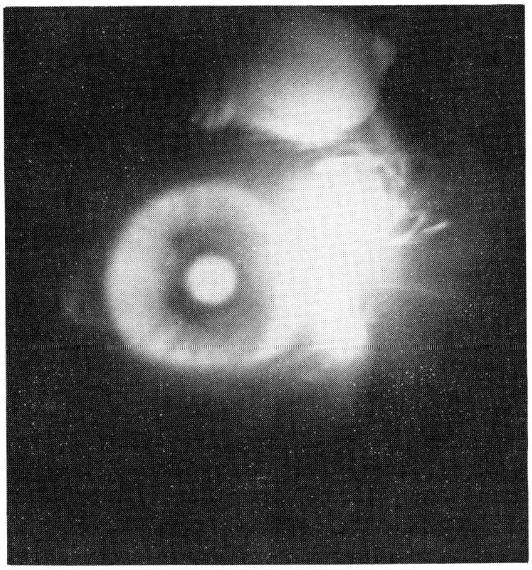

FIG 22–2.
Albinism. Iris transillumination is best seen when using the slit lamp with the beam focused on sclera near the limbus and the pupil undilated. In albinism, the entire globe may be transilluminated as well as the iris, as the pigment in the iris and retinal pigment epithelium are absent. (Courtesy of Gary Brown, M.D., and William Tasman, M.D.)

region, with a thick ganglion and nuclear cell layer instead of the normal thinning.[22] This abnormally formed macula probably does not have the ability to achieve the fine resolution needed for good central visual acuity. Nystagmus develops early in life and further compromises resolving capabilities. There is also evidence that there is abnormal optic tract decussation at the chiasm,[23] that results in misrouting of neurons from the temporal retina and disturbs the "normal" organization and spatial relationships in the cortex.

Ocular albinism (OA) is less common than the oculocutaneous type and is seen in three patterns of inheritance: X-linked (Nettleship-Falls syndrome),[24] autosomal recessive,[25] and the Chédiak-Higashi syndrome (autosomal recessive).[26] Patients with these conditions usually also manifest mild cutaneous manifestations of albinism, but the ocular abnormalities are much more striking. They are also more variable than in oculocutaneous albinims. Iris transillumination is not a constant feature and, in darkly pigmented individuals, may be absent. The iris color also varies from blue to brown, and retinal epithelial pigmentation is not uniformly reduced. A constant finding, however, is the presence of macular hypoplasia. Acuity correlates with the degree of ocular pigmentation, i.e., the more pigment, the better the acuity. Histologically, fewer than the normal number of melanosomes are noted, and most of these are normally pigmented.[21]

The X-linked form of OA shows both decreased numbers of melanosomes and abnormal types of melanosomes (macromelanosomes) on hair bulb analysis and skin biopsy. The female carrier state in Nettleship-Falls OA has characteristic ocular and cutaneous abnormalities. Partial iris transillumination is often noted, and patches of hypopigmentation are noted in the midperiphery of the retina.

The Chédiak-Higashi syndrome is OA associated with decreased bactericidal ability and a predisposition to developing a lymphoma-like syndrome. These patients have slate gray patches of skin and, on skin biopsy, have giant inclusions in all granule-producing cells.[26]

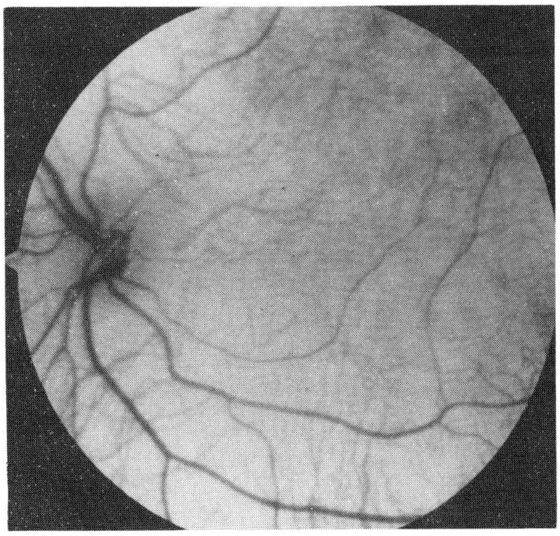

FIG 22–3.
Albinism. Foveal hypoplasia is characteristic of albinism with no foveolar reflex and no macular hyperpigmentation. The absence of normal retinal pigment makes the choroidal vasculature appear prominent.

Typical Rod Monochromatism (Typical Complete Color Blindness)

A rare form of color blindness can present within the first year of life and must be considered when confronted with an infant with subnormal vision. Typical rod monochromatism (achromatopsia) occurs in about 3 in 10,000 births and shows autosomal recessive inheritance.[27] The infant presents with nystagmus and severe photophobia so marked that the child is uncomfortable going outside during the day. Ocular examination findings are unremarkable including those of the fundus examination. An absence of the foveal reflex and some pigment stippling have, however, been reported. Pupillary reaction is slow to a light stimulus but normal during dark adaptation.[27]

Except for the ERG, functional testing of the retina to document abnormalities in infants is difficult. The ERG shows diagnostic findings of an absent photopic (light-adapted) response, a very low flicker fusion frequency, and an absence or marked diminution of the first portion of the orange-red response. These findings in association with a normal scotopic (dark-adapted) response are characteristic.

Typical rod monochromatism is a stationary defect and is not expected to worsen with age. In general, the acuity range for these children is 20/200 with better near vision than distance, and the nystagmus noted in early childhood may become less apparent in the second decade. Strabismus and astigmatism are more common in this form of color blindness than for the population as a whole.[28]

Compared with the loss of visual acuity, the disability associated with the total absence of color perception appears minor. In practical terms, the individual with complete color blindness can match different wavelengths of light (which determine the color) by merely adjusting the radiance. Thus he will be unable to discriminate the difference between stimuli on the basis of wavelength.[28]

There is also an X-linked form of incomplete achromatopsia that may present in early childhood with nystagmus, photophobia, reduced acuity, and essentially normal ocular examination results. Acuity tends to be somewhat better than in patients with the recessive form of achromatopsia. Myopia is also associated with this disorder.[29] The female carrier state in this condition can also be detected by ERG on the basis of a slightly reduced flicker fusion frequency and delayed dark adaptation.[27] Color vision testing will also reveal excessive errors on the 100-hue test.[27]

The X-linked form of incomplete achromatopsia may derive from a different mechanism at the retinal level than does typical complete achromatopsia. The defect may actually result from the combination of protanopia and deuteranopia manifested in the same individual.[27]

Coloboma of the Choroid and Retinal Detachment

Choroidal colobomas arise when the inner and outer layers of the pigment epithelium do not fuse with their identical opposing layers in the area of the fetal fissure. This fissure is located inferonasally to the disc and, during normal development, closes from the equator anteriorly and posteriorly. An area of nonpigmented sensory retina is seen in the fundus as a glistening white patch with margins that are often pigmented. The choroidal vessels develop poorly, and the retinal vessels are sparse or absent. The defect may extend to the optic nerve posteriorly and cause an optic nerve coloboma (Fig 22–4) or extend to the iris anteriorly and produce an inferonasal gap in the iris.[30]

Retinal detachment may be associated with a coloboma of the choroid soon after birth and can present a diagnostic dilemma. The membrane of retinal tissue overlying a coloboma is very thin and not attached firmly to the edges of the defect or within the defect itself. Retinal breaks in the region of the coloboma are difficult to detect in the absence of the color change associated with retinal holes over normal choroidal vasculature. Hemorrhage in the area of the coloboma may also indicate retinal tears in a region not visible ophthalmoscopically due to a posterior

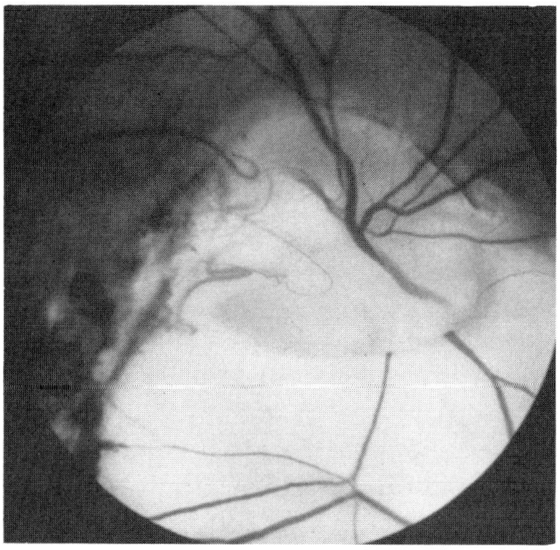

FIG 22–4.
Uveal coloboma. Uveal colobomas may extend to involve the optic nerve. (Courtesy of Gary Brown, M.D., and William Tasman, M.D.)

staphyloma or other distortion of the globe. Such breaks can lead to retinal detachment with a poor prognosis for salvaging the eye.[31]

Colobomas may occur as a sporadic finding in otherwise normal individuals or associated with chromosomal abnormalities such as trisomy 13 and other syndromes such as Goldenhar and Aicardi, and the CHARGE association.[32] Autosomal dominant inheritance with incomplete penetrance has also been documented.[33]

Retinoschisis

Congenital retinoschisis has an X-linked inheritance pattern and, as such, is manifested in males. Both posterior-pole and peripheral retinal abnormalities are seen, and both are caused by a splitting of the nerve fiber layer.[34] Posterior-pole changes in congenital retinoschisis are very common but can be subtle. Characteristically, delicate spokes of macular retinoschisis with small, superficial retinal cysts are noted (Fig 22–5). Macular edema and pucker have also been documented. The peripheral changes are more dramatic and include an elevation of the inner retinal layers, usually in the inferotemporal quadrant, that does not reach the ora serrata. Retinal vessels are frequently seen on the surface of the thin layer of retina, and holes are often present in this inner layer. If a hole develops in the outer retinal layers, a retinal detachment is likely. Vitreous veils may also be seen.[30, 35]

Schisis is rarely documented early in life, but if the posterior pole is severely affected, a marked decrease in visual acuity is likely to be accompanied by nystagmus and/or strabismus. Still the physical abnormality of the macula may be difficult to document in infants because the characteristic changes are usually documented with a contact lens and slit-lamp examination—a difficult task with a wiggling infant in the office. The ERG is clearly abnormal, with reduction of the B-wave amplitude and normal A wave reflecting the abnormality of the inner retinal layer. The natural history of congenital retinoschisis is a stationary or very slowly progressive decrease in central vision. Retinal detachment or marked elevation of a peripheral schisis cavity will likely cause decreased acuity and function.[30]

Other rare forms of hereditary retinoschisis have been described including an autosomal recessive familial foveal schisis[36] and an autosomal dominant form.[37] Traumatic retinoschisis from physical abuse should also be considered in infants with retinoschisis.[38]

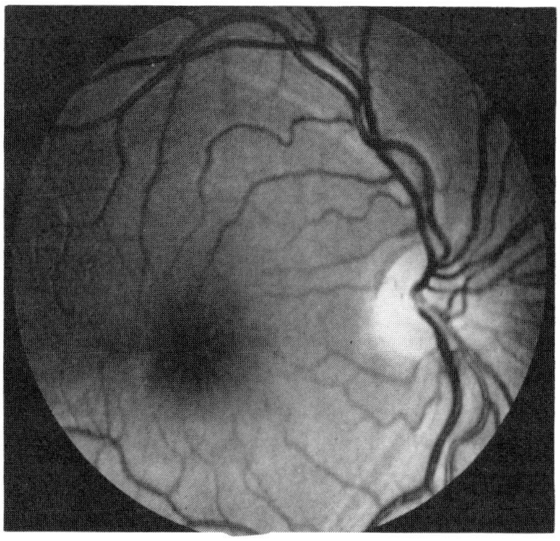

FIG 22–5.
Retinoschisis. Fine spokelike lines with small, superficial retinal cysts are noted in the macula of a patient with X-linked retinoschisis. (Courtesy of Gary Brown, M.D., and William Tasman, M.D.)

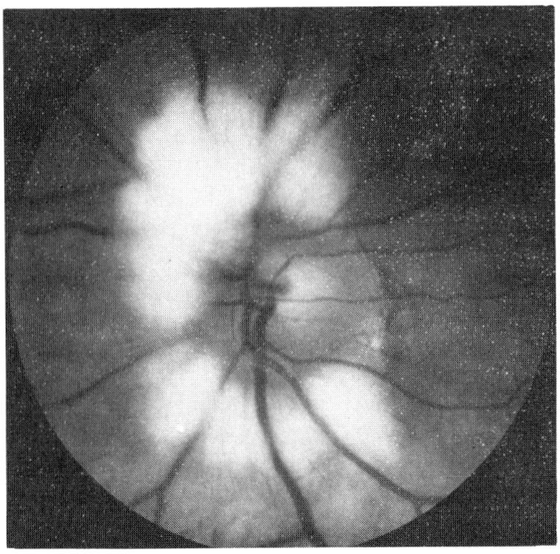

FIG 22–6.
Myelinated nerve fibers. Sprays of myelinated nerve fibers are frequently contiguous with the optic nerve head. They have feathery margins, are glistening white, and frequently obscure retinal vasculature. (Courtesy of Gary Brown, M.D., and William Tasman, M.D.)

Myelinated Nerve Fibers

Myelinated nerve fibers of the retina may be observed early in life either on ophthalmoscopic examination or as an abnormal reflex. The retina is normally transparent. However, if medullation of the optic nerve proceeds anterior to the lamina cribrosa, the superficial ganglion cell layer may be myelinated.[39] This appears as a spray of white patches that follow the course of the nerve fibers. The areas of myelination are frequently attached to the optic nerve (Fig 22–6), but they may also be separated by patches of normal retina (Fig 22–7). If the area is small and in the peripheral retina, this anomaly rarely has any serious effect on visual function, though it may produce field defects corresponding to the areas of myelinations. If extensive in the posterior pole, an accurate refraction on retinoscopy may be difficult.

Eyes with extensive myelinated nerve fibers may have decreased acuity associated with myopia, strabismus, amblyopia, and nystagmus. Straatsma et al.[40] reported four patients with extensive unilateral myelinated nerve fibers and ipsilateral myopia, amblyopia, and strabismus. These patients had profound visual impairment in the affected eye that they suggest may be at least partly organic and might be unlikely to respond to amblyopia therapy.

VITREOUS DEVELOPMENT

Hyaloid Vasculature

The hyaloid vascular system emerges early in fetal ocular development to provide a vascular supply for the primary vitreous (tunica hyaloidea propia) and the developing lens (tunica vasculosa lentis). The entire system starts to involute at about 11 weeks of gestation, with the capillaries nourishing the lens and the hyaloid artery itself being the last to atrophy.[41]

Both the tunica vasculosa lentis and the hyaloid artery may be observed in the premature infant (Fig 22–8). The degree of atrophy of the vascular supply to the lens has been well correlated with gestational age by several investigators[42, 43] and can even be used to estimate the gestational age of an infant in the first days of life.

The hyaloid artery may occasionally persist throughout life and may be blood filled or a ghost vessel. It may be segmental or seen as a vessel emerging from the optic disc and passing through the vitreous cavity toward the lens. If the insertion of the artery onto the posterior lens capsule is visible, it is called Mittendorf's dot.

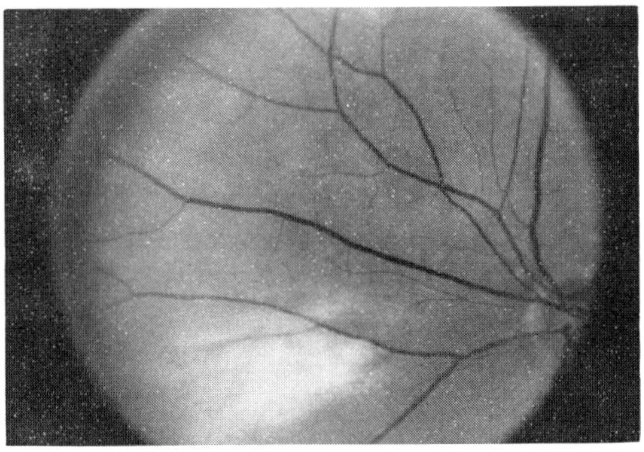

FIG 22–7.
Myelinated nerve fibers. Patches of myelinated nerve fibers may not be connected to the optic disc but may appear elsewhere in the retina.

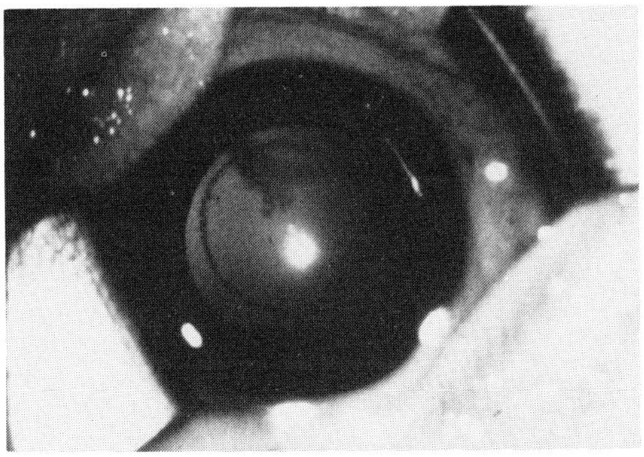

FIG 22–8.
Hyaloid vasculature. In the premature infant, remnants of the hyaloid system and tunica vasculosa lentis are frequently visible. Note the blood-filled hyaloid vessel.

Persistent Hyperplastic Primary Vitreous

Persistent hyperplastic primary vitreous (PHPV) is a developmental anomaly that may present in three forms: anterior, posterior, and combined. The abnormality is usually monocular and presents early in life with strabismus, a white reflex, or poor vision. The severity of visual disturbance is directly related to the extent of disruption from failure of the primary vitreous to regress, and findings may range from Bergmeister's papilla to marked disorganization of the eye with hemorrhage, glaucoma, and phthisis.[44]

The anterior form presents with mild microphthalmos and a shallow anterior chamber. The lens is clear early in life, and in the retrolental space, a white mass is noted. In the mass, the radial blood vessels are seen, and ciliary processes are drawn up into this mass (Fig 22–9). With time, the lens becomes cataractous with further shallowing of the anterior chamber. Vitreous hemorrhaging and further traction on the ciliary body increase the likelihood of secondary glaucoma, which is very difficult to treat.

Posterior PHPV presents with leukokoria and poor vision and is the most uncommon of the three forms.[45] Again, the lens is clear, and a dense, white vitreous band extends from the region of the disc to the periphery. Pruett and Schepens[46] reported 11 such patients and felt they were in many ways similar to the patients with a congenital retinal fold. The vitreous band became circumferential in the peripheral part of the retina and extended to the lens equator. All of these eyes had retinal folds, pigmentary disturbance, or retinal detachments. In most of these patients, the lens stayed clear, and glaucoma did not develop in the follow-up period of up to 14 years. Mann[47] suggested that this anomaly occurs because hyaloid vessels and primary vitreous can be abnormally adherent to an area of the optic cup, thereby leading to incomplete formation of the secondary vitreous with subsequent retinal folding. In a further report, Pruett[48] documented a high incidence of retinal detachment, abnormal macular function, and vitreoretinal traction. In addition, the optic nerve head appeared pale, and retinal vessels were attenuated. No other systemic or ocular anomalies were noted.

The majority of patients with PHPV have findings that are consistent with both the anterior form and posterior form and reflect the pleomorphism of this disordered development (Table 22–3). Pollard[45] reported a series of 32 patients of whom 20 had a combination of findings characteristic of anterior and posterior PHPV.

Until recently, therapy for PHPV has largely been treating secondary glaucoma and removing painful or phthisical eyes resulting from this frequent complication. In the last 15 years, however, aggressive, early management has been directed toward improving visual

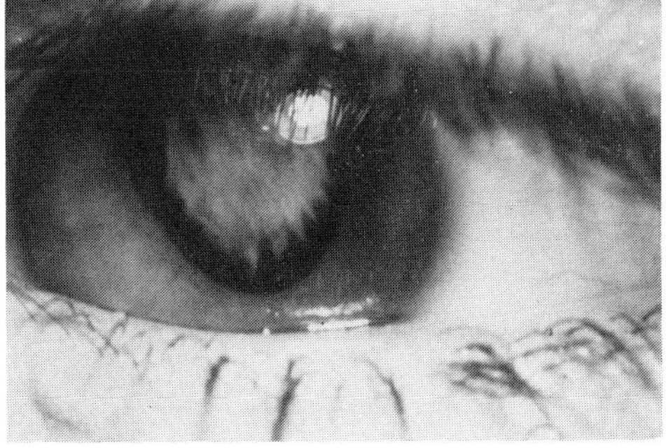

FIG 22–9.
PHPV. A white retrolental mass is noted behind a clear lens. The scalloped dark edges are the ciliary processes drawn up into the mass.

TABLE 22–3.
Persistent Hyperplastic Primary Vitreous

Common characteristics in early life	
	Mild microphthalmos
	Clear lens early on
	Leukokoria
Anterior findings that may be present	
	Retrolental whitish mass with radial vessels
	Ciliary processes visible on dilation
Posterior findings that may be present	
	Circumferential vitreous band in periphery
	Retinal folds/macular heterotopia

function. Of 32 patients seen over a 10-year period by Pollard,[45] 30 had a lensectomy with at least an anterior vitrectomy to remove the hyperplastic vitreous as a "minimum" procedure. Five of these patients have recordable visual acuities of 20/200 or better. Four patients with largely posterior surgery had a good anatomic but poor visual outcome, probably due to retinal abnormalities observed in the posterior pole. Subsequently, patients with posterior vitreous or retinal abnormalities have undergone only lensectomy with anterior vitrectomy for cosmesis and prevention of secondary glaucoma. Four of the patients in Pollard's series had bilateral PHPV.

Karr and Scott[44] reported 48 patients with a wide range of clinical manifestations of PHPV seen at the University of Iowa. Twenty-three were treated surgically, and 18 of these had aggressive optical and amblyopia therapy. Eight had acuities of 20/200 or better. The patients with better visual results tended to be operated on earlier (average age, 2.4 months) than were the infants with acuities of 20/300 or worse (average age, 4.3 months at surgery). The two groups could not be distinguished on the basis of appearance of the cataract, vascularization of the retrolental membrane, or extent of microphthalmos. The poorer visual outcome group, however, tended to have more delays in clearing the visual axis, and instituting refractive correction and amblyopia therapy. They observed that the presence of posterior-segment abnormalities, either on ophthalmoscopic or echographic examination, usually precludes successful amblyopia therapy. Surgical considerations then shift to preventing glaucoma and enucleation.

The group of nonsurgical patients in Karr and Scott's series includes two patients with a mild form of PHPV that responded to medical amblyopia management with good acuity outcome. Some ocular findings suggest that an eye will have a poor outcome: the presence of an unrecordable ERG, severe amblyopia, macular involvement, inoperable retinal detachment, phthisis, or anomalous optic nerves.

The diverse visual outcomes that may result from the broad spectrum of ocular changes seen in PHPV emphasize the importance of involving parents early because their decision will greatly affect their interaction with a new family member. The child with posterior retinal changes probably has little chance for good vision, and prior to pursuing a course of extensive optical and amblyopia therapy, the parents should be counseled. The long-term view of such surgical interventions and subsequent therapy must be emphasized.

Coloboma of the Lens and Retinal Detachment

Maldevelopment of the lens during the development of the tertiary vitreous (zonules) produces an equatorial flattening of the lens itself that is known as a lens coloboma. This rare anomaly may be associated with serious retinal problems detectable early in life. During the second trimester, a specialized area of the secondary vitreous (the marginal bundle of Druault) fails to atrophy, which causes the peripheral retina to adhere to the lens. This, in turn, prevents the retina from assuming its normal position against the retinal pigment epithelium and leads to retinal tears and detachment.[49]

Hovland and colleagues[49] reported a series of eight bilateral retinal detachments in young children that were associated with lens colobomas. Only 25% of the retinas were successfully reattached, and only 1 of 16 had better than light perception vision.

"INFLAMMATORY-LIKE" DISEASES

Familial Exudative Vitreoretinopathy

The term *Familial exudative vitreoretinopathy* (FEVR) was used by Criswick and Schepens in 1969[50] to describe a group of children with a distinct familial vitreoretinal disorder having characteristics in common with ROP, Coats' disease, peripheral uveitis, and other posterior-pole disease.[50] They described six patients from two families ranging from 3½ months to 17 years of age with similar vitreal and retinal changes. Organized vitreous membranes were present both centrally and peripherally and were adherent to the retinal surface. Macular heterotopia was usually noted, with retinal exudates and localized retinal detachment noted in the periphery. This appearance is very similar to ROP, but these patients were not premature and had no supplemental oxygen therapy or known systemic abnormalities. They also demonstrated a hereditary pattern that is not seen in ROP. In addition, new retinal vessel formation was noted at several years of age, which is not part of the abnormal vessel growth in ROP. The 3½-month-old sibling of two other affected patients had normal vision and normal external examination findings. On fundus examination, the child had small hemorrhages superotemporally that were sharply outlined and white without pressure at the vitreous base, and areas of choroidal atrophy were seen. The older children in this series had generally poor vision in at least one eye, with extensive vitreoretinal adhesions and dragging of the macula and posterior-pole vessels, and some had areas of localized retinal detachment. The investigators treated proliferating retinal vessels with photocoagulation and/or cryoapplications and retinal detachments with trap-door scleral buckling procedures.

Gow and Oliver[51] suggested dividing the spectrum of FEVR into three groups. Patients with stage 1 exhibit white with and without pressure and vitreous traction. Abnormal vascularization was not noted in this early stage. In stage 2, a peripheral fibrovascular scar is noted in the temporal periphery that is frequently associated with localized retinal detachment and macular ectopia. Stage 3 patients have advanced disease with vitreous fibrosis, a retinal detachment, and extensive subretinal exudation with secondary glaucoma and blindness. Canny and Oliver[52] subsequently documented the abnormal retinal vascular network in FEVR by using fluorescein angiography. Abrupt termination of capillaries with leakage of dye at this site was noted, which is also characteristic of other proliferative retinopathies.

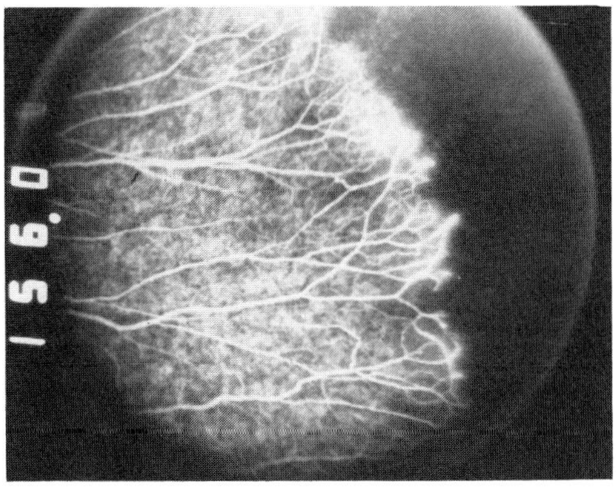

FIG 22–10.
FEVR. Fluorescein angiography of a patient with FEVR shows abrupt cessation of normal peripheral retinal vascularization with some leakage of dye at the termination of capillaries. (Courtesy of Gary Brown, M.D., and William Tasman, M.D.)

Slusher and Hutton[53] documented severe retinal abnormalities and visual loss in a 3-year-old child and emphasized the importance of early diagnosis and treatment.

Ober and colleagues[54] suggested in 1980 that the spectrum of changes included peripheral vascular abnormalities documented only by fluorescein angiography (Fig 22–10) and that this represented a subclinical manifestation of the abnormal gene. The patients had no visual complaints and did not have stage 1 findings. They also saw no progression of clinical findings in children after the second decade had passed, and while emphasizing the importance of diagnosis for genetic counseling, these authors agreed with Gitter and coworkers[55] that the disease does not progress relentlessly to visual loss in early life.

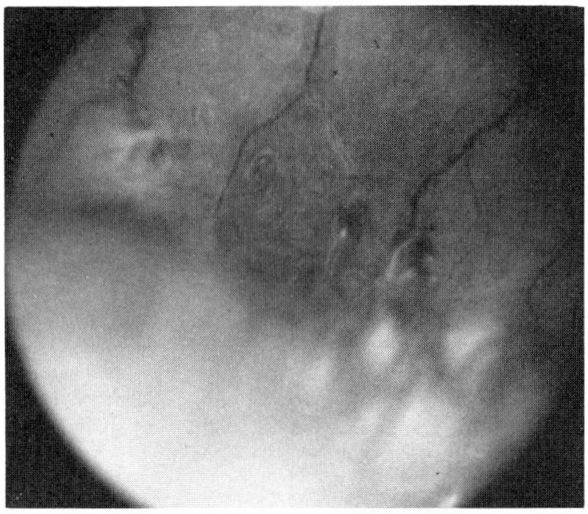

FIG 22–11.
Coats disease. Peripheral retinal vessels are telangiectatic with hemorrhage, vessel occlusion, exudate, and loss of normal retinal architecture and choroidal pattern. (Courtesy of Gary Brown, M.D. and William Tasman, M.D.)

They suggested that treatment should be administered when faced with progressive visual loss and not prophylactically in the presence of new vessel formation in the retina. Tasman and coworkers[56] reported that some 75% of those with FEVR were asymptomatic and these patients required no therapeutic intervention.

Coats Disease

Coats disease is a rare form of retinal telangiectasia with secondary subretinal exudation that may present very early in life with poor fixation, leukokoria, or strabismus. There are not usually associated systemic or ocular abnormalities, and the condition is frequently unilateral. The disease usually progresses to retinal detachment over varying periods of time. In earlier phases of the disease, telangiectatic retinal vessels can be seen on the retinal surface (Fig 22–11). The walls of these vessels are abnormally permeable, with resultant transudation of fluid (Fig 22–12), hemorrhages, and vascular occlusion.[57]

The major diagnostic dilemma confronting a clinician presented with an infant with unilateral leukokoria in a normal-sized eye is whether the process is retinoblastoma or Coats disease. Eyes with retinoblastoma may not have the characteristic calcification seen in that disease, and the serum-aqueous ratio of lactic dehydrogenase appears unreliable.[58] Enucleation of these blind eyes as a diagnostic procedure appears the most suitable alternative at present.

Ridley et al.[59] at Wills Eye Hospital reported 2 infants aged 12 months or less in a series of 41 patients in the time period from 1966 to 1980. All of these patients presented with subretinal exudation associated with retinal telangiectases of unknown cause. These investigators observed that 10 children under 4 years of age at presentation appeared to have a more virulent course that may have been influenced by early and aggressive treatment. Therapy was directed at (1) eliminating peripheral vascular telangiectasias by using cryotherapy, (2) treating dilated capillary networks and abnormal arteries and veins of the fundus behind the equator by using xenon photocoagulation, and (3) draining subretinal fluid. Re-evaluation and consideration for retreatment was done in 2 to 4 weeks until all abnormal vessels were eliminated. Three of the children in the less than 4-year-old age group presented with end-stage disease. Seven in this age group received an average of four treatments over a period of 8 to 16 months, at which time the condition stabilized. Of the 2

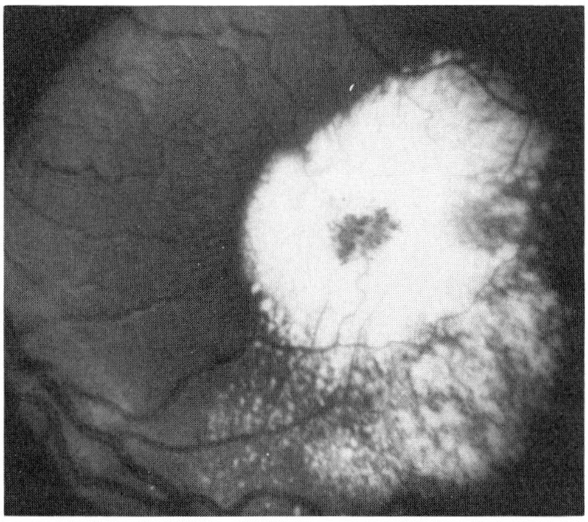

FIG 22–12.
Coats disease. Exudation in Coats disease may progress to involve the posterior pole with marked visual loss. (Courtesy of Gary Brown, M.D., and William Tasman, M.D.)

children who presented by the age of 1 year, 1 was in each of the untreatable and treated categories, one child required enucleation for neovascular glaucoma, and the other had 6/120 acuity after a 3-year follow-up. Progression of the disease was halted in the latter patient, but central vision may have been compromised by extensive subretinal gliosis and amblyopia (a particularly likely event in this unilateral problem).

TUMORS

Retinoblastoma

Retinoblastoma, the most common intraocular tumor in childhood, frequently presents in the first year of life. Tumors that are confined to the eye usually present with a white reflex (leukokoria), and/or strabismus and may be picked up on a routine examination by the infant's primary physician. Tumors that have progressed beyond the globe usually present with proptosis or distant metastases. Ellsworth[60] reports that 56% of patients present with a leukokoria, 20% with strabismus, another 12% with poor vision or a glaucomatous, painful eye, and the remainder present on routine examination (3%). Less frequent presentations include hyphema, iris heterochromia, cellulitis, and nystagmus.

Leukokoria may first be noticed by a family member or in a photograph. If the mass is in the posterior pole, it may be relatively small when the abnormal reflex is noted. Tumors that arise more peripherally, particularly near the ciliary body, may be quite large before they affect the normal red reflex. Strabismus may be the presenting sign if central vision is affected either by tumor involvement in the macula or by obscuration of the visual axis by vitreous seeding or massive tumor size (Fig 22–13). Glaucoma with redness and pain is relatively common as a presenting sign and is usually secondary to tumor hemorrhage and necrosis. Iris heterochromia or unilateral pupillary dilation are likely to be associated with extensive ocular involvement, as is hyphema when it is a presenting sign of retinoblastoma.[60]

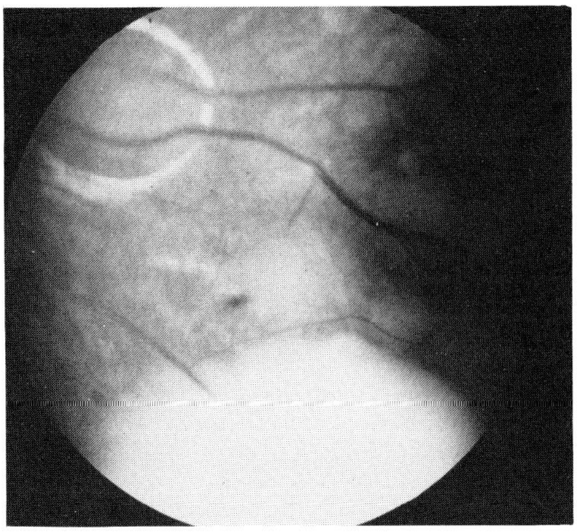

FIG 22–13.
Retinoblastoma. A large tumor mass is seen inferiorly, with several satellite tumors noted above.

This ocular tumor is highly malignant and, when advanced at presentation, is likely to be lethal.[61] Early detection, however, is associated with a survival rate around 75%.[62] The incidence of the disease varies in population studies from 1:17,000 to 1:34,000,[63] but the disease will probably become more frequent as more children with hereditary tumors survive to childbearing age and pass on the abnormal gene.

The hereditary potential of retinoblastoma has long been recognized, and exciting advances have recently been made in the laboratory diagnosis of abnormal genes and marker systems that are associated with retinoblastoma.[64] Some 60% of patients with retinoblastoma have somatic mutations without heritable predisposition; approximately 85% of these cases have unilateral disease. The remaining 40% of patients have germinal mutations and will show an autosomal dominant pattern of heredity. About 85% of the hereditary cases are bilateral or have multiple tumor foci in the same eye.[65] There is also a definite association of retinoblastoma with a deletion of the long arm of chromosome 13,[60] but most patients with retinoblastoma have "normal" chromosomes unless specialized techniques of banding, biochemical analysis, and enzymatic linkage studies are undertaken.

Knudson[66] suggested the "two-hit" hypothesis for the development of retinoblastoma in which the first mutation occurs in the retinal cell itself in nonhereditary cases or in the germinal cells in a hereditary one. The second mutation must take place before the malignancy develops, and this event is a somatic one, i.e., it takes place in the patient's retinal cells. When using restriction fragment-length polymorphism and esterase D isoenzyme linkage, Gallie and Phillips[64] found a somatic change to homozygosity with regard to the 13q14 locus in patients with retinoblastoma. They suggested that this loss of heterozygosity resulted in the loss of normal cellular differentiation and proliferation, thereby resulting in malignant change.

Although rare, congenital retinoblastoma masquerading as an opaque ectatic corneal staphyloma at birth has recently been reported by Plotsky and coworkers[67] and was similar to that in the infant reported by Zimmerman earlier.[68] Plotsky et al. reported that a corneal perforation occurred on the second day after birth and an enucleation was performed on the fourth day. After pathological examination of the specimen showed a poorly differentiated neoplasm with focal calcification consistent with retinoblastoma, a staging work-up showed no evidence of metastatic disease. Chemotherapy using cyclophosphamide, vincristine, doxorubicin (Adriamycin), and intrathecal methotrexate in conjunction with hyperfractionated radiation therapy to the orbit (3,000 rad) was administered. The tumor recurred locally within 3 months, and again a metastatic work-up was negative. Additional chemotherapy and radiation therapy had little effect, and a modified orbital exenteration was performed. Morphological and immunohistochemical studies supported a diagnosis of retinoblastoma. The child developed lethargy and vomiting 2 months later and expired shortly thereafter. The fellow eye remained unaffected during the child's lifetime.

This case is instructive for several reasons. Most unilateral tumors are nonhereditary, but Carlson and colleagues[69] state that 10% to 20% of patients with unilateral retinoblastoma will develop disease in the fellow eye, thus confirming the likelihood of a hereditary form of retinoblastoma. In addition, the clinician confronted with an abnormal blind eye at birth must consider retinoblastoma in the differential diagnosis.

Ellsworth,[60] in a series of 1,200 cases, observed no new tumor arising after 2 years and 9 months of age. If the children had been examined under anesthesia because they were in a high-risk group, the likelihood of a new tumor developing after the age of 2 years was very low.

Abramson and colleagues[62] reported an extensive series of 1,531 patients (including those just mentioned) observed over a 69-year period at the Ophthalmic Oncology Center at New York Hospital. They found that patients with unilateral disease and a positive family history were likely to have the tumor detected in early infancy (median age at diagnosis, 5 months; n = 31 for 1958 to 1983). Tumors in children with bilateral disease and a positive family history were detected somewhat later (median age at diagnosis, 11 months; n = 106 for 1958 to 1983). A negative family history increased the median age at detection to 15 months in bilateral retinoblastoma and 25 months in unilateral disease in this same time period. These workers also reported important survival rate information that is helpful when counseling family members of an affected infant. The likelihood of not dying from metastatic retinoblastoma was very similar (around 76%) in either unilateral or bilateral disease, though death, if it occurred, was more likely to happen earlier in unilateral (less than 4 years after diagnosis) than in bilateral cases (less than 8 years after diagnosis). However, they emphasized the likelihood of developing second malignancies in patients with the hereditary forms of retinoblastoma. These were not just the "radiation-induced" tumors in the field of ocular radiation therapy but also unrelated second cancers.[70] In a large series,[62] second cancers occurred within a year of the diagnosis of retinoblastoma and, after 5 years, accounted for more deaths than retinoblastoma itself. After 35 years, some 59% of patients with bilateral retinoblastoma have died of either metastatic retinoblastoma or a second tumor.

The diagnosis of retinoblastoma relies heavily on clinical history, physical examination, and careful ophthalmologic examination, and these are now supplemented by specialized diagnostic modalities. Ultrasound has been helpful in the differential diagnosis of PHPV, Coats' disease, retinoblastoma, and other diseases. B-scan ultrasound frequently demonstrates discrete, highly reflective foci, probably areas of calcification, within a tumor. This finding is common in retinoblastoma and very uncommon in other conditions.[71]

Fluorescein angiography is useful in assessing the vascularity of the mass, which carries prognostic and therapeutic implications. If massive leakage into the vitreous is noted, this suggests vitreous seeding by the tumor and that localized destruction of the tumor may be inadequate. Computerized tomography can clearly document the size of the lesion and intralesional calcification. It also delineated optic nerve abnormalities, extraocular extension, and intracranial abnormalities such as pinealoblastomas.[65]

Finally, aspiration of ocular fluids or cells from tumor masses can be useful in documenting the presence of retinoblastoma. Lactic dehydrogenase and phosphoglucose isomerase levels are frequently elevated in the aqueous humor of retinoblastoma patients and not in patients with other abnormalities. Fine-needle aspiration may also be used under carefully controlled circumstances to obtain cellular material for cytological examination.[69]

Management of patients with retinoblastoma is dependent on the status of the fellow eye and the extent of ocular involvement and extraocular extension. If there is no hope for vision, enucleation is felt to be the treatment of choice.[65] Radiation therapy including external-beam irradiation using anterior and lateral approaches and episcleral radioactive plaques are also used in selected patients. Localized ablation techniques including photocoagulation and cryotherapy are effective methods for destruction of some small tumors. Chemotherapy has been largely used in patients with metastatic disease or extraocular extension, and use in patients with only intraocular involvement remains controversial.

Phakomatoses

Phakomatosis is a term used to describe a group of diseases with ocular, intracranial, and cutaneous abnormalities. The group is diverse in symptomatology, presentation, and type of abnormally growing tissue. The tumors are hamartomas, i.e., composed of cells normally present in a specific location such as the retina, central nervous system, or skin. The phakomatoses include vascular anomalies such as Sturge-Weber syndrome, von Hippel-Lindau disease, and Wyburn-Mason syndrome and neuroectodermal disorders such as Bourneville and von Recklinghausen diseases. Each of these may be familial and presumably are present from birth, though the ocular abnormalities may not be observed until much later in life.

Sturge-Weber Syndrome

In the 1870s, Sturge[72] recognized encephalotrigeminal angiomatosis (Sturge-Weber syndrome) as a clinical entity with nevus flammeus in the distribution of the trigminal nerve, glaucoma, and hemangiomas of meninges and choroid. The nevus flammeus, or port-wine stain, is commonly unilateral with involvement of the upper and/or middle branch of the trigeminal nerve. The nevus may be subtle at birth and develop its more characteristic appearance after several months have passed.[73]

In Sturge-Weber syndrome, the most prominent ocular sign, buphthalmos due to glaucoma, is relatively common early in life, though glaucoma may also present later during childhood. The presumed etiologic mechanism for this type of glaucoma is increased venous pressure with a resultant outflow obstruction of the aqueous fluid. Surgical treatment is difficult and frequently unsuccessful.[74] Conjunctival and episcleral telangiectasis is also frequently seen. On fundus examination, a choroidal hemangioma is a common finding[75]

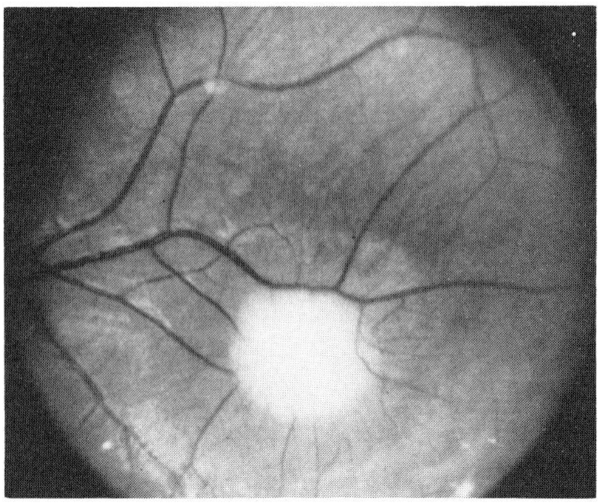

FIG 22–14.
Tuberous sclerosis. A white, smooth, and round astrocytic hamartoma is seen within the retinal vessel arcades. (Courtesy of Gary Brown, M.D., and William Tasman, M.D.)

and is characteristically elevated, circular, and darker than the surrounding uvea. Fluorescein angiography reveals a marked fluorescence during the follow-phase.

Seizures are common in Sturge-Weber syndrome patients and are related to the hemangiomatous malformations of the meninges. Calcification of gyri become visible on x-ray film after several years of life. Seizures may occur early in life and may be resistant to therapy.[76]

von Hippel-Lindau Disease

von Hippel–Lindau disease, or angiomatosis of the retina and cerebellum, has been documented histologically in the fetus[77] but is usually observed ophthalmologically in the third decade of life. von Hippel described the ocular findings in 1904,[78] and Lindau documented the association of retinal angiomatosis with visceral and central nervous system hemangiomas.[79] An autosomal dominant pattern of inheritance is suspected in less than half of the cases.[80]

The ocular tumors may occur in the pediatric age group[81] but have not yet been described in the first year of life. Ocular findings are binocular in 50% of patients. They consist initially of small, round, red lesions in the midperipheral part of the retina. A dilated retinal artery and vein are connected to the globular mass. The angiomas may enlarge and lead to hemorrhage, exudate, retinal detachment, and subsequent glaucoma and phthisis. Therapy is directed at eliminating the retinal lesions early in their development by using cryosurgery and photocoagulation.[82]

Wyburn-Mason Syndrome

Wyburn-Mason syndrome is a nonprogressive, congenital abnormality with arteriovenous malformations of the retina and midbrain.[83] Autosomal dominant inheritance is noted. Fundus examination shows marked dilation and tortuosity of retinal vessels projecting from the retinal surface, and some visual impairment should be expected.[82]

Bourneville's Disease

Tuberous sclerosis, or Bourneville disease, is characterized by multiple tumors of the central nervous system, mental deficiency, and adenoma sebaceum.[84] The ocular lesions may be observed in the course of a work-up for an infant with seizures of unknown origin and include astrocytic hamartomas of the retina and disc (Figs 22–14 and 22–15). The lesions are initially gray-white, smooth, and round, with gradual appearance of the classic mulberry-like nodules on the surface.[85] Optic nerve head drusen are also seen in tuberous sclerosis. The ocular lesions require no therapy, though with extensive hemorrhage or

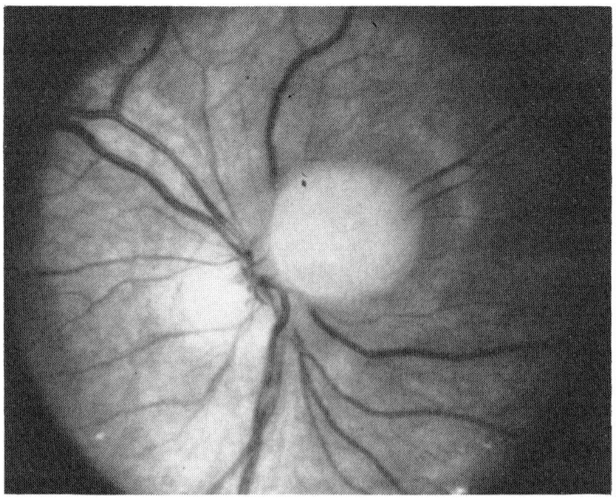

FIG 22–15.
Tuberous sclerosis. The lesion of tuberous sclerosis can also be seen near the optic nerve head. (Courtesy of Gary Brown, M.D., and William Tasman, M.D.)

secondary glaucoma they may present a diagnostic dilemma.

von Recklinghausen Disease

Neurofibromatosis (von Recklinghausen disease) is a dominantly inherited developmental abnormality with tumors of the central nervous system, bone, viscera, eye, and orbit that may present at birth.[86] The characteristic neurofibroma may develop in any area of the body and may be discreet or plexiform. Upper lid involvement with disfigurement and ptosis is common.[87] Exophthalmos may be due to a neurofibroma in the orbit, tumor of the optic nerve, or bony abnormalities of the orbit.[88] Thickened corneal nerves are observed in older children. Intraocular abnormalities include neurofibromas on the iris surface and a rarely observed retinal lesion similar to that seen in tuberous sclerosis. Congenital glaucoma is relatively common in patients with neurofibromatosis and is difficult to treat. Optic nerve gliomas occur in about 10% of patients.[82]

RETINA AND VITREOUS ABNORMALITIES SEEN EARLY IN LIFE IN SYSTEMIC DISEASE

Cherry-Red Spot

The macula may appear abnormal in color in several conditions due to the relative thinness of the retina in this region compared with the rest of the retina and the ease of visualizing the choroidal vessels. If the whole retina becomes thicker or less transparent from edema or accumulation of abnormal products, the macular area will continue to be a normal red color while the remaining retina becomes gray with an associated loss of choroidal detail and color.

In the first year of life, a cherry-red spot is usually due to storage of abnormal lipid accumulation in the ganglion cells of the nerve fiber layer. Sphingolipidoses such as Tay-Sachs, Sandhoff and Niemann-Pick diseases and mucolipidoses such as generalized gangliosidosis, Farber disease, and lipomucopolysaccharidosis usually show a cherry-red spot on fundus examination. Other ocular changes may eventually be seen in these conditions such as optic atrophy, papilledema, and pigmentary degeneration.[89]

A cherry-red spot may be associated with conditions not usually seen in infants. The most likely cause of a cherry-red spot is a central retina artery occlusion with resultant edema of the ganglion cells in the nerve fiber layer and the appearance of a red macular region. As the edema resolves, the abnormally intense cherry-red spot is no longer noted.[90]

Norrie Disease

Norrie disease was first described by Norrie in 1927 and first documented as an X-linked recessive syndrome of blindness, hearing loss, and dementia by Warburg in 1961.[91] Affected boys present in the first few months of life with a history of normal early visual development and subsequent vision abnormalities. Retrolental opacities are noted shortly after birth with total retinal detachment. Histological examination reveals retinal dysplasia and extensive hemorrhage. There is no known therapy for the ocular abnormalities.

About one third of patients with this disorder will have hearing loss at some point.[92] There is also evidence of a progressive central nervous system deterioration in some patients, and about one third are mentally retarded with normal psychomotor development early in life.[17] Dementia may also occur later in life.

The carrier state of Norrie disease does not demonstrate any ocular abnormalities, although some patients do have auditory findings. Recent work of Kivlin et al.[93] using DNA linkage studies makes prediction of the carrier state possible in informative families.

Stickler Syndrome

Stickler syndrome, relatively common in patients with high myopia, is a hereditary progressive arthro-ophthalmopathy with an autosomal dominant inheritance pattern. The systemic findings are skeletal dysplasia, cleft

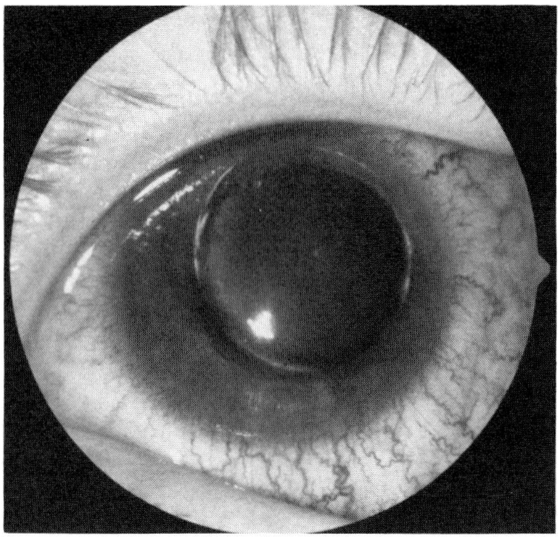

FIG 22–16.
Lens dislocation. The lens is subluxated into the anterior chamber which has resulted in acute pupillary-block glaucoma in this patient with homocystinuria.

palate, and flattened facies.[94] Occasionally, mental retardation is noted. Eye findings include high myopia, a pigmentary degeneration, and retinal detachment. Tasman[95] suggests prophylactic treatment of retinal breaks in this population because the breaks commonly occur along perivascular lattice degeneration, which makes successful repair of retinal detachment unlikely.

Spondyloepiphyseal Dysplasia Congenita

Spondyloepiphyseal dysplasia congenita (SEDC) is a rare autosomal dominant type of congenital dwarfism associated with high myopia early in life. Later in life, a high incidence of retinal detachment is documented.[96] Murray and colleagues demonstrated extensive vitreous liquefaction and detachment from the internal limiting membrane in a 5-month-old infant with SEDC.[97] Areas of vitreous attachment to the retinal surface with associated retinal traction were seen. These workers presented evidence of an abnormally small caliber of collagen fibrils in the vitreous of this patient and suggested that this abnormality may put patients with SEDC at high risk for retinal detachment.

Incontinentia Pigmenti

Incontinentia pigmenti is an autosomal dominant or sex-linked disease of abnormal skin pigmentation with associated ocular, skeletal, and central nervous system abnormalities. The skin lesions are usually the presenting sign, with bullae formation that evolve to whorl-like or linear patches of pigmentation. The Bloch-Sulzberger type of this disease presents at birth in females with epilepsy, cerebral palsy, congenital heart disease, and significant skeletal anomalies.[98] Approximately 35% of these patients have ocular abnormalities, usually a unilateral retrolental mass secondary to retinal dysplasia[99] or exudative chorioretinitis.[100] Watzke and coworkers[101] described vascular anomalies in 7 of 19 patients with this disorder. No ocular treatment has been effective, and the role of the ophthalmologist early in the patient's life is to document the ocular abnormalities and provide counseling.

Lens Dislocation

Lens dislocation due to a vitreous abnormality involving zonule formation is unlikely to present in the first year of life but is clearly congenital in nature. Patients with either homocystinuria,[102] an autosomal recessive error in amino acid metabolism, or Marfan's syndrome,[103] an autosomal dominant disorder with ocular, skeletal, and cardiovascular abnormalities, may present in the first few years of life with pupillary-block glaucoma secondary to lens dislocation (Fig 22–16). Myopia, strabismus, and retinal degeneration are also reported.[104] Glaucoma associated with aniridia, spherophakia, and the Weill-Marchesani syndrome may also present in this way.[105]

ACKNOWLEDGMENTS

I would like to thank my colleagues Gary Brown, M.D., and William Tasman, M.D., of the Wills Eye Hospital, Philadelphia, who graciously furnished the clinical photographs for

Figures 22–1, 22–2, 22–4, 22–5, 22–6, 22–10, 22–11, 22–12, 22–14, and 22–15 from their own collections.

REFERENCES

1. Leber T: Uber Retinitis pigmentosa und ungebornene Amaurose. *Graefes Arch Ophthalmol* 1869; 15:1.
2. Alstrom CH, Olsen OA: Heredo retinopathis congenitalis monohybrida recessiva autosomoalis. *Hereditas* 1957; 43:1.
3. Schroeder R, Mets MB, Maumenee IH: Leber's congenital amaurosis: Retrospective review of 43 cases and a new fundus finding in two cases. *Arch Ophthalmol* 1987; 105:356.
4. Foxman SG, Heckenlively JR, Bateman JB, et al: Classification of congenital and early onset retinitis pigmentosa. *Arch Ophthalmol* 1985; 103:1502.
5. Wagner RS, Caputo AR, Nelson LB, et al: High hyperopia in Leber's congenital amaurosis. *Arch Ophthalmol* 1985; 103:1507.
6. Ellis DS, Heckenlively JR, Martin CL, et al: Leber's congenital amaurosis associated with familial juvenile nephronophthisis and cone-shaped epiphyses of the hands (the Saldino-Mainzer syndrome). *Am J Ophthalmol* 1984; 97:233.
7. Moore A, Taylor DSI: A syndrome of congenital retinal dystrophy and saccade palsy—A subset of Leber's amaurosis. *Br J Ophthalmol* 1984; 68:421.
8. Nickel B, Hoyt C: Leber's congenital amaurosis. *Arch Ophthalmol* 1982; 100:1089.
9. Noble KG, Carr RE: Leber's congenital amaurosis: A retrospective study of 33 cases and a histopathological study of one case. *Arch Ophthalmol* 1978; 96:818.
10. Ohba N, Watanabe S, Fujita S: Primary vitreoretinal dysplasia transmitted as an autosomal recessive disorder. *Br J Ophthalmol* 1981; 65:631.
11. Shively JN, Phemister RD, Epling GP, et al: Pathogenesis of radiation induced retinal dysplasis. *Invest Ophthalmol* 1970; 9:888.
12. Silverstein AM: Retinal dysplasia and rosettes induced by experimental intrauterine trauma. *Am J Ophthalmol* 1974; 77:51.
13. Albert DM, Lahav M, Colby ED, et al: Retinal neoplasia and dysplasia. I. Induction by feline leukemia virus. *Invest Ophthalmol Vis Sci* 1977; 16:325.
14. Silverstein AM, Parshall CJ, Osburn BI, et al: An experimental, virus-induced retinal dysplasia in the fetal lamb. *Am J Ophthalmol* 1971; 72:22.
15. Preslan MW, Beauchamp GR, Zakov ZN: Congenital glaucoma and retinal dysplasia. *J Pediatr Ophthalmol Strabismus* 1985; 22:166.
16. Reese AB, Blodi FC: Retinal dysplasia. *Am J Ophthalmol* 1950; 33:23.
17. Warburg M: Norrie's disease: Differential diagnosis and treatment. *Acta Ophthalmol (Copenh)* 1975; 53:217.
18. MacRae DW, Howard RO, Albert DM, et al: Ocular manifestations of the Meckel syndrome. *Arch Ophthalmol* 1972; 88:106.
19. Fagadau WR, Heinemann MH, Cotlier E: Hermansky-Pudlak syndrome: Albinism with lipofuscin storage. *Int Ophthalmol* 1981; 4:113.
20. Auerbach VH: Inborn errors of metabolism originating in the eye, in Harley RD (ed): *Pediatric Ophthalmology*. Philadelphia, WB Saunders Co., 1975, pp 548–563.
21. O'Donnell FE, Green WR: The eye in albinism, in Duane TD (ed): *Clinical Ophthalmology*. Philadelphia, Harper & Row, Publishers, Inc. 1986.
22. Walls GL: Significance of the foveal depression. *Arch Ophthalmol* 1937; 18:912.
23. Creel DJ, Bendel CM, Weisner GL, et al: Abnormalities of the central visual pathways in Prader-Willi syndrome associated with hypopigmentation. *N. Engl J Med* 1986; 314:1606.
24. O'Donnell FE, Hambrick GW, Green WR, et al: X-linked ocular albinism: An oculocutaneous macromelanosomal disorder. *Arch Ophthalmol* 1976; 94:1883.
25. O'Donnell FE, King RA, Green WR, et al: Autosomal recessively inherited ocular albinism: A new form of ocular albinism affecting women as severely as men. *Arch Ophthalmol* 1978; 96:1621.
26. Blume RS, Wolff SM: The Chédiak-Higashi syndrome: Studies in four patients and a review of the literature. *Medicine Baltimore* 1972; 51:247.
27. Krill AE: Congenital color vision defects, in Krill AE (ed): *Krill's Hereditary Retinal and Choroidal Diseases*. Hagerstown, Md. Harper & Row, Publishers, Inc. 1977, pp 355–390.
28. Pokorny J, Smith VC, Verriest G, et al: Con-

genital color defects, in Pokorny J, Smith VC, Verriest G, et al (eds): *Congenital and Acquired Color Vision Color Defects.* New York, Grune & Stratton, 1979, pp 232–241.
29. Francois J, Verriest G, Matton-Van Leuven MT, et al: Atypical achromatopsia of sex-linked recessive inheritance. *Am J Ophthalmol* 1966; 61:1101.
30. Freeman HM: Congenital retinal diseases, in Tasman W (ed): *Retinal Disease in Children.* Philadelphia, Harper & Row, Publishers, Inc. 1971, pp 1–18.
31. Jesberg DO, Schepens CL: Retinal detachment associated with coloboma of the choroid. *Arch Ophthalmol* 1961; 65:163.
32. Pagon RA, Graham JM, Zonana J, et al: Coloboma, congenital heart disease and chonanal atresia with multiple anomalies: CHARGE association. *J Pediatr* 1981; 99:223.
33. Duke-Elder S: Normal and abnormal development. Part 2. Congenital deformities, in Duke-Elder S (ed): *System of Ophthalmology,* vol 3. St Louis, CV Mosby Co, 1963, pp 462–469.
34. Yanoff M, Rahn EK, Zimmerman LE: Histopathology of juvenile retinoschisis. *Arch Ophthalmol* 1968; 79:49.
35. Pagon RA: Ocular coloboma. *Surv Ophthalmol* 1981; 25:222.
36. Lewis RA, Lee GB, Martonyi CL, et al: Familial foveal retinoschisis. *Arch Ophthalmol* 1977; 95:1190.
37. Yassur Y, Nissenkorn I, Ben-Sira I, et al: Autosomal dominant inheritance of retinoschisis. *Am J Ophthalmol* 1982; 94:338.
38. Greenwald MJ, Weiss A, Oesterle CS, et al: Traumatic retinoschisis in battered babies. *Ophthalmology* 1986; 93:618.
39. Mann I: *Developmental Abnormalities of the Eye,* ed 2, Philadelphia, JB Lippincott, 1957.
40. Straatsma BR, Heckenlively JR, Foos RY, et al: Myelinated retinal nerve fibers associated with ipsilateral myopia, amblyopia, and strabismus. *Am J Ophthalmol* 1979; 88:506.
41. Mann I: *Development of the Human Eye.* New York, Grune & Stratton, 1969.
42. Hittner HM, Hirsch NJ, Rudolph AJ: Assessment of gestational age by examination of the anterior vascular capsule of the lens. *J Pediatr* 1977; 91:455.
43. Krishnamohan VK, Wheeler MB, Testa MA, et al: Correlation of postnatal regression of the anterior vascular capsule of the lens to gestational age. *J Pediatr Ophthalmol Strabismus* 1982; 19:28.
44. Karr DJ, Scott WE: Visual acuity results following treatment of persistent hyperplastic primary vitreous. *Arch Ophthalmol* 1986; 104:662.
45. Pollard ZF: Treatment of hyperplastic primary vitreous. *J Pediatr Ophthalmol Strabismus* 1985; 22:180.
46. Pruett RC, Schepens CL: Posterior hyperplastic primary vitreous. *Am J Ophthalmol* 1970; 69:535.
47. Mann I: Congenital retinal fold. *Br J Ophthalmol* 1935; 19:641.
48. Pruett RC: The pleomorphism and complications of posterior hyperplastic primary vitreous. *Am J Ophthalmol* 1975; 80:625.
49. Hovland KR, Schepens, Freeman HM: Developmental giant retinal tears associated with lens coloboma. *Arch Ophthalmol* 1968; 80:325.
50. Criswick VG, Schepens CL: Familial exudative retinopathy. *Am J Ophthalmol* 1969; 68:578.
51. Gow J, Oliver GL: Familial exudative retinopathy. *Arch Ophthalmol* 1971; 86:150.
52. Canny CLB, Oliver GL: Fluorescein angiography findings in familial exudative vitreoretinopathy. *Arch Ophthalmol* 1976; 94:1114.
53. Slusher MM, Hutton WE: Familial exudative vitreoretinopathy. *Am J Ophthalmol* 1979; 87:152.
54. Ober RR, Bird AC, Hamilton AM, et al: Autosomal dominant exudative vitreoretinopathy. *Br J Ophthalmol* 1980; 64:112.
55. Gitter KA, Rothschild H, Waltman DD, et al: Dominantly inherited peripheral retinal neovascularization. *Arch Ophthalmol* 1978; 96:1601.
56. Tasman W, Augsberger JJ, Shields JA, et al: Familial exudative vitreoretinopathy. *Trans Am Ophthalmol Soc* 1981; 79:211.
57. Blodi FC: Vascular anomalies of the fundus, in Duane TD (ed): *Clinical Opthalmology.* Philadelphia, Harper & Row, Publishers, Inc. 1986, pp 8–11.
58. Lifshitz T, Tessler Z, Maor E, et al: Increased aqueous lactic dehydrogenase in Coats' disease. *Ann Ophthalmol* 1987; 19:116.
59. Ridley ME, Shields JA, Brown GC, et al: Coats' disease: Evaluation and management. *Ophthalmology* 1982; 89:1381.
60. Ellsworth RM: Retinoblastoma, in Duane TD

(ed): *Clinical Ophthalmology*. Philadelphia, Harper & Row, Publishers, Inc. 1986.
61. Kodilinye HD: Retinoblastoma in Nigeria: Problem of treatment. *Am J Ophthalmol* 1967; 63:469.
62. Abramson DH, Ellsworth RM, Grumbach N, et al: Retinoblastoma: Survival, age at detection and comparison 1914–1958, 1958–1983. *J Pediatr Ophthalmol Strabismus* 1985; 22:246.
63. Francois J, Matton–van Leuven MT: Recent data on the heredity of retinoblastoma, in Boniuk M (ed): *Ocular and Adnexal Tumors, New and Controversial Aspects*. St Louis, CV Mosby Co, 1964.
64. Gallie BL, Phillips RA: Retinoblastoma: A model of oncogenesis. *Ophthalmology* 1984; 91:666.
65. Shields JA, Augsburger JJ: Current approaches to the diagnosis and management of retinoblastoma. *Surv Ophthalmol* 1981; 25:347.
66. Knudson AG Jr: Mutation and cancer: Statistical study of retinoblastoma. *Proc Natl Acad Sci USA* 1971; 68:820.
67. Plotsky D, Quinn G, Eagle R, et al: Congenital retinoblastoma: A case report. *J Pediatr Ophthalmol Strabismus* 1987; 24:120.
68. Zimmerman LE: Retinoblastoma and retinocytoma, in Spencer WH (ed): *Ocular Pathology*. Philadelphia, WB Saunders Co, 1985, pp 1292–1351.
69. Carlson EA, Letson MD, Ramsay NK, et al: Factors for improved genetic counselling for retinoblastoma based on a survey of 55 families. *Am J Ophthalmol* 1979; 87:449.
70. Shields JA, Augsberger JJ, Donoso LA: Recent developments related to retinoblastoma. *J Pediatr Ophthalmol Strabismus* 1986; 23:148.
71. Shields JA: Retinoblastoma, in *Diagnosis and Management of Intraocular Tumors*. St Louis, CV Mosby Co, 1983, pp 447–496.
72. Sturge WA: A case of partial epilepsy apparently due to a lesion of one of the vaso-motor centers of the brain. *Trans Clin Soc Lond* 1879; 12:162.
73. Walsh FB, Hoyt WF: *Clinical Neuro-ophthalmology,* ed 3. Baltimore, Williams & Wilkins, 1969, pp 1939–1989.
74. Phelps C: The pathogenesis of glaucoma in Sturge-Weber Syndrome. *Ophthalmology* 1978; 85:276.
75. Dunphy EB: Glaucoma accompanying nevus flammeus. *Trans Am Ophthalmol Soc* 1934; 32:143.
76. Behrman R, Vaughan VC, Nelson WE: *Nelson Textbook of Pediatrics,* ed 12. Philadelphia, WB Saunders Co, 1983, pp 1575–1576.
77. Rados A: Hemangioblastoma of the retina (von Hippel–Lindau disease). *Arch Ophthalmol* 1950; 43:265.
78. von Hippel E: Uber eine sehr seltene Erkrangung der Netzhaut. *Arch f Ophthalmol* 1904; 59:83.
79. Lindau A: Studien uber Kleinhircysten: Bau, Pathogenese und Beziehungen zur Angiomatosis Retinae. *Acta Pathol Microbiol Scand [Suppl]* 1926; 1:1.
80. Christopherson LA, Gustafson MB, Peterson AG: von Hippel–Lindau disease. *JAMA* 1961; 178:280.
81. Usher CH: Angiomatosis retinae. Bowman lecture. On a few hereditary eye affections. *Trans Ophthalmol Soc UK* 1935; 55:183.
82. Palena PV. Phakomatoses, in Duane TD (ed): *Clinical Ophthalmology*, vol 3. Philadelphia, Harper & Row, Publishers, Inc. 1986.
83. Wyburn-Mason R: Arteriovenous aneurysm of midbrain and retina, facial nevi and mental changes. *Brain* 1943; 66:163.
84. Bourneville DM: Sclerose tuberose des circonvolutions cerebrales: Idiote et epilepsie hemiplegique. *Arch Neurol* 1880; 1:81.
85. Martin L: Tuberous sclerosis of Bourneville, in Tasman W (ed): *Retinal Disease in Children*. Philadelphia, Harper & Row, Publishers, Inc. 1971, pp 98–103.
86. Martin L: von Recklinghausen's neurofibromatosis, in Tasman W (ed): *Retinal Disease in Children*. Philadelphia, Harper & Row, Publishers, Inc. 1971, pp 92–97.
87. Friedman MW, Ritchey CL: Unilateral congenital glaucoma, neurofibromatosis and pseudoarthrosis. *Arch Ophthalmol* 1963; 70:294.
88. Dabezies OH, Walsh FB: Pulsating enophthalmos in association with neurofibromatosis of the eyelid. *Trans Am Acad Ophthalmol Otolaryngol* 1961; 65:885.
89. Goldberg MF, Cotlier E, Fichenscher LG, et al: Macular cherry-red spot, corneal clouding, and beta-galactosidase deficiency: Clinical, biochemical, and electron microscopic study of a new autosomal recessive storage disorder. *Arch Intern Med* 1971; 128:387.
90. Henkind P, Chamber JK: Arterial occlusive

disease of the retina, in Duane TD (ed): *Clinical Ophthalmology,* vol 3, Philadelphia, Harper & Row, Publishers, Inc, 1986, p 13.
91. Warburg M: Norrie's disease. A new hereditary bilateral pseudotumor of the retina. *Acta Ophthalmol* 1961; 39:757.
92. Warburg M: Tracing and training of blind and partially sighted patients in institutions for the mentally retarded. *Dan Med Bull* 1970; 17:148.
93. Kivlin JD, Sanborn GE, Wright E, et al: Genetic counseling in Norrie's disease. Presented at the annual meeting of American Association of Pediatric Ophthalmology and Strabismus, Scottsdale, Ariz, March 1987.
94. Stickler GB, Belau PG, Farrwell EJ, et al: Hereditary progressive arthro-ophthalmopathy. *Mayo Clin Proc* 1965; 40:433.
95. Tasman W: The vitreous, in Duane TD (ed): *Clinical Ophthalmology,* vol 3, Philadelphia, Harper & Row, Publishers, Inc. 1986, p 9.
96. Spranger J, Wiedemann HR: Dysplasia spondyloepiphysaria congenita. *Helv Paediatr Acta* 1966; 21:598.
97. Murray TG, Green WR, Maumenee IH, et al: Spondyloepiphyseal dysplasia congenita. *Arch Ophthalmol* 1985; 103:407.
98. Fishbein F, Schub M, Lesko W: Incontinentia pigmenti, pheochromocytoma, and ocular abnormalities. *Am J Ophthalmol* 1972; 73:961.
99. Zwiefach P: Incontinentia pigmenti: Its association with retinal dysplasia. *Am J Ophthalmol* 1966; 62:716.
100. Leib W, Guerry D: Fundus changes in incontinentia pigmenti. *Am J Ophthalmol* 1958; 45:265.
101. Watzke R, Stevens T, Carney R: Retinal vascular changes in incontinentia pigmenti. *Arch Ophthalmol* 1976; 94:743.
102. Henkind P, Ashton N: Ocular pathology in homocystinuria. *Trans Ophthalmol Soc UK* 1965; 85:21.
103. Ramsey MS, Fine BS, Shields JA, et al: The Marfan's syndrome: A histopathologic study of ocular findings. *Am J Ophthalmol* 1973; 76:102.
104. Cross H, Jensen A: Ocular manifestations in the Marfan syndrome and homocystinuria. *Am J Ophthalmol* 1973; 75:405.
105. Motolko MA, Phelps CD: The secondary glaucomas, in Duane TD (ed): *Clinical Ophthalmology*, vol 5. Philadelphia, Harper & Row, Publishers, Inc. 1986, p 11.

23 The Pupil

Lois J. Martyn, M.D.

In infants and children, the pupil can provide important objective information about the health of the eye, the function of the visual system, and the integrity of the nervous system. The pupil may be affected by many aberrations of development and by a variety of genetic disorders and systemic diseases.

EXAMINATION TECHNIQUES

Evaluation of the pupil requires systematic assessment of pupil size, shape, and position; the direct and consensual reaction to light; the responses to reduced light; and the reaction on near gaze, with careful attention to symmetry of the pupils under all conditions.

Ideally, the pupils are first examined in moderately diffuse illumination, with the patient gazing at a distant target to control the near reflex. A bright focal light is then used to test the direct and the consensual reaction to light. Under normal conditions, both pupils should constrict fully and equally. When the light is removed or the room lights are turned off, both pupils should dilate promptly and equally. It may be necessary to use some dim indirect illumination to see the pupillary reaction in the dark. The near reaction is induced by having the patient look at an interesting accommodative target at close range; both pupils should constrict equally. If any abnormalities in size, shape, position, or reactivity are noted, careful examination of the iris and pupil margin with magnification (preferably slit-lamp biomicroscopy) should be done to look for structural defects.

In infants and very young children, the systematic examination of the pupils can be difficult owing to several factors. Babies tend to wince or blink forcefully to bright light, which allows only fleeting glimpses of the pupillary reactions. Attempts to hold the lids open often serve only to induce reflexive movements of the eyes (Bell's phenomenon), thus resulting in marked deviation of the eyes in one direction or another (usually upward), which hides the pupils from view. Attempts to control fixation of gaze long enough to differentiate the light reaction from the near response may be met with a total lack of interest in the fixation target; intense interest in the approaching light, the examiner's face, or other nearby distractions; or a frustrating bout of crying. In addition, in some babies, pupil details and reactions are difficult to visualize owing to dazzling reflections from the cornea or tear film, poor contrast between the dark pupil and brown iris in deeply pigmented babies, and the relative smallness of the pupils in infancy.

The examination is best done with the baby comfortable and content; sucking on a bottle, pacifier, or finger; and regarding an interesting target at some distance beyond the examiner. Effective fixation targets are the parent's face, a high contrast pattern (a large letter or picture acuity card, checkered pattern or stenciled "smiley face"), a bottle or other food item, or a favorite toy. The addition of appealing sound (a musical bell or gentle squeaker in the toy or mother's voice) can be helpful in attracting and maintaining the baby's attention to the target. The examiner must be in a position to control the room lights and the focal light source with facility so as not to distract or alarm the baby with sudden sweeping or jerking movements. Timing is crucial; the examiner must carefully choose the right moment to test the pupil reaction when all factors are optimal, and he must make an accurate judgment quickly before the baby shifts fixation or closes his eyes. Repeated observations often are necessary to verify the examiner's impressions, and additional help may be needed to successfully handle the baby, the lids, the lights, and the fixation target while the examiner concentrates on observing the pupil reactions. In addition, magnification and even the use of the direct or indirect ophthalmoscope can be useful. When necessary, the infant can be propped up to the slit lamp. Photographic documentation of findings, and even examination of old photographs for preexisting findings, also can be of value. In certain cases, examination of other family members may be indicated.

REVIEW OF FUNDAMENTALS

Normal Features

The pupillary aperture of the iris diaphragm normally is round or nearly round and slightly eccentric. Its center is located just inferonasal to the geometric center of the iris.

The size of the pupil varies from 1.2 to 2 mm when constricted to 7.5 to 8 or 9 mm when fully dilated. The average resting diameter is 2.5 to 4 mm. In infancy and early childhood the pupil tends to be small. The pupil is said to attain its greatest size during adolescence and to become smaller again with advancing age.

The pupil tends to be larger in females than in males and larger in myopic than in emmetropic and hyperopic individuals. These variations usually are not evident in infants, however. In addition, the pupils of individuals with lightly pigmented irides tend to be larger than those with darkly pigmented eyes.

The pupils normally are of equal or nearly equal size. Slight inequality, however, may be seen as a nonpathological variant in many individuals.

Function

The principle function of the iris diaphragm and its aperture the pupil is to regulate the amount of light that enters the eye and reaches the retina for optimal retinal and visual function. Dilatation of the pupil in the dark increases the amount of light that enters the eye and increases the ability of the rods to capture photons under scotopic conditions. Constriction of the pupil in light reduces retinal illumination and improves subsequent dark adaptation.

The pupil also plays a role in controlling the amount of chromatic and spherical aberration in the optical system of the eye. In addition, pupil size influences depth of focus. Constriction of the pupil increases the depth of focus and decreases the amount of optical aberration from the lens periphery.

Pupillary Reflexes and Normal Phenomena

The pupillary aperture is regulated by the action of the two iris muscles, the sphincter and the dilator. Constriction of the pupil is referred to as miosis, dilatation as mydriasis.

The Light Reflexes

The pupillary light reactions vary with the state of adaptation of the retina and the intensity, wavelength, and duration of the light stimulus. Normally, when either eye is stimulated with light, both pupils constrict. The response in the stimulated eye is called the direct response; that in the fellow eye is the consensual response. The pupils should constrict equally provided there is no concurrent efferent defect or iris abnormality. When light is withdrawn from the light-adapted eye, the pupil dilates in two phases—an initial rapid dilatory phase followed by a relatively slower, gradual dilatory phase.

In infancy, the pupillary reaction to light appears to be somewhat less active than it is later in childhood; at least the amplitude of excursion of the smaller pupil in infants appears to be less than that seen in older children. The course of pupil changes during dark adaptation in infants appears to be similar to that of adults.

The Near Response

As gaze is shifted from a distant object to a near object, accommodation, convergence, and miosis occur; this triad of associated changes is referred to as the near response. Although these adaptations normally occur in association, each may be affected and assessed separately. Because the near response is dependent on near effort to clear the retinal image, in children it is important to use an interesting "accommodative" target to induce a full response. The pupillary response to near may be greater than the reaction to light in certain conditions such as tonic pupil, as will be discussed.

Other Responses

Excitement and arousal, interest, joy, surprise, fear, and anxiety tend to enlarge the pupil. Also noise and pain cause the pupil to dilate. The size of the pupil tends to increase with fatigue. In sleep, the pupil usually is small. In young children, there may be dilation of the pupils and suppression of the light reaction owing to such factors, particularly anxiety and fear.

Hippus

Small-amplitude oscillations of the pupil are a normal phenomenon that is presumed to be due to fluctuations in the activity and equilibrium of the sympathetic and parasympathetic control of the pupillary muscles. The terms *physiological pupillary unrest* and *hippus* are used to describe this phenomenon. Hippus does not appear to be very apparent in the small pupil of infancy.

Pupillary Escape

When a dark-adapted eye is illuminated at subthreshold levels, the initial constriction of the pupil may be followed by a redilation to its initial size. This phenomenon is referred to as *pupillary escape*. Pupillary escape in the infant and young child should not be confused with the sign of an afferent pupillary defect, e.g., the Marcus Gunn sign.

Fine Structure and Related Developmental Features

The Sphincter Pupillae

The pupil sphincter is composed of typical smooth muscle cells arranged in an annulus that encircles the pupil in the posterior stroma of the iris. It is approximately 0.5 to 1 mm wide and 40 to 80 μm thick. The muscle fibers are bound to the surrounding tissue and dilator pupillae by connecting strands. The sphincter develops at the 65-mm stage, and is present at birth as a mass of vascularized smooth muscle. In some patients, the sphincter can be seen on slit-lamp examination as a whitish band about 1 mm wide around the pupil.

The Dilator Pupillae

The dilator is a myoepithelial layer, approximately 3 μm thick, derived from the anterior layer of the pigment epithelium of the iris. The muscle fibers extend radially from the region of the pupil to the periphery of the iris. The dilator does not appear until the sixth month of fetal life. In many babies the muscle is poorly developed at birth, and the pupil may be difficult to dilate.

The Pupil Margin

Developmentally, the margin of the pupil represents the anterior rim of the optic cup. Here the double layer of epithelium derived from the neuroectodermal layers of the cup forms a crenated border referred to as the *pupillary ruff*. In infants the crenations or radial folds of the pupil margin may be less well developed than in the adult.

Congenital accentuation of the pigment border may be seen when the pigmented epithelium extends farther around the rim of the pupil onto the anterior surface of the iris. This is referred to as congenital ectropion of the pigment border.[1]

In infants and children, the presence of significant ectropion of the pigment border, commonly referred to also as *congenital ec-*

tropion uveae, should alert one to the possibility of associated disorders, particularly neurofibromatosis, facial hemiatrophy, Rieger's anomaly, angle anomalies, and glaucoma.[2]

In some babies, small grapelike excrescences of the pigmented epithelium may be seen on examination of the pupil margin. These are referred to as flocculi. Rarely they may form cysts or partially detach.[1]

Any sectoral defect, notch, or gap in the pupil margin should alert one to the possibility of coloboma, and more extensive hypoplasia of the pupillary zone with an absence of normal structural landmarks of the margin should alert one to the possibility of aniridia (see Chapter 18).

Pupillary Pathways

Afferent Retinomesencephalic Pathway

The afferent arc of the pupillary light reflex commences in the photoreceptors of the retina. Impulses are transmitted from the rods and cones across the bipolar cells to the retinal ganglion cells. Ganglion cell axons carrying pupillary information then follow pathways similar to those for vision. They traverse the optic nerve, undergo partial decussation in the chiasm, and pass into the optic tract. Pupillary afferents do not proceed into the lateral geniculate body with the visual fibers, however, but leave the optic tract via the brachium of the superior colliculus and enter the midbrain to synapse with the pretectal nuclei.

From the pretectal nuclei fibers may (1) pass directly to the ipsilateral Edinger-Westphal nucleus, which is located in the mesencephalon anterior to the pretectal nucleus, or (2) decussate in the posterior commissure of the midbrain to synapse in the contralateral Edinger-Westphal nucleus. These fibers, forming the pretecto-oculomotor tract, are termed *intercalated neurons*.

Efferent Parasympathetic Pathway

For the sphincter pupillae, the final common pathway is a two-neuron parasympathetic arc. Fibers of the first neuron arise in the Edinger-Westphal nucleus in the mesencephalon and traverse the oculomotor nerve to the ciliary ganglion in the orbit. As they exit the brain stem, the pupillomotor fibers are situated superficially on the dorsomedial aspect of the third cranial nerve. As the third nerve proceeds toward the cavernous sinus, the pupillomotor fibers move medially. Within the cavernous sinus, the pupillomotor fibers spread out over the surface of the nerve. From the superior orbital fissue, the pupillomotor fibers follow the inferior division of the third nerve. Leaving the inferior division of the third nerve deep in the orbit, the pupillomotor fibers form the motor root of the ciliary ganglion and proceed into the ganglion where they synapse with the second-order neurons. The postganglionic fibers then traverse the eye via the short ciliary nerves; they enter the globe around the optic nerve, pass foward through the suprachoroidal space to reach the iris and ciliary body, and terminate on the sphincter pupillae.

Efferent Oculosympathetic Pathway

For the dilator pupillae, the final common pathway is a homolateral three-neuron sympathetic arc. Arising in the hypothalamus, fibers of the first order, or "central," neuron descend through the brain stem to terminate in the anterolateral column of the lower cervical and upper thoracic portions of the spinal cord (ciliospinal center of Budge). Second-order, or "preganglionic," neurons then leave the spinal cord through the ventral roots of the lower cervical and upper thoracic nerves, ascend the upper thoracic and cervical sympathetic chain, and pass over the pulmonary apex and through the stellate ganglion to terminate in the superior cervical ganglion high in the neck. Third-order, or "postganglionic," sympathetic pupillomotor fibers then traverse the nerve plexus of the internal carotid artery and course into the cavernous sinus where they join the ophthalmic division of the trigeminal nerve. Within the orbit, the sympathetic pupillary fibers follow the nasociliary branch of the fifth nerve and then the long

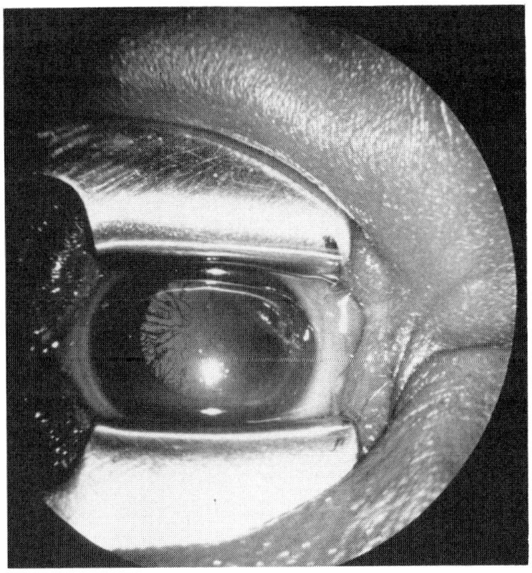

FIG 23–1.
Persistent pupillary membrane. Fine remnants of the pupillary membrane can be seen in this premature infant.

ciliary nerves to reach the iris where they terminate on the dilator pupillae.

PUPILLARY ABNORMALITIES

Persistent Pupillary Membrane

During the 4th to 5th months of gestation, the pupillary membrane forms from mesoderm in the pupillary zone. Buds from the annular vessel of the iris form arcades that grow centrally to form the anterior vascular capsule of the lens. At $6^1/_2$ to 7 months, involution of the membrane begins. Atrophy of the central arcades occurs first; the process then proceeds peripherally, leaving the minor vascular circle to supply the iris. Involution usually is complete by $8^1/_2$ months' gestation, though it is not uncommon to see some remnants of the pupillary membranes in newborns, particularly in infants born prematurely.[1,3–5] The distinctive looping pattern of the residual vascular arcades or fine weblike strands in the pupil can be visualized with the ophthalmoscope (Fig 23–1). These remnants tend to atrophy in time and usually are of no functional significance. Those that do not disappear in the first year may persist permanently, and trivial remnants of the pupillary membrane can be seen in a high percentage of normal adults. The appearance is usually that of a small tag or fine strand emanating from the iris collarette, sometimes attached to the anterior lens capsule.

When the process of involution and atrophy of the vascular arcades and associated mesodermal tissue fails to proceed normally, significant remnants of the pupillary membrane may persist in a variety of forms, sometimes preferably referred to as persistent pupillary membrane.[6] In some infants, the remnants form dense bands that traverse and distort the pupil or broad wedge-shaped sheaths of tissue that may be firmly attached to the anterior lens capsule at the apex (Fig 23–2). In others, the picture is that of an opaque hyperplastic membrane obscuring the pupil. Rarely is there patency of the vascular elements, but hyphema due to rupture of persistent vessels may occur.[7,8]

In infants with extensive persistent pupillary membrane of sufficient degree to interfere with vision in the early months, intervention must be considered to minimize deprivation amblyopia. In some cases, the use of mydriatics and occlusion therapy may be effective.[9] In others, early surgery may be needed to provide an adequate pupillary aperture.[10] The risks of surgical intervention, including infection, hemorrhage, and cataract,

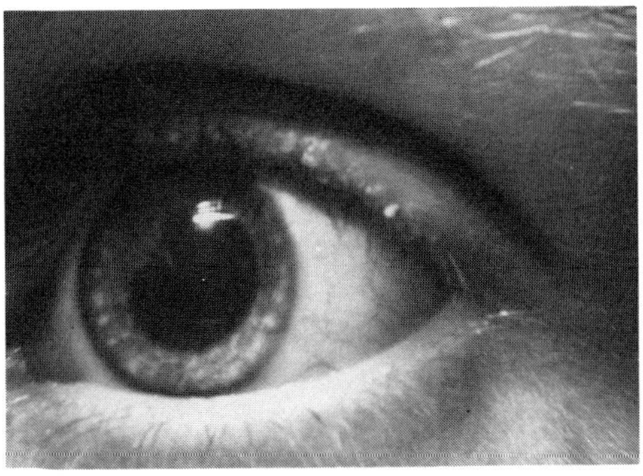

FIG 23–2.
Persistent pupillary membrane. In this child, a persistent band of pupillary membrane is adherent to the anterior capsule of the lens.

must be weighed against the probability of significant vision impairment if nothing is done.

Persistent pupillary membrane in its various forms usually occurs as a sporadic anomaly, but it may be familial and occur alone or in association with other abnormalities such as cataract, angle anomalies, or aniridia.[1,6,11] In some infants, abnormalities of the pupillary membrane such as persistence, asymmetry, or hypertrophy may be the result of congenital infection (TORCH) syndrome.[12]

Microcoria: Congenital Miosis

Absence or malformation of the dilator pupillae may result in an abnormally small pupil that is difficult to dilate. This condition is referred to as *congenital miosis* or *microcoria*.[1,13] Both sporadic and hereditary (autosomal dominant and autosomal recessive) cases have been reported.[14]

Congenital miosis may occur in association with other anomalies of the anterior segment, sometimes familially.[15]

Congenital Mydriasis

As a general rule, the primary concern in any patient with fixed dilated pupils, regardless of age, is the presence of neurological disease or injury affecting parasympathetic innervation of the pupil centrally or peripherally. One must of course also consider the possibility of pharmacological mydriasis or structural abnormality of the iris. In infants and children, there is also the possibility of a condition referred to as congenital mydriasis or familial iridoplegia.[16,17] The basis for the abnormality is not clear, though a defect of the iris musculature must be considered. In this disorder, the pupil appears dilated, does not constrict significantly to light or near, and responds minimally to miotic agents; the iris otherwise appears normal, and the affected individual is usually otherwise healthy. There is evidence for autosomal dominant, possibly X-linked dominant, transmission.

Polycoria

The term *polycoria* is used to describe the presence of more than one iris aperture having the appearance of a pupil. The openings may be round or slitlike and may appear to dilate and contract. Whether such openings are true pupils supplied with muscles or simple holes or colobomatous defects of the iris that share passively in the movements of the iris is questionable.[1] Few cases of true polycoria have been reported.[18,19]

Pseudopolycoria may be seen as the result of trauma or surgery.

Dyscoria

Abnormality in the shape or form of the pupil is referred to as *dyscoria*. The term is often used in a restricted sense to infer congenital malformation of the pupil. Secondary and acquired abnormalities of pupil shape do occur, however, and must be considered in the differential diagnosis.

A slit-shaped pupil is a rare anomaly. It is usually bilateral, rarely unilateral. The vision usually is good unless other ocular abnormalities are present. Other unusual anomalies such as rectangular, pear-shaped and hourglass-shaped pupils have also been described.[1]

Congenital irregularity in the shape of the pupil may also occur as the result of iris coloboma, persistent pupillary membrane, or inflammatory processes resulting in synechiae or segmental iris atrophy. Dyscoria may also occur in association with other anomalies of the anterior segment, as in Rieger's syndrome.[20,21]

A variety of acquired changes in pupil shape occur, some specially named. Though generally described in adults, it would be interesting to survey the incidence of similar changes in infants and children.

Peninsula pupil is an oval pupil described in residents of Newfoundland and Labrador.[22] Some affected subjects were said to have abnormal pupils from birth. Many of the affected subjects were related, and most were male, which suggests a genetic condition. The oval shape is attributed to "atrophy" of the nasal and temporal portions of the pupil sphincter.

Tadpole pupil, an intermittent peaked distortion of pupil shape, can be seen with episodic segmental spasm of the dilator.[23]

Oval pupil may occur as a temporary phase in the evolution of a third-nerve palsy, either during deterioration or recovery. This has been documented in patients suffering from severe intracranial vascular disease processes affecting the midbrain.[24]

Other distortions of pupil shape can occur with segmental palsy of the dilator or sphincter of other origins and as the result of injury or inflammation, infiltration, or mass lesions.

Corectopia

The term *corectopia* is used to describe displacement of the pupil. The abnormality may be congenital or acquired (Fig 23–3).

Congenital corectopia may occur as an isolated anomaly, sometimes as a dominant condition.[1] Alternatively it may occur in association with congenital displacement of the lens as an autosomal recessive condition known as ectopia lentis et pupillae.[25] In this disorder, the displacement of the pupil is usually opposite to that of the lens. The condition is usually bilateral and relatively symmetrical; one eye may be a mirror image of the other. In infants and children with ectopia lentis et pupillae, careful monitoring of visual development and appropriate management of associated refractive abnormalities is essential to minimize amblyopia.

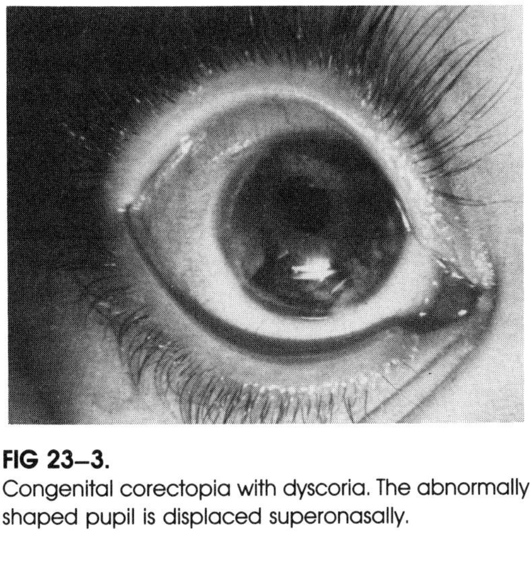

FIG 23–3.
Congenital corectopia with dyscoria. The abnormally shaped pupil is displaced superonasally.

Corectopia may be seen in association with other ocular conditions including persistent pupillary membrane, Rieger's syndrome, congenital hypoplasia of the iris stroma, and Chandler syndrome.[25–27]

Acquired displacement of the pupil may occur secondarily to intraocular inflammation and trauma. Change in pupil position has also been described in association with lesions of the midbrain.[28]

Anisocoria

The term *anisocoria* describes inequality of the pupils. Anisocoria is common, and in each case the clinician must determine its significance. In some patients, it is a sign of serious neurological or systemic disease; in others, it is the result of a local iris abnormality or a benign congenital condition. The sorting process involves answering a number of basic questions by using a systematic approach (Fig 23–4).[29–31]

The first question is which pupil is abnormal. Obviously if there is a demonstrable efferent defect in the pupillary reaction to light or if the anisocoria is greater in bright light than in dim light, the larger pupil is abnormal. In this case, the next question is whether the defect in pupillary constriction is due to an iris or sphincter abnormality, pharmacological blockade, ciliary ganglion involvement (tonic pupil), or an oculomotor (third-nerve) lesion. Careful examination of the iris with magnification (preferably slit-lamp biomicroscopy) is essential to look for developmental defects of the iris (pupillary zone hypoplasia, aniridia) and evidence of trauma (sphincter tears, synechiae) that could affect pupil size and function. The finding of segmental palsy and slow or partial contraction

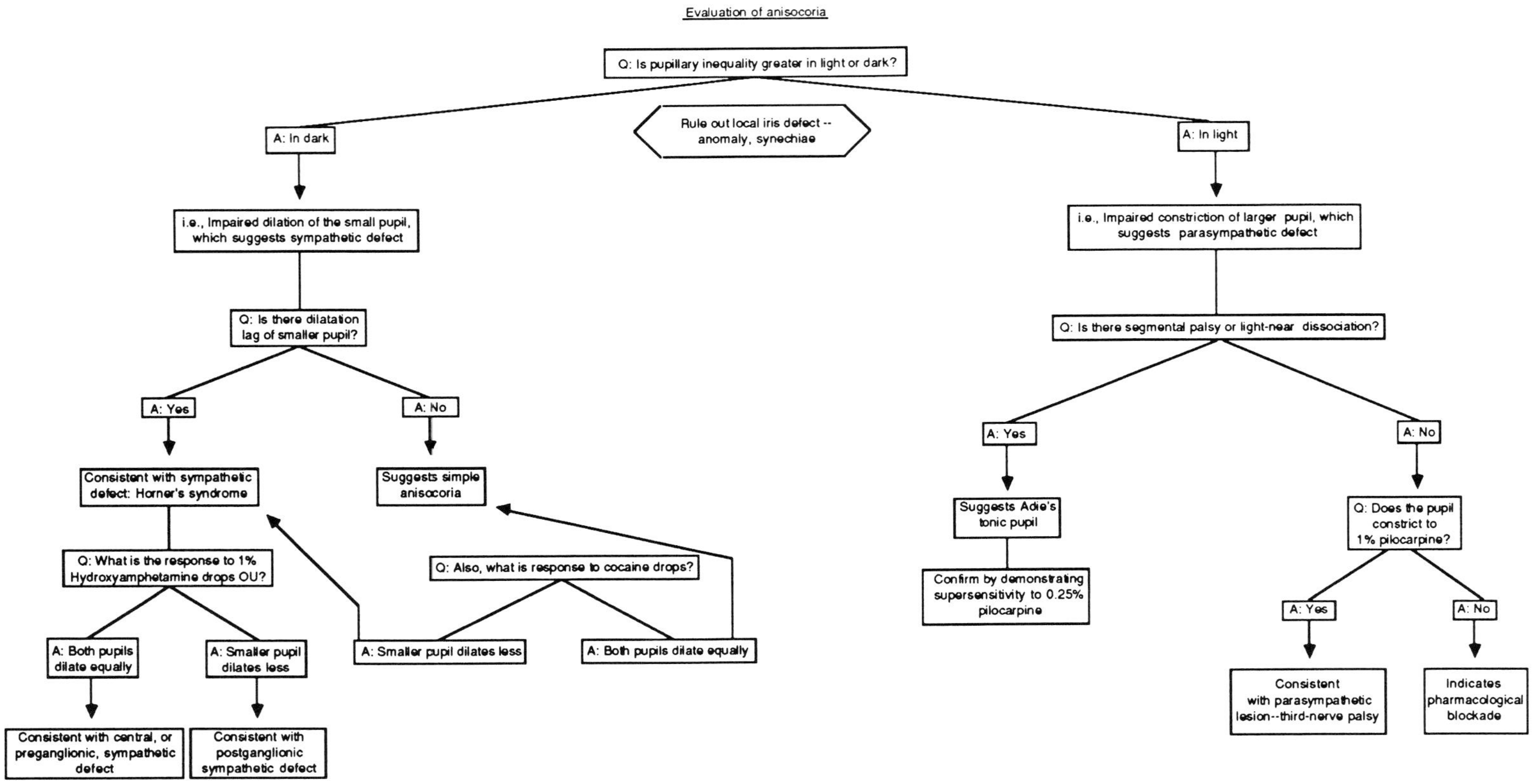

FIG 23–4.
Evaluation of anisocoria. (Adapted from Czarnecki JSC, Pilley SFJ, Thompson HS: The analysis of anisocoria: The use of photography in the clinical evaluation of unequal pupils. *Can J Ophthalmol* 1979; 14:297–302; and Weinstein JM, Zweifel TJ, Thompson HS: The clinical diagnosis of pupil disorders. *JCE Ophthalmol* 1979; 41:15–26.)

suggests tonic pupil. The diagnosis of tonic pupil is confirmed by demonstrating denervation supersensitivity to a dilute cholinergic agent, usually 0.1% pilocarpine drops topically. To differentiate pharmacological mydriasis from the iridoplegia of oculomotor palsy, testing with 0.5 to 1% pilocarpine is used. If the mydriasis is due to accidental or intentional use of an atropine-like agent (pharmacological blockade), the pupil will not constrict in response to instillation of 0.5 to 1% pilocarpine drops topically. If the mydriasis is due to oculomotor palsy, the pupil will become miotic after instillation of the pilocarpine drops. Obviously, careful clinical examination for other signs of third-nerve palsy (ptosis, impairment of eye movement, paralytic strabismus) and appropriate studies to determine the site and etiology of the palsy must be done.

If the anisocoria is greater in dim light, the smaller pupil is abnormal. In this case, the principle question is whether the patient has a sympathetic palsy (Horner's syndrome) or "simple anisocoria," though the possibility of local iris defects (dilator pupillae hypoplasia, synechiae) and pharmacological mydriasis must also be considered. Slowness of the smaller pupil to dilate when the lights are first turned off ("dilatation lag") suggests sympathetic palsy. Careful examination for other signs of Horner's syndrome (including homolateral ptosis of the upper lid and elevation of the lower lid with narrowing of the palpebral fissue and enophthalmos and in some cases heterochromia) is essential. Appropriate pharmacological testing can be done to confirm the diagnosis and to help localize the lesion (see Fig 23–4).

If the iris is structurally normal, the pupillary reactions are intact, and the responses to pharmacological testing are normal, the patient may have simple anisocoria, a benign congenital condition, rather than disease. In many patients with anisocoria, examination of old photographs can be helpful in documenting the duration of the condition.

Simple "Central" Anisocoria

Many individuals have some degree of nonpathological inequality of the pupils. That is, there is no apparent underlying neurological or ophthalmologic disease and no evidence for drug effect; the iris is structurally normal, and the pupillary reactions are intact. This benign condition is referred to as simple or central anisocoria.[32] The cause is unknown. It may be supranuclear. In some cases it is familial.[32]

The anisocoria may vary in amount from time to time. It may also vary from one eye to the other, and terms such as *springing* or *alternating* anisocoria have been applied.[32]

The incidence of simple anisocoria is about 19% to 21%.[32,33] Figures vary with the criteria and methods used in different studies.

Horner Syndrome

Interruption of the oculosympathetic pathway anywhere in its course from the hypothalamus to the orbit may result in Horner's syndrome. The familiar clinical manifestations are ipsilateral miosis, ptosis, relative enophthalmos, and in some cases anhidrosis.[34] The affected pupil is smaller than normal and exhibits dilatation lag in darkness; hence the anisocoria of oculosympathetic palsy is greater in dim light than in bright light. Pupillary reaction to light and near are unaffected. The ptosis of the upper lid, due to innervational weakness of the smooth Müller's muscle, tends to be slight (only 1 to 2 mm) and is best seen on forward gaze. It may worsen with fatigue. Levator palpebrarum action is unaffected. The lower-lid margin tends to be higher than normal ("upside down ptosis") owing to the loss of its smooth muscle tone. The result is narrowing of the palpebral fissue. Enophthalmos is more often apparent than real. Anhidrosis of the ipsilateral parts of the face and neck is associated when the lesion is proximal to the point at which fibers for sweating separate from those that serve the pupil.* Facial vas-

*Beyond the bifurcation of the carotid artery, the sympathetic fibers for sweating follow the external carotid artery.

cular dilatation also may be impaired. Straightness of the hair on the affected side has also been reported as an unusual sign of congenital Horner syndrome.[35]

Other ocular signs sometimes seen in Horner syndrome are ocular hypotony, altered amplitude of accommodation, and hypopigmentation of the affected iris.[34, 36, 37] Heterochromia is most likely to occur if sympathetic innervation is interrupted before the age of 2 years.[34, 38, 39]

Pharmacological testing is important in the confirmation of the diagnosis of Horner syndrome and in the localization of the lesion.[42] The cocaine test has traditionally been used to confirm the diagnosis of Horner's syndrome. Cocaine will dilate the pupil only when the sympathetic pathway is intact and norepinephrine is being released from the nerve endings. A drop or two of 4% to 10% cocaine is placed in each eye, and observations are made over the next 20 to 40 minutes. The affected pupil, no matter where the sympathetic lesion is located, will dilate poorly to cocaine. Demonstration of denervation supersensitivity to epinephrine, 1:1,000, or phenylephrine, 2%, can be helpful in identifying postganglionic lesions, but the hydroxyamphetamine test is generally preferred for differentiating preganglionic and postganglionic lesions, though it is not foolproof.[41–43] If the lesion causing Horner syndrome is central or preganglionic, instillation of hydroxyamphetamine, 1% (Paredrine), should produce normal mydriasis. If the lesion is postganglionic, the pupil will not dilate normally on instillation of hydroxyamphetamine.

Sweating can be judged after exercise or after the use of heat. Starch iodide can be applied to the skin to better show the response. Facial vasodilatation can be judged after exercise or during crying. In many children, it can also be assessed after instillation of cyclopentolate hydrochloride (Cyclogyl) for the fundus examination. Because this medication often produces a facial flush in infants and small children, asymmetry of the flush in Horner syndrome may be evident.

A major cause of Horner syndrome in young patients is trauma.[34, 42, 44] Many cases of congenital Horner syndrome can be attributed to birth injury, often as part of Klumpke's brachial palsy. Horner syndrome is also seen in some children following the trauma of thoracic surgery, as for congenital heart disease. Congenital Horner syndrome may occur in association with vertebral anomalies and with enterogenous cysts.[45] In some infants and children, Horner syndrome is the presenting sign of tumor in the mediastinal or cervical region, particularly neuroblastoma.[38, 44, 46, 47] Rare causes of Horner syndrome such as vascular lesions have also been reported in the pediatric age group.[44, 48] In some cases, no etiology for the Horner syndrome can be identified. Occasionally the condition is familial.[49]

When the etiology of Horner syndrome is in question, investigation including chest x-rays, computed tomography (CT) of the head and neck, and 24-hour urinary catecholamine (vanillylmandelic acid) assay are appropriate. In some cases of Horner syndrome, examination of old photographs and old records can be helpful in establishing the age of onset.

Tonic Pupil

The tonic pupil is characterized by the following[50]: it tends to be larger than normal; it reacts poorly to light; it contracts on near gaze, but the reaction is often slow and sustained; and it responds to dilute strengths of cholinergics that do not affect the normal pupil. Accommodation may be normal, impaired, or tonic. The condition is usually unilateral but may be bilateral. Tonic pupil may develop at any age and occurs in both sexes. It is more commonly seen, however, in young women, often occurring in association with abnormal (absent, diminished, or asymmetrical) deep tendon reflexes as in Adie syndrome.

Tonic pupil may develop after the acute stage of a partial or complete iridoplegia or internal ophthalmoplegia. It can be seen after trauma to the eye or orbit. It may occur in association with toxic or infectious conditions. The features of tonic pupil are explained by cholinergic supersensitivity of the sphincter following peripheral (postganglionic) denervation and imperfect reinnervation.[50, 51]

In the pediatric age group, tonic pupil is uncommon but does occur.[52] It would seem that infectious processes, primarily viral syndromes, and trauma are the primary causes. Features suggestive of tonic pupil may also be seen in infants and children with familial dysautonomia (Riley-Day syndrome), though the significance of these findings has been questioned.[53–56] Tonic pupil has also been reported in young children with Charcot-Marie-Tooth disease.[57]

Pharmacological testing can be used to demonstrate the cholinergic denervation supersensitivity and to confirm the diagnosis of tonic pupil. Instillation of 0.1% pilocarpine drops in each eye usually will produce constriction of the tonic pupil but will not affect the normal pupil.

Marcus Gunn Pupillary Sign

The Marcus Gunn pupillary sign is indicative of an asymmetrical afferent conduction defect of the anterior visual pathways. In most cases, it indicates that the site of the lesion is anterior to the chiasm and involves either the ipsilateral optic nerve or retina. There is evidence, however, that a relative afferent pupillary defect may also occur with contralateral tract lesions.[58, 59]

The sign is usually demonstrated by the so-called swinging flashlight or alternating light test.[60] The test is best done in dim room light with the patient gazing at a distant target to control the near reflex. Using a good source of direct focal illumination, the examiner alternately stimulates each eye in turn by repeatedly swinging the light back and forth from one eye to the other several times while carefully observing the direct and consensual response to each stimulus. On direct stimulation of the normal or better eye, both pupils will constrict fully and equally. On stimulation of the affected eye, relative redilation of both pupils will occur owing to the impaired conduction.

In infants and young children, the Marcus Gunn phenomenon is of special value because it provides objective evidence of pregeniculate visual pathway dysfunction, even when the visual acuity or field cannot be measured accurately, when the ophthalmoscopic fundings appear normal or are of eqivocal significance, or when the fundus cannot be seen. For example, in the infant with strabismus or unilateral or asymmetrical nystagmus, the Marcus Gunn pupil sign may be the primary clue to an underlying lesion such as an optic glioma or birth injury even before disc changes are visible. Similarly, the Marcus Gunn pupil sign can be useful in the diagnosis of optic neuritis and in differentiating organic from nonorganic vision disorders.

When assessing for afferent pupil defects in the clinical setting, it is important to remember that the presence or absence of the Marcus Gunn sign does not necessarily directly reflect the degree of visual acuity loss per se but varies with the amount of visual field loss.[61] Also, a small relative afferent defect can be seen in some patients with amblyopia.[62, 63]

Paradoxical Pupil Reaction

Paradoxical constriction of the pupil to darkness has been observed in children with congenital stationary night blindness and congenital achromatopsia and in occasional patients with optic nerve disease.[64–66] The phenomenon is best seen on going from moderate light (room illumination) to darkness. There is an initial brisk constriction of the pupils when the lights are turned off; the pupils then redilate slowly. The response to direct-light stimulation and the near response usually are normal.

The mechanism is not clear, but paradoxical constriction of the pupil to darkness can be a useful clinical sign in the detection of congenital retinal disease in infants and children with poor vision.

REFERENCES

1. Duke-Elder S: Normal and abnormal development. Congenital deformities, in Duke-Elder S (ed): *System of Ophthalmology,* vol 3. St. Louis, CV Mosby Co, 1963.
2. Ritch R, Forbes M, Hetherington Jr J, et al: Congenital ectropion uveae with glaucoma. *Ophthalmology* 1984; 91:326–330.
3. Duke-Elder S: Normal and abnormal development. Embryology, in Duke-Elder S (ed): *System of Ophthalmology*, vol. 3. St. Louis, CV Mosby Co, 1963.
4. Hittner HM, Hirsch NJ, Rudolph AJ: Assessment of gestational age by examination of the anterior vascular capsule of the lens. *J Pediatr* 1977; 91:453–458.
5. Hittner HM, Gorman WA, Rudolph AJ: Assessment of gestational age in infants small for gestational age. *J Pediatr Ophthalmol Strabismus* 1981; 18:52–54.
6. Merin S, Crawford JS, Cardarelli J: Hyperplastic persistent pupillary membrane. *Am J Ophthalmol* 1971; 72:717–719.
7. McLean DW: An unusual case of intra-ocular haemorrhage. *Br J Ophthalmol* 1946; 30:758.
8. Martyn LJ: Personal observation.
9. Miller SD, Judisch GF: Persistent pupillary membranes. Successful medical management. *Arch Ophthalmol* 1979; 97:1911–1913.
10. Reynolds JD, Hiles DA, Johnson BL, et al: Hyperplastic persistent pupillary membrane—Surgical management. *J Pediatr Ophthalmol Strabismus* 1983; 20:159–162.
11. Cassady JR, Light A: Familial persistent pupillary membrane. *Arch Ophthalmol* 1957; 55:438–448.
12. Hittner HM, Speer ME, Rudolph AJ: Examination of the anterior vascular capsule of the lens. III. Abnormalities in infants with congenital infection. *J Pediatr Ophthalmol Strabismus* 1981; 18:55–60.
13. Holth S, Berner O: Congenital miosis or pinhole pupils owing to developmental faults of the dilator muscle. *Br J Ophthalmol* 1923; 7:401–419.
14. Polomeno RC, Milot J: Congenital miosis. *Can J Ophthalmol* 1979; 14:43–46.
15. Veirs ER, Brown W: Congenital miosis. Associated with a narrow angle of the anterior chamber and abnormally placed iris tissue. *Arch Ophthalmol* 1961; 65:59–60.
16. Caccamise WC, Townes PL: Bilateral congenital mydriasis. *Am J Ophthalmol* 1976; 81:515–519.
17. Hersh JH, Douglas C, Houston J, et al: Familial iridoplegia. *J Pediatr Ophthalmol Strabismus* 1987; 24:49–50.
18. Giri DV: A case of secondary pupil. *Br J Ophthalmol* 1918; 2:275–277.
19. Jaffe NJ, Knie P: True polycoria. *Am J Ophthalmol* 1952; 35:253–255.
20. MacRae A: Bilateral congenital dyscoria. *Trans Ophthalmol Soc UK* 1937; 57:346.
21. von Noorden GK, Baller RS: The chamber angle in split-pupil. *Arch Ophthalmol* 1963; 70:598–602.
22. Bosanquet RC, Johnson GJ: Peninsula pupil. Anomaly unique to Newfoundland and Labrador. *Arch Ophthalmol* 1981; 99:1824–1826.
23. Thompson HS, Zackon DR, Czarnecki JSC: Tadpole-shaped pupils caused by segmental spasm of the iris dilator muscle. *Am J Ophthalmol* 1983; 96:467–477.
24. Fisher CM: Oval pupils. *Arch Neurol* 1980; 37:502–503.
25. Cross HE: Ectopia lentis et pupillae. *Am J Ophthalmol* 1979; 88:381–384.
26. Mathur SP: Unilateral corectopia. *Br J Ophthalmol* 1960; 44:574–575.
27. Cross HE, Maumenee AE: Progressive spontaneous dissolution of the iris. *Surv Ophthalmol* 1973; 18:180–199.
28. Selhorst JB, Hoyt WF, Feinsod M, et al: Midbrain corectopia. *Arch Neurol* 1976; 33:193–195.
29. Thompson HS, Pilley SFJ: Unequal pupils: A flow chart for sorting out the anisocoria. *Surv Ophthalmol* 1976; 21:45–48.
30. Czarnecki JSC, Pilley SFJ, Thompson HS: The analysis of anisocoria. The use of photography in the clinical evaluation of unequal pupils. *Can J Ophthalmol* 1979; 14:297–302.
31. Weinstein JM, Zweifel TJ, Thompson HS: The clinical diagnosis of pupil disorders. *JCE Ophthalmol* 1979; 41:15–26.
32. Lowenfeld IE: "Simple central" anisocoria: A common condition seldom recognized. *Trans Am Acad Ophthalmol Otolaryngol* 1977; 83:832–839.
33. Lam BL, Thompson HS, Corbett JJ: The prevalence of simple anisocoria. *Am J Ophthalmol* 1987; 104:69–73.
34. Giles CL, Henderson JW: Horner's syndrome: An analysis of 216 cases. *Am J Ophthalmol* 1958; 46:289–296.

35. Shewmon DA: Unilateral straight hair in congenital Horner's syndrome. *Ann Neurol* 1983; 13:345–346.
36. Cogan DC: Accommodation and the autonomic nervous system. *Arch Ophthalmol* 1938; 18:739–766.
37. Weisfeld L, Streeten BW: Horner's syndrome with ipsilateral accommodative paresis. *Am J Ophthalmol* 1978; 86:114–117.
38. Jaffe N, Cassady R, Filler RM, et al: Heterochromia and Horner syndrome associated with cervical and mediastinal neuroblastoma. *J Pediatr* 1975; 87:75–77.
39. Maloney WF, Younge BR, Moyer NJ: Evaluation of the causes and accuracy of pharmacologic localization in Horner's syndrome. *Am J Ophthalmol* 1980; 90:394–402.
40. Thompson HS: Diagnosing Horner's syndrome. *Trans Am Acad Ophthalmol Otolaryngol* 1977; 83:840–842.
41. Thompson HS, Mensher JH: Adrenergic mydriasis in Horner's syndrome. Hydroxyamphetamine test for diagnosis of postganglionic defects. *Am J Ophthalmol* 1971; 72:472–480.
42. Weinstein JM, Zweifel TJ, Thompson HS: Congenital Horner's syndrome. *Arch Ophthalmol* 1980; 98:1074–1077.
43. Newman NM: Testing the pupil in Horner's syndrome. *Arch Neurol* 1987; 44:471.
44. Sauer C, Levinsohn MW: Horner's syndrome in childhood. *Neurology* (NY) 1976; 26:216–220.
45. Robinson GC, Dikrainian DA, Roseborough GF: Congenital Horner's syndrome and heterochromia iridum. Their association with congenital foregut and vertebral anomalies. *Pediatrics* 1965; 35:103–107.
46. Beckerman BL, Seaver R: Congenital Horner's syndrome and thoracic neuroblastoma. *J Pediatr Ophthalmol Strabismus* 1978; 15:24–25.
47. Musarella MA, Chan HSL, De Boer G, et al: Ocular involvement in neuroblastoma: Prognostic implications. *Ophthalmology* 1984; 91:936–940.
48. Gilchrist AG: Aneurysm of the internal carotid artery. *J Laryngol Otol* 1973; 87:501–505.
49. Durham DG: Congenital hereditary Horner's syndrome. *Arch Ophthalmol* 1958; 60:939–940.
50. Lowenfeld IE, Thompson HS: The tonic pupil: A re-evaluation. *Am J Ophthalmol* 1967; 63:46–48.
51. Lowenfeld IE, Thompson HS: Mechanism of tonic pupil. *Ann Neurol* 1981; 10:275–276.
52. Agbeja AM, Dutton GN: Adie's syndrome as a cause of amblyopia. *J Pediatr Ophthalmol Strabismus* 1987; 24:176–177.
53. Goldberg MF, Payne JW, Brunt PW: Ophthalmologic studies of familial dysautonomia. The Riley-Day syndrome. *Arch Ophthalmol* 1968; 80:732–743.
54. Thrush DC: Autonomic dysfunction in four patients with congenital insensitivity to pain. *Brain* 1973; 96:591–600.
55. Korczyn A, Rubenstein AE, Yahr MD, Axelrod FB: The pupil in dysautonomia. *Neurology* (NY) 1981; 3:628–629.
56. Gadoth N, Schlaen N, Maschlowski D, Becker M: The pupil cycle time in familial dysautonomia. Further evidence for denervation hypersensitivity. *Metab Pediatr Syst Ophthalmol* 1983; 7:131–134.
57. Keltner JL, Swisher CN, Gay AJ, et al: Myotonic pupils in Charcot-Marie-Tooth disease. *Arch Ophthalmol* 1975; 93:1141–1148.
58. Bell RA, Thompson HS: Relative afferent pupillary defect in optic tract heminopsias. *Am J Ophthalmol* 1978; 85:538–540.
59. O'Connor PS, Kasdon D, Tredici TJ, et al: The Marcus Gunn pupil in experimental tract lesions. *Ophthalmology* 1982; 89:160–164.
60. McCrary JA III: Light reflex anatomy and the afferent pupil defect. *Trans Am Acad Ophthalmol Otolaryngol* 1977; 83:820–826.
61. Thompson HS, Montague P, Cox TA, et al: The relationship between visual acuity, pupillary defects, and visual field loss. *Am J Ophthalmol* 1982; 93:681–688.
62. Greenwald MJ, Folk ER: Afferent pupillary defects in amblyopia. *J Pediatr Ophthalmol Strabismus* 1983; 20:63–67.
63. Portnoy JZ, Thompson HS, Lennarson L, Corbett JJ: Pupillary defects in amblyopia. *Am J Ophthalmol* 1983; 96:609–614.
64. Barricks ME, Flynn JT, Kushner BJ: Paradoxical pupillary responses in congenital stationary night blindness, in Smith JL (ed): Neuro-Ophthalmology Update. New York, Masson Publishing USA, Inc, 1977, pp 31–38.
65. Flynn JT, Kazarian E, Barricks M: Paradoxical pupil in congenital achromatopsia. *Int Ophthalmol* 1981; 3:91–96.

66. Price MJ, Thompson HS, Judisch GF, Corbett JJ: Pupillary constriction to darkness. *Br J Ophthalmol* 1985; 69:205–211.

PART III

Acquired Ocular Disorders of the Newborn

24 Ocular Trauma

Sherwin J. Isenberg, M.D.

With the loving care parents naturally bestow upon newborn babies, it is almost unimaginable to consider the topic of trauma occurring to these beautiful and helpless beings. Yet, there are two circumstances when such trauma may occur. The first, unintended birth trauma, is outside the usual control of anyone. The second, child abuse (or, in our situation, battering of babies), occurs when there is a tragic aberration of the biologic love parents give their offspring. In both these situations, prompt diagnosis can prevent early deprivation amblyopia and legal blindness.

BIRTH TRAUMA

Some form of neonatal ocular or adnexal injury, ranging from trivial to serious, has been estimated to occur in as many as 25% of normal and 50% of difficult deliveries.[1] A more recent survey found the frequency in India to be 12% of all deliveries.[2] The injuries have usually involved the retina, but other ocular and adnexal structures have been affected.

Eyelids and Orbit

In a series of over 2,000 deliveries, the eyelids were found to be ecchymotic in five cases.[2] The eyelids are also frequently found to be edematous following birth. These changes are generally not considered to be of consequence to visual development.

However, there are congenital eyelid problems that are of more significance. Sachs and colleagues reported a freshly cut marginal eyelid laceration discovered at birth that was allegedly caused by the episiotomy scissors.[3] Ptosis of the eyelid has also been reported as a result of birth trauma.[4] We must be cautious in cases of neonatal eyelid closure from any cause since Hoyt and colleagues reported that axial myopia may result.[5] They found the eye with a history of neonatal eyelid closure secondary to obstetric trauma to have an increased axial length of 1.7 to 2.6 mm and greater myopia of about 3 to 5 D compared with the fellow eye. This asymmetry may certainly lead to amblyopia.

A potentially more frightening disorder is congenital eversion of the eyelid. In this disorder, the eyelids are completely everted, with the conjunctival suface exposed to the environment (Fig 24–1). With time, the conjunctiva becomes dry, ulcerated, and infected. There appears to be an increased frequency and severity of this entity in trisomy 21,[6] children of multiparous mothers, and black infants.[7] The etiology of this disorder has been attributed to many different structural anomalies of the lateral canthus, orbicularis oculi, eyelid skin, epicanthus, and vertical dimension of the upper eyelid. The only proven anatomic etiology has been a lack of fusion of the orbital septum to the levator palpebrae aponeurosis that is caused either by delayed structural development or by birth trauma.[8] This dysjunction allows the orbital fat to move inferiorly and anteriorly through the levator-septal defect. This is probably exacerbated by the newborn squeezing and grimacing during delivery and also by orbital pressure being elevated by uterine contractions and head molding during the act of delivery. The advancing orbital fat can cause the tarsus to evert.

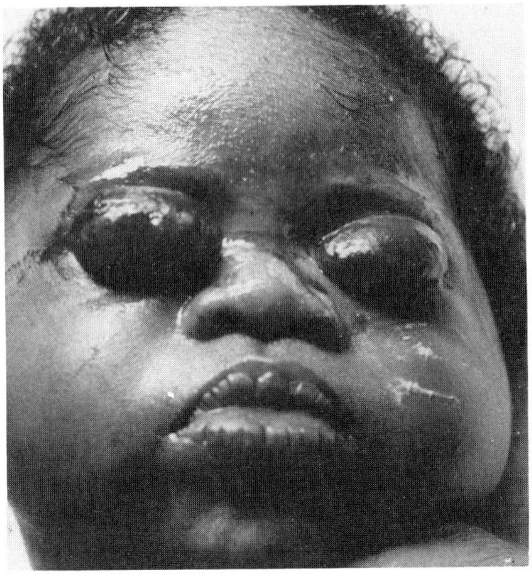

FIG 24–1.
The eyes are hidden behind these edematous congenitally everted eyelids. (From Isenberg SI: An anatomical etiology of congenital eyelid eversion. *Ophthalmic Surg* 1984; 15:111. Used with permission.)

The treatment for congenital eyelid eversion is at first conservative. The condition will usually spontaneously resolve within weeks, possibly because of postnatal growth of the orbital septum onto the levator aponeurosis that prevents further adipose tissue from dislocating anteriorly. Until the spontaneous resolution, the physician should keep the exposed conjunctiva moist with lubricated eyelid dressings and other lubricants and perform an adhesive strip tarsorrhaphy to attempt to revert the eyelid. If the conjunctiva shows signs of worsening such as infected ulcerations despite conservative management or if the cornea becomes affected, surgery should be considered. Previously, surgical procedures have involved the lateral canthus[9] or the placement of skin grafts to the upper eyelids.[10] We have been successful with removal of a spindle of conjunctiva, excision of anteriorly displaced adipose tissue after clamp and cautery were applied, suturing the orbital septum to the levator aponeurosis, and a horizontal eyelid shortening with a full-thickness pentagon resection.[8]

The globe as a whole may be injured during birth. At least 30 cases of luxation or subluxation of the globe in newborns have been reported in the literature.[11] This is usually attributed to the delivery forceps engaging the posterior orbit and forcing the globe anteriorly. Other causes of this phenomenon include a finger placed in the birth canal by the obstetrician and anatomic abnormalities of the maternal pelvis. Some cases have occurred in normal spontaneous vaginal deliveries. Once displaced, the globe is usually maintained in an abnormal anterior location by the closed eyelids behind the globe. One should apply gentle and steady pressure to replace the globe. If that is impossible, a tarsorrhaphy should be attempted.[12]

The orbit can also be affected by birth trauma. These injuries are usually related to an abnormally difficult and prolonged labor. Currently, this type of labor is often terminated by cesarean section, which makes these injuries quite rare. Hemorrhage within the orbit can be sufficiently severe to cause ecchymosis and even proptosis. Conservative management, as that described earlier for congenital eyelid eversion and luxation of the globe, is usually all the treatment required. The extraocular muscles (usually the lateral rectus) may become damaged, thereby result in strabismus if fibrosis occurs. Orbital fractures may rarely be caused by the delivery or prolonged labor. Because newborns have a very strong tendency to develop conjunctival chemosis with even mild insults (including the physician's examination), one should suspect orbital injury if a neonate has chemosis without a satisfactory explanation.

Conjunctiva

Conjunctival hemorrhages in neonates have been noted to occur as frequently as in 13% of births. Neonatal conjuctival hemorrhages have been shown to be associated with large head circumference, large birth weight, increased gestational age, maternal multiparity, and increased speed of the second stage of labor.[13] These generally clear without sequelae.

Cornea

While many ocular injuries may go unnoticed at birth, a cloudy cornea will be appreciated because of its prominent location and resemblance to congenital glaucoma. These injuries are caused by the delivery forceps engaging at least part of the globe during delivery and possibly pushing it against the orbital walls. The damage is almost always unilateral. The cornea presents with a diffuse steamy appearance (Fig 24–2). Within a period of two weeks, the cornea usually is healed and appears transparent.

When such a child presents, the ophthalmologist is usually concerned about the possibility of congenital glaucoma, although there is a long differential diagnosis of cloudy corneas in infants (see Chapter 7). There are a few characteristics that distinguish a cloudy cornea caused by birth trauma from other etiologies. Most important is a history of a forceps or an otherwise traumatic delivery. Second are the accompanying ocular and adnexal signs that indicate trauma such as conjunctival hemorrhage (see Fig 24–2) and chemosis with eyelid edema and ecchymosis. Third are signs found directly on the cornea including linear opacities, usually oriented somewhat vertically, which are caused by ruptures in Descemet's membrane, and short parallel lines of blood found within the corneal stroma.[14] Measurement of the intraocular pressure and corneal diameter as well as ophthalmoscopy of the optic nerve, when possible, should confirm the absence of glaucoma.

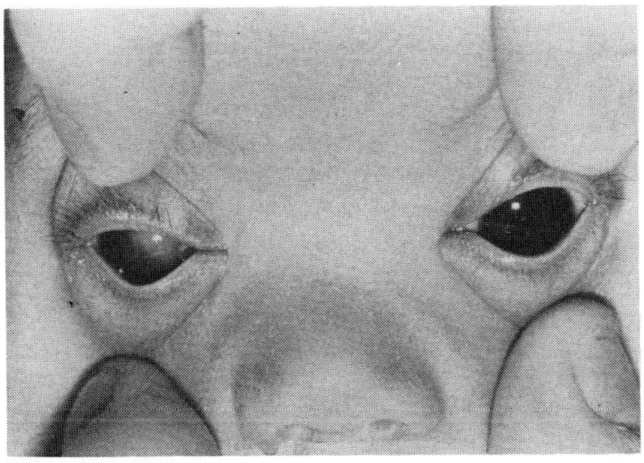

FIG 24–2.
Unilateral corneal edema from birth trauma.

The long-term sequelae of the corneal opacity largely depends on involvement of Descemet's membrane. Permanent corneal opacities other than the linear kind are quite rare. If Descemet's membrane is not ruptured, the cornea generally heals without sequelae. However, if Descemet's membrane is ruptured, astigmatism that can exceed 10 D or high myopia of greater than 8 D may result. The axis of the astigmatism generally follows the orientation of the Descemet's membrane ruptures. These refractive changes can cause amblyopia and subsequent strabismus. Therefore, even if the corneal stroma appears to clear completely, these children should be followed for the possible development of amblyopia and secondary strabismus.[15] A rigid contact lens may be used on such a cornea with severe astigmatism in conjunction with intermittent occlusion of the unaffected eye to combat amblyopia and maximize vision in the traumatized eye.[16]

Although even less common than Descemet's membrane ruptures, the cornea has been reported to spontaneously perforate at or shortly before birth in infants not delivered by instruments.[17] Other ocular structures may extrude through the corneal opening (Fig 24–3).[18] These perforations have been attributed to infectious, structural, and inflammatory etiologies.

Anterior Chamber and Vitreous

Hemorrhage within the anterior chamber, known as hyphema, has been reported in a small number of cases. This may or may not result from a forceps delivery, especially in the presence of residual tunica vasculosa lentis vessels. In all the reported cases, the hyphema cleared within a few weeks without specific treatment.[19] This and vitreous hemorrhage are forms of intraocular hemorrhage that can appear in the newborn. Dense bilateral vitreous hemorrhages existent at birth have been associated with a deficiency in protein C.[20] Because retinal hemorrhage occurs

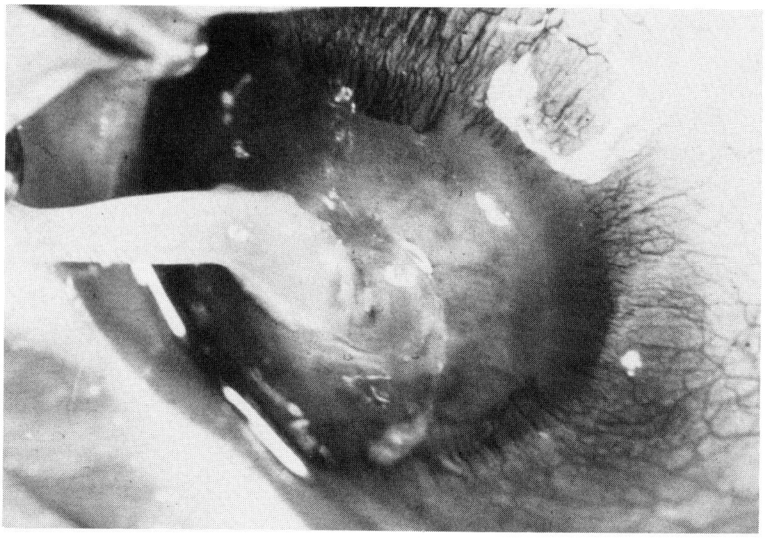

FIG 24–3.
Congenital corneal perforation with intraocular material exuding from the perforation site. (From Heckenlively JR, Kielar R: Congenital perforated cornea in Peter's anomaly. *Am J Ophthalmol* 1979; 88:63. Used with permission.)

more than 100 times as frequently as does hyphema in newborns and is potentially more threatening to vision, the topic of intraocular hemorrhages will be further considered with retinal hemorrhages.[2]

Retina

Undoubtedly, retinal hemorrhage is the most frequent type of ocular injury caused by the birth process (Fig 24–4). It has been found in as many as 59% of all births. Most of the inconsistency in the reported incidence of congenital retinal hemorrhages probably results from the variation in time of examination following birth. More recent studies found the incidence to be about 40%[21, 22] within 1 hour of birth and decrease to 11% within 72 hours following birth.[2]

It has been suggested that these retinal hemorrhages are caused by compression of the head within the birth canal, thereby increasing intracranial pressure. Indirect evidence suggests that either a slow increase or a sudden decompression in intracranial pressure increases the likelihood of retinal hemorrhage.[20] The incidence of retinal hemorrhages is similar whether the baby is delivered spontaneously or by instruments but is significantly lower in cesarean section and breech deliveries. An Israeli study found that the frequency of retinal hemorrhages in cases of induced labor may be dependent on the

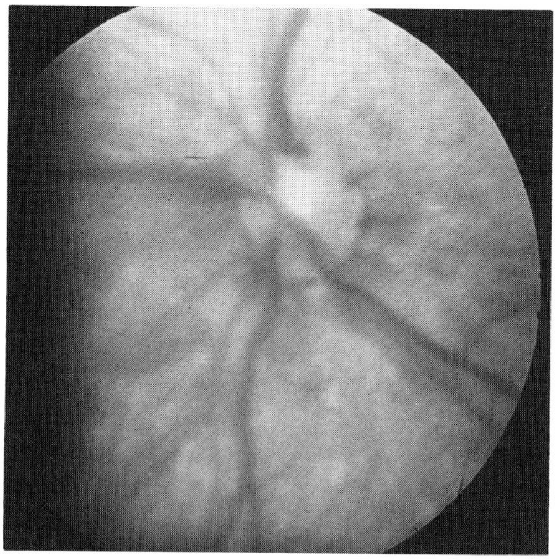

FIG 24–4.
Retinal hemorrhages from birth trauma. A vitreous hemorrhage obscures the view of the fundus.

choice of inducing agent.[23] They reported the incidence to be 28% in oxytocin-induced deliveries and 40% in dinoprostone-induced deliveries and attributed the difference to the prostaglandin properties of dinoprostone. Retinal hemorrhages are more frequent when the mother is toxemic or primiparous or when the first stage of labor exceeds 1 hour. Retinal hemorrhages have been found to be more frequent in infants treated with parenteral vitamin E (tocopherol) for prophylaxsis for retinopathy of prematurity.[24]

In a study of 400 newborn eyes, von Barsewisch found 30% to have at least one retinal hemorrhage within 24 hours of birth.[25] He found most of the hemorrhages to be intraretinal in the nerve fiber layer (flame shaped), the internal plexiform layer (granular or dot shaped), or beneath the internal limiting membrane (dome shaped). In addition, he found extraretinal hemorrhages to be located in the subretinal space, between the internal limiting membrane and the hyaloid membrane, or in the vitreous.

The hemorrhages generally resorb within 10 days of birth. The flame-shaped hemorrhages appear to resorb faster. Macular hemorrhages, which are particularly slow to resorb, pose a therapeutic problem when they do not resorb within a few weeks. Von Barsewisch examined 62 eyes 6 to 7 years after congenital macular hemorrhages and found none to have poor vision that could be attributed to the macular hemorrhage.[22] However, I have two patients with unilateral congenital macular hemorrhage whom I observed and have followed. These patients later presented with amblyopia of the eye with the resorbed macular hemorrhage that did not respond to occlusion therapy. An organic foveal change caused by congenital retinal hemorrhages is unlikely because the foveal area lacks blood vessels. Foveal hemorrhages result from bleeding perimacular vessels. But if a hemorrhage remains beneath the internal limiting membrane for a few weeks, deprivation amblyopia could result. It should be remembered that macular hemorrhages can be found in about 4% of all births, which greatly exceeds the frequency of amblyopia. Thus, if a congenital retinal hemorrhage involves the macula, the ophthalmologist should give the parents an optimisic but guarded prognosis until amblyopia can later be ruled out. Otherwise, congenital retinal hemorrhage is not dangerous. In fact, follow-up studies have found children who had congenital retinal hemorrhages to develop normally.[20]

Ophthalmologists are faced with an occasional therapeutic problem when a congenital vitreous hemorrhage is present. The work-up should include ocular ultrasound and computerized tomography to rule out retinal pathology that may require more immediate therapy. If the work-up indicates no intrinsic retinal problem other than the possible presence of retinal hemorrhage, a dilemma remains. On one hand, conservative therapy, consisting of observation with anticipation of spontaneous resolution of the media opacity, may be appropriate. However, if the opacity remains too long, deprivation amblyopia will develop. On the other hand, surgical intervention consisting of vitrectomy to remove the opacity may be in order. But this procedure may cause cataract, glaucoma, rubeosis iridis, macular edema, or other complications. Unfortunately, it is difficult to know when such a media opacity should be removed. At the current state of knowledge, it would be safe to consider a unilateral congenital, visually significant, vitreous hemorrhage analogous to a unilateral congenital cataract and remove it before 2 to 3 months of age.

An unusual retinal lesion that has occasionally been attributed to birth trauma is massive retinal gliosis. In this disorder, the retina and most of the posterior segment is totally or partially replaced by glial tissue proliferation. It has been associated with congenital ocular infections and also with microphthalmos. The mass, which presents as a solid tumor underlying a detached retina, may resemble an intraocular malignancy. Calcium deposition and metaplastic bone, which have been found histologically, can cause confusion between this entity and retinoblastoma. Thus, it is not surprising that these eyes have

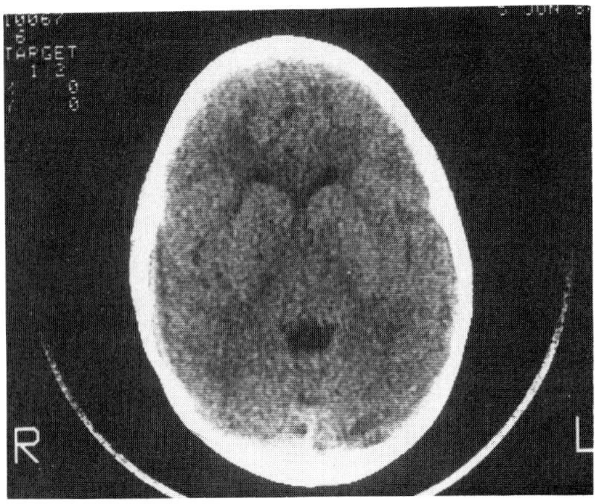

FIG 24–5.
Computerized tomogram showing occipital hypodensities in a child with 20/200 vision.

been enucleated in the belief that a malignancy was present. Yanoff and colleagues felt that this massive glial proliferation represented a nonneoplastic tissue response to retinal injury.[26]

The Central Nervous System

While the general topic of birth injuries to the central nervous system is beyond the scope of this chapter, damage to the visual cortex should be considered. Such injuries may be a direct result of congenital fractures of the skull or intracranial vascular events. Skull fractures, especially the linear type, are relatively common in newborns and may cause trauma to the brain directly or through a vascular mechanism. There are many causes of hemorrhages, hypoxia, and ischemia in the perinatal central nervous system, and it is often difficult to definitely attribute the etiology to birth trauma in a specific case.

With the advent of computerized tomography and cranial ultrasonography, it is easier to diagnose cerebral injuries that may have resulted from birth injury. Neonatal hypoxic and ischemic brain injuries secondary to asphyxia are a frequent cause of neurological dysfunction. Typically, the infants become lethargic or comatose and may develop seizures.[27] Computerized tomography shows the ischemic or infarcted areas of brain tissue as hypodensities. Magnetic resonance imaging can detect these changes before they become evident by computerized tomography. Electroencephalography is frequently helpful. The ophthalmic sequelae include cortical blindness, hemianopia, and strabismus.

Occasionally, the question of poor vision arises in a child who is already a number of years old. The radiological findings permit this diagnosis even a number of years after birth. Figure 24–5 demonstrates the computed tomogram of a 4-year-old girl who had poor vision with a normal electroretinogram and depressed visually evoked response. The figure shows hypodensities of the occipital cortex, presumably caused by perinatal ischemia, possibly from birth trauma. In premature infants, hypodensities may not be pathological, but only represent unmyelinated nerve fibers. These hypodensities will generally vanish as the child matures.

Periventricular and intraventricular hemorrhages, common in preterm infants, are rare in term newborns. They usually occur in the subependymal margin of the lateral ventricles but can occur elsewhere and affect the visual pathways.[28] In infants with a birth weight under 1,500 gm, the incidence of these hemorrhages has been reported to be as high as 58% when diagnosed by ultrasound or computerized tomography. The use of vitamin E (tocopherol) in low–birth weight infants may increase the incidence of these hemorrhages.[24] Computerized tomography shows a hyperdensity at the site of hemorrhage. As many as a third of surviving children with these hemorrhages will have multiple handicaps including blindness.

A last topic to consider is facial nerve palsy. The facial nerve is the most common cranial nerve to be affected by birth trauma, damage to it occurring in about 6% of forceps and natural deliveries.[29] This birth injury usually results from the pressure of either the maternal sacral spine when the baby is in an occiput transverse position or, less commonly, a forceps on the area of the stylomastoid foramen. The ophthalmologist becomes involved in managing these infants by treating any exposure conjunctivitis and keratitis with appropriate moistening agents. The vast majority of these palsies improve without specific treatment.

Ocular Perforation During Amniocentesis

Amniocentesis, which is usually performed in midtrimester for prenatal genetic studies, occasionally has resulted in needle puncture of the fetus. The incidence of fetal puncture from midtrimester amniocentesis is approximately 3%. This puncture has usually resulted in a cutaneous scar. However, more significant complications such as hemiparesis, persistent amniotic fluid leakage, and porencephalic cysts have been reported.

Among these are reports of ocular perforation during amniocentesis in midtrimester or as late as the 37th week of gestation. In these cases, the immediate damage was to the anterior segment of the eye. In all reported cases but one, the visual result has been a blind or eviscerated eye. Isenberg and Heckenlively reported a case of puncture to the sclera and retina that resulted in useful vision, although the child did require occlusion therapy, and a contact lens for amblyopia and unilateral high myopia.[30] The other cases in the literature have involved a cornea that was perforated and/or edematous, vascularization or hyphema in the anterior chamber, and synechia of the iris. Segmental unilateral chemosis (Fig 24–6) or corneal edema should alert physicians to the possibility of ocular trauma having occurred either at the time of delivery or while in utero caused by an amniocentesis needle. The ophthalmologist must then close the perforation, and repair the eye as soon as possible. Attention must be paid to the potential development of amblyopia in the damaged eye.

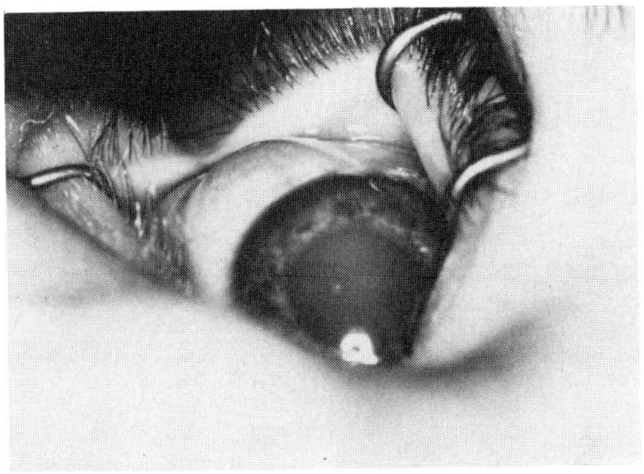

FIG 24–6.
Segmental chemosis overlying a scleral perforation caused by an amniocentesis needle.

BATTERED BABIES AND OCULAR DAMAGE

In recent years, physicians and the general public are becoming more aware of the terrible social disorder of child abuse. It is particularly pathetic when the injuries are inflicted on a helpless infant. In fact, most child abuse is inflicted on children under 3 years old. Initially, the diagnosed injuries were primarily fractures of the long bones and subdural hematomas. As more knowledge about this disorder has been gained, it is becoming apparent that the eyes are frequently involved.[31] Although many of the ocular manifestations of infant battering resolve without sequelae, Harcourt and Hopkins reported 8 of 11 babies in their series to have permanent visual impairment due to optic atrophy, retinal detachment, macular scarring, or cortical blindness.[32]

In general, one may think of the ocular injuries falling into three circumstances: (1) the eye is directly assaulted, (2) the eye itself is not assaulted but is affected indirectly by cranial trauma, and (3) the eye is injured by violent shaking or whiplash to the child's head. It must be recognized that there is overlap among these three categories.

Direct Assault On the Eye

In general, the most frequent ocular findings in cases of child abuse are ecchymoses of the orbit and eyelids and various retinal abnormalities. However, it must be recognized that the anterior segment of the eye can be involved, especially in cases of direct ocular trauma. Conjunctival hemorrhage and chemosis may be present. The cornea may have opacities from current or previous traumatic ruptures. I have examined infants with clean circular corneal abrasions caused by thermal damage from a lit cigarette. The lens has been found in a few cases to be dislocated or cataractous.[28] Hyphemas have also been observed. Retinal hemorrhages may appear as found in the other two categories of trauma as will be subsequently described.

It should be remembered that in direct trauma the anterior segment is often affected as well as the retina. In the other two categories of indirect ocular injury, the damage is usually limited to the posterior segment and spares the cornea and other anterior structures. This makes the diagnosis of indirect ocular injury secondary to abuse difficult for the nonophthalmologist to make. Pupillary responses may be secondarily impaired by significant posterior segment injuries.

Involvement of the Eye Secondary to Cranial Injury

In these cases, the head is directly battered and the eye is affected by the head trauma. Among the types of cranial trauma observed are subdural hematomas, subarachnoid hemorrhages, cavernous sinus thromboses, meningoceles, hydrocephalus, and various bruises, contusions, and lacerations of the surface of the head. The ocular injury resulting from child abuse to receive the most study has been retinal hemorrhages. They have been reported to occur in 30% to 60% of cases of infant abuse and are often associated with subdural hematomas and/or cranial fractures.[33] Characteristically, the intraocular hemorrhages are intraretinal and preretinal. They may break through the inner limiting membrane and result in a vitreous hemorrhage. In more severe cases, retinal hemorrhages have been found in all layers, especially the nerve fiber and outer plexiform layers. In addition, retinal tears and detachment over subretinal hemorrhage have also been reported.[34]

A less common type of retinal hemorrhage that can result from abuse is Purtscher's retinopathy. This form of hemorrhagic angiopathy, presenting with retinal exudates as well as hemorrhage, usually results from sudden compression of the thorax or from automobile accidents when there is an acute transmission of high intravascular pressure to the eyes. Although usually recognized in adults, this retinopathy has been reported in battered infants with a history of seizures and chest injury.[35]

In addition to the retina, papilledema has been found secondary to an elevated intracranial pressure from subdural hematoma or intracranial hemorrhage. Proptosis and esotropia have also been reported.

Ocular Injury by Violent Shaking of the Head

In 1974, Caffey reported that some abused infants were not battered but actually severely and repeatedly shaken.[36] They are subject to these injuries because the relatively heavy infantile head with its soft brain is supported by weak cervical muscles. The repeated, rapid, to-and-fro flexions of the head has resulted in intracranial and intraocular hemorrhages and traction lesions of the long bones. Absent from these infants are fractures and contusions of the cranium and long bones. Sometimes, shaking of the infant has not been intended for abusive purposes but to "resuscitate" or "awaken" a lethargic child. Mushin and Morgan examined the eyes of a shaken infant who died.[37] They described extensive intraretinal, subhyaloid, and vitreous hemorrhages as well as myelin extrusion from the disc.

In addition to retinal and vitreous hemorrhages, Greenwald and associates reported a series of infants with retinal cysts filled with blood or clear fluid as in retinoschisis.[38] Poor vision resulted if the cysts involved the macula. Electroretinographic evidence indicated that the visual loss was primarily caused by damage to the inner retinal layers. They suggested that head shaking placed traction on the retina by transmission through the lens and vitreous humor. The tugging on the retina separated retinal tissue and caused different forms of hemorrhage, including cystic lesions.

Conclusions

While birth trauma and child abuse may never totally disappear, there are measures that can be taken to decrease their frequency. Better methods of obstetric care have already decreased the incidence of birth trauma. Since many battered infants sustain ocular injuries, the ophthalmologist is often in a position to decide whether an injury was accidental or possibly secondary to child abuse. When in doubt, the physician is morally and legally obligated to report any cases of suspected child abuse to the proper legal authorities. Indeed, by bearing the signs of child abuse in mind, all physicians can contribute to the welcome demise of this vile disorder.

REFERENCES

1. Duke-Elder S: *System of Ophthalmology,* vol 14, St Louis, CV Mosby Co, 1972, pp 9–17.
2. Jain IS, Singh YP, Grupta SL, et al: Ocular hazards during birth. *J Pediatr Ophthalmol Strabismus* 1980; 17:14.
3. Sachs D, Levin PS, Dooley K: Marginal eyelid laceration at birth. *Am J Ophthalmol* 1986; 102:539.
4. Crawford, JS: Ptosis as a result of trauma. *Can J Ophthalmol* 1974; 9:244.
5. Hoyt CS, Stone RD, Fromer C, et al: Monocular axial myopia associated with neonatal eyelid closure in human infants. *Am J Ophthalmol* 1981; 91:197.
6. Gilbert HD, Smith RE, Berlow MH, et al: Congenital upper eyelid eversion and Down's syndrome. *Am J Ophthalmol* 1973; 75:469.
7. Lu LW, Bansal RK, Katzman B: Primary congenital eversion of the upper lids. *J Pediatr Ophthalmol Strabismus* 1979; 16:149.
8. Blechman B, Isenberg S: An anatomical etiology of congenital eyelid eversion. *Ophthalmic Surg* 1984; 15:111.
9. Hartman DC: Congenital anomalies of the lids. *Int Ophthalmol Clin* 1964; 4:73.
10. Forbes D: Congenital eversion of upper eyelids: A case report. *Br J Plast Surg* 1965; 18:180.
11. Friedenwald H: Luxation and avulsion of eyeball during birth. *Am J Ophthalmol* 1918; 1:10.
12. Dutescu M, Lappe A: Luxation of the eyeball in the newborn. *J Pediatr Ophthalmol* 1974; 11:82.
13. Baum JD, Bulpitt CJ: Retinal and conjunctival haemorrhage in the newborn. *Arch Dis Child* 1970; 45:344.
14. Sugar HS, Airala MA: Birth injuries of the cornea. *J Pediatr Ophthalmol* 1971; 8:26.
15. Angell LK, Robb RM, Berson FG: Visual prognosis in patients with ruptures on Descemet's membrane due to forceps injuries. *Arch Ophthalmol* 1981; 99:2137.
16. Stein RM, Cohen EJ, Calhoun JH, et al: Corneal birth trauma managed with a contact lens. *Am J Ophthalmol* 1987; 103:596.
17. Heckenlively JR, Kielar R: Congenital perforated conea in Peter's anomaly. *Am J Ophthalmol* 1979; 88:63.
18. Backes DO, Makley TA, Rogers GL, et al: Spontaneous corneal perforation with expulsion of the lens and retina in a premature infant. *J Pediatr Ophthalmol Strabismus* 1980; 17:242.
19. Wu G, Behrens MM: Hyphema in the newborn: Report of a case. *J Pediatr Ophthalmol Strabismus* 1982; 19:56.
20. Pilido JS, Lingua RW, Cristol S, et al: Protein C deficiency associated with vitreous hemorrhage in a neonate. *Am J Ophthalmol* 1987; 104:546.
21. Levin S, Janive J, Mintz M, et al: Diagnostic and prognostic value of retinal hemorrhages in the neonate. *Obstet Gynecol* 1980; 55:309.
22. Giles CL: Retinal hemorrhages in the newborn. *Am J Ophthalmol* 1960; 49:1006.
23. Schoenfeld A, Buckman G, Nissenkorn I, et al: Retinal hemorrhages in the newborn following labor induced by oxytocin or dinoprostone. *Arch Ophthalmol* 1985; 103:932.
24. Rosenbaum AL, Phelps DL, Isenberg SJ, et al: Retinal hemorrhages in retinopathy of prematurity associated with tocopherol treatment. *Ophthalmology* 1985; 92:1012.
25. von Barsewisch B: *Perinatal Retinal Haemorrhages.* Berlin, Springer-Verlag, 1979.

26. Yanoff M, Zimmerman LE, Davis RL: Massive gliosis of the retina. *Int Ophthalmol Clin* 1971; 11:211.
27. Volpe JJ: *Neurology of the Newborn*. Philadelphia, WB Saunders Co, 1981, pp 180–237.
28. Towbin A: Cerebral intraventricular hemorrhage and sub-ependymal matrix infarction in the fetus and premature newborn. *Am J Pathol* 1968; 52:121.
29. Hepner WR: Some observations on facial paresis in the newborn infant: Etiology and incidence. *Pediatrics* 1951; 8:494.
30. Isenberg SJ, Heckenlively JR: Traumatized eye with retinal damage from amniocentesis. *J Pediatr Ophthalmol Strabismus* 1985; 22:65.
31. Friendly DS: Ocular manifestations of physical child abuse. *Trans Am Acad Ophthalmol Otolaryngol* 1971; 75:318.
32. Harcourt B, Hopkins D: Ophthalmic manifestations of the battered baby syndrome. *Br Med J* 1971; 3:398.
33. Eisenbrey AB: Retinal hemorrhage in the battered child. *Child's Brain* 1979; 5:40.
34. Ober RR; Hemorrhagic retinopathy in infancy: A clinicopathological report. *J Pediatr Ophthalmol Strabismus* 1980; 17:17.
35. Tomasi LG, Rosman NP: Purtscher retinopathy in the battered child syndrome. *Am J Dis Child* 1975; 129:1335.
36. Caffey J: The whiplash shaken infant syndrome: Manual shaking by the extremities with whiplash-induced intracranial and intraocular bleedings, linked with residual permanent brain damage and mental retardation. *Pediatrics* 1974; 54:396.
37. Mushin A, Morgan G: Ocular injury in the battered baby syndrome. *Br J Ophthalmol* 1971; 55:343.
38. Greenwald MJ, Weiss A, Oesterle CS, et al: Traumatic retinoschisis in battered babies. *Ophthalmology* 1986; 93:618.

25 Infectious Diseases

Gary N. Holland, M.D.

A variety of infectious diseases pose serious risks to the newborn eye and ocular adnexa. Congenital infections acquired in utero may cause severe ophthalmic disease, and pathogens encountered during delivery may result in isolated ocular surface disease or disseminated infections with intraocular involvement. Early recognition and therapy is necessary for preservation of sight, but even appropriate therapy may not prevent the loss of vision, which emphasizes the important role of disease prevention.

ACQUIRED INFECTIOUS DISEASES

Infection of the Ocular Surface (Ophthalmia Neonatorum)

Neonates may be exposed to a variety of normal and pathogenic organisms during birth. Subsequent infection of the ocular surface can result in an inflammatory disorder termed *ophthalmia neonatorum.* Infection may be asymptomatic or transient, but in its most severe forms, ophthalmia neonatorum results in permanent damage to the eyes and blindness.

The widespread use of prophylaxis against infection (discussed later) has reduced the risk of ophthalmia neonatorum but has not eliminated it as a problem. Molgaard and associates reported that 16.6% of newborns required antibiotic therapy for conjunctivitis despite prophylaxis in most cases,[1] but most investigators report a much lower incidence. Stenson and associates reported 3.0 cases of ophthalmia neonatorum per 1,000 live births,[2] and Watson and associates reported a 2.6% incidence.[3] Armstrong and associates reported 302 cases of ophthalmia neonatorum among 35,047 births (transmission rate, 0.9%) in an inner-city hospital following chemical prophylaxis.[4] The nature of the study, a retrospective review of perinatal medical records, may have resulted in an underreporting of cases, especially of those with delayed onset. Prolonged rupture of membranes increases the risk of ophthalmia neonatorum due to ascending infection.[4] Some studies have found an increased incidence of ophthalmia neonatorum in premature infants,[5] although other investigators have found no association between prematurity or low birth weight and infection.[4]

Causes

A variety of organisms have been implicated as causes of ophthalmia neonatorum (Table 25–1). The types and incidence of neonatal infection vary with the locale and the populations studied.

Neisseria Gonorrhoeae.—The most serious form of ophthalmia neonatorum is keratoconjunctivitis caused by *Neisseria gonorrhoeae.* In the 1800s, gonococcal infection was a major cause of childhood blindness; Crede reported a 10% incidence of infection.[15] Following his introduction of silver nitrate prophylaxis, the incidence of gonococcal conjunctivitis was sharply reduced. Nearly one quarter of admissions to schools for the blind

TABLE 25–1.
Frequency of Bacterial and Chlamydial Isolation in Cases of Infectious Ophthalmia Neonatorum*

Pathogen	Reported Incidence (%)	References
Chlamydia trachomatis	10–43	1–10
Staphylococcus aureus	5–27	2, 4, 7–9, 11, 12
Neisseria gonorrhoeae	4–14	2, 3, 5
Streptococcus sp, viridans group	1–29	2, 9, 11, 12
Hemophilus species	5–14	2, 7, 9, 11
Streptococcus pneumoniae	5–6	2, 9
Escherichia coli	2–5	11, 12
Branhamella catarrhalis	1–5	2, 9
Mycoplasma hominis	3	13
Streptococcus sp, group D	3	9
Corynebacterium sp	2	9
Pseudomonas aeruginosa	1	2

*Includes pathogens isolated from cases of ophthalmia neonatorum in the absence of other organisms and that have been reported in more than one series or identified in more than one patient in single large series.

in the early 20th century were attributed to ophthalmia neonatorum, but the percentage had dropped to 0.3% by 1959.[16] The incidence of ophthalmia neonatorum attributed to *Neisseria gonorrhoeae* is currently reported to be in the range of 0.14% to 0.26% of live births.[17–19] It appears to have risen in recent years, which parallels the increase in adult infections. In 1970 the incidence of neonatal gonococcal conjunctivitis at Duke University jumped to 265 per 100,000 live births from 18 per 100,000 for the previous 10-year period.[17]

The majority of neonatal infections are due to exposure of the newborn to *Neisseria gonorrhoeae* in the birth canal when the mother has unrecognized or inadequately treated gonorrhea. Ascending infections resulting in gonococcal amnionitis also have been reported.[20, 21] Thus, even newborns delivered by cesarean section may develop gonococcal conjunctivitis.[6, 22, 23] Prolonged rupture of membranes will increase the chance of gonococcal infection.[22, 23] Ocasionally, infants are infected postnatally by inadvertant exposure to contaminated secretions on the hands of family members. Infected infants are highly contagious, and nosocomial infections also can occur in the nursery.

The onset of the clinical signs of gonococcal infection can occur from 1 to 21 days after birth.[4, 6, 17, 18, 22] In most series, the majority of cases have developed a discharge following day 4.[6, 18, 22, 24] Infection therefore may not become apparent until after the newborn leaves the hospital. Most infections acquired at birth will progress to clinical disease by day 6. The cases occurring after 1 week may be postnatally acquired.

The risk of gonococcal conjunctivitis in neonantes born to mothers with untreated gonorrhea is not known. A report by Davidson and associates described seven pregnant women with positive cultures for *Neisseria gonorrhoeae* who were allowed to complete their pregnancy without treatment.[25] Four women had cultures performed again before delivery, and two of their four offsprings had positive cultures at birth. The remaining three neonates did not have cultures done. All seven received prophylaxis against *Neisseria gonorrhoeae*, and none developed ophthalmia neonatorum. This study frequently has been cited inaccurately as the source of a widely quoted but unsubstantiated statistic that 28% of infants born to mothers with gonorrhea will develop gonococcal conjunctivitis.[26–28] Others have estimated a 16% to 17% risk of gonococcal conjunctivitis in newborns with infected mothers.[29]

Gonococcal conjunctivitis in neonates may be an indolent infection, less severe than that seen in adults and older children. In its worst form, however, it can have devastating consequences. Severe gonococcal conjunctivitis is characterized by a marked inflammatory response with eyelid swelling, chemosis (conjunctival edema), and copious purulent discharge that can be blood tinged (Fig 25–1). The conjunctiva may balloon out between the eyelid margins, and membrane or pseudomembrane formation can occur. Concomitant infection of the cornea can result in necrosis with scarring or perforation and loss of the eye. Approximately three quarters of cases are bilateral.[4]

Gonococcal conjunctivitis is the most common clinical form of neonatal *Neisseria gonorrhoeae* infection. At birth infected newborns usually will have no signs of systemic disease. Rarely, however, gonococcal infection can lead to disseminated disease with genital, pharyngeal, meningeal, and joint involvement.

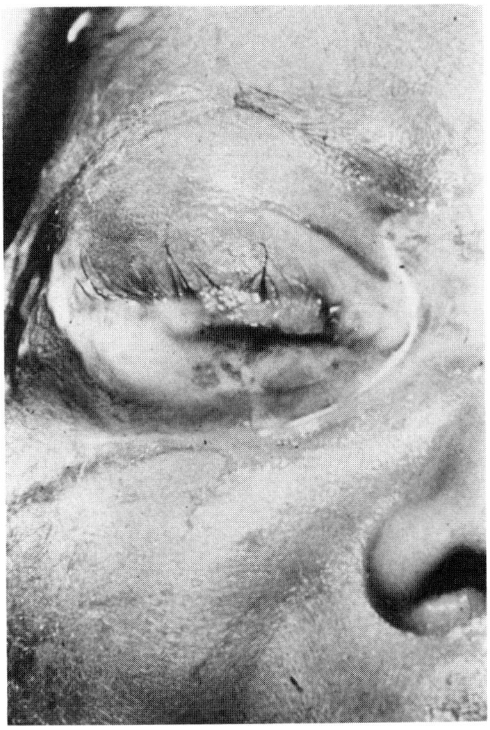

FIG 25–1.
Purulent discharge in a newborn with gonococcal conjunctivitis. (From the Francis I. Proctor Foundation teaching collection, courtesy of Mario Valenton, M.D.)

Chlamydia trachomatis.—Chlamydial conjunctivitis ("inclusion blenorrhea") is currently the most common form of infectious ophthalmia neonatorum. It has an incidence of 3 to 8 per 1,000 live births[12, 30] and accounts for 10% to 46% of all cases of neonatal conjunctivitis.[6–11] *Chlamydia trachomatis* (serotypes D, E, F, G, H, I, J, K) is the most common sexually transmitted pathogen in the United States where an estimated 4 million individuals are infected each year.[31] Also known as the "TRIC agent" *TR*achoma-*I*nclusion *C*onjunctivitis), it is an obligate intracellular bacteria-like organism that infects the epithelium of mucous membranes. It is the leading cause of nongonorrheal ("nonspecific") urethritis in males and can infect the cervix, endometrium, urethra, and fallopian tubes of females.

The reported incidence of cervical infections with *Chlamydia* in pregnant women varies from 2% to 18%,[19, 30, 32–35] but most investigators place it at approximately 5%.[30] Mardh and associates found that the incidence of positive cervical cultures varied between 4% and 24% depending on the age of the patient, with the highest incidence among females under 20 years of age in the puerperal period.[34] Most series have found infection to be more common in young, unmarried females of low socioeconomic status.[10, 32, 33] It is not, however, restricted to that group.

Twenty-eight to 70% of neonates exposed to *Chlamydia* at birth will develop culture or serological evidence of chlamydial infection.[30, 31, 33–35] With prolonged rupture of membranes, chlamydial conjunctivitis also may develop in newborns delivered by cesarean section due to ascending infection.[6, 7] Conjunctivitis is the most common site of chlamydial disease in neonates and occurs in as many as 74% of those infected[35]; it develops in 18% to 50% of infants exposed at birth.[1, 19, 30–34, 36] Subclinical infection of the conjunctiva is unusual.[35]

Some authors have found prematurity to

be associated with chlamydial conjunctivitis.[7] Although a greater percentage of cases may be identified in premature infants due to their longer hospitalization, chlamydial infection was felt to have a causal relationship to prematurity by some investigators.[6] Others, however, have found no correlation with prenatal or perinatal complications including prematurity, Apgar scores, birth weight, or congenital malformations.[10, 33, 35]

Chlamydial infection of the conjunctiva can result in a spectrum of diseases from mild redness to severe purulent conjunctivitis. In general, though, it is much less severe than gonococcal conjunctivitis. Infection usually is characterized by mild lid swelling, chemosis, hyperemia, and a papillary conjunctivitis with scant discharge (Fig 25–2). More severe cases can result in pseudomembrane formation. Corneal involvement is unusual, although a mild keratitis with residual peripheral scarring and superficial vascularization (micropannus) can occur.[3, 37–40] Even mild or transient cases of ophthalmia neonatorum can cause conjunctival scar and micropannus formation. Early treatment may decrease the incidence of scarring.[37] Scarring is never severe enough to result in visual loss.

Sixty-four to 69% of cases were unilateral in some series,[4, 8] while the majority of cases were bilateral in others.[10] Signs of disease usually occur between 4 and 12 days after birth, with the majority appearing on approximately day 7 or 8.[4, 6, 7, 10, 34, 41, 42] Chlamydial conjunctivitis can occur within the first 5 days of life with the purulent discharge usually attributed to gonococcal disease.[39] An onset as early as the first day of life may be due to prolonged rupture of membranes.[4] Delayed onset also is seen, with some infants developing clinical signs as late as weeks 5 to 6.[32]

Even untreated, infection is self-limited, with low-grade inflammation lasting 2 to 12 months.[7] The average infection will last $4^1/_2$ months, if left untreated,[42] but occasionally it persists for as long as 2 years.[39] If infection remains untreated for 3 to 6 weeks, infants will develop the follicular conjunctivitis characteristic of adult chlamydial conjunctivitis; younger infants are incapable of mounting a follicular response.

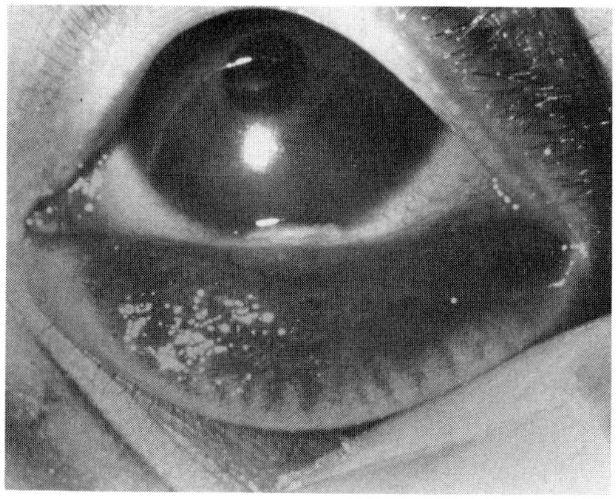

FIG 25–2.
Papillary conjunctivitis with scant mucopurulent discharge caused by *Chlamydia trachomatis* infection in a newborn. (Courtesy of Peter A. Rapoza, M.D.)

Chlamydia also can infect the respiratory and gastrointestinal tracts of newborns; late pneumonia occurs in 10% to 20% of newborns exposed to *Chlamydia* at birth.[31] Chlamydial pneumonia develops gradually after the second or third week of life. It is characterized by nasal obstruction and discharge, tachypnea, and a characteristic staccato cough.[43, 44] The eye has been hypothesized as a possible portal of entry for respiratory infections.[35, 44] Although extension from a conjunctival focus may occur in some cases, the respiratory tract can be infected separately.[44] It has been found that conjunctivitis does not precede most cases of chlamydial pneumonia.[19, 31]

Herpes Simplex Virus.—Infection with herpes simplex virus (HSV) can cause neonatal keratoconjunctivitis with lid swelling, conjunctival injection, corneal clouding, and typical dendritic staining of the corneal epithelium when fluorescein is applied. In most cases ocular infection is only one manifestation of disseminated herpetic disease. Rarely, however, herpetic keratoconjunctivitis occurs without other sites of infection or before other lesions develop. Neonatal HSV infections are discussed in greater detail later in the section on disseminated infections.

There is no evidence that any other viruses are important causes of natally acquired conjunctivitis. Coxsackie A9 virus has been isolated in a newborn who also had chlamydial keratoconjunctivitis.[10] It is possible, however, to transmit adenovirus to newborns in the postnatal period with development of epidemic keratoconjunctivitis (EKC). Dawson and associates reported the development of EKC caused by adenovirus, serotype 8, in a newborn in the second week of life.[45] The infection was characterized by bilateral redness, exudate, and pseudomembrane formation. Chlamydial disease was included in the differential diagnosis; the presence of EKC in other family members, however, provided clues to the correct diagnosis.

Other.— Numerous bacteria have been cultured from eyes of neonates with ophthalmia neonatorum (Table 25–2). Frequently multiple isolates are obtained. Nongonococcal, nonchlamydial conjunctivitis is usually of later onset.[10,46] The significance of positive cultures is uncertain since the same organisms are frequently isolated from neonates without evidence of disease as well. Positive bacterial cultures have been reported in up to 72% of all newborns.[1] In one series where bacteria was isolated from 10.7% of newborns cultured, the majority were *Staphylococcus* species and *Escherichia coli*.[25] Ophthalmia neonatorum was attributed to *Staphylococcus* species in 10% of cases from another series.[4] The role of staphylococci in the pathogenesis of neonatal conjunctivitis has been questioned, however.[8,12,13] In one study, 57 infants had positive cultures for *Staphylococcus aureus*, but of these, only 2 had conjunctivitis.[1] Pierce and associates have shown that *Staphylococcus aureus*, cultured from 9.5% of their cases with ophthalmia neonatorum, was isolated just as frequently from control infants without disease.[12] Using the same techniques, the authors showed a statistically significant association between other bacteria, such as *Streptococcus viridans*, and disease. In contrast, Sandstrom and associates did find a statistical difference in the incidence of *Staphylococcus aureus* infection between neonates having ophthalmia neonatorum and those without disease.[9] Prentice and associates compared cultures taken from 104 cases of ophthalmia neonatorum to 104 matched controls.[13] *Staphylococcus aureus, Streptococcus viridans*, and *Escherichia coli* were isolated with significantly increased frequency in disease cases. The presence of *Staphylococcus aureus* was significantly different, however, only when bilateral cases were compared with control patients; there was no statistically significant difference when cultures from unilateral cases were compared with cultures taken from opposite, uninvolved eyes. It is unclear therefore whether *Staphylococcus* species are causative agents for ophthalmia neonatorum or, if they are causes, what factors lead to the development of overt clinical disease in only certain newborns.

TABLE 25–2.
Bacteria Isolated From Cases of Ophthalmia Neonatorum With Uncertain Significance

Staphylococcus aureus
Staphylococcus epidermidis
Pseudomonas aeruginosa
Streptococcus pneumoniae
Aerobacter species
Hemophilus species
Streptococcus faecalis
Klebsiella pneumoniae
Enterobacter species
Proteus species
Acinetobacter sp (*Mima polymorpha*)

Although gram-negative bacteria are isolated frequently from normal infants, other laboratory and clinical evidence has led Armstrong and associates to conclude that these bacteria may cause conjunctivitis in certain cases.[4] Also, they found that cases of ophthalmia neonatorum attributed to *Pseudomonas aeruginosa* were more likely to be associated with sepsis than those due to other organisms such as *Neisseria gonorrhoeae*.

Mycoplasma hominis was isolated from 8 of 250 cases of purulent ophthalmia neonatorum in one series without other apparent causes of disease.[14] Based on the high incidence of maternal infection, a 1% to 2% transmission rate was hypothesized. In another large series, no cases of *Mycoplasma* species infection were identified although specifically sought.[13]

Other infections that cause neonatal sepsis, including group B streptococci (*Streptococcus agalactiae*) and *Listeria monocytogenes*, can cause a purulent conjunctivitis in affected newborns.[47–49] Howard and McCracken reported an isolated purulent conjunctivitis in 1 of 71 infants with group B streptococcus infection. The infection resolved with penicillin therapy, and permanent damage to the eyes did not occur.[50]

Sterile cultures have been reported in 6% to 87% of neonates with ophthalmia neonatorum in various series.[4,9,12,13] These cases are frequently self-limited without ophthalmic sequelae. It has been suggested that anaerobic organisms not identified by routine culture techniques may play a greater role in the pathogenesis of ophthalmia neonatorum than heretofore realized and may account for some of these cases.[51] The significance of such infections and their proper management will require further investigation.

Chemical Conjunctivitis

Silver nitrate, when used as prophylaxis against ophthalmia neonatorum is irritating to mucous membranes and can cause a chemical conjunctivitis that is sometimes confused with infection. The incidence of redness, conjunctival edema and mild watery or mucopurulent discharge attributable to silver nitrate varies widely among published series. Armstrong reported chemical conjunctivitis in 5 of 302 cases (1.6%) studied retrospectively[4]; mild or transient cases may have been missed. Others report its incidence to be approximately 49%.[25] It may be as high as 90% during the first 6 hours of life, but signs rapidly resolve, with only 7% still having conjunctivitis at 24 hours.[52] The signs and time course may overlap with infectious ophthalmia neonatorum. In general, however, one should always suspect an infectious cause with early purulent discharge or catarrhal inflammation lasting greater than 3 days. Chemical conjunctivitis does not appear to increase the incidence of secondary infections.[52]

The use of prophylaxis may delay the clinical onset of an established infection.[4] The early signs of redness and conjunctival edema in such cases may be misdiagnosed as chemical conjunctivitis. All cases of conjunctival inflammation therefore should be followed closely for late development of signs indicating infection.

Prophylaxis

The introdution of silver nitrate prophylaxis against gonococcal ophthalmia neonatorum by Crede in 1880 was a milestone in the history of preventive medicine. By instilling 1 drop of 2% (later 1%) silver nitrate onto the newborn eye, he was able to reduce the incidence of gonococcal keratoconjunctivitis from 10% to 0.3%. Prophylaxis is now required by law in most states. The continued need for prophylaxis in all newborns, however, has been questioned by some. In recent times, the incidence of gonococcal ophthalmia neonatorum has been low even in many populations where routine prophylaxis is not used.[26] In England where prophylaxis is not required, Pierce and associates reported a 12% incidence of ophthalmia neonatorum,[12] and Prentice and associates reported an 8.4% incidence,[13] but no cases of *Neisseria gonorrhoeae* were reported in either series. With the growing problem of sexually transmitted diseases in modern society and the emergence of drug-resistant strains of *Neisseria gonorrhoeae,* however, few doubt the wisdom of continued prophylactic treatment at birth. The importance of prophylaxis was demonstrated at Columbia Presbyterian Medical Center in New York during a 6-month period in 1957 when prophylaxis was discontinued; there was a marked increase in cases of neonatal gonococcal conjunctivitis.[53] In a study comparing two similar maternity services where one used silver nitrate prophylaxis and one used no prophylaxis, the percentage of infections caused by *Neisseria gonorrhoeae* were 0% and 7% respectively.[29] Prophylaxis decreased the incidence of other bacterial infections as well.

The agent of choice for prophylaxis has become a matter of debate. The emergence of *Chlamydia trachomatis* as the leading cause of infection has resulted in a reassessment of prophylactic procedures. Since its introduction by Crede, silver nitrate has been the standard technique. It continues to be highly effective against *Neisseria gonorrhoeae*, the most serious cause of ophthalmia neonatorum, as well as other bacteria including *Staphylococcus aureus* and *Escherichia coli*. It is not active against *Chlamydia trachomatis*, however. Current recommendations therefore include the use of 0.5% erythromycin or 1% tetracycline ointments, agents effective against both *Neisseria gonorrhoeae* and *Chlamydia trachomatis*, as alternative forms of prophylaxis.

Experience at some institutions suggests that the use of these antibiotics rather than silver nitrate has been associated with an increased failure rate and an increased incidence of late ophthalmia neonatorum.[52] It also is feared that antibiotic usage may result in the emergence of drug-resistant strains of organisms. Stenson and associates reported an increased incidence of ophthalmia neonatorum, including gonococcal infections, when tetracycline was used instead of silver nitrate for prophylaxis.[2] In a randomized study comparing erythromycin and silver nitrate prophylaxis, however, both drugs were equally effective, and erythromycin was less irritating to the conjunctiva.[54] In a review of several published series, Bernstein and associates also found that both tetracycline and erythromycin were as effective as silver nitrate against *Neisseria gonorrhoeae*.[55] Rothenberg, in fact, states that tetracycline and erythromycin may be more effective than silver nitrate for prophylaxis against *Neisseria gonorrhoeae*, although their efficacies have not specifically been tested in high-risk groups.[26]

Of the two drugs, there is evidence that tetracycline is less effective than erythromycin in prevention of disease.[56] Cases of chlamydial conjunctivitis following tetracycline prophylaxis have been reported.[41] Agents such as sulfonamides and bacitracin are not considered adequate for prophylaxis due to unacceptably high failure rates.[26]

The emergence of penicillinase-producing *Neisseria gonorrhoeae* has created new concerns regarding prophylaxis of newborns. Tetracycline and erythromicin may not be as effective as silver nitrate for protection against these organisms.[57] Infants born in areas with a high incidence of penicillinase producing *Neisseria gonorrhoeae* infection should be monitored closely.

Penicillin has been shown to be a highly effective topical agent for prophylaxis against *Neisseria gonorrhoeae*[25, 26] but is not used because of the potential for sensitization to the drug, its lack of efficacy against *Chlamydia trachomatis*, and the emergence of penicillinase-producing strains of *Neisseria gonorrhoeae*.[27]

On the basis of accumulated experience with neonatal infections, the Centers for Disease Control (CDC) and the American Academy of Pediatrics have published guidelines for prophylaxis against ophthalmia neonatorum.[28, 58] A 1% silver nitrate solution or an ointment containing 1% tetracycline or 0.5% erythromycin should be instilled in both eyes of all infants following birth. Single-dose containers should be used; contamination of drugs, errors in compounding silver nitrate, or evaporation of silver nitrate resulting in increased concentrations of the solution that can produce severe ocular surface burns can thereby be avoided.

Prophylactic agents should not be flushed from the eye. The efficacy of prophylaxis following flushing has not been adequately studied and probably does not decrease the incidence of chemical conjunctivitis.[52] Prophylaxis may be instilled up to 1 hour after birth to facilitate initial maternal-infant bonding. Because prophylaxis may be ineffective in established infections, longer delays are not acceptable.

Infants born by cesarean section also should receive prophylaxis. Although most infections are acquired during passage through the birth canal, ascending infections can occur with or without rupture of membranes.

Even with proper prophylactic techniques there is a small but definite risk of ophthalmia neonatorum in infants born to mothers with untreated vaginal infections. Thompson and associates reported 2 cases of gonococcal conjunctivitis among 29 infants born to mothers with untreated disease despite prophylaxis.[22] Larger series place this incidence between 0.06% and 2%.[4,5] A review of 24 series since 1930 revealed a 0.6% risk for failure of silver nitrate prophylaxis.[26] Prophylaxis may be ineffective if instilled incorrectly or if there has been prolonged rupture of membranes with establishment of infection before birth. In some cases, "prophylactic failures" may actually represent postnatal transmission from contact with infected family members.

Prophylaxis is not a substitute for identification and treatment of sexually transmitted disease in pregnant women. Armstrong and associates found a 10.9% incidence of positive cultures for *Neisseria gonorrhoeae* in the labor and delivery suites.[4] The cervicitis may be asymptomatic. Not only may established infections in neonates be inadequately treated by prophylactic measures, but postnatal infection of infants who escape infection at delivery can occur via late contact with contaminated secretions from the mother.

Prenatal screening has been effective in reducing the incidence of ophthalmia neonatorum.[4,22] Screening programs will continue to be less than 100% effective, however, because of subclinical infections, falsely negative cultures, inadequate treatment, or reinfection before delivery. Also, those women at highest risk for sexually transmitted diseases are the least likely to have had antenatal care. Prophylaxis therefore will continue to be an important public health measure.

When an infant is born to a mother having previously untreated gonorrhea, prophylaxis alone is considered inadequate, whether or not there are signs of conjunctivitis. Such infants should receive 50,000 units (20,000 units for low-birth weight infants) of intravenous or intramuscular aqueous crystalline penicillin G,[28] and infants should be isolated for 24 hours to prevent the possible spread of infection.

Proper hygiene of the newborn eyelids was an important feature of Crede's original prophylaxis. Direct exposure of the conjunctiva is required for bacterial or chlamydial infection. Immediate cleaning of the face at birth with removal of blood and secretions from the closed eyelids may help to minimize the incidence of infection by preventing infected secretions from contacting the ocular surface.

Because respiratory tract infections are not always a sequelae of chlamydial conjunctivitis, even successful prophylaxis against chlamydial conjunctivitis will not eliminate respiratory infections.[19] One disadvantage of prophylaxis against *Chlamydia trachomatis* in the viewpoint of some clinicians, therefore, is that it eliminates ocular infection as an early indicator of infants at risk for chlamydial pneumonitis (a later and much more serious condition) and of mothers at risk for chlamydial endometritis.

None of the current recommended techniques of prophylaxis are effective against HSV. Maternal screening therefore is critical; if viral shedding is present in the mother, babies should be delivered by cesarean section, as discussed in greater detail in a later section. Some investigators have instilled vidarabine ointment empirically four to five times daily for 5 days in the eyes of infants born to mothers with genital HSV without apparent adverse effect as a means of prophylaxis.[59] The efficacy of this procedure is unknown.

Diagnosis

Adequate therapy for ophthalmia neonatorum requires early and accurate diagnosis. Delayed or inappropriate management may have severe consequences. Failure to recognize gonococcal keratoconjunctivitis can result in blindness. Early recognition of HSV, *Chlamydia trachomatis*, or other bacterial infections of the eye will alert the clinician to the possible need for treatment of serious associated nonocular infections. Because of overlap in the signs and onset of disease among various forms of ophthalmia neonatorum, diagnosis on clinical grounds alone is not reliable. Also, it has been reported that in 72% of nonchlamydial and in 50% of chlamydial conjunctivitis cases multiple agents can be identified.[10] Infection with both *Neisseria gonorrhoeae* and *Chlamydia trachomatis* has been reported frequently.

All infants with ocular surface inflammation, whether or not they have had prophylaxis, should be thoroughly evaluated by laboratory techniques. Bacterial, viral, and chlamydial (if available) cultures should be performed. Conjunctival scraping should be obtained and stained with Gram and Giemsa stains. Gram staining and culture have been reported to have equal sensitivity for identification of *Neisseria gonorrhoeae* infections.[4] *Neisseria gonorrhoeae* can be seen as gram-negative intracellular diplococci in exudative material. In addition to cultures for *Neisseria gonorrhoeae*, antibiotic sensitivity testing is necessary due to the emergence of penicillin-resistant strains.

Giemsa-stained scrapings are examined for the presence of csytological changes. Multinucleate giant cells and intranuclear inclusions are characteristic of HSV infections. Chlamydial infections produce large purple intracytoplasmic inclusions, usually found adjacent to the nucleus, from which the name inclusion blenorrhea was derived (Fig 25–3). They are much more common in neonatal infections than in the adult counterpart.[42] In trained hands, cytological examination for inclusions and their components, free elementary and initial bodies, can be a highly sensitive method of diagnosis in neonatal infections.[60] Because chlamydiae are obligate intracellular organisms, scrapings must contain epithelial cells for diagnosis. Study of exudative material alone is inadequate. The highest yield is obtained from the lower tarsal conjunctiva.[42] Inclusion conjunctivitis is also characterized by a mixed inflammatory response with abundant polymorphonuclear leukocytes.[61]

Chlamydiae can be grown in tissue culture systems. Isolation of organisms may be related to the time of sampling; cultures may be negative in exposed infants during the first 3 to 6 days of life.[30,36]

Fluorescein-conjugated monoclonal antibody staining of McCoy cell cultures is considered to be the test of choice for chlamydial infections by some investigators.[10,62] Cell culture techniques, however, are expensive and

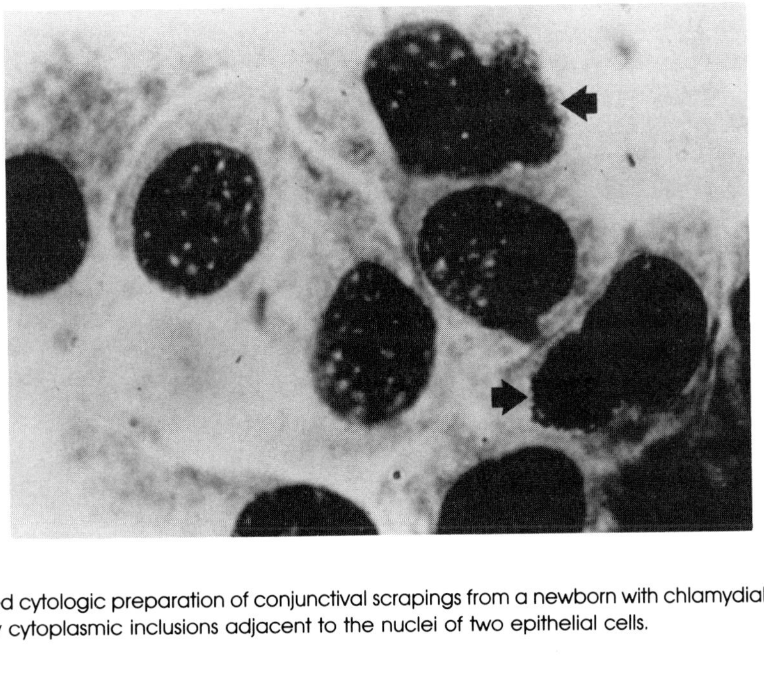

FIG 25–3.
Geimsa-stained cytologic preparation of conjunctival scrapings from a newborn with chlamydial conjunctivitis. *Arrows* identify cytoplasmic inclusions adjacent to the nuclei of two epithelial cells.

TABLE 25–3.
Ophthalmia Neonatorum: Summary of Treatment Guidelines*

Chlamydia trachomatis	Oral erythromycin syrup: 50 mg/kg/day in 4 divided doses for 2 wk. Reinstate therapy for recurrences (1–2 wk)
Neisseria gonorrhoeae	Isolate newborns for 24 hr after start of therapy
Neonates at risk due to exposure	50,000 units aqueous crystalline penicillin G, IM or IV (20,000 units for low–birth weight infants)
Neonates with ophthalmia neonatorum	100,000 units/kg/day aqueous crystalline penicillin G in 4 divided doses for 7 days
Penicillinase-producing *Neisseria gonorrhoeae*	Cefotaxime, IV 25 mg/kg, every 8 to 12 hr for 7 days (the efficacy of tetracycline and erythromycin has not been established)

*Adapted from Centers for Disease Control: 1985 Standard treatment guidelines. *MMWR* 1985; 34 (suppl): 75–108. Anonymous: Treatment of sexually transmitted diseases. *Med Lett Drugs Ther* 1986; 28: 23–28. Abbreviations: IM = intramuscular; IV = intravenous.

of limited availability, and results will be delayed several days. Immunocytochemical techniques can be used to identify chlamydiae on tissue scrapings as well. Rapoza and associates have shown direct immunofluorescent antibody staining of conjunctival scrapings to be 100% specific and 94% sensitive.[63] Immunocytochemical techniques are also available for diagnosis of HSV infections.

A thorough history of *both* parents regarding urethral or vaginal discharge, genital vesicles, or known history of sexually transmitted diseases may provide important clues to the cause of ophthalmia neonatorum.

Until treated, infants with all forms of ophthalmia neonatorum should be considered highly contagious and maintained in isolation to prevent nosocomial spread of disease.

Treatment

With appropriate therapy, all forms of ophthalmia neonatorum can resolve without sequelae. Ophthalmia neonatorum caused by *Neisseria gonorrhoeae* or *Chlamydia trachomatis* requires systemic antimocrobial therapy (Table 25–3). Neonates with gonococcal conjunctivitis should be treated with aqueous crystalline penicillin G, 100,000 units/kg/day in four doses for 7 days.[58] The recommended dose is based on cumulative experience[26]; it has not been tested in formal drug trials. Topical therapy alone is insufficient.[4, 27] With systemic therapy, topical antibiotics provide no added therapeutic benefit, but exudative material should be removed frequently with saline irrigation. An alternative therapy in cases of penicillinase-producing *Neisseria gonorrhoeae* is cefotaxime, a long-acting cephalosporin, 25 mg/kg every 8 to 12 hours for 7 days.[64] Single-dose cefotaxine (125 mg intramuscularly) has been investigated and found effective as the sole treatment of gonococcal conjunctivitis in underdeveloped countries where follow-up care of infected neonates may be difficult.[65] The same investigators found single-dose kanamycin (75 or 150 mg) combined with topical gentamicin or tetracycline ointment also to be effective,[65, 66] although there is some concern for ototoxicity with kanamycin.

Even in the absence of clinical disease, neonates born to mothers with known gonococcal infections should receive a single intravenous or intramuscular injection of 50,000 units of aqueous crystalline penicillin G (20,000 units for low–birth weight infants). Lossick recommends using 20,000 units/kg for infants weighing less than 2,000 gm because they have been found to have lower peak serum levels of drug for a given dose than normal-weight infants.[24]

Infants must be isolated with wound precautions during the first 24 hours of treatment to prevent spread of infection in the nursery. Ophthalmic consultation is important during the period of treatment. Infants who demonstrate signs of nonocular gonococcal infection in addition to ophthalmia neonatorum should receive higher doses of drug under the supervision of a pediatric infectious disease specialist.

Topical therapy for chlamydial conjunctivitis with sulfacetamide or tetracycline has been reported to be successful.[4,67] Clinical signs of disease may resolve rapidly, but therapy may be only partially effective and does not treat nonocular sites of disease. There may be persistent evidence of inflammatory cells on cytological examination of scrapings despite resolution of clinical signs.[38,41] Recent studies have confirmed that topical therapy alone has a high failure rate.[6,8,30,34,39,56] Up to 75% of treated infants will develop recurrent, albeit usually milder disease. Some failures may be attributed to the difficulty experienced by mothers with instillation of ointment.

Systemic therapy is currently recommended for all infants with chlamydial conjunctivitis. It also will successfully treat nonocular sites of infection including nasopharyngeal and lung infections.[68] Current recommendations call for treatment with erythromycin (12.5 mg/kg orally or intravenously four times a day for 14 days).[58,64] Heggie and associates found that this regimen caused resolution of conjunctival disease in 14 of 15 infants (93%) compared with resolution in only 4 of 14 infants (29%) treated with topical sulfacetamide alone in a randomized study.[46] Higher failure rates have been reported with oral therapy when lower doses or shorter courses were used.[56,68] Rapoza and associates, however, have reported a 19% failure rate following one course of treatment, even using current CDC recommendations.[10] Sixty percent also had persistence of disease after a second course of therapy. Failures may have beeen due to incorrect administration of drug, inadequate levels due to nausea and emesis caused by oral erythromycin, reinfection, or possible resistence of the organism to erythromycin. All patients responded to a third course of trimethoprim-sulfamethoxazole (0.5 mL/kg/day in two divided doses for 2 weeks) and topical tetracycline applied four times daily for 1 week.

Although tetracycline is an effective treatment for adult chlamydial infection, it should not be used systemically in children due to its effect on teeth and bone. Both parents of infants with gonococcal or chlamydial conjunctivitis must receive treatment as well.

All nongonococcal, nonchlamydial infections respond to topical therapy alone.[10] Instillation of gentamicin ointment four times daily for 1 week is reported to be effective therapy for conjunctivitis attributed to gram-negative organisms. Mild cases of conjunctivitis not attributable to *Neisseria gonorrhoeae* or *Chlamydia trachomatis* frequently resolve with lid hygiene alone.[11]

Infectious Dacryocystitis

Thirty to 75% of newborns have an imperforate membrane at the distal end of the nasolacrimal duct.[69] In most cases, the condition resolves spontaneously, although 1.75% to 6% of newborns may have persistent congenital nasolacrimal obstruction.[70] Infection of the nasolacrimal sac and its contents may result. Signs of dacryocystitis include purulent reflux from the puncta and epiphora. In the majority of cases, disease develops within the first 6 days of life.[69] It is bilateral in approximately one third of cases.[69]

Dacryocystitis frequently is associated with conjunctivitis. Seventeen percent of newborns with conjunctivitis had dacryocystitis in one series.[11] There was a strong correlation between failure of nonchlamydial conjunctivitis to respond to antibiotic therapy and obstruction of the nasolacrimal duct. Nineteen (51%) of 37 patients considered clinical failures had obstructions, while only 3 (6%) of 47 clinical cures had obstruction.[11]

There was an association between conjunctivitis caused by *Hemophilus* species or *Streptococcus pneumoniae* and nasolacrimal duct obstruction in one series. Three of 6 infants with conjunctivitis attributed to one of these two pathogens had obstruction while only 2 of 22 infants with conjunctivitis attributed to other organisms had obstruction.[9,26] In another study by the same authors, however, there was no association between nasolacrimal duct obstruction and specific organisms. *Staphylococcus aureus, Streptococcus viridans, Hemophilus influenza,* and *Branhamella* species were all isolated from patients with dacryocystitis. Rapoza and associates discovered dacryocystitis in 4 of 100 infants with conjunctivitis. In each case, *Streptococcus epidermidis* or *Streptococcus viridans* was isolated.[10]

Antibiotic therapy will cause temporary improvement in dacryocystitis, but complete resolution will occur only after patency of the nasolacrimal duct is established. The obstruction is frequently relieved by massage over the nasolacrimal system.[70] In cases where patency is not established by conservative therapy, probing of the nasolacrimal duct is indicated. The age at which probing should occur remains a subject of debate. Various authors recommend waiting anywhere from 2 to 12 months before probing.[11,69,70] Early probing is advocated by some clinicians to relieve epiphora and persistent drainage of mucopurulent material and to avoid the development of more serious infections including periorbital cellulitis and lacrimal abscesses. Ffooks reported lacrimal abscess formation in 7 (1.6%) of 440 infants with chronic nasolacrimal duct obstruction.[71] Infection was caused by *Streptococcus pyogenes* in those cases where an infectious agent was identified. Others argue against early probing because of the high frequency with which spontaneous resolutions occur. By waiting, the procedure with its associated risks and discomfort can be avoided. Cases of dacryocystitis associated with chronic conjunctivitis unresponsive to antibiotic therapy should be probed early.

Disseminated Infections

Some perinatally acquired infections result in disseminated disease with serious ophthalmic sequelae. Group B streptococci (*Streptococcus agalactiae*) are a leading cause of serious disseminated bacterial infections in newborns, occurring in 1.3 to 3 per 1,000 live births.[47] These bacteria can be isolated from cervicovaginal cultures in 4.6% to 26% of pregnant females, and prospective studies indicate a transmission rate of 65% to 72% in neonates born to colonized mothers.[48] Only 1% to 2% of these neonates will develop invasive infection, however. Infection usually occurs during the first 3 days of life but may occur up to 3 months later. Some late cases may be the result of nosocomial transmission of bacteria.

Ophthalmic manifestations of neonatal group B streptococcal disease include conjunctivitis and endogenous endophthalmitis.[47,48,50] Meningitis, the most common site of late disseminated infection, can result in permanent neurological deficits with ophthalmic sequelae including cortical blindness and cranial nerve palsies.[48]

Herpes Simplex Virus Infections

HSV infections are a cause of severe neonatal morbidity. Infection may remain localized to the skin, mouth, or ocular surface. HSV, however, is life-threatening if it causes localized central nervous system (CNS) disease or disseminated infection involving liver, adrenals, respiratory tract, gastrointestinal tract, pancreas, spleen, heart, and bone marrow. In only rare instances will infection be asymptomatic. The majority of infected infants die or are left with severe neurological and ocular sequelae; there is a 70% to 80% incidence of mortality or severe brain damage.[67,72]

Signs of HSV disease usually become apparent between 3 days and 3 weeks after birth.[59,67,73–75] In 90% of newborns disease will be apparent within 2 weeks, with a mean onset of 7 days.[73] When infection first becomes apparent, infants may have localized skin, mouth, or ocular surface lesions as the only manifestation; 70% of such babies, however, eventually will develop disseminated disease.[76] Signs of disseminated disease may not become apparent until 1 to 3 weeks after birth. Skin vesicles are the hallmark of HSV disease but occur in only one third of neonatal infections. The initial signs of disease may be nonspecific rather than localized; anorexia, vomiting, lethargy, and fever can be mistaken for bacterial sepsis.

Most newborns acquire infection at the time of birth when they encounter virus in the maternal genital tract. It therefore is recommended that infants be delivered by cesarean section if the mother is shedding virus at the time of delivery. With prolonged rupture of membranes, however, an ascending infection can occur, and cesarean section will not always prevent neonatal disease.[77] In a study of females with HSV infection after 32 weeks' gestation, there was an overall risk of 10% for neonatal infection.[78] The risk increased to 40% to 60% if infants were not delivered by cesarean section within 4 hours of membrane rupture.

Infants born to mothers with primary genital herpes are at greatest risk.[67, 78] Brown and associates have reported that serious perinatal morbidity occurred in 6 (40%) of 15 infants born to mothers with primary infection vs. none of 14 infants born to mothers with genital herpes who had serological evidence of prior, asymptomatic infection.[79] The higher risk is attributed to the fact that in primary infections there is a greater incidence of persistent, asymptomatic shedding of virus from the cervix. The risk, therefore, is increased further when primary maternal infection occurs during the third trimester.

Although cesarean section is recommended for pregnant women with known active genital herpetic lesions, symptomatic genital disease at the time of delivery actually is infrequent in mothers of newborns with HSV infection. As many as 70% may have asymptomatic mothers,[76] and in only 65% will there be a history of genital herpetic lesions in either the mother or the father.[80] Clinicians therefore must maintain a high clinical suspicion of HSV infection in infants even in the absence of a positive maternal history of genital disease.

The incidence of neonatal HSV infection has risen in recent years as a consequence of the increased incidence of genital herpetic infections in women of childbearing age. In King County, Washington, the incidence of neonatal HSV infection rose from 2.6 per 100,000 live births in the years 1966 through 1969 to 12 per 100,000 in the years 1978 through 1981 to 28.2 per 100,000 in 1982.[80] It is more common in infants born to young mothers of low socioeconomic status. HSV is more common in premature infants, which reflects the fact that there is an increased risk of early delivery in mothers with genital herpes (especially those with primary disease) after 20 weeks of gestation.[78]

There are two HSV serotypes. HSV, type I, is the most common cause of "cold sores" on the lips and corneal disease in adults. HSV, type II, is the most common cause of genital herpetic lesions in adults. Because of its association with genital herpes, most neonatal infections have been due to HSV, type II, although HSV, type I, can be a cause of neonatal HSV disease as well. It is believed that most infants infected with HSV, type I, acquire virus from nongenital or nonmaternal sources[80, 81]; exposure to maternal HSV type I lesions on the lips is one potential source of infection, and it is suspected that virus can be carried between infants in the nursery by health care workers who do not observe proper precautions to prevent nosocomial transmission of disease.[82]

Occasionally, newborns already have vesicles, disseminated disease, CNS infection, or ocular lesions at birth, thus suggesting in utero infection by a transplacental route.[67, 74, 75, 80, 83–88] Such infants also have developmental deformities,[86] hepatic calcifications,[87] and osseous lesions.[87] Rare cases of presumed transplacental infection early in gestation have resulted in microcephaly, micrencephaly with intracranial calcifications, microphthalmos, and intraocular developmental abnormalities, which suggests that HSV, type II, may have neurotropic teratogenic potential.[84]

In utero infections must be differentiated from the other congenital infectious diseases discussed later. The presence of skin vesicles will assist in diagnosis, but they may not be present. A sexual history from the infant's parents may provide important clues for correct diagnosis but also may be negative, as discussed previously.

Ocular disorders, including conjunctivitis, keratitis, retinopathy, and cataracts, occur in 16% to 23% of newborns with HSV infection.[76, 89] There may be no ocular lesions when patients are first examined, however. Of 28 infants with progressive HSV disease, 4 developed eye involvement after the onset of disease.[76]

Conjunctivitis, characterized by lid swelling, conjunctival injection, and serosanguineous discharge, may be the initial or only manifestation of HSV infection.[90] If characteristic HSV vesicular lesions are not present on the eyelids, conjunctivitis can be mistaken for other forms of opthalmia neonatorum. Corneal infection can occur with a variety of manifestations including the characteristic dendritic lesions of adult HSV epithelial keratitis, geographic epithelial defects, or diffusely cloudy corneas. It is likely that newborns with seemingly isolated ocular surface disease subsequently will develop dissemination of infection.[91]

Retinopathy is the most serious of the HSV-associated disorders. Viral infection causes retinal necrosis, seen as patches of retinal whitening on ophthalmoscopic examination. There also may be retinal vasculitis and hemorrhage. In most cases of intraocular disease, only the retina becomes infected; iris and choroid infections are less common.[92] In survivors, the necrotic retina heals with gliotic scarring and mottled pigmentation. Infants are left blind or with severely reduced vision depending on which area of the fundus is involved. Retinitis may not develop until many months after birth.[59] Infants with HSV retinitis frequently have cataracts as well, and virus can be isolated from these lenses.[93, 94]

HSV, types I and II, causes a similar spectrum of neonatal disease with the exception of retinitis.[89] HSV type I retinitis in newborns has been reported rarely,[95] but HSV retinitis in newborns is almost exclusively due to HSV, type II.

The frequent association between HSV retinopathy and encephalitis suggests that virus reaches the retina by neural spread from the brain.[89, 92] Nevertheless, retinitis can develop without neurological disease[93, 94]; it is possible that virus reaches the eye hematogenously in those cases.

In a randomized, controlled study, vidarabine (15 mg/kg/day over 12 hours for 10 days) was shown to decrease the mortality of babies with localized CNS or disseminated HSV infection.[96] The severity of disease sequelae was reduced in surviving infants who had localized ocular or CNS disease. Nevertheless, even with treatment, the majority of infants were not normal at 1 year of age. Although acyclovir has been shown to be more effective than vidarabine for treatment of HSV encephalitis in older patients,[72] preliminary results from studies in infants have not indicated that one drug is superior to the other.

Candidiasis

Newborns with perinatal illnesses that require medical or surgical intervention are at risk for disseminated candidiasis with endogenous candidal chorioretinitis and endophthalmitis.[97–99] *Candida albicans* is the most common species to cause disease. Disseminated candidiasis in infants results in respiratory deterioration, abdominal distension, guaiac-positive stools, carbohydrate intolerance, meningitis, erythematous rash, temperature instability, and hypotension.[99] The mean onset of symptoms is 33 days after birth.[99]

Organisms reach various organs hematogenously. Factors that predispose to candidemia include indwelling catheters, abdominal surgery, bacterial sepsis, the prolonged use of broad-spectrum antibiotics, debilitating diseases, or a combination of these factors.[100] Baley and associates reported a series of eight infants with disseminated candidiasis seen over a 1-year period in which all had low birth weight, evidence of sepsis, indwelling catheters, and antibiotic usage.[101] These infants made up 4% of all newborns weighing less than 1,500 gm during that period. Four of the eight developed retinal and vitreous infections. Low birth weight has been associated with candidal chorioretinitis by other investigators as well, although it also may occur in full-term, normal–birth weight infants who require prolonged hospitalization.[98]

Organisms initially infect the richly vascularized choroid in most cases. Infection eventually spreads to involve the retina and vitreous. Early lesions appear as discrete, densely yellow-white opacities that may resemble cotton-wool spots. There usually is an overlying haze of inflammatory cells in the vitreous. Histopathologically lesions are composed of organisms surrounded by dense infiltration of acute and chronic inflammatory cells. Newborn and preterm infants have been shown to have a deficiency in the candidacidal ability of leukocytes, which may enhance the severity of candidal endophthalmitis.[102]

Anterior ocular structures are not involved early in the course of infections, and the external eye may appear normal. Any infant with candidal sepsis therefore should have a careful fundus examination. Most lesions appear in the macular area, but indirect ophthalmoscopy should be performed since lesions occasionally appear first in the peripheral retina.

Infection of the eye usually is associated with invasive infection of other organs. In a large autopsy study of adults, Edwards and associates found that 80% of patients with candidal endophthalmitis had tissue-invasive infection of other organs.[100] The same is assumed to be true in neonates. The kidneys and heart are the most common sites of nonocular tissue-invasive infections.[100]

Aggressive antifungal therapy is warranted because untreated infection can lead to a loss of the eye. Spontaneous resolution of candida chorioretinitis in adults following withdrawal of the source of candidemia has been reported but is rare. Spontaneous improvement is less likely in infants because of their defect in cell-mediated immunity.

Successful treatment of neonatal candidal chorioretinitis has been reported; Baley and associates observed clearing of ocular lesions in three neonates who received treatment consisting of intravenous amphotericin B and 5-fluorocytosine.[101] This drug combination has synergistic activity against *Candida albicans* in vitro and is considered by many investigators to be the treatment of choice for candidal chorioretinitis. Severe nephrotoxicity with oliguria and anuria is common in neonates receiving amphotericin B. Although doses up to 1 mg/kg/day may be used, it has been recommended that the daily dosage not exceed 0.5 mg/kg/day in neonates to reduce renal toxicity.[103] 5-Fluorocytosine is given in a dosage of 150 mg/kg/day.[101] In adults with extensive vitreous involvement, vitrectomy and injection of amphotericin B into the vitreous cavity has been necessary for control of infection.

Reactivation of infection several months after apparently successful amphotericin B treatment has been reported.[97] Lesions should be followed closely therefore after completion of drug therapy.

CONGENITAL INFECTIOUS DISEASES

In the 1970s, Nahmias and colleagues popularized the concept of the TORCH complex, a group of congenital and perinatally acquired infectious diseases caused by agents that usually are of low pathogenicity in adults but can cause severe morbidity in newborns.[104] It may be difficult to differentiate between these diseases—*TO*xoplasmosis, *R*ubella, *C*ytomegalic inclusion disease (CID, caused by cytomegalovirus [CMV]), and *H*SV infections—and others, including congenital syphilis, on clinical grounds alone.

The use of "TORCH titers" has been advocated as a diagnostic aid to differentiate these infections but serological diagnosis has many potential pitfalls and is not a substitute for isolation and identification of pathogens. IgG antibodies in newborns during the perinatal period may be of maternal origin, passed transplacentally to the fetus. Persistence or elevation of antibody levels after the first few months of life when concentrations of maternally derived antibodies should be falling may indicate active neonatal infection, but it is in the perinatal period that institution of appropriate antimicrobial therapy is crucial. TORCH remains a useful concept, however, for remembering important life- and sight-threatening neonatal infections.

Toxoplasmosis

Toxoplasma gondii is a common protozoan parasite. The cat is the definitive host, but infection can occur in other animals and humans who then retain infectious cysts in muscle and other tissues. The infection is acquired by humans through ingestion of undercooked meat or ingestion of oocytes excreted by cats that contaminate the environment. Women who are first infected by *Toxoplasma gondii* during pregnancy can transmit parasites transplacentally to the fetus. Maternal infection may result in a mild systemic illness with lymphadenopathy but usually is asymptomatic.[105–107] In most series, congenital infection develops in 30% to 50% of infants born to mothers with serological evidence of newly acquired *Toxoplasma gondii* infection during pregnancy.[107–110]

The incidence of congenital toxoplasmosis varies with social and economic factors. Societies in which there is an increased consumption of raw or undercooked meat and areas with poor sanitation have higher rates. In the United States where approximately 70% of women of childbearing age are at risk for primary infection,[106] it is reported that congenital toxoplasmosis occurs in 1 of 750 to 1 of 3,000 live births.[105, 111]

Maternal immunity protects against fetal transmission; thus, women infected before pregnancy are at little or no risk for delivering a child with congenital toxoplasmosis, and women who deliver one child with congenital toxoplasmosis are at little or no risk of having a second infected child.[105–109, 112] Although fetal infections with *Toxoplasma gondii* in consecutive pregnancies of an infected mother have been reported,[113] most cases of toxoplasmosis in multiple siblings, especially when discovered at an older age, probably are attributable to acquired disease.

Congential toxoplasmosis originally was described by the classic triad of retinochoroiditis hydrocephalus, and intracranial calcifications. It is now known that neonatal disease can have a broad spectrum of clinical manifestations. The majority of infections result in no clinically apparent disease; 65% to 90% of infected infants are asymptomatic.[105, 107, 108, 111, 114]

The incidence of fetal infection is greatest when maternal infection occurs in the later stages of pregnancy, but those fetal infections that do occur early in gestation are more likely to produce clinically apparent disease.[105, 107, 108, 112] Patients with clinically apparent disease fall into two broad categories. In the first group, infants appear normal at birth but after several weeks or months develop signs and symptoms attributable to CNS infection including hydrocephalus, intracranial calcifications, deterioration of intellect, deafness, and retinochoroidal lesions. In the second group, which is less common, infants have disseminated infection that is evident at birth and characterized by splenomegaly, jaundice, hepatomegaly, fever, anemia, lymphadenopathy, pneumonitis, vomiting, and diarrhea. Microcephaly and other neurological manifestations also may be apparent in this group. The prognosis is poor for patients symptomatic at birth; the mortality rate is 12%, and only 10% of surviving infants are left without debilitating sequelae.[115]

Ocular infection occurs in 70% to 80% of all patients with congenital toxoplasmosis.[111, 112, 114] Eichenwald found that the incidence of retinochoroiditis was related to the type of congenital disease; 94.4% of patients with neurological disease alone had ocular

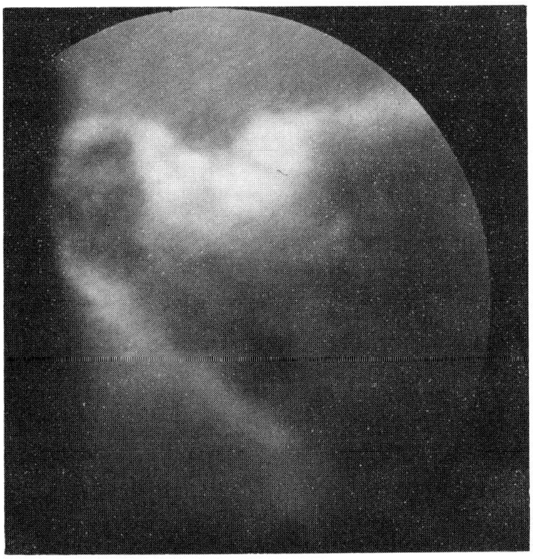

FIG 25–4.
Active toxoplasmic retinochoroiditis in a newborn.

lesions while only 65.9% of infants with disseminated disease at birth had ocular lesions.[115] Ocular infection may be the only manifestation of congenital toxoplasmosis; 10% of patients have ocular lesions without evidence of disease in other organs.[111, 116, 117]

The retina is the primary site of *Toxoplasma gondii* infection in the eye. It causes a focally destructive lesion with intense surrounding inflammation and an overlying vitreous inflammatory haze (Fig 25–4). The choroid is secondarily inflamed but is not a site of infection. Retinochoroidal lesions are self-limited; frequently they are not identified until after resolution of the inflammation and in fact may already have healed at birth. Resolution of the inflammation leaves a discrete yellow-white atrophic scar with hyperpigmented borders (Fig 25–5).

Live organisms may persist in quiescent lesions for many years after birth; reactivation of these organisms can cause recurrent episodes of retinochoroidal inflammation in older children and adults.[118] In fact, because recurrent toxoplasmic retinochoroiditis in adults usually occurs at the borders of retinochoroidal scars typical of those seen in congenital toxoplasmosis, it is believed that the vast majority of adult cases are recurrent congenital infections in persons without other manifestations of congenital disease.[116, 117]

It was assumed by many early investigators that retinochoroidal lesions in congenital toxoplasmosis were always bilateral and involved the maculae, but Hogan and associates have shown that macular lesions are found in only 46% of patients.[119] When unilateral disease or peripheral lesions only occur, they

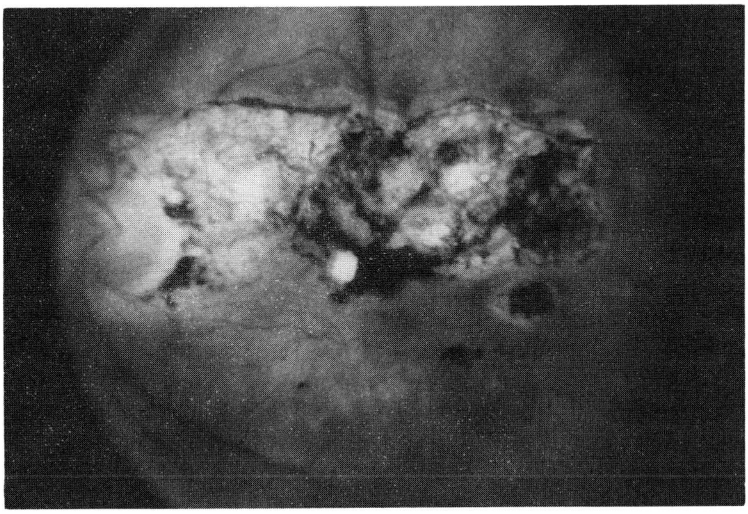

FIG 25–5.
Inactive macular retinochoroidal scar in a patient with congenital ocular toxoplasmosis.

may be asymptomatic and are easily missed on newborn examinations. Also, lesions are not always present at birth: they often develop months or years later.[105, 108, 109, 114] In a study of 12 patients with congenital toxoplasmosis, Loewer-Sieger and associates found that 4 had retinochoroidal lesions at the age of 1. By the age of 18, 9 of 11 had lesions, 4 of whom had visual loss.[110]

Microphthalmos is an uncommon manifestation of congenital toxoplasmosis.[107, 116, 117] Other ophthalmic disorders, including nystagmus and strabismus, most likely are due to sensory deprivation resulting from extensive retinal infection.

Pyrimethamine and sulfonamides are the most commonly used antimicrobial agents for treatment of newborns with congenital toxoplasmosis.[106–112, 115] Pyrimethamine inhibits folic acid metabolism of the proliferative form of *Toxoplasma gondii* but also is toxic to human cells and can result in bone marrow suppression. Patients therefore are given folinic acid to counteract the toxic effects of the drug; exogenous folinic acid can be used in folic acid metabolism by human but not parasitic cells. Treatment may prevent further progression of ocular lesions[111] and shorten the course of active disease[115] but does not prevent late recurrences.[110]

Rubella

Maternal rubella infection during the first trimester of pregnancy can result in serious disease of the newborn. The congenital rubella syndrome (CRS) consists of cardiac defects (the most common being patent ductus arteriosus with pulmonary stenosis), hearing loss, psychomotor and growth retardation, lesions of the long bones, dental deformities, thrombocytopenia with purpura, microcephaly, and inflammatory lesions of the CNS. Ocular manifestations of CRS include cataracts, glaucoma, pigmentary retinopathy, shallowing of the anterior chamber, microphthalmos, corneal clouding with or without elevations in intraocular pressure, and anterior uveal disease. There is a strong correlation between the presence of ocular and cardiac defects.[120] Estimates of the risk of fetal damage with maternal infection range from 10% to 50%.[121, 122] Seventy percent of infected newborns may be asymptomatic; of these however, 70% will develop clinically apparent disease, primarily hearing loss, by the age of 5.[105] Rubella acquired in the early postnatal period is not associated with severe disease.[105]

A great deal was learned about CRS in the last major rubella epidemic to occur in the United States, that of 1963 and 1964. There were 12.5 million cases; 52,500 cases involved women during their first trimester of pregnancy, and 10,500 infants were born with moderate to severe CRS.[122]

Since rubella vaccine became available in 1969, the incidence of this disease has declined by 99%, with an associated drop in cases of CRS.[123] Fifty-seven cases of CRS were reported to the CDC in 1979, while only 2 were reported in 1985. There were 12 cases in 1986 however, reversing a consistent downward trend since 1982.[123] Eight of the cases were in New York City, but these figures probably underestimate the true incidence of CRS nationwide because of the passive rather than active surveillance system of reporting. Clinicians must consider the possibility of CRS in newborns with congenital ocular disease, even without a maternal history of infection, since rubella in pregnancy can be subclinical.[120]

In a prospective study of CRS that followed 328 patients for as long as 7 years, Wolff identified 175 (53%) who had one or more ocular lesions.[122] Geltzer and associates reported a 49% incidence of ocular lesions among 49 infants with serological or culture evidence of rubella infection.[120] Ocular involvement is bilateral in 70% of cases.[121]

Cataracts, the most common ocular lesion in CRS, occur in 31% to 75% of infants.[120–122] They characteristically are dense nuclear opacities, although total opacification of the lens can occur.[122] Cataracts may develop after birth and progress over time[124]; Murphy and associates reported that in 12 of 23 patients with rubella cataracts opacities developed after 4 weeks of age.[125] Live virus can be recovered from rubella cataracts for as long as 35 months after birth.[122, 125] In fact, the lens is the most common ocular tissue from which virus can be isolated. The presence of virus in the lens may explain the severe intraocular inflammation that occurs in some patients following cataract extraction.[122]

Glaucoma occurs in approximately 10% of infants with CRS.[122, 126] It may be identical to isolated cases of congenital glaucoma, with persistent elevations in pressure and evidence of developmental abnormalities in the anterior chamber angle, or it may be transient, which suggests decreased aqueous outflow, possibly due to inflammation.[126] Persistent glaucoma tends to be severe; 8 of 15 patients reported by Wolff were blind by the age of 7.[122]

Some investigators have reported that glaucoma and cataracts rarely occur in the same infant with CRS,[126, 127] possibly because they result from viral injury at different times during embryogenesis.[127] Wolff, however, has shown that they are not mutually exclusive; he found that the incidence of their concurrent development in infants with CSR is equal to that predicted by the independent frequency of each.[122]

Damage to the retinal pigment epithelium causes a pigmentary retinopathy that is a hallmark of CRS (Fig 25–6). Most investigators place its incidence between 25% and 60%,[120–122, 124] but it may be more common than reported since it cannot be visualized through opaque ocular media in many cases. It also may develop and progress after birth.[122, 128] Rubella retinopathy is characterized by pigmentary mottling similar to that seen with congenital syphilis. Involvement may be unilateral or bilateral and focal or diffuse; it usually involves the posterior pole but can involve the periphery as well.[122, 124] Retinal vessels remain normal.[124] In most cases, retinal function is not impaired, and visual acuity will be normal in the absence of other ocular lesions.[122, 124]

Corneal clouding is associated with glaucoma in CRS but also can occur with normal intraocular pressure; edema in these cases may be transient. Histopathologic examination of such a case revealed absent Descemet's membrane, interstitial keratitis, and swelling, derangement, and focal absence of endothelial cells.[129] It has been hypothesized that these changes are the result of direct viral damage during embryogenesis.[129]

Lesions of the iris include stromal atrophy

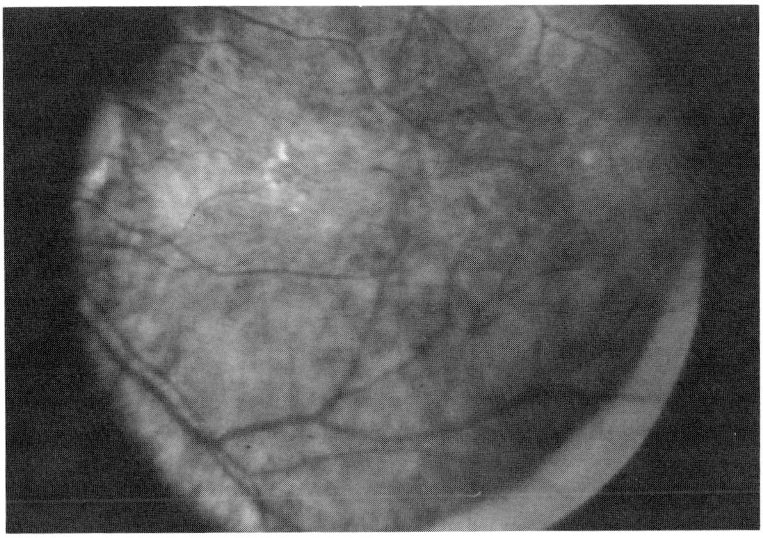

FIG 25–6.
Faint pigmentary mottling associated with rubella retinopathy.

and hypoplasia, vacuolization and necrosis of the pigment epithelium, and partial or complete absence of dilator muscles. Necrosis of the ciliary body produces a characteristic histopathologic appearance.[127] These changes have been attributed to a direct viral cytopathic affect.[122] Autopsy studies also reveal infiltration of the iris and ciliary body with lymphocytes and plasma cells, although clinical signs of iridocyclitis are not a prominent manifestation of the disease.[122]

Microphthalmos occurs in 17% to 39% of cases.[122, 125] It is recognized clinically by microcorneas but can be missed easily; very severe microphthalmos does not occur. The associated horizontal corneal diameters rarely are less than 5 to 8 mm.[121] When cataract or glaucoma develops in association with microphthalmos, there is an increased risk of complications following surgical therapy.[122]

Strabismus and nystagmus have been associated with CRS but in most cases probably are secondary to sensory deprivation by other ocular disorders.[122]

Children with CRS may shed virus persistently for many months.[105] Newborns with CRS are contagious and should be isolated to prevent the spread of rubella to those at risk, including nonimmune health care workers.

Cytomegalic Inclusion Disease

CMV is the most common pathogen to cause intrauterine infections and occurs in 0.5% to 2.4% of live births.[105, 130–132] There are an estimated 33,000 infants born with congenital CMV infections in the United States each year.[133] Ninety percent of them have subclinical infection at birth[105, 133]; only 5% have typical CID. The reticuloendothelial system and the CNS are the major sites for development of congenital disease; characteristic findings include hepatomegaly (the most common finding at birth), splenomegaly, jaundice, petechiae, respiratory distress, and intracranial calcifications, which makes differentiation from congenital toxoplasmosis difficult in many cases.[105, 130, 134] Congenital heart disease has been reported in CID but is not common.[130] A unique histopathologic finding in tissues infected by CMV is the presence of giant, or cytomegalic, cells with intranuclear and intracytoplasmic viral inclusions. Infants with CID have persistent defects in cell-mediated immunity, as indicated by a decreased in vitro lymphocyte blastogenic response to CMV antigens.[135, 136]

Intrauterine growth retardation and prematurity are common, but clinical findings may not be apparent within the first 24 hours of life.[105, 130] There is a 30% mortality rate among patients with symptomatic CID.[132] Of survivors, approximately 90% will have damage to the CNS or organs of perception during the first few years of life.[105, 132] Although intelligence may develop normally, mental retardation varying from mild to severe is very common.[130] Other CNS disorders include seizures, microcephaly, motor disabilities, and behavioral disorders.[130, 131, 134] Deafness is also a major problem. Five to 15% of infants with subclinical disease at birth will go on to develop CNS damage later in childhood.[131–133, 136–138]

Unlike toxoplasmosis or rubella, neonatal CMV infection can result from either primary or recurrent maternal infection during pregnancy.[105] Infection during pregnancy may occur by sexual or nonsexual routes of transmission.[137] It may result in a mononucleosis-like illness but is asymptomatic in the majority of pregnant women.[136, 138] With primary maternal infections, there is an increased incidence of symptomatic neonatal disease that is estimated to be 30% to 50%.[133, 136, 138] Five (15%) of 33 neonatal infections that followed primary maternal infection in pregnancy were symptomatic in one series.[136] Neonatal infection resulting from recurrent maternal CMV infection, in contrast, is rarely symptomatic. Symptomatic disease also is more frequent when maternal infection occurs earlier in pregnancy.[138]

Among CMV-infected women, transplacental transmission of virus with fetal infection is more common in those from lower socioeconomic groups for unknown reasons. Also, a greater proportion of women from lower

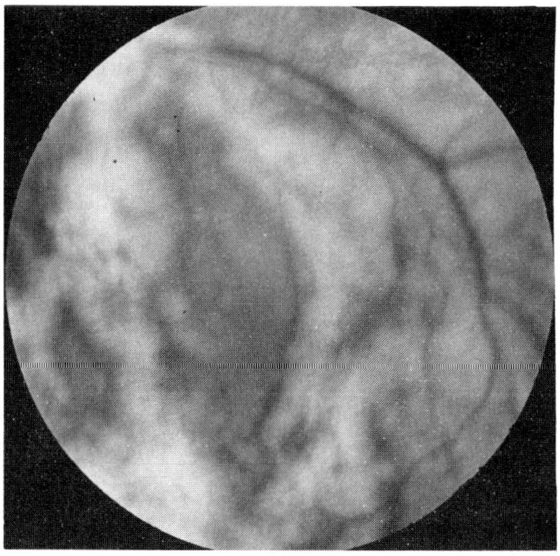

FIG 25–7.
CMV retinopathy in a newborn. Areas of perivascular retinal necrosis appear white.

socioeconomic groups have antibodies to CMV, thus indicating prior infection.[136] The incidence of neonatal infection, therefore, is higher in lower socioeconomic groups. Infants with neonatal infections are more likely to be symptomatic, however, when born to mothers in higher socioeconomic groups because a greater proportion of these pregnant women are susceptible to primary CMV infections.[136] The risk of neonatal CMV infection is reported to be higher in second and third pregnancies due to the increased risk of maternal infection from young children within the household who may have been infected with the virus at school or day-care facilities.[137, 138]

Newborns can also develop CMV infections following blood transfusions from CMV antibody-positive donors.[139] Such infections can result in fatal or severe neonatal disease as occurs with intrauterine transmission. Perinatally acquired CMV infections from exposure to cervical infections or nongenital sources may occur but usually does not result in severe disease.

In 1947, Kalfayan reported the presence of cytomegalic cells with nuclear inclusions at the "sclerocorneal junction," in episcleral tissue, and in ciliary body tissue of an infant that, in retrospect, probably had CID.[140] As more clinical experience was gained with congenital CID in the 1950s and 1960s, however, it was learned that the retina was the primary site of ocular disease in infants with disseminated CMV infection.[141–145]

CMV retinopathy is characterized by full-thickness necrosis of the retina, similar to what occurs with HSV infection. Cytomegalic cells with typical viral inclusions may be seen in all retinal layers. On clinical examination, patients may have one or more discrete patches of retinal whitening that correspond to areas of necrosis (Fig 25–7). It is commonly reported to occur in the peripheral retina, but may develop anywhere in the fundus. The borders of lesions are feathered and indistinct in contrast to those of toxoplasmosis. Retinal hemorrhages and vascular sheathing may be associated findings.[145] Infection reaches the eye hematogenously. Cells with viral inclusions have been seen in choroidal and retinal vasculature.[146] Infection also may involve the optic nerve,[143, 145] and optic atrophy is a common finding.[114, 132, 147]

Five to 30% of newborns with clinically apparent congenital CMV infection will develop CMV retinopathy.[114, 130, 132, 134, 147] Retinal "hyperpigmentation" also has been reported.[114, 130, 147] This finding may represent foci of healed disease; the incidence of retinal infection therefore may be higher than reported. Retinopathy usually develops in infants with clinically apparent disseminated CMV infection at birth but has been reported as the only manifestation of CMV infection.[134] Most investigators state that retinal disease will be seen only if present at birth.[114, 148] Cases have been reported, however, in which retinal disease develops several weeks after birth.[149] Furthermore, Alford and associates[135] state that 2% of subclinically infected newborns may develop late "chorioretinitis," but they provide no details about these cases, and development of retinopathy in previously uninfected eyes has not been reported as a long-term complication of CID in other series. CMV retinopathy has not been seen in perinatally acquired CMV infection, even among infants who develop symptomatic disease.[114]

In immunodeficient adults, CMV retinopathy progresses continuously until immunocompetence can be restored; lesions expand until the entire retina is destroyed and replaced by glial scar tissue. The natural history of CMV retinopathy in congenital CID is less well understood. In a study of 12 patients with CID who were followed for 3 to 12 years after birth, Berenberg and Nankervis noted that 4 of 12 "continued to have retinal involvement."[148] No information was given about the activity of these lesions or changes that occurred during serial examinations. They may simply have observed scarring from old sites of infection. On the basis of isolated case reports, lesions apparently may continue to be active for many months, during which time extensive areas of the retina can be destroyed. Lesions eventually become quiescent and leave areas of atrophy and scarring.[149, 150] Hyperpigmentation may occur and give the fundus a finely mottled appearance.

Until recently there have been no medications useful for the treatment of human CMV infections. An experimental antiviral drug, ganciclovir, appears to be effective for halting or reducing the spread of CMV retinopathy in immunodeficient adults.[151] The drug has been used in children as young as 32 months,[152] but experience with the drug in neonates with congenital CID has not been reported.

Infection of tissues other than the retina and optic nerve are uncommon. Uveal tissue may be secondarily inflamed,[143–145] but spread of viral infection to the choroid, iris, and ciliary body occurs rarely if at all. Sundmacher and colleagues reported a case of disciform-like corneal clouding and increased intraocular pressure that they hypothesized to be the result of CMV corneal endotheliitis and trabeculitis on the basis of isolation of CMV from aqueous humor and conjunctiva.[153] Histopathologic confirmation of tissue infection was not obtained, however.

Developmental anomalies reported to be associated with CID include microphthalmos,[143, 154] optic nerve hypoplasia, optic nerve colobomas,[154] anophthalmia,[147] and Peter's anomaly.[147] Strabismus and nystagmus have been seen in patients with CID, but a causal relationship has not been established.[114] Dvorak-Theobald reported cataracts in a stillborn infant with CMV retinopathy.[141]

Infected infants excrete CMV into nasopharyngeal secretions and urine for many months or years, but there is no evidence that health care workers who have contact with these infants are at increased risk for CMV infection when compared with the general population.[155]

CMV retinopathy is the most common opportunistic infectious disease of the eye in adults with the acquired immunodeficiency syndrome (AIDS) and has occurred in children with AIDS. Congenital infections of the eye have not been reported in infants at birth as manifestations of in utero infection with human immunodeficiency virus, however.

Other Herpetic Infections

Other members of the Herpesviridae group also have been implicated as rare causes of congenital infections, but little is known about the ocular disorders that they are reported to produce. Herpes zoster virus, the cause of varicella (chickenpox) and zoster (shingles), is believed to result in a group of disorders collectively termed the *congenital varicella syndrome* in rare infants born to mothers with varicella in pregnancy. Ocular disorders including microphthalmos, intraocular developmental abnormalities, cataract, "chorioretinitis," and hyperpigmentation of the retina have been reported in patients with this syndrome.[156, 157] The pathogenesis of the fundus changes are unknown. Charles and associates discovered a focus of apparent chorioretinal scarring, consistent with an inflammatory lesion, in a 13-month-old child with the syndrome, but there was no activity at the time of examination.[157] Other reports provide little clinical information about the ocular lesions they report.

Epstein-Barr virus is a ubiquitous agent that causes infectious mononucleosis, and most adults are infected with this virus. A few reports have claimed that congenital infection with multiple disorders, including cataract formation, can occur after infectious mononucleosis in the first trimester of pregnancy.[133] Proof of viral causation has not been obtained.

Syphilis

The incidence of congenital syphilis fell after benzathine penicillin therapy became available in the 1950s, and little has been written in the medical literature about its ocular manifestations in recent years. It remains a potentially serious neonatal disease, however. The number of congenital syphilis cases per year in the United States among patients less than 1 year old rose between 1978 and 1985 from 108 to 268 cases, which reflects a similar rise in syphilis rates for women of childbearing age.[158]

The fetus is at risk for infection with *Treponema pallidum* between the fifth and ninth months of pregnancy.[159] The incidence of infection increases when maternal disease is of less than 2 years' duration and has been reported to be as high as 95%.[159]

Physicians must be alert for congenital syphilis even in babies born to mothers who have already been treated. Nineteen percent of congenital syphilis cases reported to the CDC were due to failure of prenatal antibiotic treatment; 69% of the failures were related to treatment in the third trimester of pregnancy or to treatment with erythromycin in penicillin-allergic mothers.[158]

Infection can involve all tissues of the body. Bone, liver, kidneys, and pancreas were the most common organs of involvement in a review of autopsies performed on newborns with congenital syphilis at the Johns Hopkins Hospital between 1940 and 1970.[160] Only a minority of cases in this series had clinical features at birth that are considered "classic" for congenital syphilis: saddle-nose deformities, "snuffles" due to mucosal inflammation, and desquamation of the skin with shiny, reddened palms and soles. Many common features of congenital syphilis including prematurity, failure to thrive, hepatomegaly, splenomegaly, anemia, thrombocytopenia, and petechial rash are nonspecific, thus leading to confusion with infections in the TORCH complex. However, osteochondritis and periostitis produce roentgenographic changes in long bones that may be helpful in the differential diagnosis.

Congenital syphilis may escape detection at birth; only 30% of newborns with syphilis reported to the CDC in recent years had signs suggestive of the disease.[158] Twleve percent were asymptomatic, and diagnosis was made only after evaluation was initiated because of positive maternal serological test results.[158]

Treponema pallidum infects all tissues of the eye; organisms have been identified in choroid, retina, vitreous, aqueous humor, and lens cortex.[161, 162] Most frequently, it is found in tissues around blood vessels.[163, 164] Live treponemes have been found in the eye of a newborn after the administration of penicillin therapy in dosages considered to be adequate, and the organisms were not drug resistant.[164] This finding suggests the possibility of persistent ocular disease despite treatment.

The most common ocular manifestation of early congenital syphilis is a pigmentary retinopathy believed to be the consequence of fetal or early infantile choroidal and retinal inflammation (Fig 25–8). The most common

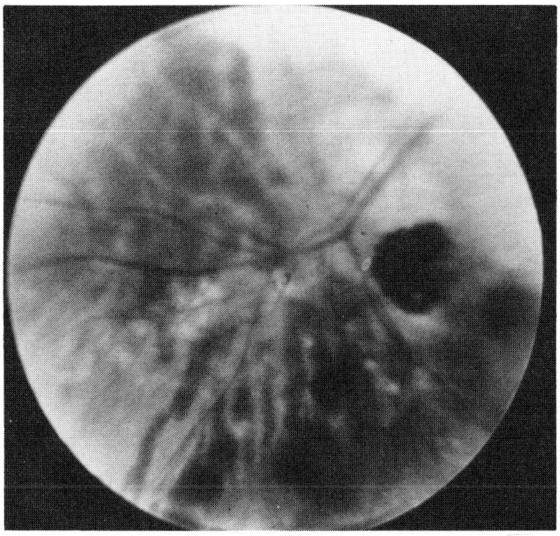

FIG 25–8.
Coarse pigmentary mottling associated with the retinopathy of congenital syphilis.

appearance is a diffuse pigmentary mottling in the peripheral fundus that gives rise to the descriptive term *salt-and-pepper retinopathy*. Other pattens of chorioretinal disease also may be present, however, including discrete foci of dense pigmentary clumping. Affected patients may have normal vision unless severe pigmentary changes involve the maculae.

In 1953, a review by Klauder and Meyer of the existing literature on chorioretinitis associated with congential syphilis found that the reported incidence varied between 3% and 75%.[165] Patients of all ages from infancy to adulthood were studied. Although pigmentary retinopathy may be seen at birth, chorioretinitis apparently is more common in adults with a history of congenital syphilis, which indicates that it is progressive or may develop late.

Other ocular disorders associated with congenital syphilis include sheathing, attenuation, and obliteration of retinal vessels that is attributed to perivascular inflammation, and optic atrophy.[165] Inflammation of the iris, choroid, and ciliary body are observed frequently at autopsy,[161, 163, 164] but the degree of inflammation is mild and probably clinically inapparent in most cases. Atrophy of the iris also has been reported.[159]

Many of the characteristic features of congenital syphilis develop or become apparent many years after birth. Deafness is a late manifestation of disease. There may be pathognomonic abnormalities of teeth in older individuals including "mulberry" molars and Hutchinson's teeth (peg-shaped upper incisors with central notching in the secondary dentition). Interstitial keratitis, an immunologic reaction to *Treponema pallidum* that occurs in 20% to 52% of patients,[159] is a hallmark of congenital syphilis but does not develop until late childhood or adolescence. It is a self-limited disorder characterized by dense inflammation of the corneal stroma, perilimbal injection, lacrimation, and photophobia. Blood vessels that invade the corneal stroma give it a pink color during the active phase of disease and result in ghost vessels after resolution of inflammation.

CONCLUSION

Ophthalmic infectious diseases continue to be a major problem in neonatal medicine. Despite more than 100 years of prophylaxis and study, ophthalmia neonatorum remains a problem. Some infections, including rubella and congenital syphilis, have become uncommon but continue to be important because of the severe morbidity of ocular involvement in cases that do occur. As new treatments increase survival of infants with congenital and disseminated infectious diseases such as HSV infection, the long-term sequellae of ocular involvement will be an increasingly important public health problem.

To allow early recognition and appropriate therapy, physicians should be aware of the signs and symptoms of neonatal ophthalmic infections, the groups at greatest risk for these diseases, and the factors that predispose to infection such as prolonged rupture of membranes. New drugs provide some hope for better treatment of ocular infections, but the mainstay of therapy will remain prevention. Public health and education measures to prevent sexual and nonsexual disease transmission will be critical.

REFERENCES

1. Molgaard IL, Nielsen PB, Kaern J: A study of the incidence of neonatal conjunctivitis and of its bacterial causes including *Chlamydia trachomatis*. Clinical examination, culture and cytology of tear fluid. *Acta Ophthalmol* 1984; 62:461–471.
2. Stenson S, Newman R, Fedukowicz H: Conjunctivitis in the newborn: Observations on incidence, cause and prophylaxis. *Ann Ophthalmol* 1981; 13:329–334.
3. Watson PG, Gairdner D: TRIC agent as a cause of neonatal eye sepsis. *Br Med J* 1968; 3:527–528.
4. Armstrong JH, Zacarias F, Rein MF: Ophthalmia neonatorum: A chart review. *Pediatrics* 1976; 57:884–892.
5. Pearson HE: Failure of silver nitrate prophylaxis for gonococcal ophthalmia neonatorum. *Am J Obstet Gynecol* 1957; 73:805.
6. Rees E, Tait IA, Hobson D, et al: Neonatal

conjunctivitis caused by *Neisseria gonorrhoeae* and *Chlamydia trachomatis*. *Br J Vener Dis* 1977; 53:173–179.
7. Hobson D, Rees E: Maternal genital chlamydial infection as a cause of neonatal conjunctivitis. *Postgrad Med J* 1977; 53:595–597.
8. Rowe DS, Aicardi EZ, Dawson CR, et al: Purulent ocular discharge in neonates: Significance of *Chlamydia trachomatis*. *Pediatrics* 1979; 63:628–632.
9. Sandstrom KI, Bell TA, Chandler JW, et al: Microbial causes of neonatal conjunctivitis. *J Pediatr* 1984; 105:706–711.
10. Rapoza PA, Quinn TC, Kiessling LA, et al: Epidemiology of neonatal conjunctivitis. *Ophthalmology* 1986; 93:456–461.
11. Sandstrom I: Treatment of neonatal conjunctivitis. *Arch Ophthalmol* 1987; 105:925–928.
12. Pierce JM, Ward ME, Seal DV: Ophthalmia neonatorum in the 1980s: Incidence, aetiology and treatment. *Br J Ophthalmol* 1982; 66:728–731.
13. Prentice MJ, Hutchinson GR, Taylor-Robinson D: A microbiological study of neonatal conjunctivae and conjunctivitis. *Br J Ophthalmol* 1977; 61:601–607.
14. Jones DM, Tobin B: Neonatal eye infections due to *Mycoplasma hominis*. *Br Med J* 1968; 3:467–468.
15. Crede CSF: Reports from the obstetrical clinic in Leipzig. Prevention of eye inflammation in the newborn. *Am J Dis Child* 1971; 121:3–4.
16. Barsam PC: Medical intelligence current concepts. Specific prophylaxis of gonorrheal ophthalmia neonatorum. *N Engl J Med* 1966; 274:731–741.
17. Snowe RJ, Wilfert CM: Epidemic reappearance of gonococcal ophthalmia neonatorum. *Pediatrics* 1973; 51:110–114.
18. Pierog S, Nigam S, Marasigan DC, et al: Gonococcal ophthalmia neonatorum. Relationship of maternal factors and delivery room practices to effective control measures. *Am J Obstet Gynecol* 1975; 122:589–592.
19. Hammerschlag MR, Chandler JW, Alexander ER, et al: Erythromycin ointment for ocular prophylaxis of neonatal chlamydial infection. JAMA 1980; 244:2291–2293.
20. Rothbard MJ, Gregory T, Salerno LJ: Intrapartum gonococcal amnionitis. *Am J Obstet Gynecol* 1975; 121:565–566.
21. Nickerson CW: Gonorrhea amnionitis. *Obstet Gynecol* 1973; 42:815–817.
22. Thompson TR, Swanson RE, Wiesner PJ: Gonococcal ophthalmia neonatorum. Relationship of time of infection to relevant control measures. *JAMA* 1974; 228:186–188.
23. Strand CL, Arango VA: Gonococcal ophthalmia neonatorum after delivery by cesarean section: Report of a case. *Sex Transm Dis* 1979; 6:77–78.
24. Lossick JG: Prevention and management of neonatal gonorrhea. *Sex Transm Dis* 1979; 6(suppl):192–194.
25. Davidson HH, Hill JH, Eastman NJ: Penicillin in the prophylaxis of ophthalmia neonatorum. JAMA 1951; 145:1052–1055.
26. Rothenberg R: Ophthalmia neonatorum due to *Neisseria gonorrhoeae*: Prevention and treatment. *Sex Transm Dis* 1979; 6(suppl):187–191.
27. Oriel JD: Ophthalmia neonatorum: Relative efficacy of current prophylactic practices and treatment. *J Antimicrob Chemother* 1984; 14:209–220.
28. American Academy of Pediatrics: Prophylaxis and treatment of neonatal gonococcal infections. *Pediatrics* 1980; 65:1047–1048.
29. Seedorf HH: Is prophylactic treatment of the eyes of newborn infants still necessary? *Dan Med Bull* 1960; 7:128–132.
30. Schachter J, Grossman M, Sweet RL, et al: Prospective study of perinatal transmission of *Chlamydia trachomatis*. JAMA 1986; 255:3374–3377.
31. Schachter J, Grossman M: Chlamydial infections. *Annu Rev Med* 1981; 32:45–61.
32. Chandler JW, Alexander ER, Pheiffer TA, et al: Ophthalmia neonatorum associated with maternal chlamydial infections. *Trans Am Acad Ophthalmol Otolaryngol* 1977; 83:302–308.
33. Frommell GT, Rothenberg R, Wang S-P, et al: Chlamydial infection of mothers and their infants. *J Pediatr* 1979; 95:28–32.
34. Hammerschlag MR, Anderka M, Semine DZ, et al: Prospective study of maternal and infantile infection with *Chlamydia trachomatis*. *Pediatrics* 1979; 64:142–148.
35. Heggie AD, Lumicao GG, Stuart LA, et al: *Chlamydia trachomatis* infection in mothers and infants. *Am J Dis Child* 1981; 135:507–511.
36. Mardh P-A, Helin I, Bobeck S, et al: Colonisation of pregnant and puerperal women and neonates with *Chlamydia trachomatis*. *Br J Vener Dis* 1980; 56:96–100.
37. Mordhorst CH, Dawson C: Sequelae of neo-

natal inclusion conjunctivitis and associated disease in patients. *Am J Ophthalmol* 1971; 71:861–867.
38. Goscienski PJ, Sexton RR: Follow-up studies in neonatal inclusion conjunctivitis. *Am J Dis Child* 1972; 124:180–182.
39. Freedman A, Al-Hussaini MK, Dunlop EMC, et al: Infection by TRIC agent and other members of the Bedsonia group with a note on Reiter's disease. II. Ophthalmia neonatorum due to TRIC agent. *Trans Ophthalmol Soc UK* 1966; 86:313–320.
40. Forster RK, Dawson CR, Schachter J: Late follow-up of patients with neonatal inclusion conjunctivitis. *Am J Ophthalmol* 1970; 69:467–472.
41. Goscienski PJ: Inclusion conjunctivitis in the newborn infant. *J Pediatr* 1970; 77:19–26.
42. Thygeson P, Stone W Jr,: Epidemiology of inclusion conjunctivitis. *Arch Ophthalmol* 1942; 27:91–122.
43. Beem MO, Saxon EM,: Respiratory-tract colonization and a distinctive pneumonia syndrome in infants infected with *Chlamydia trachomatis*. *N Engl J Med* 1977; 296:306–310.
44. Harrison HR, English MG, Lee CK, et al: *Chlamydia trachomatis* infant pneumonitis. Comparison with matched controls and other infant pneumonitis. *N Engl J Med* 1978; 298:702–708.
45. Dawson C, Jawetz E, Hanna L, et al: A family outbreak of adenovirus 8 infection (epidemic keratoconjunctivitis). *Am J Hyg* 1960; 72:279–283.
46. Heggie AD, Jaffe AC, Stuart LA, et al: Topical sulfacetamide vs oral erythromycin for neonatal chlamydial conjunctivitis. *Am J Dis Child* 1985; 139:564–566.
47. Anthony BF, Okada DM: The emergence of group B streptococci in infections of the newborn infant. *Annu Rev Med* 1977; 28:355–369.
48. Baker CJ: Group B streptococcal infections. *Adv Intern Med* 1980; 25:475–501.
49. Robertson MH: Listeriosis. *Postgrad Med J* 1977; 53:618–622.
50. Howard JB, McCracken GH Jr,: The spectrum of group B streptococcal infections in infancy. *Am J Dis Child* 1974; 128:815–818.
51. Isenberg SJ, Apt L, Yoshimori R, et al: Bacterial flora of the conjunctiva at birth. *J Pediatr Ophthalmol Strabismus* 1986; 23:284–286.
52. Nishida H, Risemberg HM: Silver nitrate ophthalmic solution and chemical conjunctivitis. *Pediatrics* 1975; 56:368–373.
53. Mellin GW, Kent MP: Ophthalmia neonatorum. Is prophylaxis necessary? *Pediatrics* 1958; 22:1006–1015.
54. Christian JR: Comparison of ocular reactions with the use of silver nitrate and erythromycin ointment in ophthalmia neonatorum prophylaxis. *J Pediatr* 1960; 57:55–60.
55. Bernstein GA, Davis JP, Katcher ML: Prophylaxis of neonatal conjunctivitis. An analytic review. *Clin Pediatr* 1982; 21:545.
56. Rees E, Tait IA, Hobson D, et al: Persistence of chlamydial infection after treatment for neonatal conjunctivitis. *Arch Dis Child* 1981; 56:193–198.
57. Washington AE: Update on treatment recommendations for gonococcal infections. *Rev Infect Dis* 1982; 4(suppl):758.
58. Centers for Disease Control: 1985 Standard treatment guidelines. *MMWR* 1985; 34(suppl):75–108.
59. Gammon JA, Nahmias AJ: Herpes simplex ocular infections in the newborn, in Darrell RW (ed): *Viral Diseases of the Eye*. Philadelphia, Lea & Febiger, 1985, pp 46–58.
60. Schachter J, Dawson CR: Comparative efficiency of various diagnostic methods for chlamydial infection, in Holmes KK, Hobson D (eds): *Nongonococcal Urethritis and Related Infections*. Washington, DC, American Society for Microbiology, 1977, pp 337–341.
61. Naib ZM: Cytology of TRIC agent infection of the eye of newborn infants and their mothers' genital tracts. *Acta Cytol* 1970; 14:390–395.
62. Stephens RS, Kuo C-C, Tam MR: Sensitivity of immunofluorescence with monoclonal antibodies for detection of *Chlamydia trachomatis* inclusions in cell culture. *J Clin Microbiol* 1982; 16:4–7.
63. Rapoza PA, Quinn TC, Kiessling LA, et al: Assessment of neonatal conjunctivitis with a direct immunofluorescent monoclonal antibody stain for chlamydia. *JAMA* 1986; 225:3369–3373.
64. Anonymous: Treatment of sexually transmitted diseases. *Med. Lett Drugs Ther* 1986; 28:23–28.
65. Laga M, Naamara W, Brunham RC, et al: Single-dose therapy of gonococcal ophthalmia neonatorum with ceftriaxone. *N Engl J Med* 1986; 315:1382–1385.
66. Fransen L, D'Costa L, Ronald AR, et al: Sin-

gle-dose kanamycin therapy of gonococcal ophthalmia neonatorum. *Lancet* 1984; 2:1234–1237.
67. Csonka GW, Coufalik ED: Chlamydial, gonococcal, and herpes virus infections in neonates. *Postgrad Med J* 1977; 53:592–594.
68. Patamasucon P, Rettig PJ, Faust KL, et al: Oral v. topical erythromycin therapies for chlamydial conjunctivitis. *Am J Dis Child* 1982; 136:817–821.
69. Ffooks OO: Dacryocystitis in infancy. *Br J Ophthalmol* 1962; 46:422–434.
70. Kushner BJ: Congenital nasolacrimal system obstruction. *Arch Ophthalmol* 1982; 100:597–600.
71. Ffooks OO: Lacrimal abscess in the newborn. A report of seven cases. *Br J Ophthalmol* 1961; 45:562–565.
72. Whitley RJ, Alford CA, Hirsch MS, et al: Vidarabine versus acyclovir therapy in herpes simplex encephalitis. *N Engl J Med* 1986; 314:144–149.
73. Witzleben CL, Driscoll SG: Possible transplacental transmission of herpes simplex infection. *Pediatrics* 1965; 36:192–199.
74. Sieber OF, Fulginiti VA, Brazie J, et al: In utero infection of the fetus by herpes simplex virus. *J Pediatr* 1966; 69:30–34.
75. Hutchison DS, Smith RE, Haughton PB: Congenital herpetic keratitis. *Arch Ophthalmol* 1975; 93:70–73.
76. Whitley RJ, Nahmias AJ, Visintine AM, et al: The natural history of herpes simplex virus infection of mother and newborn. *Pediatrics* 1980; 66:489–494.
77. Light IJ, Linnemann CC: Neonatal herpes simplex infection following delivery of cesarean section. *Obstet Gynecol* 1974; 44:496–499.
78. Nahmias AJ, Josey WE, Naib ZM, et al: Perinatal risk associated with maternal genital herpes simplex virus infection. *Am J Obstet Gynecol* 1971; 110:825–837.
79. Brown ZA, Vontver LA, Benedetti J, et al: Effects on infants of a first episode of genital herpes during pregnancy. *N Engl J Med* 1987; 317:1246–1251.
80. Sullivan-Bolyai J, Hull HF, Wilson C, et al: Neonatal herpes simplex virus infection in King County, Washington. Increasing incidence and epidemiologic correlates. *JAMA* 1983; 250:3059–3062.
81. Light IJ: Postnatal acquisition of herpes simplex virus by the newborn infant: A review of the literature. *Pediatrics* 1979; 63:480–482.
82. Francis DP, Herrmann KL, MacMahon JR, et al: Nosocomial and maternally acquired herpesvirus hominis infections. A report of four fatal cases in neonates. *Am J Dis Child* 1975; 129:889–893.
83. Mitchell JE, McCall FC: Transplacental infection by herpes simplex virus. *Am J Dis Child* 1963; 106:207–209.
84. South MA, Tompkins WAF, Morris CR, et al: Congenital malformation of the central nervous system associated with genital type (type 2) herpesvirus. *J Pediatr* 1969; 75:13–18.
85. Florman AL, Gershon AA, Blackett PR, et al: Intrauterine infection with herpes simplex virus. Resultant congenital malformations. *JAMA* 1973; 225:129–132.
86. Montgomery JR, Flanders RW, Yow MD: Congenital anomalies and herpesvirus infection. *Am J Dis Child* 1973; 126:364–366.
87. Chalhub EG, Baenziger J, Feigen RD, et al: Congenital herpes simplex type II infection with extensive hepatic calcification, bone lesions and cataracts: complete postmortem examination. *Dev Med Child Neurol* 1977; 19:527–534.
88. Komorous JM, Wheeler CE, Briggaman RA, et al: Intrauterine herpes simplex infections. *Arch Dermatol* 1977; 113:918–922.
89. Nahmias AJ, Dowdle WR, Josey WE, et al: Newborn infection with herpesvirus hominis types 1 and 2. *J Pediatr* 1969; 75:1194–1203.
90. Bobo CB, Antine B, Manos JP: Neonatal herpes simplex infection limited to the cornea. *Arch Ophthalmol* 1970; 84:697–698.
91. Berkovich S, Ressel M: Neonatal herpes keratitis. *J Pediatr* 1966; 69:652–653.
92. Yanoff M, Allman MI, Fine BS: Congenital herpes simplex virus, type 2, bilateral endophthalmitis. *Trans Am Ophthalmol Soc* 1977; 75:325–326.
93. Hagler WS, Walters PV, Nahmias AJ: Ocular involvement in neonatal herpes simplex virus infection. *Arch Ophthalmol* 1969; 82:169–176.
94. Cibis A, Burde RM: Herpes simplex virus–induced congenital cataracts. *Arch Ophthalmol* 1971; 85:220–223.
95. Reersted P, Hansen B: Chorioretinitis of the

newborn with herpes simplex virus type 1. Report of a case. *Acta Ophthalmol (Stockh)* 1979; 57:1096–1100.
96. Whitley RJ, Nahmias AJ, Soong S-J, et al: Vidarabine therapy of neonatal herpes simplex virus infection. *Pediatrics* 1980; 66:495–501.
97. Hill HR, Mitchell TG, Matsen JM, et al: Recovery from disseminated candidiasis in a premature neonate. *Pediatrics* 1974; 53:748–752.
98. Palmer EA: Endogenous *Candida* endophthalmitis in infants. *Am J Ophthalmol* 1980; 89:398–395.
99. Baley JE, Kliegman RM, Fanaroff AA: Disseminated fungal infections in very low birth weight infants: Clinical manifestations and epidemiology. *Pediatrics* 1984; 73:144–152.
100. Edwards JE, Foos RY, Montgomerie JZ, et al: Ocular manifestations of candida septicemia: Review of seventy-six cases of hematogenous candida endophthalmitis. *Medicine (Baltimore)* 1974; 53:47–75.
101. Baley JE, Annable WL, Kliegman RM: *Candida* endophthalmitis in the premature infant. *J Pediatr* 1981; 98:458–461.
102. Xanthou M, Valassi-Adam E, Kintzonidou E, et al: Phagocytosis and killing ability of *Candida albicans* by blood leucocytes of healthy term and preterm babies. *Arch Dis Child* 1975; 50:72–75.
103. Baley JE, Kliegman RM, Fanaroff AA: Disseminated fungal infections in very low birth weight infants: Therapeutic toxicity. *Pediatrics* 1984; 73:153–157.
104. Nahmias AJ, Walls KW, Stewart JA, et al: The TORCH complex—Perinatal infection with toxoplasma and rubella, cytomegalo- and herpes simplex viruses. *Pediatr Res* 1971; 5:405–406.
105. Alford CA Jr: Chronic congenital infections of man. *Yale J Biol Med* 1982; 55:187–192.
106. Kimball AC, Kean BH, Fuchs F: Congenital toxoplasmosis: A prospective study of 4,048 obstetric patients. *Am J Obstet Gynecol* 1971; 111:211–218.
107. Desmonts G, Couvreur J: Toxoplasmosis in pregnancy and its transmission to the fetus. *Bull NY Acad Med* 1974; 50:146–159.
108. Desmonts G, Couvreur J: Congenital toxoplasmosis. A prospective study of 378 pregnancies. *N Engl J Med* 1974; 290:1110–1116.
109. Koppe JG, Kloosterman GJ, de Roever-Bonnet H, et al: Toxoplasmosis and pregnancy, with a long-term follow-up of the children. *Eur J Obstet Gynecol Reprod Biol* 1974; 4:101–110.
110. Loewer-Sieger DH, Rothova A, Koppe JG, et al: Congenital toxoplasmosis, a prospective study based on 1821 pregnant women, in Saari KM (ed): *Uveitis Update.* Amsterdam, Elsevier Science Publishers, 1984, pp. 203–207.
111. Alford CA Jr., Stagno S, Reynolds DW: Congenital toxoplasmosis: Clinical, laboratory, and therapeutic considerations, with special reference to subclinical disease. *Bull NY Acad Med* 1974; 50:160–181.
112. Couvreur J, Desmonts G: Congenital and maternal toxoplasmosis. A review of 300 congenital cases. *Dev Med Child Neurol* 1962; 4:519–530.
113. Garcia AGP: Congenital toxoplasmosis in two successive sibs. *Arch Dis Child* 1968; 43:705–710.
114. Stagno S, Reynolds, DW, Amos CS, et al: Auditory and visual defects resulting from symptomatic and subclinical congenital cytomegaloviral and *Toxoplasma* infections. *Pediatrics* 1977; 59:669–678.
115. Eichenwald HF: A study of congenital toxoplasmosis with particular emphasis on clinical manifestations, sequellae and therapy, in Siim JC (ed): *Human Toxoplasmosis.* Baltimore, Williams & Wilkins, 1959, pp 41–49.
116. Fair JR: Congenital toxoplasmosis. Chorioretinitis as the only manifestation of the disease. *Am J Ophthalmol* 1958; 46:135–154.
117. Fair JR: Clinical eye findings in congenital toxoplasmosis. *Surv Ophthalmol* 1961; 6:923–935.
118. Hogan MJ, Zweigart PA, Lewis A: Recovery of toxoplasmosis from a human eye. *Arch Ophthalmol* 1958; 60:548–554.
119. Hogan MJ, Kimura SJ, O'Connor GR: Ocular toxoplasmosis. *Arch Ophthalmol* 1964; 72:592–600.
120. Geltzer AI, Guber D, Sears ML: Ocular manifestations of the 1964–65 rubella epidemic. *Am J Ophthalmol* 1967; 63:221–229.
121. Alfano JE: Ocular aspects of maternal rubella syndrome. *Trans Am Acad Ophthalmol Otolaryngol* 1966; 70:235–266.
122. Wolff SM: The ocular manifestations of con-

genital rubella. *Trans Am Ophthalmol Soc* 1972; 70:577–614.
123. Centers for Disease Control: Rubella and congenital rubella—United States, 1984–1986. *MMWR* 1987; 36:664–675.
124. Krill AE: The retinal disease of rubella. *Arch Ophthalmol* 1967; 77:445–449.
125. Murphy AM, Reid RR, Pollard I, et al: Rubella cataracts. Further clinical and virologic observations. *Am J Ophthalmol* 64:1109–1119.
126. Sears ML: Congenital glaucoma in neonatal rubella. *Br J Ophthalmol* 1967; 51:744–748.
127. Boniuk M, Zimmerman LE: Ocular pathology in the rubella syndrome. *Arch Ophthalmol* 1967; 77:455–473.
128. Collins WJ, Cohen DN: Rubella retinopathy. A progressive disorder. *Arch Ophthalmol* 1970; 84:33–35.
129. Deluise VP, Cobo LM, Chandler D: Persistent corneal edema in the congenital rubella syndrome. *Ophthalmology* 1983; 90:835–839.
130. McCracken GH, Shinefield HR, Cobb K, et al: Congenital cytomegalic inclusion disease. A longitudinal study of 20 patients. *Am J Dis Child* 1969; 117:522–539.
131. Hanshaw JB: Congenital cytomegalovirus infection: A fifteen year perspective. *J Infect Dis* 1971; 123:555–561.
132. Pass RF, Stagno S, Myers GJ, et al: Outcome of symptomatic congenital cytomegalovirus infection: Results of long-term longitudinal follow-up. *Pediatrics* 1980; 66:758–762.
133. Stagno S, Whitley RJ: Herpesvirus infections of pregnancy. Part I: Cytomegalovirus and Epstein-Barr virus infections. *N Engl J Med* 1985; 313:1270–1274.
134. Weller TH, Hanshaw JB: Virologic and clinical observations on cytomegalic inclusion disease. *N Engl J Med* 1962; 266:1233–1244.
135. Alford CA, Pass RF, Stagno S: Early and late developmental abnormalities associated with congenital cytomegalovirus and *Toxoplasma* infections. *Prog Clin Biol Res* 1985; 163:343–349.
136. Stagno S, Pass RF, Dworsky ME, et al: Congenital cytomegalovirus infection. The relative importance of primary and recurrent maternal infection. *N Engl J Med* 1982; 306:945–949.
137. Pass RF, Little EA, Stagno S, et al: Young children as a probable source of maternal and congenital cytomegalovirus infection. *N Engl J Med* 316:1366–1370.
138. Stagno S, Pass RF, Cloud G, et al: Primary cytomegalovirus infection in pregnancy. *JAMA* 1986; 256:1904–1908.
139. Yeager AS, Grumet FC, Hafleigh EB, et al: Prevention of transfusion-acquired cytomegalovirus infections in newborn infants. *J Pediatrics* 1981; 98:281–287.
140. Kalfayan B: Inclusion disease of infancy. *Arch Pathol* 1947; 44:467–476.
141. Dvorak-Theobald G: Cytomegalic inclusion disease. Report of a case. *Am J Ophthalmol* 1959; 47:52–56.
142. Manschot WA, Daamen CBF: A case of cytomegalic inclusion disease with ocular involvement. *Ophthalmologica* 1962; 143:137–140.
143. Miklos G, Orban T: Ophthalmic lesions due to cytomegalic inclusion disease. *Ophthalmologica* 1964; 148:98–106.
144. Smith ME, Zimmerman LE, Harley RD: Ocular involvement in congenital cytomegalic inclusion disease. *Arch Ophthalmol* 1966; 76:696–699.
145. Tarkkanen A, Merenmies L, Holmstrom T: Ocular involvement in congenital cytomegalic inclusion disease. *J Pediatr Ophthalmol* 1972; 9:82–86.
146. Christensen L, Beeman HW, Allen A: Cytomegalic inclusion disease. *Arch Ophthalmol* 1957; 57:90–99.
147. Frenkel LD, Keys MP, Hefferen SJ, et al: Unusual eye abnormalities associated with congenital cytomegalovirus infection. *Pediatrics* 1980; 66:763–766.
148. Berenberg W, Nankervis G: Long-term follow-up of cytomegalic inclusion disease of infancy. *Pediatrics* 1970; 46:403–410.
149. Guyton TB, Ehrlich F, Blanc WA, et al: New observations in generalized cytomegalic-inclusion disease of the newborn. Report of a case with chorioretinitis. *N Engl J Med* 1957; 257:803–807.
150. Burns RP: Cytomegalic inclusion disease uveitis. Report of a case with isolation from aqueous humor of the virus in tissue culture. *Arch Ophthalmol* 1959; 61:376–387.
151. Holland GN, Sidikaro Y, Kreiger AE, et al: Treatment of cytomegalovirus retinopathy with ganciclovir. *Ophthalmology* 1987; 94:815–823.
152. Rosecan LR, Laskin OL, Kalman CM, et al:

Antiviral therapy with ganciclovir for cytomegalovirus retinitis and bilateral exudative retinal detachments in an immunocompromised child. *Ophthalmology* 1986; 93:1401–1407.
153. Sundmacher R, Neumann-Haefelin D, Mattes A, et al: Connatal monosymptomatic corneal endothelitis by cytomegalovirus, in Sundmacher R (ed): *Herpetische Augenerkrankungen (Herpetic Eye Diseases),* Munich, JF Bergmann, 1981, pp 501–504.
154. Hittner HM, Desmond MM, Montgomery JR: Optic nerve manifestations of human congenital cytomegalovirus infection. *Am J Ophthalmol* 1976; 81:661–665.
155. Dworsky ME, Welch K, Cassady G, et al: Occupational risk for primary cytomegalovirus infection among pediatric health-care workers. *N Engl J Med* 1983; 309:950–953.
156. Paryani SG, Arvin AM: Intrauterine infection with varicella-zoster virus after maternal varicella. *N Engl J Med* 1986; 314:1542–1546.
157. Charles NC, Bennett TW, Margolis S: Ocular pathology of the congenital varicella syndrome. *Arch Ophthalmol* 1977; 95:2034–2037.
158. Centers for Disease Control: Congenital syphilis—United States, 1983–1985. *MMWR* 1986; 35:625–628.
159. Robinson RCV: Congenital syphilis. *Arch Dermatol* 1968: 99:599–610.
160. Oppenheimer EH, Hardy JB: Congenital syphilis in the newborn infant: Clinical and pathological observations in recent cases. *Johns Hopkins Med J* 1971; 129:63–82.
161. Contreras F, Pereda J: Congenital syphilis of the eye with lens involvement. *Arch Ophthalmol* 1978; 96:1052–1053.
162. Nicol WG, Rios-Montenegro EN, Smith JL: Congenital ocular syphilis. *Am J Ophthalmol* 1969; 68:467–472.
163. Friedenwald JS: Ocular lesions in fetal syphilis. *Trans Am Ophthalmol Soc* 1929; 27:203–218.
164. Ryan SJ, Hardy PH, Hardy JM, et al: Persistence of virulent *Treponema pallidum* despite penicillin therapy in congenital syphilis. *Am J Ophthalmol* 1972; 73:258–261.
165. Klauder JV, Meyer GP: Chorioretinitis of congenital syphilis. *Arch Ophthalmol* 1953; 49:139–157.

26A Retinopathy of Prematurity: A Neonatologist's Perspective

Dale L. Phelps, M.D.

Retinopathy of prematurity (ROP) is a disorder that occurs in a small but significant number of neonatal intensive care survivors. Not only is the possibility of blindness a severe blow to loving family and nursery staff, but each case also raises fears of possible litigation. Enormous sums of money have been awarded to some affected children and their families by well-intentioned juries misled to believe that blindness occurs only when there has been medical malpractice. Neonatologists express feelings of helplessness and rage when "found guilty of malpractice" after providing what they believe to have been optimal care. The need to understand and control this disorder has resulted in a welcome resurgence of investigative effort.[1]

CHARACTERISTICS OF INFANTS WHO DEVELOP RETINOPATHY OF PREMATURITY

Incidence

As in earlier years, surveys done in the 1970s and 1980s confirm that ROP is a disease of premature infants and that the incidence rises as the infant's birth weight becomes smaller.[2–9] Such surveys have recorded that, on average, 40% of infants 1 to 1.5 kg will develop ROP of some degree and that this may be as high as 80% to 100% of infants born weighing less than 1 kg.[3, 4] Fortunately, in most cases the retinopathy does regress so that only 5% to 8% of infants under 1 kg and 0.5% of infants weighing 1 to 1.5 kg experience severe loss of vision. An increasing survival of infants weighing less than 1,500 gm at birth throughout the 1980s, however, means that if the weight-adjusted incidence of ROP remains the same there will be an increasing absolute number of visually handicapped survivors each year.[10] Survival for infants under 1 kg has risen from around 35% in 1979 to over 50% in 1986. Projected into 1987, these data would predict that 563 infants will experience severe loss of vision from ROP annually in the United States (Table 26A–1).

Causation and Correlations

As a disorder involving abnormal growth of immature retinal vessels, ROP occurs almost exclusively in premature infants and at a rate proportional to the degree of retinal vascular immaturity at the time of birth. Thus prematurity is normally a prerequisite for the disorder, although it is not sufficient alone to cause the problem since many premature infants do not develop ROP. (On rare occasion ROP appears to begin in utero, an unusual circumstance that leads to interesting ques-

TABLE 26A–1.
Projected Number of Infants With Severe Vision Loss From ROP

Infant Characteristic	Year of Projection 1979*	1987
<1 kg birth weight		
Number of births	16,602	18,555
Survival (%)	5,811 (35%)	9,277 (50%)
"Blind" from ROP (%)	465 (8%)	464 (5%)
1–1.5 kg birth weight		
Number of births	20,080	22,442
Survival (%)	16,264 (81%)	19,749 (88%)
"Blind" from ROP (0.5%)	81	99
Total "blind"	546	563

*From Phelps DL: Retinopathy of prematurity: An estimate of vision loss in the United States—1979. *Pediatrics* 1981: 67:924. Used with permission.

tions for study.[11] These cases are distinguished from familial exudative retinopathy, a recently described, dominantly inherited retinopathy of variable penetrance that closely imitates ROP.[12]) While cause and effect cannot be established by survey and case control methodology, the Randomized, Controlled, Cooperative study published in 1956[13] could demonstrate a "cause-and-effect" link between prolonged oxygen administration and retrolental fibroplasia (RLF—an earlier name for ROP). The severe stages of RLF or ROP with residual vitreoretinal scars occurred in 23% of infants randomized to receive the then routine oxygen treatment (4 weeks of greater than 50% oxygen) while it developed in only 7% of those who received curtailed oxygen administration (supplemental oxygen decreased to room air as soon as the infant no longer became cyanotic without it). The study design of that trial is shown in Figure 26A–1. It is important to note that the trial was conducted entirely in infants under 1,500 gm birth weight and before the availability of blood gas monitoring or artificial ventilation. Therefore, although there were over 700 infants in the trial, relatively few were under 1 kg birth weight, and most infants in the routine oxygen treatment group probably had very high arterial partial pressures of oxygen for 2 to 4 weeks. In addition, note that this study began only at 48 hours of life and therefore that oxygen use during the first 2 days was not controlled by the study design.

Thus, the prolonged (4 weeks) administration of oxygen without clinical evidence for its need causes the risk of ROP to rise. Case control studies have additionally revealed several correlations with severe ROP. When one matches for birth weight and gestational age, those infants who develop severe ROP more frequently have the most complicated hospital courses, i.e., asphyxia at birth, respiratory distress syndrome requiring mechanical ventilation, pneumothoraces, patent ductus arteriosus, cerebral intraventricular hemorrhage, sepsis, and other complications commonly associated with prematurity. Therefore any laboratory value or hospital course variable caused by a prolonged, complicated neonatal intensive care stay correlates positively with ROP. Examples would be the number of blood gas analyses performed, the number of arterial PaO_2 or $PaCO_2$ values outside the normal range, the number of blood transfusions given, duration of oxygen supplements, and duration of artificial ventilation or hospitalization,[2–9] and although it has not been published, I am quite certain that the number of pages in the hospital record would also correlate positively. Significant correlations are not evidence of causation, (i.e., having a thick hospital record does not cause ROP), and Sachs and colleagues have shown that, if the length of time that an infant requires oxygen supplementation is controlled (a good general indicator of degree of illness), blood transfusions no longer predict those infants who develop severe ROP.[14] These correlations are extremely valuable nonetheless because they guide research efforts to understand why medical complications should combine with prematurity and lead to the disordered growth of retinal blood vessels.

To minimize the incidence of ROP in premature infants, it appears that medical complications should be minimized insofar as possible and oxygen should be given only as needed. Some specific maneuvers to prevent ROP have recently been tested (to be dis-

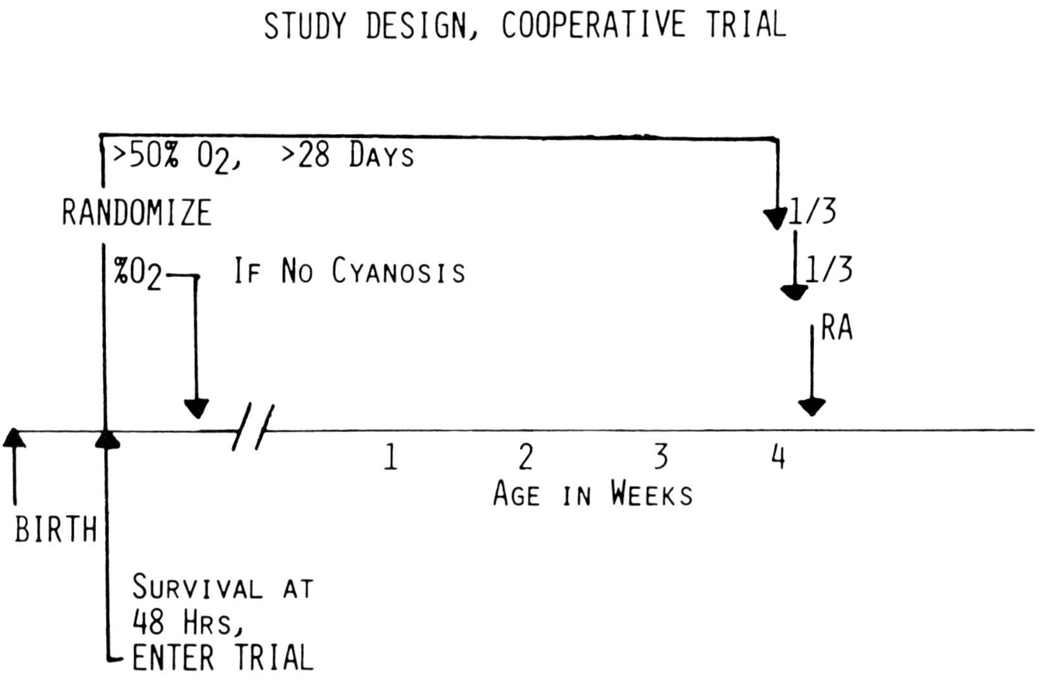

FIG 26A–1.
The study design for the cooperative study of RLF and the use of oxygen.[13] Infants under 1,500 gm birth weight were entered into the trial if they survived for 48 hours. At that point in time, they were radomized to receive routine oxygen or curtailed oxygen. Routine oxygen was over 50% inspired oxygen for 28 days, after which it was reduced by one third on day 29, one third on day 30, and stopped on day 31. Curtailed oxygen meant that added oxygen was given only if the infant was judged by the physician to be critically in need of it, and then only the minimum was given, not to exceed 50% oxygen.

cussed in the following section), but none has yet proved to be effective.

PATIENT MANAGEMENT AIMED AT PREVENTING RETINOPATHY OF PREMATURITY

Controlling Oxygen Administration

Some unfortunate policies evolved and were followed in the years after the release of the cooperative trial of oxygen administration to premature infants. The ones of most concern stated that "RLF can be either completely or almost completely eliminated by administering oxygen only at times of clinical need and then for as brief periods as possible and at concentrations less than 40 percent."[15] Widely accepted,[16] this doctrine was followed by apparent increases in cerebral palsy[17] and infant mortality[18] that were thought to be a result of withholding high oxygen concentrations from cyanotic infants who needed greater than 40% inspired oxygen. The ability to measure arterial oxygen tensions (PaO_2) on microquantities of blood in the late 1960s released physicians from this dilemma. Although arterial levels of oxygen that are safe in regard to causing ROP were not then known (and still are not), it became possible to administer oxygen based on the infants' ability to transport it into the bloodstream. Gradually, oxygen use ceased to be controlled by the "40% oxygen rule" and was based on patient need. However, that "rule" has haunted pediatricians for years. During the late 1950s, 1960s and even into the 1970s, if an infant was blinded by ROP, it seemed a foregone conclusion that "too much oxygen had been given" and that the physician, nurses, and nursery were liable. We now know that some infants can develop this disorder without the administration of any supplemental oxygen.[19] Many infants do develop ROP despite meticulous monitoring. Therefore the only prudent course is to give oxygen on the basis of need, and the results must be monitored as frequently as indicated by the infant's changing condition.

Continuing technological achievements have permitted micromeasurements in smaller quantities of blood, continuous measurements of PaO_2 or oxygen saturation from indwelling catheters, and noninvasive continuous measurements of transcutaneous PaO_2 and pulse oximetry (arterial oxygen saturation). Figure 26A–2 shows a premature infant with many of these monitors in place. Increasingly, it is becoming possible to know what a particular infant's oxygenation status is at any moment. Unfortunately, to date neither arterial PaO_2 monitoring[20] nor transcutaneous oxygen monitoring[21] has made it possible to eliminate ROP. No safe level of arterial oxygen concentration, PaO_2, has been identified. Neonatologists manage infants today with what seem to be "reasonable" levels rather than "proven safe" levels. The Fetus and Newborn Committee of the American Academy of Pediatrics (AAP) recommended in 1977 that arterial PaO_2 be kept at 50 to 70 mm Hg and not higher than 80 mm Hg.[22] However, the most recent AAP 1983 guidelines have recognized that we do not yet understand what levels of oxygen are safe and that maintaining infants in a range to be expected in healthy infants, i.e., a PaO_2 of 50 to 90 mm Hg may be more prudent.[23] Pulse oximetry has not yet been evaluated sufficiently to relate to "safe levels" for ROP. However, many centers are using saturation goals of 80% to 95% in premature infants, which corresponds to arterial PaO_2 levels of 40 to 80 mm Hg 94% of the time.[24] The pulse oximeter is becoming extremely popular because the probe does not require heating, gives a nearly instantaneous readout when applied, and is more accurate than capillary oxygen measurements obtained by puncture, a painful procedure that alters the infants' respirations and blood gases while drawing the sample. It will be important to study the use of this new instrument in relation to ROP.

Maintaining Homeostasis

Since most complications of prematurity are associated with increases in the incidence of ROP, it would follow that the smoother the

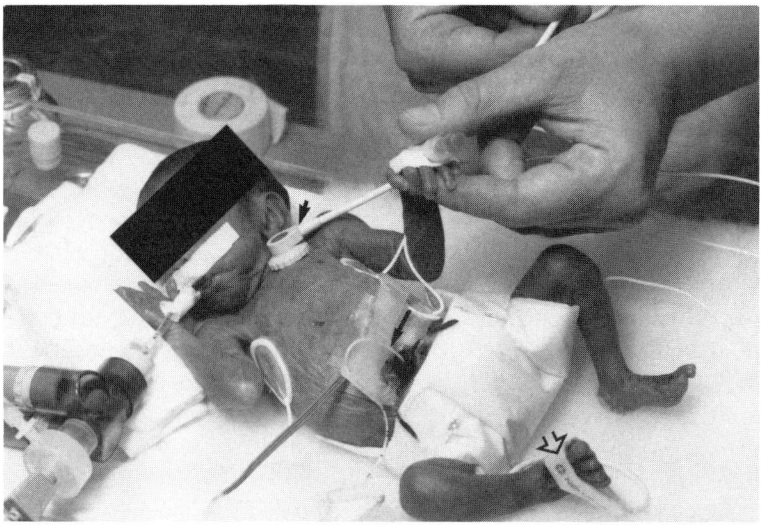

FIG 26A–2.
Extremely premature infant with multiple monitors in place. *Short black arrow* indicates the transcutaneous oxygen monitor; *long black arrow,* the umbilical artery line; and *open arrow,* a pulse oximeter.

hospital course, the lower the number of complications and, subsequently, the lower the risk of ROP. These goals are in keeping with the basic principals to optimize homeostasis for all neonates. Premature infants in utero require careful monitoring for signs of fetal distress. Trauma at delivery should be minimized. Specially trained resuscitation teams should attend each delivery, with prompt attention to ventilation, oxygenation, circulation, warmth, fluids, and glucose homeostasis. Increasing abilities of intensive care nurseries to optimize nutrition and minimize skin trauma, pulmonary barotrauma, and other stress as well as fluid and electrolyte shifts have all contributed to the increased survival of these infants. The combined effect of these approaches has reduced the incidence of severe intracranial hemorrhage and other complications and thus should reduce the incidence of ROP as well. Ideally, these advances will eventually invalidate the calculations made in Table 26A–1.

Vitamin E

Vitamin E has a long association with ROP beginning in 1949 and is now considered of possible benefit by some investigators because of its antioxidant properties.[25] However, while the 1981 study of Hittner and colleagues observed a reduced incidence of severe ROP (from 10% to 0%) in the treated infants, the incidence was exceptionally high in their control group and has not been observed elsewhere.[26] Despite several subsequently reported clinical trials, the results remain inconclusive as to its efficacy in the smallest infants.[5, 6, 27, 28] At best it may reduce the incidence of severe disease in those infants over 27 weeks' gestation at birth.[26] Lack of good pharmacological data on the dose and dosage formulation of tocopherol, either parenterally or orally, currently limits its potential usefulness since significant morbidity (sepsis, necrotizing enterocolitis, cerebral hemorrhage) and mortality have been reported with prolonged high doses, particularly when it has been given parenterally.[6, 29–32]

Ambient Light

Bright light falling on the premature retina was considered a possible cause of ROP in the 1940s. However specific studies to investigate this possibility failed to find an adverse effect of either ambient nursery lighting at that time or the brighter lights used intermittently during direct ophthalmoscopy.[33] More recently, it has been recognized that the sample size in these earlier studies was too small to be reasonably certain to have detected small effects of light, and it was reasoned that incident light may generate oxygen-free radicals exceeding the capacity of the retina to protect itself from activated oxygen, thus triggering the retinopathy. Glass and coworkers found that reducing light exposure did reduce the incidence of ROP from one year to the next in two nurseries.[4] However, the sequential design of that study (therefore neither masked nor concurrently controlled) and the exceptionally high incidence of ROP in the control period (85% and 100% in infants under 1 kg) have raised methodological questions about that report.

Penicillamine

Lakatos and coworkers in Hungary noted a lower incidence of ROP among premature infants who had been enrolled in a penicillamine treatment program to reduce hyperbilirubinemia.[34, 35] These investigators then progressed to a prospective, randomized, and masked controlled trial and were able to replicate their findings.[36] Further testing of the heavy-metal–binding antioxidant D-penicillamine is certainly warranted.

Cryotherapy

Once ROP has become established, it may regress and heal or progress to various degrees of retinal scarring and vision loss. Cryotherapy is an ablative procedure proposed for use in severe active ROP. It is aimed at destroying avascular peripheral retina in order to stop the rapidly growing vessels that are presumably being driven to grow by an angiogenic factor released by the peripheral avascular retina. Currently this treatment is undergoing a controlled multicenter test that will both document the natural course of ROP by using the new international classification of ROP[37] and test the safety and efficacy of the treatment, both short term and long term.[38]

Current Neonatal Precautions

Each of these possible interventions require further testing, and it is comforting to know that multicenter trials of vitamin E supplementation, light restriction, and cryoablative therapy are being conducted. However, infants born today under our present care will not be able to benefit from the results of those trials. Each day, neonatologists must make working decisions in caring for present patients while awaiting the outcome of further testing. Optimizing homeostasis and minimizing direct bright light to the face of premature infants appear to be, as best we can judge, benign procedures to institute. However, the administration of high doses of D-penicillamine or vitamin E or even the severe restriction of ambient light clearly requires further study before widespread application.

EYE EXAMINATIONS

Timing of the First Examination

During the early hospital course of a premature infant, neonatologists and families have frequent conversations regarding the clinical course and likely outcomes. The possibility of ROP (as well as other adverse sequelae) often arises during these discussions; however, the timing of fundus examinations has a profound effect on the resolution of the anxiety such conversations provoke. If the first examination is done on the day of discharge from the unit (about 10 weeks after birth in the typical 26-week–gestation infant), a report of severe active retinopathy or retinal detachment comes as an excruciatingly cruel blow to a family that has survived 10 weeks of the tribulations of intensive care and is now excitedly dressing the infant for the first ride home. Unfortunately this scenario has been all too common because there is a reluctance to perform earlier (and therefore more likely multiple) examinations since the examinations are time-consuming and the ophthalmologist's time is limited. In addition, there is no proven treatment to arrest the retinopathy when it is discovered, so many physicians see little point in early examinations for information only.

On the other hand, ROP is nearly always manifested by 4 to 7 weeks postpartum, and this is a useful time to perform the first examination.[25,39] If the retinal vasculature is complete, then the parents may be reassured. If it is incomplete (immature), they can be counseled that a risk of retinopathy still exists, even if there is no ROP present. If significant retinopathy is present, discussion can proceed early and in a more anticipatory manner. The practice described in Table 26A–2 is one that has worked well in our nursery and is in compliance with AAP guidelines.[23]

In premature infants over 1 kg birth weight, discharge dates may occur before the recommended 4 to 7 weeks of age; however, the examination should still be performed for two reasons. First, infants may be lost to follow-up after discharge, but if distinctly abnormal findings are present, this will serve as an additional motivator for some parents to

TABLE 26A–2.
Examination Schedule for Fundoscopic Examination of Premature Infants to Rule out ROP as Used at the University of Rochester in 1987

Infants who require examination
33–36 weeks' gestation if >6 hours of supplemental oxygen
<33 weeks' gestation or <1,500 gm irrespective of oxygen history
Timing of examinations
All infants prior to discharge from the hospital
All infants by 6 weeks after birth if sufficiently stable
Schedule of repeat examinations:
Fully vascularized retina, no ROP: No repeat examinations needed for ROP
No ROP but immature: Repeat as indicated by degree of retinal immaturity
ROP present: Repeat as indicated by the severity of the disease

return. Second, many infants have a mature retinal vasculature with no ROP on their first examination, and they may then be discharged from further ophthalmologic follow-up for ROP. As cryotherapy or other future treatments prove to be efficacious in arresting active ROP, earlier examinations become essential to permit detection in time for treatment.

Risks of Examination

As smaller and smaller infants survive, first examinations done at approximately 4–6 weeks of age will be occurring in infants of lower weights than ever before. Problems that may occur during examinations and issues of safety are important considerations in weighing the potential benefit of early first examinations. The transient corneal, lens, and vitreous haze seen soon after birth may persist in such infants and interfere with a clear view of the retina.

Apnea and Bradycardia

Infants under 34 weeks' gestation are subject to spontaneous apnea and bradycardic episodes that are also common during their eye examinations. The oculocardiac reflex, seen at all ages, is similar to these episodes and may be particularly severe and prolonged.[40] The mechanism of the reflex has been studied in children having strabismus surgery and was found to be precipitated most consistently by sudden stretches on the extraocular muscles.[41] The reflex was common in unmedicated infants, was exacerbated under conditions of hypercarbia, and could largely be prevented with anticholinergic drugs such as atropine. If a particularly unstable infant must be examined, atropine is often helpful (usually 0.05 to 0.10 mg intramuscularly). When bradycardic episodes do occur, whether they are normal apneic episodes or the oculocardiac reflex, interrupting the examination for a few moments is usually the only therapy needed. If this is not sufficient, increased ventilation and oxygen may need to be given as well.

Hypoxia

Crying and breath holding during the examination may cause hypoxemia; this is particularly true if an infant's oxygenation status is marginal. Individuals responsible for observing the infant during the examination must be able to monitor the infant's color as well as the heart rate and respiration, a task made difficult with the room lights darkened. Anytime the observer (usually one of the intensive care unit nurses) asks for the examination to be interrupted, the ophthalmologist should comply promptly, provide light for the observer, and continue the examination only when the infant has stabilized. In some particularly unstable cases, means of directly measuring the infant's continuous oxygen status such as pulse oximetry should be considered.

Hypertension

Hypertension has been a concern of neonatologists because of its possible link with intracerebral hemorrhage, a major complication in extremely premature infants. However, the vast majority of intracranial hemorrhages occur within the first 3 days after delivery. The smallest infants may develop intracranial hemorrhages or extensions of their initial hemorrhage into the second and third weeks after birth, but it would be exceptional to have this occur as late as 6 weeks of age when the eye examination is to be done. Therefore transient increases in blood pressure with crying should not be a major concern; however, if an infant has had medical complications with hypertension, the neonatologist and ophthalmologist should discuss the risks, benefits, and timing of the examination and take into account the type of eye drops used as well.

Dilating Drops

Phenylephrine eye drops in a concentration of 2.5% to 10% have been demonstrated to cause a significant increase in blood pressure in premature infants.[42] Blanching of the thin facial skin around the eyes of these infants alerted physicians to the likelihood that systemic absorption of these eye drops was occurring. The authors who described this went on to test 0.5% cyclopentolate alone or in combination with 0.5% tropicamide (Mydriacyl) and 0.2% cyclopentolate with 1% phenylephrine. None of these lower concentrations of drugs caused a change in blood pressure, and all gave good dilation results in most infants.[43] The 0.2% cyclopentolate–1% phenylephrine gave the greatest and most prolonged dilation. In addition, studies on the gastric secretory effects of cyclopentolate eyedrops have demonstrated that concentrations of 0.5% decreased gastric acid production volume and concentration but 0.25% had no measurable effect.[44] Nurses administering the drops should be taught how to compress the nasolacrimal duct and wipe excess fluid from the eyelids to minimize systemic absorption. Parents and staff should be forewarned to expect possible blanching of the periorbital skin from the dilating drops.

Conjunctivitis

After the eye examination, some edema and erythema of the lids is to be expected since a lid speculum and scleral depressor are commonly used. Occasionally small conjunctival hemorrhages also occur. Each of these findings as well as a mild conjunctivitis are common sequelae. At times, however, the conjunctivitis is not minor, so cultures must be obtained and local antibiotics given. Hand washing and thorough cleansing and rinsing of the instruments between infants is critical to minimize this problem, which can be due to true infection, chemical irritation from cleansing agents, or trauma of the examination.

Discussions With Families

Ophthalmologists must often examine premature infants at times inconvenient for the parents to be present. Because of this, the responsibility of communicating the findings to the family often falls on the neonatologist or house staff. This is beneficial in some ways since the families are normally well known to the pediatricians and communication is efficient. However, in order for this route to succeed, it is necessary for ophthalmologists to legibly and completely record the results of the retinal examination on the chart and to teach their pediatric colleagues how to interpret their report. Figure 26A–3 is a family's information sheet used in our nursery to help parents understand the need for examination and to facilitate discussion. This was modified from the CRYO-ROP Study Manual of Operations.[38]

The examination may show mature vessels, immature vessels without ROP, ROP of some severity, or other findings. The new ROP classification is described in the following chapter. Based upon this classification, more specific prognostic information will soon become available. However, at this time the prognostic implications of the findings can generally be thought about as follows. (1) If there are *mature vessels* at or adjacent to the ora serrata and there is no ROP present now, none will develop. The parents can be reassured that ROP will not affect their infant's vision. (2) If *immaturity of the vessels* can be seen, but there is no ROP now, it could develop, and the parents should be told that ROP remains a risk and that more examinations will be needed. (3) If *ROP is present* (or other findings), in these cases the ophthalmologist should communicate the level of concern warranted directly to the parents and/or pediatricians.

SUMMARY

In summary, increasing numbers of immature infants are surviving with incompletely developed retinal vessels at risk for ROP. Since adverse perinatal events seem closely associated with the more severe forms of the disorder, neonatologists may be able to contribute most to the reduction of ROP if they can optimize the neonatal course of these infants. However, to date no particular intervention has been proved to be efficacious in preventing ROP. Neonatologists are eager to be educated about this disorder, to commu-

ABOUT PREMATURE BABY'S EYES

TO: To Parents of ______________________ DATE: ______________

FROM: Dr. ______________________

At the request of the pediatricians looking after your baby, an eye examination has been performed on your infant because of prematurity at birth. This pamphlet explains the reasons why this eye examination was necessary.

WHAT IS RETINOPATHY OF PREMATURITY

The retina is the inner lining of the eyeball that receives light and turns it into visual messages that are sent to the brain. If one thinks of the eye as being like a camera, the retina functions as the film. Blood vessels that supply the retina are one of the last structures of the eye to mature, and have barely completed growing when a full term baby is born. This means that a premature infant's retina is still incompletely developed.

For reasons not yet fully understood by medical science, the blood vessels in the immature part of the retina may develop abnormally in some premature infants, especially the very smallest babies. This is called Retinopathy of Prematurity (abbreviated ROP or RLF). Current technology in newborn intensive care units allows us to provide the best available care for premature infants, but in spite of this, we still cannot prevent the development of ROP in certain infants.

When ROP develops, one of three different things can happen:

1) In the large majority of babies who develop ROP (80%), the abnormal blood vessels will heal themselves completely, usually during the first year of life.

2) In some babies the abnormal blood vessels heal only partially. In these infants nearsightedness (myopia) commonly develops. Glasses may be required early in life. These children may be more prone to developing lazy eye (amblyopia) or a wandering eye (strabismus). Infants who develop these findings need to have regular eye examinations and treatment to assure that they develop the best possible vision. In some cases a scar may be left in the retina resulting in vision problems which are not entirely correctable with glasses; patients with these scars need life long ophthalmic care. The residual scars of incompletely healed ROP are referred to as Retrolental Fibroplasia (RLF), which may be mild or severe.

3) In the most severe cases, the retinal blood vessels continue developing abnormally and form scar tissues which pull the retina out of its normal position in the back of the eye. This severe problem results in serious loss of vision. Fortunately, only a small percent (less than 5%) of babies develop severe eye abnormalities.

WHAT ABOUT YOUR BABY'S EYES?

___ Your infant's eyes have mature blood vessels and he / she needs only routine follow up according to your regular doctor.

___ Your infant requires another examination because he / she:

  ___ Has a normal examination but could develop problems later, because the eye blood vessels are still not fully developed.

  ___ Has early ROP that will need further examination to watch for possible serious developments.

The next eye examination is recommended: ______________________

This is your copy to keep.

The pediatricians taking care of your infant can give you more information and will arrange a meeting with an ophthalmologist for additional details if you wish.

____
Examining Ophthalmologist

FIG 26A–3.
Family's information sheet used at Strong Children's Medical Center. A modified version of the parent's information pamphlet "About a Premature Infant's Eyes" from the CRYO-ROP Multicenter Study Group Manual of Operations is shown. (Modified from Palmer EA, Biglan AW, Hardy RJ: Retinal ablative therapy for active proliferative retinopathy of prematurity: History, current status and prospects, in Silverman WA, Flynn JT (eds): *Contemporary Issues in Fetal and Neonatal Medicine 2. Retinopathy of Prematurity.* Boston, Blackwell Scientific Publications, Inc, 1985; p 207.)

nicate the results of timely examinations to infants' families, to participate with ophthalmologists in the ongoing ophthalmic care of these tiny survivors, and to investigate means to prevent ROP.

REFERENCES

1. Silverman WA, Flynn JT: *Contemporary Issues in Fetal and Neonatal Medicine 2. Retinopathy of Prematurity.* Boston, Blackwell Scientific Publications, 1985.
2. Reisner SH, Amir J, Shohat M, et al: Retinopathy of prematurity: Incidence and treatment. *Arch Dis Child* 1985; 60:698.
3. Majima A: Studies on retinopathy of prematurity I. Statistical analysis of factors related to occurrence and progression in active phase. *Jpn J Ophthalmol* 1977; 21:404.
4. Glass P, Avery GB, Subramanian KNS, et al: Effect of bright light in the hospital nursery on the incidence of retinopathy of prematurity. *N Engl J Med* 1985; 313:401.
5. Schaffer DB, Johnson L, Quinn GE, et al: Vitamin E and retinopathy of prematurity. Follow-up at one year. *Ophthalmology* 1985; 92:1005.
6. Phelps DL, Rosenbaum AL, Isenberg SJ, et al: Tocopherol efficacy and safety for preventing retinopathy of prematurity: A randomized, controlled, double-masked trial. *Pediatrics* 1987; 79:489.
7. Merritt JC, Kraybill EN: Retrolental fibroplasia: A five-year experience in a tertiary perinatal center. *Ann Ophthalmol* 1986; 18:65.
8. Gunn TR, Easdown J, Outerbridge EW, et al: Risk factors in retrolental fibroplasia. *Pediatrics* 1980; 65:1096.
9. Purohit DM, Ellison RC, Zierler S, et al: Risk factors for retrolental fibroplasia: Experience with 3,025 premature infants. *Pediatrics* 1985; 76:339.
10. Phelps DL: Retinopathy of prematurity: An estimate of vision loss in the United States—1979. *Pediatrics* 1981; 67:924.
11. Kushner BJ, Gloeckner E: Retrolental fibroplasia in full-term infants without exposure to supplemental oxygen. *Am J Ophthalmol* 1984; 97:148.
12. Criswick VG, Schepens CL: Familial exudative vitreoretinopathy. *Am J Ophthalmol* 1969; 68:578.
13. Kinsey VE: Cooperative study of retrolental fibroplasia and the use of oxygen. *Ophthalmology* 1956; 56:481.
14. Sachs LM, Schaffer DB, Anday E, et al: Retrolental fibroplasia and blood transfusion in very low–birth-weight infants. *Pediatrics* 1981; 68:770.
15. Guy LP, Lanman JT, Dancis J: The possibility of total elimination of retrolental fibroplasia by oxygen restriction. *Pediatrics* 1956; 17:247.
16. Silverman WA, Flynn JT: Overview: A "developmental" retinopathy reconsidered, in Silverman WA, Flynn JT (eds). *Contemporary Issues in Fetal and Neonatal Medicine 2. Retinopathy of Prematurity.* Boston, Blackwell Scientific Publications, 1985, p xi.
17. McDonald AD: Neurological and ophthalmic disorders in children of very low birth weight. *Br. Med J* 1962; 1:895.
18. Cross KW: Cost of preventing retrolental fibroplasia? *Lancet* 1973; 2:954.
19. Lucey JF, Dangman B: A reexamination of the role of oxygen in retrolental fibroplasia. *Pediatrics* 1984; 73:82.
20. Kinsey VE, Arnold HJ, Kalina RE, et al: PaO_2 levels and retrolental fibroplasia: A report of the cooperative study. *Pediatrics* 1977; 60:655.
21. Bancalari E, Flynn J, Goldberg RN, et al: Influence of transcutaneous oxygen monitoring on the incidence of retinopathy of prematurity (ROP). *Pediatrics* 1987; 79:663.
22. American Academy of Pediatrics: *Standards and recommendations for hospital care of newborn infants.* Evanston, Ill, 1977.
23. American Academy of Pediatrics and American College of Obstetricians and Gynecologists: *Guidelines for Perinatal Care.* Evanston, Ill, and Washington, DC, 1983.
24. Deckhardt R, Steward DJ: Noninvasive arterial hemoglobin oxygen saturation versus transcutaneous oxygen tension monitoring in the preterm infant. *Crit Care Med* 1984; 12:935.
25. Hittner HM, Godio LB, Rudolph AJ, et al: Retrolental fibroplasia: Efficacy of vitamin E in a double-blind clinical study of preterm infants. *N Engl J Med* 1981; 305:1365.
26. Phelps DL: Vitamin E and retinopathy of prematurity, in Silverman WA, Flynn JT (eds): *Contemporary Issues in Fetal and Neonatal Medicine 2. Retinopathy of Prematurity.* Boston, Blackwell Scientific Publications, 1985, p 181.

27. Puklin JE, Simon RM, Ehrenkranz RA: Influence on retrolental fibroplasia of intramuscular vitamin E administration during respiratory distress syndrome. *Ophthalmology* 1982; 89:96.
28. Finer NN, Schindler RF, Grant G, et al: Effect of intramuscular vitamin E on the frequency and severity of retrolental fibroplasia: A controlled trial. *Lancet* 1982; 1:1087.
29. Johnson L, Bowen FW, Abbasi S, et al: Relationship of prolonged pharmacologic serum levels of vitamin E to incidence of sepsis and necrotizing enterocolitis in infants with birth weights 1,500 grams or less. *Pediatrics* 1985; 75:619.
30. Finer NN, Peters KL, Hayek Z, et al: Vitamin E and necrotizing enterocolitis. *Pediatrics* 1984; 73:387.
31. Rosenbaum AL, Phelps DL, Isenberg SJ, et al: Retinal hemorrhages in retinopathy of prematurity associated with tocopherol treatment. *Ophthalmology* 1985; 92:1012.
32. Martone WJ, Williams WW, Mortensen ML, et al: Illness with fatalities in premature infants: Association with an intravenous vitamin E preparation. E-Ferol. *Pediatrics* 1986; 78:591.
33. Locke JC, Reese AB: Retrolental fibroplasia. The negative role of light, mydriatics, and the ophthalmoscopic examination in its etiology. *Arch Ophthalmol* 1952; 48:44.
34. Lakatos L, Hatvani I, Oroszlan G, et al: D-penicillamine in the prevention of retrolental fibroplasia. *Acta Paediatr Hung* 1982; 23:327.
35. Lakatos L, Hatvani I, Oroszlan G, et al: Prevention of retrolental fibroplasia in very low birth weight infants by D-penicillamine. *Eur J Pediatr* 1982; 138:199.
36. Lakatos L, Hatvani I, Oroszlan G, et al: Controlled trial of D-penicillamine to prevent retinopathy of prematurity. *Acta Paediatr Hung* 1986; 27:47.
37. An international classification of retinopathy of prematurity. *Pediatrics* 1984; 74:127.
38. Palmer EA, Biglan AW, Hardy RJ: Retinal ablative therapy for active proliferative retinopathy of prematurity: History, current status and prospects, in Silverman WA, Flynn JT: *Contemporary Issues in Fetal and Neonatal Medicine 2. Retinopathy of Prematurity.* Boston, Blackwell Scientific Publications, 1985, p 207.
39. Palmer EA: Optimal timing of examination for acute retrolental fibroplasia. *Ophthalmology* 1981; 88:662.
40. Clarke WN, Hodges E, Noel LP, et al: The oculocardiac reflex during ophthalmoscopy in premature infants. *Am J Ophthalmol* 1985; 99:649.
41. Blanc VF, Hardy JF, Milot J, et al: The oculocardiac reflex: A graphic and statistical analysis in infants and children. *Can Anaesth Soc J* 1983; 30:360.
42. Rosales T, Isenberg S, Leake R, et al: Systemic effects of mydriatics in low weight infants. *J Pediatr Ophthalmol Strabismus* 1981; 18:42.
43. Isenberg S, Everett S, Parelhoff E: A comparison of mydriatic eyedrops in low-weight infants. *Ophthalmology* 1984; 91:278.
44. Isenberg, SJ, Abrams C, Hyman PE: Effects of cyclopentolate eyedrops on gastric secretory function in pre-term infants. *Ophthalmology* 1985; 92:698.

26B Retinopathy of Prematurity: An Ophthalmologist's Perspective

Paul T. Urrea, M.D., M.P.H.
Arthur L. Rosenbaum, M.D.

DESCRIPTION OF THE DISORDER

Introduction

Retinopathy of prematurity (ROP), formerly called retrolental fibroplasia (RLF), is a vasoproliferative retinal disorder of the newborn that, since its recognition, has produced blindness in tens of thousands of premature infants. Each year in the United States, it is estimated that retinopathy of prematurity is responsible for producing some degree of visual loss in approximately 1,300 children and severe visual loss in 450 to 500 children.[1–3]

History

ROP was not recognized until the initial report of Theodore Terry in 1942 that described blindness and extreme prematurity in five infants.[4] During a 3-year period following his original paper, Terry collected and reported on slightly over 100 cases of RLF.[4–9] Based on Terry's anatomic observations and incomplete understanding of the pathology, the disorder came to be known as RLF.[10] In the year's following his early reports, sporadic cases of RLF were reported in the literature.[11–13] Toward the latter part of the decade, however, the incidence of RLF was noted to be on the rise. In his early publications, Terry correctly observed that prematurity was important to the development of the disease.[4–9] In other reports, many additional related factors were proposed.[5, 12, 14–16] Prior to 1950, however, no one factor other than prematurity was found to be unequivocably associated with the development of the disease. By 1949, the incidence of RLF was noted to have greatly increased, and the disease was found to be responsible for 30% of blindness reported in preschool children in the United States.[17, 18] By 1950, the incidence of RLF mushroomed and was found to have reached frightening, epidemic proportions (Fig 26B–1).

No true light was shed upon other risk factors associated with the development of RLF until the report of Campbell in 1951.[19] In this important report, the association between the use of high levels of oxygen and the development of RLF in premature infants was first noted. This initial report was followed soon thereafter by similar reports from investiga-

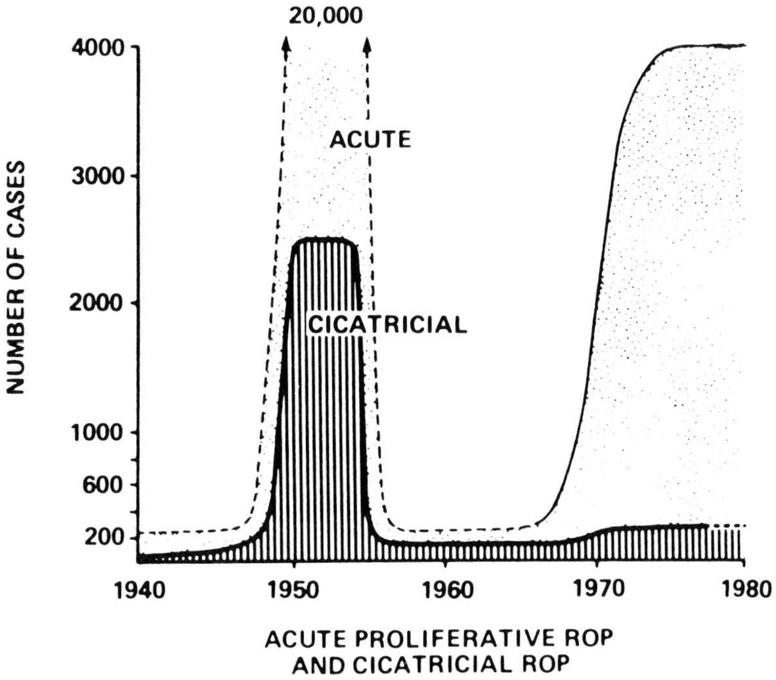

FIG 26B–1.
The incidence of ROP in prematures in the United States. (From Patz A, Payne JW: Retinopathy of prematurity (retrolental fibroplasia), in Duane TD, Jaeger EA (eds): *Clinical Ophthalmology*, vol 3. Philadelphia, Harper & Row, Publishers, Inc, 1987, pp 1–19; and Payne JW, Patz A: Current status of retrolental fibroplasia: The retinopathy of prematurity. Review article. *Ann Clin Res* 1979; 11:205. Used with permission.)

tors throughout the world that linked oxygen use and RLF.[20, 21] In subsequent randomized, controlled, and multicenter studies by various investigators,[22–24] the association between RLF and supplemental oxygen exposure was confirmed. Laboratory studies using animals to reproduce RLF[25–28] provided additional early support to the notion that oxygen therapy played an important role in the etiology of this devastating disease.

As a consequence of these findings, stringent curtailment of the use of oxygen in premature infants was instituted. The resultant incidence of RLF was noted to drop dramatically (see Fig 26B–1).[1] Based on a study by Lanman et al[23] and subsequent studies by other investigators,[29–31] it was optimistically concluded that protection against the development of RLF could be ensured if oxygen use was limited to inspired concentrations of 40% or less.[32] In retrospect it can now be seen that a single clinical trial involving only 85 infants and purporting to demonstrate that "under 40% is safe" was too small a sample size to justify this sweeping claim.[33] However, by the end of the 1950s, based upon implementation of these recommendations, the incidence of RLF did dramatically fall.[34] But, by the 1960s it was recognized that stringent curtailment of oxygen use was a double-edged sword because the morbidity from cerebral palsy[35] and mortality from respiratory distress syndrome ("hyaline membrane disease") rose in inverse relation to the falling incidence of RLF.[32, 36–38] One investigator estimated that 16 infants died in the United States from hyaline membrane disease for every case of prevented blindness from RLF.[39] As a consequence, between the mid-1960s and early 1970s, there evolved a gradual trend toward liberalization of oxygen use in premature nurseries,[1,32] and in that period of time there was a measurable increase in the incidence of RLF (Fig 26B–2).[1]

Retinopathy of Prematurity vs. Retrolental Fibroplasia

The term *RLF* had been used almost exclusively in reference to this disease since its introduction by Terry and Messenger in 1944.[10] After the invention of the indirect ophthalmoscope allowed the identification of previously unobserved "acute" proliferative changes in the peripheral part of the retina, a term permitting a broader definition of the disease was needed. The term *ROP* was first coined in 1951[40] but did not come into widespread use until recently. With the recognition that identification of early acute changes of the disease may have prognostic significance (see later), the term *ROP* was adopted as the all-encompassing term. ROP denotes the entire spectrum of acute and cicatricial retinal pathology. The term *RLF* serves as a well-known descriptor of the destructive, late cicatricial phases of the disease, and its continued use is appropriate only for this phase.[4–9]

Incidence

Since the late 1960s and early 1970s with the ability to recognize early phases of the disease, the incidence of acute ROP has been observed to increase dramatically (see Fig 26B–1).[1,41] Fortunately, because most cases of acute ROP undergo spontaneous regression and do not progress to cicatrization, the incidence of cicatricial ROP (i.e., RLF), although on the rise, has not increased as markedly as during the epidemic of 3 decades ago. Premature infants

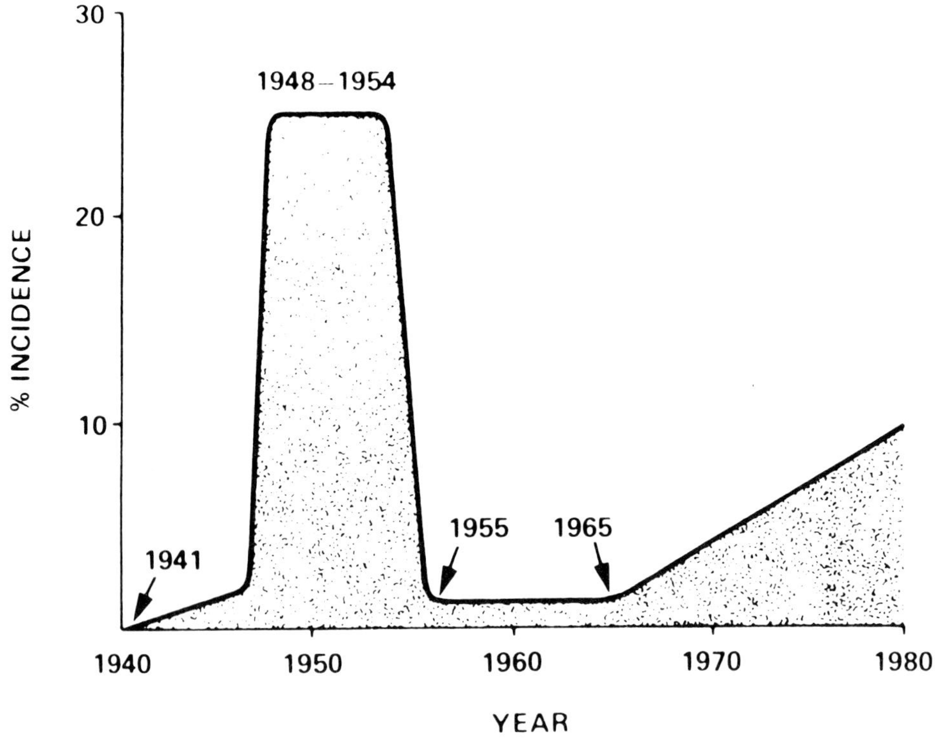

FIG 26B–2.
The incidence of acute proliferative and cicatricial ROP in prematures in the United States. (From Patz A, Payne JW: Retinopathy of prematurity (retrolental fibroplasia), in Duane TD, Jaeger EA (eds): *Clinical Ophthalmology,* vol 3. Philadelphia, Harper & Row, Publishers, Inc, 1987, pp 1–19; and Payne JW, Patz A: Current status of retrolental fibroplasia: The retinopathy of prematurity. Review article. *Ann Clin Res* 1979; 11:205. Used with permission.)

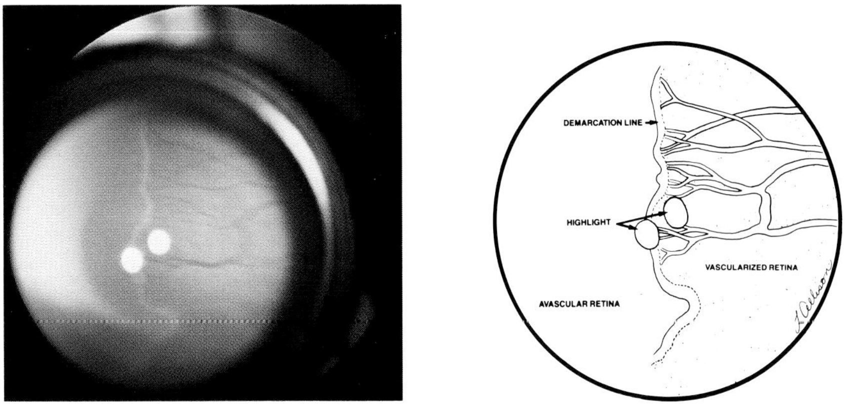

PLATE 1.—Fundus photograph and line drawing show demarcation lines of stage 1 ROP. (From Flynn JT: An international classification of retinopathy of prematurity, in Silverman WA, Flynn JT (eds): *Retinopathy of Prematurity II. Contemporary Issues in Fetal and Neonatal Medicine.* Boston, Blackwell Scientific Publications, 1985, pp 1–17; and Committee for the Classification of Retinopathy of Prematurity: An international classification of retinopathy of prematurity. *Arch Ophthalmol* 1984; 102:1130–1134. Used with permission.)

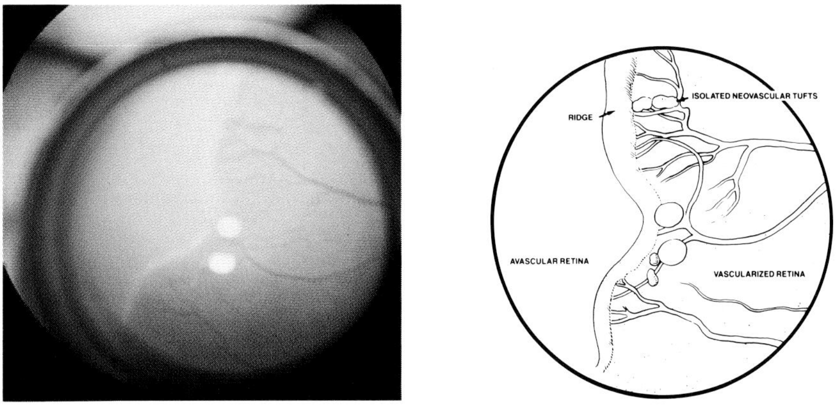

PLATE 2.—Fundus photograph and line drawing show the development of a ridge characteristic of stage 2 ROP. (From Flynn JT: An international classification of retinopathy of prematurity, in Silverman WA, Flynn JT (eds): *Retinopathy of Prematurity II. Contemporary Issues in Fetal and Neonatal Medicine.* Boston, Blackwell Scientific Publications, 1985, pp 1–17; and Committee for the Classification of Retinopathy of Prematurity: An international classification of retinopathy of prematurity. *Arch Ophthalmol* 1984; 102:1130–1134. Used with permission.)

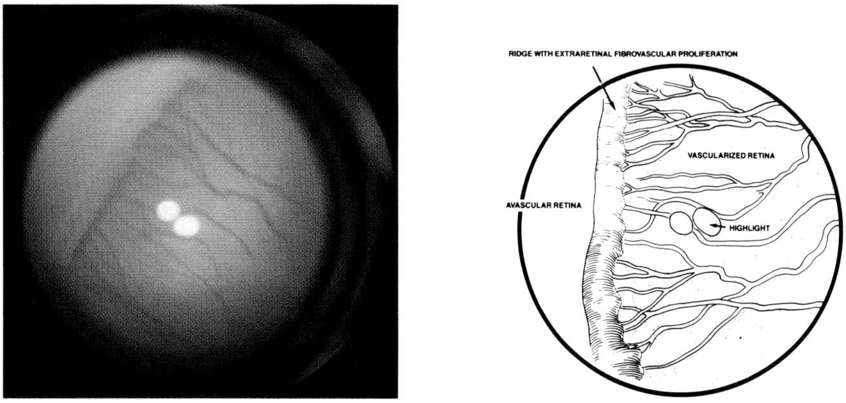

PLATE 3.—Fundus photograph and line drawing of extraretinal fibrovascular proliferative tissue of stage 3 ROP. (From Flynn JT: An international classification of retinopathy of prematurity, in Silverman WA, Flynn JT (eds): *Retinopathy of Prematurity II. Contemporary Issues in Fetal and Neonatal Medicine.* Boston, Blackwell Scientific Publications, 1985, pp 1–17; and Committee for the Classification of Retinopathy of Prematurity: An international classification of retinopathy of prematurity. *Arch Ophthalmol* 1984; 102:1130–1134. Used with permission.)

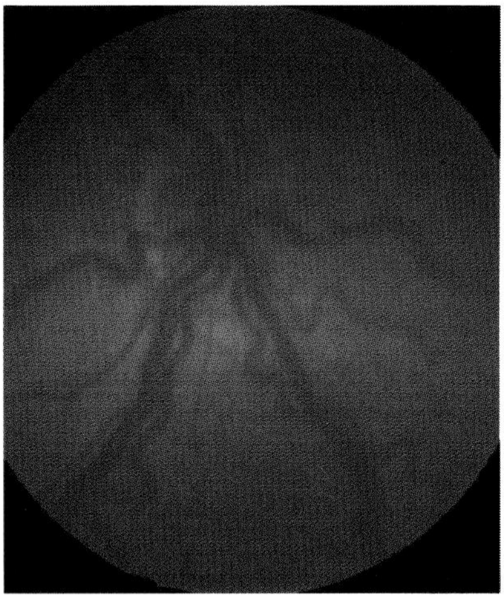

PLATE 4.—Fundus photograph of posterior venous dilation and arteriolar tortuosity characteristic of "plus" disease. (From Flynn JT: An international classification of retinopathy of prematurity, in Silverman WA, Flynn JT (eds): *Retinopathy of Prematurity II. Contemporary Issues in Fetal and Neonatal Medicine.* Boston, Blackwell Scientific Publications, 1985, pp 1–17; and Committee for the Classification of Retinopathy of Prematurity: An international classification of retinopathy of prematurity. *Arch Ophthalmol* 1984; 102:1130–1134. Used with permission.)

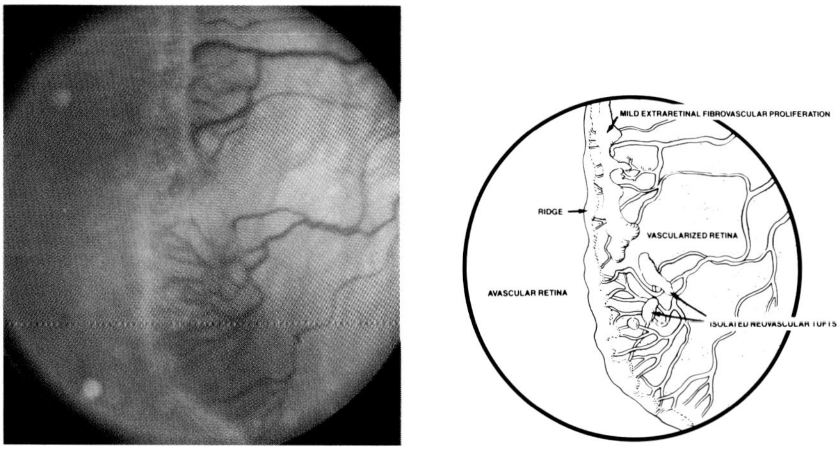

PLATE 5.—Fundus photograph and line drawing show the amount of extraretinal fibrovascular proliferative tissue judged to be mild stage 3 ROP. (From Flynn JT: An international classification of retinopathy of prematurity, in Silverman WA, Flynn JT (eds): *Retinopathy of Prematurity II. Contemporary Issues in Fetal and Neonatal Medicine.* Boston, Blackwell Scientific Publications, 1985, pp 1–17; and Committee for the Classification of Retinopathy of Prematurity: An international classification of retinopathy of prematurity. *Arch Ophthalmol* 102:1130–1134, 1984; 102:1130–1134. Used with permission.)

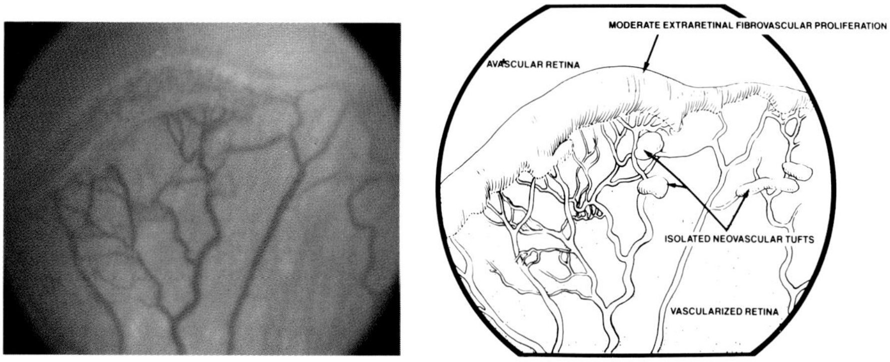

PLATE 6.—Fundus photograph and line drawing of moderate proliferation of extraretinal fibrovascular proliferative tissue from ridge. (From Flynn JT: An international classification of retinopathy of prematurity, in Silverman WA, Flynn JT (eds): *Retinopathy of Prematurity II. Contemporary Issues in Fetal and Neonatal Medicine.* Boston, Blackwell Scientific Publications, 1985, pp 1–17; and Committee for the Classification of Retinopathy of Prematurity: An international classification of retinopathy of prematurity. *Arch Ophthalmol* 1984; 102:1130–1134. Used with permission.)

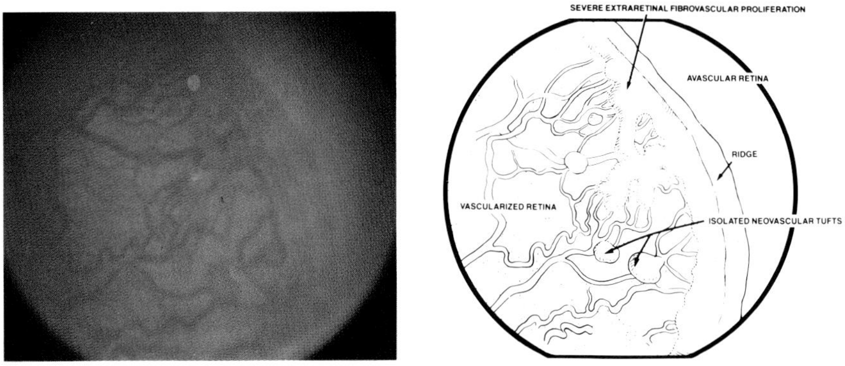

PLATE 7.—Fundus photograph and line drawing of extraretinal fibrovascular proliferation of amounts of tissue judged to be characteristic of severe stage 3 ROP. (From Flynn JT: An international classification of retinopathy of prematurity, in Silverman WA, Flynn JT (eds): *Retinopathy of Prematurity II. Contemporary Issues in Fetal and Neonatal Medicine.* Boston, Blackwell Scientific Publications, 1985, pp 1–17; and Committee for the Classification of Retinopathy of Prematurity: An international classification of retinopathy of prematurity. *Arch Ophthalmol* 1984; 102:1130–1134. Used with permission.)

of very low birth weight sustain the highest risk of developing acute and cicatricial ROP.[1, 43–52] The incidence of acute ROP in infants weighing less than 1,500 gm ranges from 4% to 65%.[1] In survivors weighing less than 1,000 gm at birth, the incidence of acute ROP ranges from 40% to 77%.[1] Cicatricial ROP (i.e., RLF) and blindness probably occurs in 5% or fewer of infants with active ROP and is estimated to affect up to 500 infants yearly in the United States.[1]

The apparent resurgence of ROP has been attributed not only to better screening and detection but also to modern technological advances. Neonatalogists are achieving remarkable success in saving the lives of very low birth weight premature infants who would perish were it not for the use of sophisticated life support systems. Phelps has estimated that the survival rate of premature infants with birth weights less than 1,000 gm has increased from 8% in 1950 to approximately 35% in 1980.[53, 54] The current resurgence of ROP cannot be explained by the simple notion of the past that prematurity combined with supplemental oxygen invariably results in ROP.[55] The etiology of ROP is surely much more complex. According to Silverman and Flynn,[55] "The treatment history of today's affected infant is strikingly different from the medical experience of past victims. The number of possible influences [on the development of ROP] has increased markedly."

The association between the use of supplemental oxygen and the development of ROP had been accepted as valid. An implicit assumption developed that the risk of ROP was believed to be directly related to the degree of elevated arterial Po_2. According to Silverman and Flynn[55] this assumption was translated into an official statement by the American Academy of Pediatrics[56] that "when the normal oxygen tension is exceeded, there is an increased risk of RLF." There, of course, was no definitive proof at that time to directly correlate the risk of developing RLF with the level of arterial Po_2.[57] With the introduction in the 1960s and 1970s of intravascular and transcutaneous measurement techniques to monitor the infant's state of oxygenation, it was hoped that with continuous monitoring the maintenance of normal oxygen tension would provide a safeguard against hyperoxia and the development of RLF.[57–64] Recent evidence indicates that this may be true in infants weighing greater than 1,000 gm at birth.[65] But in infants weighing less than 1,000 gm, the occurrence of cicatricial disease continues to occur more frequently and with much greater severity despite careful monitoring of the infant's state of oxygenation.[66]

A correlation between duration of oxygen therapy and the development of ROP has been demonstrated in premature infants,[19–24] but the exact role of oxygen in the pathophysiology of ROP remains to be elucidated. Researchers have been unable to establish either a critical blood level of oxygen that induces ROP or a regimen of care for preventing its development.[67] It is unclear whether hyperoxia is coupled with other potential factors such as hypoxia, hypercarbia, acidemia, prostaglandins, fetal hemoglobin, etc., to produce the disease.[55] Although skillful neonatal intensive care is considered vital to maintaining an optimal balance between hyperoxia and hypoxia, increasing numbers of specialists are concerned that the best of care may never be sufficient to prevent ROP in all instances.[67]

According to Patz and Payne,[1]

> Presently, there appears to be an irreducible minimum incidence of ROP in spite of the most careful blood gas monitoring.[43] It would seem that prematurity per se may be responsible for most of the current cases of ROP, in contrast to the overuse of oxygen as the major cause in the epidemic years. Because an immature retina is fundamental to the pathogenesis of the disease, excess oxygen can be considered the major precipitating factor only.

Further research is needed to elucidate the basic mechanisms that lead to the clinical manifestations of arrested retinal vasculogenesis, neovasculariation, and in severe cases, destructive proliferative vitreoretinal pathology.

Pathophysiology

According to Ashton's[68] theory of normal vasculogenesis of the human retina, the first blood vessels appear in the retina in the fourth month of gestation in the form of mesenchymal cells. This mesenchyme, representing vascular precursor, emanates from the disc, proliferates into the inner layers of the retina, and extends peripherally. With normal vasculogenesis the retinal vessels reach the nasal ora serrata by the 7th to 8th months of gestation and reach the temporal ora serrata by the 9th month or slightly after birth in the full-term infant. The greater distance from the optic disc to the temporal periphery than to the nasal periphery is the reason for the delay in vascularization of the temporal retina and probably accounts for the greater susceptibility of the temporal retina to develop ROP.

The classic pathogenesis of ROP as proposed by Patz[69–71] involves the following events: (1) vasoconstriction of the immature retinal vessels triggered by significantly elevated arterial Po_2 levels from supplemental oxygen administration; (2) vascular closure and subsequent permanent vascular occlusion if vasoconstriction is sustained; (3) upon return of the arterial Po_2 to levels from inspired ambient air, there is marked endothelial proliferation from residual vascular complexes adjacent to the vessels closed during the period of hyperoxia; (4) subsequent extension of these vasoproliferative elements within the retina and, in some cases, into the vitreous produces hemorrhage and promotes fibrous and glial tissue ingrowth with subsequent vitreoretinal traction and retinal detachment.

An alternative theory proposed by Kretzer et al, and Hittner et al,[72–77] postulates the induction of retinal and vitreal neovascularization by spindle cells in the following sequence: (1) an oxidative insult to spindle cells, the precursors of intraretinal vessels, by elevated arterial Po_2 levels; (2) intracellular biochemical alterations in the spindle cells that halt normal vasculogenesis and trigger "gap junction" formation which promotes the synthesis and secretion of angiogenic factors; (3) neovascularization from endothelial cells that arises from residual vascular complexes with migration of myofibroblasts into the vitreous body; and (4) subsequent vitreoretinal traction and retinal detachment if "downmodulation" of the gap junctions fails to occur.

TECHNIQUE AND FREQUENCY OF EXAMINATION

Role of the Ophthalmologist

The primary role of the ophthalmologist in the nursery is the screening of premature infants for ROP. Important data from the patient history that should be noted by the consulting ophthalmologist include birth weight, gestational age, degree of exposure to supplemental oxygen, and multiple births. Additional relevant factors include exposure of the mother to drugs, ionizing radiation, or infectious agents during gestation; complications during pregnancy; type of delivery; and complications during delivery. Postnatal clinical information such as the presence of respiratory distress syndrome, cardiovascular and other congenital anomalies, anemia, septicemia, intraventricular hemorrhage, and treatment with therapeutic agents such as vitamin E should also be reviewed.

Ocular Examination

An examination of the external lids, adnexal structures, and anterior segment of the eye—including the appearance of the cornea, depth of the anterior chamber, appearance and vascularity of the iris, appearance of the pupils, and pupillary reactions—should precede dilation of the pupils for fundus examination. Dilation of the pupils may be achieved by the use of a topical parasympatholytic agent such as cyclopentolate hydrochloride, 0.5% (Cyclogyl), or tropicamide hydrochloride,

0.5% (Mydriacyl), in conjunction with a sympathomimetic agent, namely, phenylephrine hydrochloride, 2.5% (Neo-Synephrine). The use of phenylephrine hydrochloride, 10%, is strictly avoided because this high a concentration is not necessary for adequate pupillary dilation and can be harmful due to toxic systemic effects.[78, 79] The use of less concentrated combination drops containing both cyclopentolate, 0.2%, and phenylephrine, 1.0% (Cyclomydril), limits the risk of systemic side effects and is preferred because adequate pupillary dilation with fewer risks can be achieved.[80, 81] In order to decrease possible systemic side effects from absorption of any of these medications through the nasolacrimal system, punctal occlusion in the medial region of the eyelids by simple digital pressure may be used.[82] After dilation, a topical anesthetic such as proparacaine (Ophthaine or Ophthetic) is recommended prior to placement of a Sauer-type lid speculum. Because most infants will react to placement of the speculum by attempting to remove it with their hands, an assistant such as a nurse or nurse's aide should be present to gently but firmly hold the infant.

Examination of the fundus should be performed with the use of a binocular indirect ophthalmoscope. The presence of lens opacities, persistant hyaloid vascular remnants, and congenital optic nerve head abnormalities and/or retinal colobomas should be noted.[83] Attention to both the posterior pole and peripheral part of the retina is of paramount importance. Tortuosity of the posterior pole vessels or straightening of the vascular arcades should be noted as well as any heterotropia of the macula. In most instances, the posterior pole will have a normal appearance. If vascularization has proceeded beyond the equator of the globe, careful attention must be paid to the peripheral portion of the retina. Although vascularization of the nasal retina out to the ora serrata will occur earlier than in the temporal periphery, it is nonetheless important to examine both hemispheres. The use of a 20- or 28-D condensing lens enhanced by the technique of scleral depression is invaluable for visualization of the peripheral part of the retina. Retinal changes as described in the following section on the international classification of ROP (ICROP) should be carefully documented as to stage, extent, and location. Often in the first few weeks of life the ocular media is hazy, and visualization of retinal detail may be suboptimal. If adequate examination is not possible or the infant is unable to tolerate the examination, the infant should be reexamined in 2 weeks' time.[67]

It is important for the examiner to be aware of the possible adverse reactions to manipulation of the globe during examination. Premature infants of very low birth weight may become hypoxic during examination because the stimulus of the examination may produce apnea and tax the ability of the immature respiratory system to adequately oxygenate the blood. Cardiac arrythmias, secondary to oculocardiac reflex from manipulation of the globe during placement or movement of the lid speculum or, more likely, during scleral depression, should be kept in mind as the examination is being performed.[84]

Timing and Frequency of Examination

Various recommendations regarding the timing of ocular examination of infants deemed to be at risk of ROP developing are present in the literature. In 1974, the American Academy of Pediatrics[85] made the recommendation that

> A person experienced in recognizing retrolental fibroplasia should examine the eyes of all infants born at less than 36 weeks gestational age, or weighing less than 2000 grams (4.4 lbs.), who have received oxygen therapy. This examination should be made at discharge from the nursery and at three to six months of age.

Palmer has recommended that if the ophthalmologist is able to examine the infant only once prior to discharge from the nursery the optimal age for detecting signs of ROP is between 7 and 9 weeks postpartum.[86] He points

TABLE 26B–1.
Criteria for Frequency and Timing of Ocular Examinations According to Brown et al.*

1. Examine all infants with birth weights less than 1,600 gm
2. Examine all infants with birth weights greater than 1,600 gm if supplemental oxygen is administered for greater than 50 days
3. Optimal time for examination is between 6 to 7 weeks of life
4. If the retina is not fully vascularized, examine weekly until the "fundus is mature" (i.e., vessels extend to far retinal periphery)

*From Brown DR, Biglan AW, Stretabsky MAM: Screening criteria for the detection of retinopathy of prematurity in patients in a neonatal intensive care unit. *J Pediatr Ophthalmol Strabismus* 1987; 24:213–214. Used with permission.

out that ROP is rarely manifested prior to 9 weeks of age and that retinal detachment seldom occurs beforehand.[67] He states that screening examinations during the first month of life therefore are of little advantage and in fact are disadvantageous in light of the aforementioned potential complications. Patz and Payne state that if early disease is detected during the initial examination re-examination at 2- to 3-week intervals during the active phase of the disease is recommended. Orellana[87] points out that continued follow-up examinations are crucial and that extensive changes can occur in a matter of days. Examinations done too infrequently can overlook significant progression of pathology and thereby deny the infant the opportunity of early treatment or surgical intervention, as will be discussed later.

Brown et al.[88] have recently recommended a modification of the guidelines for screening infants at risk for developing ROP. Based on a recent report involving nearly 3,000 infants with birth weights less than 2,000 gm who were examined for ROP and had received supplemental oxygen, their recommendations are (1) all infants with birth weights of less than 1,600 gm should be examined, and (2) infants with birth weights above 1,600 gm should be examined only if they are exposed to greater than 50 days of supplemental oxygen. They recommend that the optimal time for performing examinations in these infants should be at 6 to 7 weeks of life. Brown and coworkers suggest that these modifications should benefit the family economically by preventing unnecessary examinations and benefit the infant by avoiding complications resulting from excessive instrumentation (Table 26B–1).

Flynn[89] concurred with the updated recommendations by Brown and associates. In addition, Flynn recommended that the "conceptual age" of the baby be used in determining the proper time of screening for ROP. Conceptual age is defined by Flynn as the gestational age of the baby at birth plus the age following birth. Flynn points out that this method of delineating the neonate's age puts every baby on the same time axis. In a single-center randomized trial of oxygen monitoring by Flynn, the diagnosis of ROP was made in 85% of 214 infants between 35 and 45 weeks of conceptual age. On the basis of these findings, Flynn suggests examination of neonates between 35 and 45 weeks of conceptual age for proper diagnosis.

In addition, Brown et al[88] indicated in their study that any patient whose peripheral portion of the fundus was not completely vascularized at the time of initial examination was re-examined weekly "until the fundus was mature" (i.e., until complete vascularization of the peripheral part of the retina was noted). In response, Flynn[89] recommended that if an infant were noted to have vascularization up to the nasal ora serrata and temporal peripheral retina it would be very unlikely for that baby to go on to develop any serious acute complications from ROP. If vascularization has extended this far peripherally, Flynn recommends that follow-up be postponed for 6 months in order to check for the development of amblyopia, myopia, etc. If normal retinal vascularization is noted to extend out to the retinal periphery, anterior to the equator but not quite out to the nasal ora (outer zone II by ICROP), then Flynn recommends that follow-up examinations be performed every month. If, however, normal retinal vascularization has extended only out to the region just anterior to the equator, then follow-up examinations should be performed every week because there is a larger area of retina at risk for progression of the disease to cicatricial stages (Table 26B–2).

USE AND INTERPRETATION OF INTERNATIONAL CLASSIFICATION OF RETINOPATHY OF PREMATURITY*

*Portions of the text and figures that follow here are published with permission of *Archives of Ophthalmology*[90, 91] and Drs. Silverman and Flynn.[92]

The early classification of ROP by Reese and colleagues was based upon observations made with the use of the direct ophthalmoscope.[93] With the introduction of the indirect ophthalmoscope, improved visualization of the retina permitted more detailed observations of the early stages of ROP. Much of what has been learned during the past 2 decades about acute ROP fails to fit within classification system of Reese et al.[93] Furthermore, the real incidence of the ROP may be increasing, although the evidence for this is not conclusive. Treatment of the disease in its active and cicatricial form has been advocated, but it is not always clear which disease stage is being treated and what the results of such treatment are. Given our improved ability to diagnose earlier stages of the disease and rapidly evolving basic and clinical research in the area of potentially beneficial therapies, the need for a new classification system of the acute stages of ROP has become apparent.

Classification

The system presented by the Committee for the Classification of Retinopathy of Prematurity differs from previous systems in that it permits the examiner to specify at the outset two parameters of the disease not recognized in other classification systems. These are the *location* of the disease in the retina and the *extent* of the developing vasculature involved. In addition, the examiner grades the retinopathy according to a system more consistent with current clinical observations.

Location

For the purpose of defining the variable of location, three zones of retinal involvement are recognized (Fig 26B–3). Each zone is centered on the optic disc rather than the macula, contrary to standard retinal drawings. The new scheme was selected because normal retinal vascular growth proceeds outward from the disc toward the ora serrata in an orderly fashion. The first two zones occupy that portion of the fundus that lies within a circle drawn by using the disc as the center and the distance to the nasal ora serrata at the horizontal meridian as its radius. Therefore, any ROP that is circumferential must, by definition, fall into one of these two posterior zones.

Zone I.—The posterior pole, or inner zone, consists of a circle (see Fig 26B–3) whose radius subtends an angle of 30 degrees and extends from the disc to twice the distance from the disc to the center of the macula. The limits of the zone are consequently defined as twice the disc-fovea distance in all directions from the optic disc (i.e., an arc of 60 degrees).

TABLE 26B–2.
Additional Criteria Regarding Frequency and Timing of Ocular Examinations According to Flynn*

1. Conceptual age (measured in weeks) = gestational age at birth + age postpartum
2. Conceptual age places all infants on same time axis
3. Greatest likelihood of diagnosing ROP is between 35 and 45 weeks' conceptual age (85% of diagnoses are made during this time period)
4. If vascularization is noted up to nasal ora serrata and temporal periphery, probability of developing serious acute complications from ROP is rare. Follow-up in 6 months recommended
5. If vascularization extends to retinal periphery anterior to equator but not quite to nasal ora (outer zone II by ICROP), recommends monthly follow-up examinations
6. If vascularization extends only to region anterior to equator (inner zone II by ICROP), recommends weekly follow-up examinations because large area of retina is at risk for progression of disease to cicatricial stages

*From Flynn JT: Discussion of "Screening criteria for the detection of retinopathy of prematurity in patients in a neonatal intensive care unit." *J Pediatr Ophthalmol Strabismus* 1987; 24:215. Used with permission.

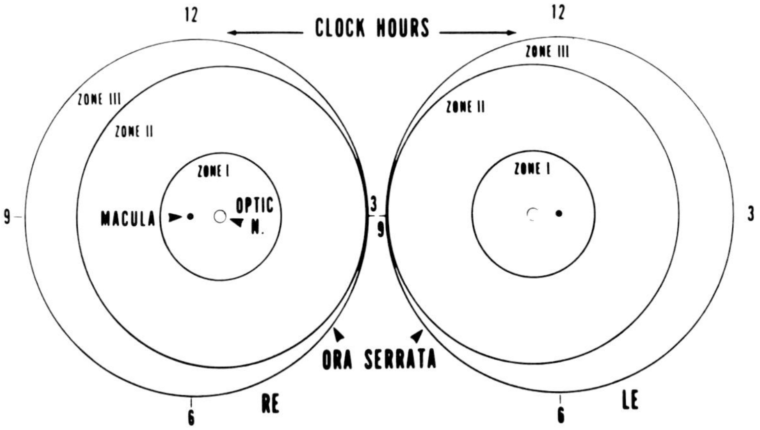

FIG 26B–3.
Scheme of the retinas of the right eye (RE) and the left eye (LE). Note the zone borders and clock hours used to describe the location and extent of ROP. (From Flynn JT: An international classification of retinopathy of prematurity, in Silverman WA, Flynn JT (eds): *Retinopathy of Prematurity II. Contemporary Issues in Fetal and Neonatal Medicine.* Boston, Blackwell Scientific Publications, 1985, pp 1–17; and Committee for the Classification of Retinopathy of Prematurity: An international classification of retinopathy of prematurity. *Arch Ophthalmol* 1984; 102:1130–1131. Used with permission.)

Zone II.—The middle area extends from the edge of zone I peripherally to a position tangential to the nasal ora serrata (at 3 o'clock in the right eye, 9 o'clock in the left eye) and around to an area near the temporal anatomic equator. The temporal edge of zone II cannot be defined with precision in clinical practice because the anatomic landmarks needed to determine the equator in a premature infant are obscured. Indeed, these landmarks are sufficiently varied in humans to render precise location difficult at any age.

Zone III.—The outermost area is the residual crescent of retina anterior to zone II. This is the zone that is vascularized last in the eyes of premature infants and is the most frequently involved with ROP.

Extent of the Disease

Extent of the involvement is specified by hours of the clock. As the observer looks at each eye, 3 o'clock is nasal (to the right) in the right eye and temporal in the left eye, and 9 o'clock is temporal (to the left) in the right eye and nasal in the left eye (see Fig 26B–3).

Staging the Disease

In addition to the two aforementioned parameters of classification, the final one to be specified is the severity of abnormal vascular response observed. Four stages are recognized, and staging for the eye as a whole is by the most severe manifestation present. However, for purposes of recording the complete examination, the extent of each stage is defined by clock hours.

Stage 1: Demarcation Line.—The initial feature of ROP is a thin but definite structure that separates the avascular retina anteriorly from the vascularized retina posteriorly (Plate 1). There are recognizable abnormal branching or arcading of vessels leading up to the demarcation line. It is relatively flat, lies within the plane of the retina, and is white in color.

Stage 2: Ridge.—The demarcation line of stage 1 now has grown, has height and width, occupies a volume, and extends up out of the plane of the retina (Plate 2). The ridge may change in color from white to pink, and vessels may leave the plane of the retina to enter the new elevated structure. Small isolated tufts of new vessels lying on the surface of the retina may be seen posterior to the ridge. Such tufted vascular lesions do not constitute the fibrovascular growth that is a necessary condition for stage 3.

Stage 3: Ridge With Extraretinal Fibrovascular Proliferation.—At the next level of severity, extraretinal fibrovascular proliferative tissue is added to the ridge of stage 2 (Plate 3). The characteristic locations where the new proliferating tissue may be found are (1) continuous with the posterior aspect of the ridge, which causes a ragged appearance of the ridge as proliferation becomes more extensive; (2) immediately posterior to the ridge but not always appearing to be connected with it; and (3) into the vitreous perpendicular to the retinal plane. Fibrovascular proliferation may be seen in any or all of these locations in stage 3 ROP.

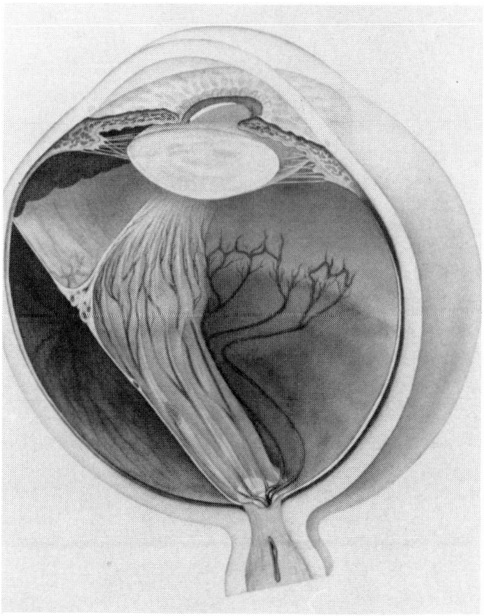

FIG 26B–5.
Artist's rendering of stage 4: subtotal retinal detachment including the fovea. (From International Committee for the Classification of the Late Stages of Retinopathy of Prematurity: International classification of retinopathy of prematurity II. The classification of retinal detachment. *Arch Ophthalmol* 1987; 105:906–912. Used with permission.)

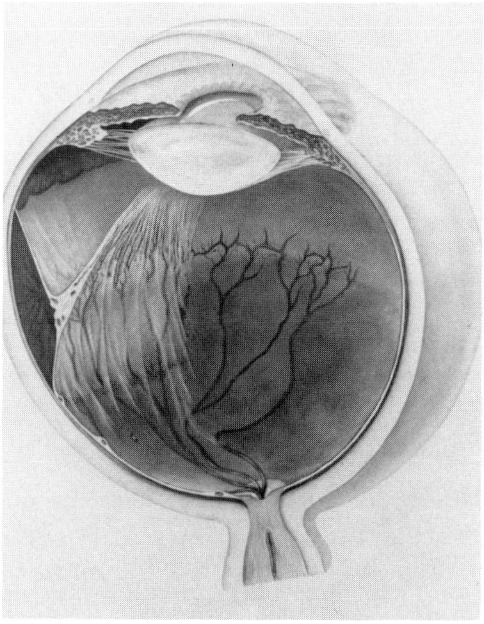

FIG 26B–4.
Artist's rendering of stage 4 ROP: subtotal retinal detachment that remains outside of the fovea. (From International Committee for the Classification of the Late Stages of Retinopathy of Prematurity: International classification of retinopathy of prematurity II. The classification of retinal detachment. *Arch Ophthalmol,* 1987; 105:906–912. Used with permission.)

Stage 4: Retinal Detachment.—At the next level of severity there is evidence of unequivocal detachment of the retina (Figs 26B–4 and 26B–5). The change may be caused by an exudative effusion of fluid, traction, or both, even in this early stage.

Stage 4A, *Extrafoveal Retinal Detachment* (see Fig 26B–4), is a concave, traction type of detachment that occurs in the periphery without involvement of the macula. The prognosis of vision, in the absence of extension posteriorly, is relatively good. Generally these detachments are located in the anterior parts of zone II or zone III. They may be circumferential, in which case they extend for 360 de-

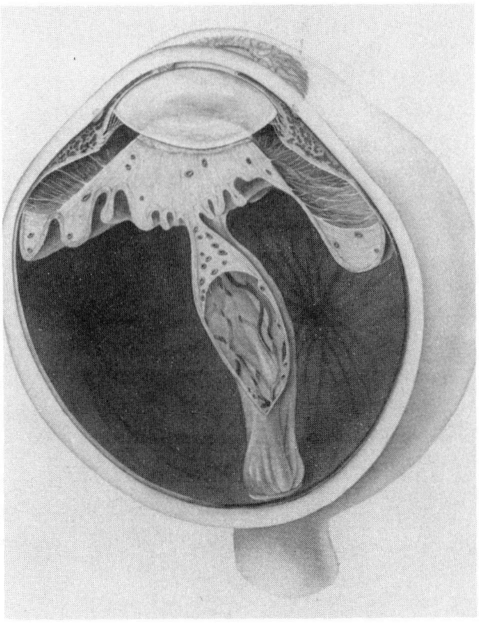

FIG 26B–6.
Artist's rendering of stage 5: total retinal detachment extending posteriorly in a narrow funnel to the optic disc. (From International Committee for the Classification of the Late Stages of Retinopathy of Prematurity: International classification of retinopathy of prematurity II. The classification of retinal detachment. *Arch Ophthalmol* 1987; 105:906–912. Used with permission.)

grees, or segmental and occupy only a portion of the circumference of the periphery.[91]

Stage 4, *Partial Retinal Detachment* including the fovea (see Fig 26B–5), is segmental and usually extends in the form of a fold from the disc through zone I to involve zone II and zone III. The prognosis for vision in this second segmental type of subtotal retinal detachment is poor.[91]

Stage 5: Total Retinal Detachment.—Stage 5, total retinal detachment (Fig 26B–6), is always funnel shaped. The configuration of the funnel itself permits a subdivision of this stage. For descriptive purpose, the committee divided the funnel into an anterior and posterior part. When open both anteriorly and posteriorly, the detachment has a concave configuration and extends to the optic disc. A second frequent configuration is one in which the funnel is narrow in both its anterior and posterior aspects and the detached retina is located just behind the lens. A third less common type is one in which the funnel is open anteriorly but narrowed posteriorly. Least common is a funnel that is narrow anteriorly and open posteriorly. These more unusual configurations of the funnel-shaped detachment of stage 5 ROP can sometimes be appreciated by ultrasonography.[91]

Serial examinations may be required to be certain of a true detachment. It should be emphasized that the presence of elevated retinal vessels running from the retinal plane to the height of the ridge does not constitute a posterior detachment.[91]

"Plus" Disease.—Progressive vascular incompetence accompanying the changes described at the edge of the abnormally developing retinal vasculature is characterized by increasing dilation and tortuosity of the peripheral retinal vessels, iris vascular engorgement, pupillary rigidity, and vitreous haze. The designation "plus" should be added only when and if the vascular changes are so marked that the posterior veins are enlarged and the arterioles tortuous (Plate 4). For example, the ridge of stage 2 ROP combined with posterior vascular dilation and tortuosity would be written stage 2+ ROP. When the ROP is located in zone I or posterior zone II and "plus" disease is present, the disorder may progress very rapidly.

Recording the Results

A detailed computer-compatible examination record for detailing the ophthalmic examination results has been developed (Fig 26B–7). Should the disease be amenable to surgical therapy, the examination record may be adapted to permit preoperative, intraoperative, and postoperative recording of observations on a single form.

The more posterior the disease and the greater the amount of involved retinal vascular tissue, the more serious the disease. This is the unifying principle underlying the inter-

A

RETINOPATHY OF PREMATURITY (ROP) OPHTHALMIC EXAMINATION RECORD II

BIOGRAPHICAL DATA

Name_______________________________ Hospital # __ __ __ __ __ __

Birthdate (MM/DD/YY) __ __/__ __/__ __ Sex (M=1, F=2) __

Birthweight (grams) __ __ __ __ Gestational Age (weeks) __ __

Multiple Births (Single-1, Twin=2, Triplet=3) __

EXAMINATION:

Date of Exam __ __/__ __/__ __ Examiner's Initials or # __ __ __

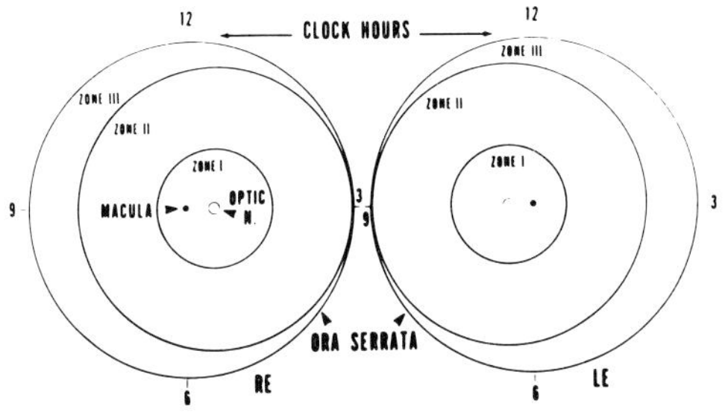

B

O.D. (Z I: 11-12, 10-11, 9-10, 8-9, 7-8, 6-7 | 12-1, 1-2, 2-3, 3-4, 4-5, 5-6; Z II; Z III)

O.S. (Z I: 11-12, 10-11, 9-10, 8-9, 7-8, 6-7 | 12-1, 1-2, 2-3, 3-4, 4-5, 5-6; Z II; Z III)

0 = No view possible
1 = Demarcation line
2 = Ridge
3 = Ridge plus extraretinal proliferation
4 = Stage 4A, subtotal R.D. without macula detachment
5 = Stage 4B, subtotal R.D. with macula detachment
6 = Stage 5, total detachment, open funnel
7 = Stage 5, total detachment, narrow funnel
8 = Stage 5, type undetermined
9 = Avascular, retina attached

Other Findings

O.D. O.S.

__ If Stage 3: 0=no info, 1=mild, 2=moderate, 3=severe __
__ Dilatation/tortuosity posterior vessels: 0=no information, 1=yes, 2=no __

O.D. O.S.

NATURE OF DETACHMENT

__ 1. Type of detachment present __
0 = no information
1 = none
2 = traction
3 = exudative
4 = combined
5 = rhegmatogenous

__ 2. Macula __
0 = no information
1 = attached
2 = shallow detachment
3 = high detachment

__ 3. Peripheral Trough __
1 = not visible
2 = present

__ 4. Subretinal fluid __
0 = no information
1 = clear
2 = bloody
3 = exudate

C

ANTERIOR SEGMENT
(0 = no information, 1 = yes, 2 = no)

O.D. O.S.

1. Cornea
   - __ Clear __
   - __ Cloudy __
2. Anterior chamber
   - __ Normal depth __
   - __ Shallow __
   - __ Absent __
3. Iris
   - __ Normal __
   - __ Active vasculature __
   - __ Atrophy __
   - __ Synechiae __
4. Pupil
   - __ Normal __
   - __ Fixed __
   - __ Secluded __
5. Lens
   - __ Clear __
   - __ Cataract __
6. Retrolental space
   - __ Clear __
   - __ Vascularized membrane __
   - __ Opaque membrane __
7. Vitreous
   - __ Clear __
   - __ Hemorrhage __

REGRESSED ROP
(0 = no information, 1 = Present, 2 = Absent)

A. Peripheral Changes

Vascular

O.D. O.S.

__ Failure to vascularize to ora __
__ Abnormal branching __
__ Vascular arcades __
__ Telangiectatic vessels __

Retinal

__ Pigmentary changes __
__ V-R interface changes __
__ Thin retina __
__ Peripheral folds __
__ Vitreous membranes __

D

B. Posterior Changes

Vascular

O.D. O.S.

__ Tortuosity __
__ Straightening of vessels __
__ Decrease in angle of insertion of major temporal arcade __

Retinal

__ Pigmentary changes __
__ Distortion/ectopia of macula __
__ Fold of retina __
__ V-R interface changes __
__ Vitreous membranes __
__ Dragging of retina over disc __
__ Traction/rhegmatogenous retinal detachment __

FIG 26B–7.
Ophthalmic examination form for ROP. (From International Committee for the Classification of the Late Stages of Retinopathy of Prematurity: International classification of retinopathy of prematurity II. The classification of retinal detachment. *Arch Ophthalmol* 1987; 105:906–912. Used with permission.)

national classification system. The staging of the disease at any given location expresses the natural history and evolution of events at the border between vascularized and avascular retina. The classification system is designed to permit the examiner full latitude in transcribing his observations so that they will be immediately intelligible to another examiner who may not have had the opportunity to examine the specific infant.

Problems Confronted

The committee recognized that no classification, including the present one, is perfect. During deliberations, problem areas were encountered for which interim solutions were developed. The following problems occurred.

Definition of Zone

Defining anatomic landmarks, apart from the optic disc and ora serrata, are difficult to discern in the eye of the premature infant. The boundaries of zones I and II, for example, are only approximate. The same can be said of zones II and III; although when vascular development has reached the nasal ora, any disease found elsewhere is by definition in zone III. The committee recommended that when doubt exists as to the appropriate zone to locate the disease it be classified as lying on the posterior side of a debated boundary.

Stage 3 Disease Problems

The committee clearly recognized the need to further subdivide stage 3 disease for its potential prognostic significance. It chose as its yardstick the amount of fibrovascular proliferative tissue present. The presence of only limited amounts would constitute mild stage 3 (see Plate 5). If, on the other hand, significant amounts of tissue are seen infiltrating the vitreous and proliferating posteriorly from the ridge, moderate stage 3 would be present (Plate 6). Finally, if massive infiltration of the tissues surrounding the ridge is occurring, the threshold for severe stage 3 has been reached (Plate 7).

Differential Diagnosis

Occasionally vitreous hemorrhage may be observed at the time of examination. In such cases one should consider the possibility that the vitreous hemorrhage resulted from trauma at birth or a hemorrhagic diathesis rather than ROP. Similarly, the presence of a complete congenital retinal detachment should bring to mind the possibility of Norrie's disease for consideration in the differential diagnosis. Other causes of leukokoria must also be considered such as persistent hyperplastic primary vitreous, retinal dysplasia, Coats' disease, or retinoblastoma (see Chapters 7 and 22). In older children, peripheral retinal abnormalities typical of ROP must be distinguished from familial exudative vitreoretinopathy as well as from myopic, traumatic, and inflammatory conditions that may produce peripheral retinal disorders.[67]

TREATMENT

An effective means for the prevention and treatment of ROP remains to be found. At the present time there is no universally accepted therapy for acute or cicatricial ROP. Several investigations examining various treatment methods have been pursued. The three areas of greatest research for the treatment of ROP are (1) the use of vitamin E for prophylaxis and possible prevention of progression of acute ROP, (2) the use of cryotherapy and photocoagulation for treating severe acute ROP, and (3) surgical intervention by means of scleral buckling for retinal detachment from ROP and/or intraocular vitreoretinal surgery using mechanical vitreous cutting instruments for the treatment of severe cicatricial disease.

Vitamin E Therapy

Vitamine E (tocopherol) is a lipophilic substance that is distributed in the lipid bilayer of cell membranes. It is believed that vitamin E plays an important role in maintaining cell membrane integrity by functioning as a "scavenger" of oxygen free radicals that inhibit the oxidation of membrane lipids and prevent cell lysis.[94] Tissue levels of tocopherol in newborn infants are initially low in comparison to levels found in adults. Once nursing has begun, however, the levels of tocopherol normally reach or exceed normal levels found in adults.[95] In premature infants tocopherol levels are lower than those found in full-term infants and remain subnormal until feedings are initiated.[96, 97]

The first report on the possible role of vitamin E in the development of ROP was by Owens and Owens in 1949.[15] The hypothesis of these investigators was that since many premature infants were supplemented with fat-soluble vitamins A, D, and K because of difficulty absorbing fats the failure of clinicians to provide supplementation with vitamin E might be responsible for the development of ROP. Their report on the use of orally administered tocopherol acetate provided encouraging results on the possible benefits of vitamin E in preventing ROP. Investigators at other institutions, however, were unable to repeat their results,[98, 99] and for many years the use of vitamin E in the premature was abandoned.

In the 1970s, with the improved sophistication of life support technology for premature infants and the accompanying rapid rise in survival of very low–birth weight infants,[100] the number of neonates developing visual loss from ROP multiplied.[53,101] In a renewed vitamin E trial by Johnson and colleagues[102] in 1974 using intramuscular tocopherol acetate ester, positive results were also reported. A considerable number of clinical and experimental studies have followed on the use of supplemental vitamin E to counterbalance body deficiencies that may contribute to the development of ROP.[103–118] Many of these studies have strongly suggested that vitamin E deficiency may be a contributing factor in developing visual loss from ROP. However, combining the results of various studies to obtain statistically significant numbers to evaluate the efficacy of vitamin E in preventing ROP has been hindered by differences in study design, differences in classification schemes for categorizing ROP, and variation between studies in routes of administration, drug formulation, and dosages of administered vitamin E.

Three hypotheses regarding the etiology of ROP that incorporate a therapeutic role for the use of vitamin E are (1) the oxygen injury hypothesis, (2) the embryonic or flow hypothesis, and (3) the spindle cell hypothesis.

In the *oxygen injury hypothesis*, the initial injury to immature retinal capillaries and arterioles is believed to be the result of oxidative damage from oxygen-derived free radicals. When premature infants are exposed to supplemental oxygen administration, there is an abrupt rise in arterial Po_2 levels. Because of low tissue levels of tocopherol in the newborn premature infant, direct oxygen-related injury to retinal vessel cell membranes may occur. Because tocopherol is the primary antioxidant in cell membranes, administration of tocopherol before cellular injury occurs could theoretically reduce the possibility of developing ROP from retinal vessel injury.[100]

In the *embryonic or flow hypothesis*, it is postulated that the failure of forward blood flow in retinal vessels due to constriction of arterioles in response to elevated Po_2 levels results in interference with the normal organization and remodeling of growing endothelium.[100] In this hypothesis, the injury to immature retinal vessels is ascribed to the disruption of normal vascular growth from irreversible vasoconstriction rather than to cell membrane damage. If the initial injury is secondary to ischemia resulting from hypoperfusion, tocopherol could theoretically be expected to modulate the extent of injury by suppressing auto-oxidation in damaged tissue.[119]

In the *spindle cell hypothesis*, the precursors of endothelial cells (i.e., spindle cells) are postulated to sustain oxidative injury from the elevation of levels of arterial Po_2. Resultant intracellular biochemical alterations are believed to halt normal vascular growth and trigger the formation of gap junctions between spindle cells, with subsequent secretion of angiogenic factors and development of ROP. In this hypothesis, the early administration of tocopherol downmodulates the biochemical perturbation of the spindle cells and diminishes the likelihood of developing neovascularization and ROP.[104, 120]

A number of recent studies have demonstrated numerous deleterious side effects from the clinical use of vitamin E in premature infants. These negative side effects have included the development of retinal hemorrhages,[121] necrotizing enterocolitis,[122] sepsis,[123] intraventricular hemorrhage,[124] and death from intravenous administration.[125] Such reports of severe infant morbidity and mortality from the administration of tocopherol emphasizes the importance of establishing safe and acceptable dosages and methods of administration of vitamin E in premature infants. The optimal levels of tocopherol for the body and the ideal form of administration for correcting its deficiency remain obscure and in need of further clarification.[67] At the present time, the risks of developing complications from the use of vitamin E as compared with the benefits of potentially diminishing the incidence of ROP remain controversial and subject to debate.[67] Further basic research on tocopherol pharmacology and on the pathophysiology of ROP must be done prior to the design of a definitive large multicenter clinical trial that could provide clinical recommendations on the role of vitamin E in the prophylaxis and treatment of ROP.

Cryotherapy and Photocoagulation

Prior to the introduction of the technique of retinal ablation by means of cryotherapy or photocoagulation, no treatment was considered effective in arresting the progression of severe ROP. Several reports on the use of cryotherapy and photocoagulation in the treatment of ROP have appeared in the literature over the past several years.[126–145] Encouraging results from a number of medical centers in Japan,[146–157] Canada,[159, 160] and Israel[131] have suggested that ablative therapy may be beneficial in selected cases of ROP. The treatment rationale is that ablation of nonvascularized ischemic retinal tissue can minimize abnormal preretinal vasoproliferative tissue in ROP (as in diabetes). As a result of these studies, cryotherapy—which is technically much easier to perform in the nursery than light photocoagulation—is being used for the treatment of acute stage III ROP in several countries throughout the world. The objective of treatment of stage III ROP with cryotherapy is the prevention of retinal detachment during the active phase of the disease.

It is important to note that some studies have indicated that cryotherapy is not always useful in the treatment of acute ROP.[133] In addition, a few reports have suggested deleterious effects from the use of cryotherapy in ROP.[132, 157] Furthermore, because of the high rate of spontaneous regression of ROP without intervention, it is difficult to objectively evaluate the effectiveness of cryotherapy in the treatment of ROP without a controlled therapeutic study. It is known that cryotherapy does not always prevent blindness.[140] In addition, the use of cryotherapy is not risk free because there are risks from general anesthesia and cardiac arrythmias.[145]

Multicenter Trial of Cryotherapy for ROP (CRYO-ROP)

In the United States, the use of cryotherapy in infants with ROP is currently the subject of a multi-center clinical trial. The Multicenter Trial of Cryotherapy for Retinopathy of Prematurity (CRYO-ROP)[141, 142] has been designed to take advantage of the fact that ROP usually progresses in a symmetric fashion. Consequently, enrollees in the study will receive the experimental application of cryotherapy in one eye while the untreated fellow eye will serve as a control. The trial is designed so that no enrolled patient will receive cryotherapy to both eyes. Twenty-three regional medical centers throughout the United States are participating in this study. It is anticipated that within the next two to three years, the results of the study should provide sufficient information to objectively determine whether or not cryotherapy is helpful for treating selected acute stages of ROP.

Of note, a recent interim report on preliminary 3-month outcome data of the multicenter trial indicates that cryotherapy is indeed effective in reducing the risk of visually unfavorable retinal pathology that may develop from progression of a dangerous threshold level of stage 3 ROP.[161] An unfavorable outcome—defined as a posterior retinal detachment, a retinal fold involving the macula, or retrolental tissue—was found to be significantly less frequent in eyes undergoing cryotherapy (21.8%) as compared with eyes that remained untreated (43%). These preliminary data, at least at 3 months after treatment, indicate that cryotherapy reduces the risk of developing unfavorable retinal outcomes in ROP in approximately 50% of selected cases that have a high potential for producing severe visual loss. It is important to note that at the time of this writing the follow-up of these patients remained incomplete and that there was insufficient long-term data to permit conclusive recommendations regarding the efficacy of applying cryotherapy to *both* eyes of a patient with significant bilateral ROP. However, the preliminary data do justify the recommendation that cryotherapy be applied to at least one eye of symmetric cases that meet the study criteria of the dangerous threshold level of stage 3 ROP. Subsequent reports of the CRYO-ROP Study should provide clinically significant long-term data regarding the safety and efficacy of bilateral cryotherapy in the treatment of the potentially blinding stages of this disorder.[162]

Surgery for Retinopathy of Prematurity

Retinal detachment in active ROP commonly occurs by means of the following two mechanisms, occurring alone or in combination: (1) vitreoretinal "traction," which produces partial or total retinal detachment, and (2) subretinal serous exudation producing fluid accumulation that results in an "exudative" retinal detachment. The former two types of retinal detachment are referred to as "nonrhegmatogenous" retinal detachment because there is no "hole" or "break" in the retina. In older children who have had previous ROP without blinding sequelae, a late-onset rhegmatogenous retinal detachment may occur as a result of a retinal hole or break. The treatment of this latter type of retinal detachment (i.e., rhegmatogenous) is commonly accomplished by means of scleral buckling surgery.[160–166] The role of scleral buckling surgery in the former type of retinal detachment (i.e., nonrhegmatogenous) in acute ROP is controversial, although many authors have reported favorable results when using this technique.[165–174] According to Palmer,[67] although at least 50% of ROP patients with scleral buckling for nonrhegmatogenous retinal detachment reportedly respond well to this surgery, a satisfactorily controlled study has yet to be conducted in these patients. Because partial nonrhegmatogenous retinal detachments spontaneously resolve in a significant number of infants with acute ROP, the therapeutic value vs. the risks of early surgical intervention from scleral buckling requires careful consideration.[67]

Surgery for severe retinal detachment occurring in advanced cicatricial stages of ROP consists of "closed" and "open-sky" vitrectomy techniques. Eyes that undergo surgery with these techniques, most of which have stage 5 RLF with total retinal detachment and leukokoria, in the past were relegated to complete blindness. Understandably, surgeons feel an obligation to intervene in an attempt to salvage any potential vision. Nonetheless, controversy exists as to the advantages and disadvantages of various techniques.

In the closed vitrectomy technique as advocated by Charles,[175] after removal of the lens by ultrasonic fragmentation, the vitreous or hyaloid membranes that lie in the retrolental space are segmented by making pie-shaped cuts. Preretinal membranes are then delaminated or removed from the surface of the retina and are circumscribed peripherally near the ora serrata to eliminate anterior "loop" traction. Charles has reported anatomic reattachment in 45% of over 400 consecutive cases,[176] with similar success reported by other surgeons using closed vitrectomy techniques.[181–183]

In the open-sky vitrectomy technique as advocated by Hirose and Schepens,[184, 185] the cornea is removed and stored during the surgery in tissue culture fluid. The lens is then removed by intracapsular extraction with a cryoprobe, and the retrolental membrane is incised, dissected, and excised 360 degrees from the surface of the retina. Vitreous remnants are removed, and hyaluronic acid (Healon) is injected to flatten the retina, after which the cornea is sutured back to its original place. Hirose and Schepens report an overall success rate similar to that of Charles, with anatomic reattachment of 38% in well over 150 cases.[184] Visual success in Charles' series was reported at about 36%.[176] The minimum criteria for a visually successful outcome as defined by Charles was the "unequivocal ability to pick up small objects and ambulate in familiar surroundings without striking obstacles."[175]

Reports of successful anatomic reattachment with some useful postoperative vision pays tribute to the enormous strides that retina-vitreous surgery has made in instrumentation, microscopic technique, and intraocular illumination over the past several years. Despite the anatomic success, according to Silverman and Flynn,[55]

> There [remains] a real and compelling question to be answered before an all-out surgical campaign is mounted against ROP. For each infant we must ask, will this infant see better for a longer time as the result of the proposed surgical intervention? It will take not only the best efforts of surgeons but also the application of the highest state-of-the-art skills of physiologists, psychologists and ophthalmologists interested in the development of vision to answer the current questions about surgical treatment of cicatricial ROP.

According to Palmer,[67] surgeons at several medical centers are presently developing techniques to more effectively manage the dreaded complication of blindness resulting from ROP. Investigators are planning collaborative studies of safety and efficacy of these combined procedures.

DISCUSSION WITH FAMILY AND PEDIATRICIANS

The discussion between the ophthalmologist and family and neonatologist and/or pediatrician should encompass the various aspects of the diagnosis and pathology of ROP as well as acute therapeutic options, alternatives, and potential outcomes. The ophthalmologist must work closely with the primary-care pediatric provider and be prepared to render the necessary care as well as support and advice to the infant's family. If specialized care is required that is not within the scope of practice of the consulting ophthalmologist, the patient should be referred to a qualified subspecialist knowledgeable in the diagnosis and treatment of ROP. In all instances of ROP, the need for long-term follow-up should be stressed.

Infants with ROP will vary in degree of disease severity and subsequent visual outcome. Familiarity with developmental, emotional, and social issues relevant to infants with severe visual impairment enables the physician to provide needed support and advice to the infant's family at a time of emotional shock and confusion. Furthermore, of relevance to physicians responsible for rendering care to infants with ROP is an understanding of medicolegal issues germane to the maintenance of high standards of care and avoidance of unnecessary litigation.

Therapeutic Options and Alternatives

It is the task of the ophthalmologist to present the findings of his examination to the primary-care provider and family. The various therapeutic options and alternatives including oxygen monitoring, vitamin E therapy, cryotherapy, photocoagulation, and surgery for

ROP were discussed in the previous section as well as in Chapter 26A by Dr. Phelps. The benefits, alternatives, and risks of therapy must be clearly explained. Because of the investigational nature of certain therapies (e.g., vitamin E and cryotherapy), informed consent is of paramount importance and in all instances should be obtained.

Long-Term Outcome and Follow-up Care

It is estimated that approximately 22,000 infants with birth weights of less than 1,500 gm survive annually in the United States.[55] As previously noted, ROP is responsible for producing significant vision impairment in approximately 1,300 and severe visual loss in 450 to 500 of these infants each year.[1–3]

Significant and Severe Visual Impairment

Although a full discussion of the developmental, emotional, and social implications of infants with significant and severe visual impairment from ROP is beyond the scope of this chapter, certain key issues require attention.

Parents of children blinded by ROP often experience frustration and anxiety after learning of their child's condition. In general, although information regarding their child's visual impairment is presented to them by the physician in a compassionate and sympathetic manner, the parents nonetheless are often left with many unanswered questions and unresolved fears.[186] While ophthalmologists and pediatricians do not generally have formal training in the developmental styles of blind children or in techniques related to their education, an understanding of certain general principles serves to foster improved communication with the families and appropriate referral for developmental intervention.[186]

According to Teplin,[186] Fraiberg,[187] Gesell and colleagues,[188] and Warren,[189] there are differing developmental pathways of blind and sighted children. By prolonged visual tracking of people and objects, a sighted infant learns important concepts such as object permanence and causal relationships.[186–188] Similarly, visually cued imitation promotes learning and facilitates advances in mobility, language, and socialization.[186] The absence of normal vision impacts the development of blind or severely visually impaired children. Moreover, children with blindness and severe visual impairment may also be handicapped in approximately 35% to 70% of cases by associated mental retardation, cerebral palsy, hearing impairment, and epilepsy.[186, 190, 191, 192] Many of these children, as a consequence of other associated diseases (e.g., respiratory illness and cardiac disease), may require multiple hospitalizations including surgery. Taken together with their visual handicap, these additional impediments work to adversely affect development.[186]

Research on blind infants without other handicaps has demonstrated their capability of developing through the same stages and along remarkably similar timetables as sighted infants with the assistance of actively involved parents as initial mediators of the environment.[186] However, important differences in timing and sequence are observed in the development process.[186]

Factors such as guilt, stress, feelings of inadequacy, and tenuous bonding often overwhelm the parents, which may lead to infant emotional and developmental problems. Parental underexpectation and despair may give rise to parental overprotection and/or withdrawal, with resultant understimulation and withdrawal of the infant. This process may cause a viscious cycle of delayed development and/or emotional problems[186, 192] that further exacerbates parental feelings of withdrawal and emotional despair.

Physician awareness of parental needs and anxieties allows appropriate counseling and referral. All too frequently physician communication styles focus on describing pathological conditions and skim over or ignore emotional, developmental, and social issues.

According to Stetten,[194] a physician who wrote poignantly of his own deteriorating vision, as quoted by Teplin.[186]

> If after all [of the diagnostic and therapeutic manipulations of the patient's eyes] the patient still has a serious visual impairment, the ophthalmologist is missing an extraordinary opportunity if he or she fails to direct the patient's attention to . . . the aids and agencies designed to improve the quality of life of the visually handicapped person.

Proper communication with the infant's parents regarding social and developmental issues can be of vital importance to the parent's subsequent outlook and coping strategies. Both the pediatrician and ophthalmologist should be prepared to engage in a dialogue with the family to encourage them to express their questions and fears.

> Frequently the pediatrician or family physician assumes that since the ophthalmologist is the eye specialist, he or she will know how to answer the mother's questions about how best to raise her blind child and where intervention services are located. But most ophthalmologists, rigorously trained as surgical subspecialists, have little or no training in counseling parents on these developmental issues.
>
> Blindness is a tragic handicap. However, physicians can greatly enhance the quality of the lives of their visually impaired young patients and their families. An appreciation of the impact of blindness on normal development, a knowledge of the community and national services available, and a willingness to confront and overcome physician attitudinal barriers are the necessary ingredients for effectively helping parents in encouraging optimal development of their visually impaired children.[186]

Less Severe Ocular Sequelae of Retinopathy of Prematurity

In addition to infants with severe vision impairment, there are greater numbers of infants with regressed ROP who, as they mature, are at risk for developing more subtle but no less significant visual problems that require attention by the pediatrician and ophthalmologist.

The less severe but more common forms of ocular and visual impairment from ROP result in children with mild to moderate residual cicatricial changes of ROP. However, ocular sequelae can occur in cases with near total regression and even in cases with ophthalmoscopically confirmed totally regressed ROP.[194] Infants with regressed ROP are susceptible to developing: refractive errors,[195–197] amblyopia,[195] strabismus,[197,198] nystagmus,[197] glaucoma,[199] cataracts,[200] corneal changes,[201,202] and retinal and vitreous abnormalities[177] (Table 26B–3).

According to Kushner,[194] all children who have been diagnosed as having ROP, even if it totally regresses, should be monitored at least until they are literate and until amblyopia and strabismus can be definitely ruled out.

> Followup must include streak retinoscopy after adequate cycloplegia, and should be carried out by an ophthalmologist comfortable with making those determinations in preliterate children.
>
> The presence of amblyopia or strabismus should be treated vigorously in affected children and the ophthalmologist should not conclude that the problem cannot be corrected because of the presence of "RLF."
>
> Any patient that develops any significant degree of peripheral retinal cicatrization should be advised to have continued and regular ophthalmologic care throughout their life.
>
> All patients with any significant degree of

TABLE 26B–3.
Possible Sequelae of Regressed ROP According to Kushner*

1. Refractive errors
2. Amblyopia
3. Strabismus
4. Nystagmus
5. Glaucoma
6. Cataracts
7. Corneal pathology
8. Retinal and vitreous abnormalities

*From Kushner BJ: The sequelae of regressed retinopathy of prematurity, in Silverman WA, Flynn JT (eds): *Retinopathy of Prematurity II. Contempory Issues in Fetal and Neonatal Medicine.* Boston, Blackwell Scientific Publications, 1985, pp 239–247. Used with permission.

peripheral retinal cicatricial changes should be warned of the possibility of developing acute narrow angle glaucoma, or retinal detachment, and they should be alerted to the signs of those conditions.[194]

Medicolegal Aspects of Retinopathy of Prematurity

According to Bettman,[203] the number of medicolegal claims related to ROP is significant. In one analysis of 500 claims from all classifications in ophthalmology, 29 cases (5.8%) were found to be based upon ROP.[204]

In the aforementioned cases, claims were filed for reasons not always related to alleged substandard medical care. The role that oxygen administration and degree of prematurity played in the filing of these claims was only one facet of the problem. Related socioeconomic factors that contributed to making ROP a target of medicolegal claims included poor communication between physician and parent, the sympathetic emotional impact that a ROP patient could have upon a jury, and a history of large awards to plaintiffs in ROP cases.

The etiology of ROP is multifactorial, and at the present time we have no way to establish precisely the duration or concentration of oxygen required so as to determine that oxygen is the principal cause of ROP.[205] In instances of extreme prematurity, despite meticulous monitoring and expert neonatal care, we cannot be certain that oxygen was the important contributory factor.[1,43] At the present time we are not yet able to accurately define the degree of prematurity that makes ROP likely.[1–3,203] Factors that impinge upon the decision to administer oxygen or not must take into consideration a risk-benefit determination that weighs the risks of developing respiratory distress, cerebral palsy, or possible death vs. the benefit of avoiding the development of ROP. These decisions fall within the realm of the neonatologist and pediatrician who should seek consultation and support from the ophthalmologist.[203] In the opinion of Bettman,[204] "a medicolegal claim in the name of one with apparent ROP should be pursued only if there has been a history of oxygen having been used for [a] significant period [of time] in amounts not required."

In a court of law the legal merits of a claim in ROP are based upon a medical standard that must be established by qualified experts willing to present necessary scientific knowledge.[205–207] Claims for damages could arise, for example, from a determination that improper oxygen therapy was administered, when death or hepatic failure has occurred as a result of improper (not Food and Drug Administration [FDA] approved) prophylactic vitamin E administration, or when there is a delay in obtaining ophthalmologic consultation that precludes possibly useful elective therapy, etc.[205] Whether liability is imposed under specific circumstances remains under the purview of a chosen jury.[205]

Assuming that "good medical care"[205] is rendered, the parental decision as to whether to file a claim or not essentially depends upon the nature and quality of the physician-parent relationship. The positive nature of this relationship in large measure is based upon human compassion and the sensitive conveyance of accurate information.

Insight regarding improving parental communication in cases of ROP can be gained from Bettman[203]:

> After a successful struggle to keep a tiny premature infant alive, the parents [generally] are permitted to take home a live and apparently healthy child. [The parents] might be unaware of the risk of blindness, the need for supplemental oxygen, or do not fully understand this. The unpleasant surprise of possible blindness [not communicated to the parents] results in anger that, in turn, brings the thought of suit to their minds.
>
> The timing of communication is important. If the risk of blindness is mentioned soon after birth, the parents can have a feeling of rejection. They might say, "I would rather have the baby dead than blind." Instead of stating the risk then, the physician should stress that the eyes will have to be carefully examined. The parents must be told of the threat of blindness, but this can be done two or three weeks

after birth, at which time [bonding has occurred and the likelihood that] they will want the infant [is higher].

With regard to other socioeconomic variables that may affect the decision to file a claim or not (i.e., the sympathetic emotional impact upon a jury and a history of large wards), one must keep in mind that claims may be filed even though there has been no evidence of substandard practice.[203]

> The sight of a blind child who has enophthalmos can influence a jury to award large sums—even though they have been presented with little or no evidence of substandard care. . . .
>
> This, plus the sympathy factor, has encouraged some attorneys to file claims and to persevere. These claims are occasionally successful. The court's rulings are not always based upon what might be substandard practice. Consider the following quotation from an associate justice of the Washington State Supreme Court: there is "a strong and growing tendency, where there is blame on neither side, to ask, in view of the exigencies of social justice, who can best bear the loss and hence to shift the loss by creating liability where there has been no fault."[203]

Guidelines developed by Bettman for physicians involved in the care of patients with ROP to reduce the incidence of medicolegal claims are as follows[204]:

I. Render good pediatric care with careful evaluation of oxygen need and proper monitoring of oxygen, pH, and CO_2.
II. Give full disclosure to the family with an open discussion of risks and alternative.
III. Complete documentation of the above. Documentation in cases in which there is a high risk of medicolegal claim is best accomplished by the following methods:
   A. Fully explain the risks, reasons for the risks, and the alternative.
   B. Ask for feedback to be certain that this is understood.
   C. Hand the patient's chart to the parents and have them write on the chart what they do understand.
   D. Correct any misunderstandings.
IV. Refer the high-risk pregnant mother to a tertiary-care center before delivery or the neonate to such a center if the circumstances permit.

CONCLUSION

In the preceding sections an overview of the condition of ROP has been given from the perspective of the ophthalmologist. The disorder was described, and recommendations were made regarding the technique and frequency of examination. Use and interpretation of the ICROP was summarized, and currently accepted as well as experimental treatment modalities were presented. Moreover, a perspective regarding fruitful interaction between the ophthalmologist and family and pediatrician was shared.

The literature regarding these and other aspects of ROP is vast. The reader is encouraged to bear in mind that additional study by further reading as outlined in the references and staying abreast of the rapidly evolving literature is necessary in order to maintain a proper perspective of this rapidly expanding area of both clinical and basic science research.

REFERENCES

1. Patz, A, Payne, JW: Retinopathy of prematurity (retrolental fibroplasia), in Duane TD, Jaeger EA (eds): *Clinical Ophthalmology,* vol 3. Philadelphia, Harper & Row, Publishers, Inc. 1987, pp 1–19.
2. Patz A: Symposium on retrolental fibroplasia: Summary. *Ophthalmology* 1979; 86:1761–1763.
3. Tasman W: The natural history of active retinopathy of prematurity. *Ophthalmology* 1984; 91:1499–1503.
4. Terry TL: Extreme prematurity and fibroplastic overgrowth or persistent vascular sheath behind each crystalline lens. I. Preliminary report. *Am J Ophthalmol* 1942; 25:203–205.
5. Terry HL: Fibroplastic overgrowth of persistent tunica vasculosa lentis in infants born prematurely. III. Studies in development and

regression of hyaloid artery and tunica vasculosa lentis. *Am J Ophthalmol* 1942; 25:1409–1423.

6. Terry HL: Fibroplastic overgrowth of persistent tunica vasculosa lentis in premature infants. II. Report of cases—Clinical aspects. *Arch Ophthalmol* 1943; 29:36–53.
7. Terry TL: Fibroplastic overgrowth of persistent tunica vasculosa lentis in premature infants. IV. Etiologic factors. *Arch Ophthalmol* 1943; 29:54–68.
8. Terry HL: Retrolental fibroplasia in premature infants. V. Further studies on fibroplastic overgrowth of persistent tunica vasculosa lentis. *Arch Ophthalmol* 1945; 33:203–208.
9. Terry HL: Ocular maldevelopment in extremely premature infants: Retrolental fibroplasia; general considerations. *JAMA* 1945; 138:582–585.
10. Silverman WA: A new affliction in premature infants, in *Retrolental Fibroplasia: A Modern Parable*. New York, Grune & Stratton, 1980.
11. Krause AC: Congenital encephalo-ophthalmic dysplasia. *Arch Ophthalmol* 1946; 36:387–444.
12. Unsworth AC: Retrolental fibroplasia. A preliminary report. *Arch Ophthalmol* 1948; 40:341–346.
13. Galloway NPR: Fibrosis of the posterior vascular sheath of the lens. *Proc R Soc Med* 1948; 4:724.
14. Kinsey VE, Zacharias L: Retrolental fibroplasia. *JAMA* 1949; 139:572–578.
15. Owens WC, Owens EU: Retrolental fibroplasia in premature infants. II. Studies on the prophylaxis of the disease: The use of alpha tocopheryl acetate. *Am J Ophthalmol* 1949; 32:1631–1637.
16. Silverman WA: Appendix A: Causes of RLF first ten years (1942–1952), in *Retrolental Fibroplasia: A Modern Parable*. New York, Grune & Stratton, 1980.
17. Orellana J: Identification of Retinopathy of prematurity/retrolental fibroplasia, in McPherson AR, Hittner HM, Kretzer FL (eds): *Retinopathy of Prematurity: Current Concepts and Controversies*. Toronto, BC Decker, Inc, 1986, pp 1–9.
18. Heath P: Pathology of retinopathy of prematurity: Retrolental fibroplasia. *Am J Ophthalmol* 1951; 43:1249–1259.
19. Campbell K: Intensive oxygen therapy as a possible cause of retrolental fibroplasia: A clinical approach. *Med J Aust* 1951; 2:48–50.
20. Ryan H: Retrolental fibroplasia. A clinicopathologic study. *Am J Ophthalmol* 1952; 35:329–342.
21. von Goldman H, Tobler W: Etiology of retrolental fibroplasia. *Schweiz Med Wochenschr* 1952; 82:381–385.
22. Patz A, Hoeck LE, DeLaCruz E: Studies on the effect of high oxygen administration in retrolental fibroplasia. Nursery observations. *Am J Ophthalmol* 1952; 27:1248–1253.
23. Lanman JT, Guy LP, Dancis J: Retrolental fibroplasia and oxygen therapy. *JAMA* 1954; 155:223–226.
24. Kinsey VE: Retrolental fibroplasia: Cooperative study of retrolental fibroplasia and the use of oxygen. *Arch Ophthalmol* 1956; 56:481–543.
25. Gyllensten LH, Hellstrom BD: Retrolental fibroplasia: Animal experiments—the effect of intermittently administered oxygen on the postnatal development of the eyes of full-term mice. A preliminary report. *Acta Paediatr Scand* 1952; 42:577–582.
26. Ashton N, Ward B, Serpell G: Direct observation of the effect of oxygen on developing vessels. Preliminary report. *Br J Ophthalmol* 1953; 38:513–520.
27. Ashton N, Cook C: Direct observation of the effect of oxygen on developing vessels. Preliminary report. *Br J Ophthalmol* 1954; 38:433–440.
28. Patz A, Eastham A, Higgingotham DH, et al: Oxygen studies in retrolental fibroplasia. II. The production of microscopic changes of retrolental fibroplasia in experimental animals. *Am J Ophthalmol* 1953; 36:1511–1522.
30. Guy LP, Lanman JT, Dancis J: The possibility of total elimination of retrolental fibroplasia by oxygen restriction. *Pediatrics* 1956; 17:247–251.
31. Slobody LB, Wasserman WE: *Survey of Clinical Pediatrics*. New York, McGraw-Hill International Book Co, 1963, p 160.
32. Flynn JT: Retrolental fibroplasia: Update, in *Pediatric Opthalmology and Strabismus. Transactions of the New Orleans Academy of Ophthalmology*. New York, Raven Press, 1986.
33. Lanman JT, Guy LP, Dancis J: Retrolental fibroplasia and oxygen therapy. *JAMA* 1954; 155:223–226.
34. Silverman WA: *Dunham's Premature Infants*, ed 3. New York, PB Hoeber, 1961.
35. McDonald AD: Cerebral palsy in children of

very low birth weight. *Arch Dis Child* 1963; 38:579.
36. Avery MD, Oppenheimer EH: Recent increase in mortality from hyaline embrane disease. *J Pediatr* 1960; 57:553.
37. Warley MA, Gairdner D: Respiratory distress syndrome of the newborn: Principles in treatment. *Arch Dis Child* 1962; 37:455.
38. McDonald AD: Cerebral palsy in children of very low birth weight. *Arch Dis Child* 1963; 38:579.
39. Cross KW: Cost of preventing retrolental fibroplasia? *Lancet* 1973; 2:954–956.
40. Heath P: Pathology of the retinopathy of prematurity: Retrolental fibroplasia. *Am J Ophthalmol* 1951; 34:1249–1268.
41. Patz A: Retrolental fibroplasia (retinopathy of prematurity). *Am J Ophthalmol* 1982; 94:552–554.
42. Alberman ED: Epidemiology of retinopathy of prematurity, in Silverman WA, Flynn JT (eds): *Retinopathy of Prematurity II. Contemporary Issues in Fetal and Neonatal Medicine.* Boston, Blackwell Scientific Publications, 1985, pp 249–266.
43. Kinsey VE, Arnold, Kalina RE, et al: Pao_2 levels and retrolental fibroplasia: A report of the cooperative study. *Pediatrics* 1977; 60:655.
44. Kingham JD: Acute retrolental fibroplasia. *Arch Ophthalmol* 1977; 95:39.
45. Gunn TR, Easdown J, Outerbridge EW, et al: Risk factors in retrolental fibroplasia. *Pediatrics* 1980; 6:1096.
46. Doray BH, Orquin J: Incidence of retinopathy of prematurity in *Syllabus: Retinopathy of Prematurity Conference,* vol 1. Washington, DC, Dec 4–6, 1981, pp 477–487.
47. Hittner HM, Godio LB, Rudolph AJ, et al: Retrolental fibroplasia: Efficacy of vitamin E in a double-blind clinical study of preterm infants. *N Engl J Med* 1981; 305:1365.
48. Kalina RE, Karr DJ: Retrolental fibroplasia: Experience over two decades in one institution, in *Syllabus: Retinopathy of Prematurity Conference,* vol 1. Washington, DC, Dec 4–6, 1981, pp 328–345.
49. Palmer EA: Natural history of retinopathy of prematurity, in *Syllabus: Retinopathy of Prematurity Conference,* vol 2. Washington, DC, Dec 4–6, 1981, pp 441–448.
50. Petersen RA: Six years of experience with retrolental fibroplasia in the joint program for neonatology at Harvard Medical School, in *Syllabus: Retinopathy of Prematurity Conference,* vol 1. Washington, DC, Dec 4–6, 1981, pp 346–351.
51. Procianoy RS, Garcia-Prats JA, Hittner HE, et al: An association between retinopathy of prematurity and intraventricular hemorrhage in very low birth weight infants. *Acta Paediatr Scand* 1981; 70:473.
52. Yamanouchi I, Igarashi I, Ouchi E: Incidence and severity of retinopathy of prematurity in low birth weight infants monitored by continuous transcutaneous oxygen monitoring, in *Syllabus: Retinopathy of Prematurity Conference,* vol 2. Washington, DC, Dec 4–6, 1981, pp 505–525.
53. Phelps DL: Vision loss due to retinopathy of prematurity. *Lancet* 1981; 1:606.
54. Phelps DL: Retinopathy of prematurity: An estimate of vision loss in the United States, 1979. *Pediatrics* 1981; 67:924.
55. Silverman WA, Flynn JT: Overview: A "developmental" retinopathy reconsidered, in Silverman WA, Flynn JT (eds): *Retinopathy of Prematurity II. Contemporary Issues in Fetal and Neonatal Medicine.* Boston, Blackwell Scientific Publications, 1985, pp xi–xxiii.
56. American Academy of Pediatrics. *Standards and Recommendations for Hospital Care of Newborn Infants,* ed 5. Evanston, Ill, American Academy of Pediatrics, 1971.
57. Horbar JD: Monitoring and controlling neonatal oxygen therapy, in Silverman WA, Flynn JT (eds): *Retinopathy of Prematurity II. Contemporary Issues in Fetal and Neonatal Medicine.* Boston, Blackwell Scientific Publications, 1985, pp 153–180.
58. Finer NN, Stewart AR: Continuous transcutaneous oxygen monitoring in the critically ill neonate. *Crit Care Med* 1980; 8:319–323.
59. Huch R, Huch A, Lubbers DW: *Transcutaneous Po_2.* New York, Thieme-Stratton, Inc, 1981.
60. Kilbride HW, Merenstein GB. Continuous oxygen monitoring in acutely ill preterm infants. *Crit Care Med* 1984; 12:121–124.
61. Lubbers DW: Cutaneous and transcutaneous Po_2 and Pco_2 and their measuring conditions. *Birth Defects* 1979; 15:13–31.
62. Lucey JF: Clinical uses of transcutaneous oxygen monitoring. *Adv Pediatr* 1981; 28:27–56.
63. Cassidy G: Transcutaneous monitoring in the newborn infant. *J Pediatr* 1983; 103:837–848.
64. Pasnick M, Lucey JF: Practical uses of continu-

ous transcutaneous oxygen monitoring. *Pediatr Rev* 1983; 5:5–12.
65. Bancalari E, Flyn JT, Cassady J, et al: Influence of continuous transcutaneous oxygen monitoring on the incidence of retinopathy of prematurity (ROP) (abstract). *Pediatr Res* 1985; 19:332.
66. Bancalari E, Flynn J, Goldberg RN, et al: Influence of transcutaneous oxygen monitoring on the incidence of retinopathy of prematurity. *Pediatrics* 1987; 79:663–669.
67. Palmer EA: *Module 12: Retinopathy of prematurity. Focal Points 1984: Clinical Modules for Ophthalmologists.* San Francisco, American Academy of Ophthalmology, 1984.
68. Ashton NW: Oxygen and the growth and development of retinal vessels. *Am J Ophthalmol* 1966; 62:412–435.
69. Patz A: Current therapy of retrolental fibroplasia. *Ophthalmology* 1983; 90:425–427.
70. Patz A: Current concepts of the effects of oxygen on the developing retina. *Curr Eye Res* 1984; 3:159–163.
71. Patz A: Retinal neovascularization: Early contributions of Professor Michaelson and recent observations. *Br J Ophthalmol* 1984; 68:42–46.
72. Kretzer FL, Hittner HM, Johnson AT, et al: Vitamin E and retrolental fibroplasia: Ultrastructural support of clinical efficacy. *Ann NY Acad Sci* 1982; 393:145–166.
73. Kretzer FL, Hunter DG, Mehta RS, et al: Spindle cells as vasoformative elements in the developing human retina: Vitamin E modulation, in Coates PW, Markwad RR, Kenney AD (eds): *Developing and Regenerating Vertebrate Nervous Systems.* New York, Alan R. Liss, Inc, 1983, pp 199–210.
74. Kretzer FL, Mehta RS, Johnson AT, et al: Vitamin E protects against retinopathy of prematurity through action on spindle cells. *Nature* 1984; 309:793–795.
75. Hittner HM, Rudolph AJ, Kretzer FL: Suppression of severe retinopathy of prematurity with vitamin E supplementation: Ultrastructural mechanism of clinical efficacy. *Ophthalmology* 1984; 91:1512–1523.
76. Hittner HM, Kretzer FL: Retinopathy of prematurity: Pathogenesis, prevention, and treatment, in Chiswick ML (ed): *Recent Advances in Perinatal Medicine,* vol 2. London, Churchill Livingston, Inc, 1985, pp 145–163.
77. Kretzer FL, Hittner HM: Initiating events in the development of retinopathy of prematurity, in Silverman WA, Flynn JT (eds): *Retinopathy of Prematurity II. Contemporary Issues in Fetal and Neonatal Medicine.* Boston, Blackwell Scientific Publications, 1985.
78. Borromeo-McGrail V, Bordiuk JM, Keitel H: Systemic hypertension following ocular administration of 10 percent phenylephrine in the neonate. *Pediatrics* 1973; 51:1032–1036.
79. Fraunfelder FT, Scafidi AF: Possible adverse effects from topical ocular 10 percent phenylephrine. *Am J Ophthalmol* 1978; 85:447–453.
80. Isenberg SJ, Everett S, Parelhoff E: A comparison of mydriatic eyedrops in low-weight infants. *Ophthalmology* 1984; 91:278–279.
81. Isenberg SJ, Abrams C, Hyman PE: Effects of cyclopentolate eyedrops on gastric secretory function in pre-term infants. *Ophthalmology* 1985; 92:698–700.
82. Bauer CR, Trottier MCT, Stern L: Systemic cyclopentolate (Cyclogel) toxicity in the newborn infant. *J Pediatr* 1973; 82:501–505.
83. Alden ER, Kalina RE, Hodson WA: Transient cataracts in low–birth-weight infants. *J Pediatr* 1973; 82:314–318.
84. Clark WN, Hodges E, Noel LP, et al: The oculocardiac reflex during ophthalmoscopy in premature infants. *Am J Ophthalmol* 1985; 99:649–651.
85. Graven SN: Oxygen therapy in the newborn infant: A statement of the Committee on Fetus and Newborn by the American Academy of Pediatrics. *Wis Med J* 1971; 70:224.
86. Palmer EA: Optimal timing of examination for acute retrolental fibroplasia. *Ophthalmology* 1981; 88:662–668.
87. Orellana J: Examination of the premature infant, in McPherson AR, Hittner HM, Kretzer FL (eds): *Retinopathy of Prematurity: Current Concepts and Controversies.* Toronto, BC Decker, Inc, 1986, pp 11–15.
88. Brown DR, Biglan AW, Stretabsky MAM: Screening criteria for the detection of retinopathy of prematurity in patients in a neonatal intensive care unit. *J Pediatr Ophthalmol Strabismus* 1987; 24:213–214.
89. Flynn JT: Discussion of "Screening criteria for the detection of retinopathy of prematurity in patients in a neonatal intensive care unit." *J Pediatr Ophthalmol Strabismus* 1987; 24:215.
90. Committee for the Classification of Retinopa-

thy of Prematurity: An international classification of retinopathy of prematurity. *Arch Ophthalmol* 1984; 102:1130–1134.

91. International Committee for the Classification of the Late Stages of Retinopathy of Prematurity: International classification of retinopathy of prematurity II. The classification of retinal detachment. *Arch Ophthalmol* 1987; 105:906–912.
92. Silverman WA, Flynn JT: *Retinopathy of Prematurity II. Contemporary Issues in Fetal and Neonatal Medicine.* Boston, Blackwell Scientific Publications, 1985.
93. Reese AB, King MJ, Owens WC. A classification of retrolental fibroplasia. *Am J Ophthalmol* 1953; 36:1333–1335.
94. Machlin LJ (ed): *Vitamin E: A Comprehensive Treatise.* New York, Marcel Dekker Inc, 1980, pp 289–306.
95. Bucher JR, Roberts RJ: Alpha tocopherol (vitamin E) content of lung, liver, and blood in the newborn rat and human infant: Influence of hyperoxia. *J Pediatr* 1981; 98:806–811.
96. Filer LJ: Introductory remarks; symposium on hemolytic anemia in the premature infant. *Am J Clin Nutr* 1968; 21:3–6.
97. Mino M, Nishino H, Yamaguchi T, et al: Tocopherol level in human fetal and infant liver. *J Nutr Sci Vitaminol (Tokyo)* 1977; 23:63–69.
98. Laupus WE, Bousquet FP Jr: Retrolental fibroplasia: The role of hemorrhage in its pathogenesis. *Am J Dis Child* 1951; 81:617–626.
99. Reese AB, Blodi FC: Retrolental fibroplasia. *Am J Ophthalmol* 1951; 34:1–24.
100. Phelps DL: Vitamin E and retinopathy of prematurity, in Silverman WA, Flynn JT (eds): *Retinopathy of Prematurity II. Contemporary Issues in Fetal and Neonatal Medicine.* Boston, Blackwell Scientific Publications, 1985, pp 181–205.
101. Phelps DL: Retinopathy of prematurity: An estimate of vision loss in the United States—1979. *Pediatrics* 1981; 67:924–926.
102. Johnson L, Schaffer D, Boggs TR Jr: The premature infant, vitamin E deficiency and retrolental fibroplasia. *Am J Clin Nutr* 1974; 27:1158–1173.
103. Phelps DL, Rosenbaum AL: The role of tocopherol in oxygen-induced retinopathy: Kitten model. *Pediatrics* 1977; 59(suppl):998–1005.
104. Kretzer FL, Mehta RS, Johnson AT, et al: Vitamin E protects against retinopathy of prematurity through action on spindle cells. *Nature* 1984; 309:793–795.
105. Phelps DL, Rosenbaum AL: Vitamin E in kitten oxygen-induced retinopathy II. Blockage of vitreal neovascularization. *Arch Ophthalmol* 1979; 97:1522–1526.
106. Phelps DL, Rosenbaum AL: Effects of marginal hypoxemia on recovery for oxygen-induced retinopathy in the kitten model. *Pediatrics* 1984; 73:1–6.
107. Phelps DL, Rosenbaum AL: Variable oxygenation during recovery from oxygen induced retinopathy in the kitten model (abstract). *Pediatr Res* 1984; 18:340.
108. Hittner HM, Godio LB, Rudolph AJ, et al: Retrolental fibroplasia: Efficacy of vitamin E in a double-blind clinical study of preterm infants. *N Engl J Med* 1981; 305:1365–1371.
109. Finer NN, Shindler RF, Grant G, et al: Effect of intramuscular vitamin E on the frequency and severity of retrolental fibroplasia: A controlled trial. *Lancet* 1982; 1:1087–1091.
110. Puklin JE, Simon RM, Ehrenkranz RA: Influence on retrolental fibroplasia of intramuscular vitamin E administration during respiratory distress syndrome. *Ophthalmology* 1982; 89:96–103.
111. Phelps DL, Rosenbaum AL, Isenberg SJ, et al: Effect of IV tocopherol on retinopathy of prematurity (ROP) (abstract). *Pediatr Res* 1985; 19:375.
112. Milner RA, Watts JL, Paes B, et al: RLF in 1500 gram neonates: Part of a randomized clinical trial on the effectiveness of vitamin E, in *Retinopathy of Prematurity Conference Syllabus*, vol 2, Washington, DC, Dec 4–6, 1981, pp 703–716.
113. Hittner HM, Godio LB, Speer ME, et al: Retrolental fibroplasia: Further clinical evidence and ultrastructural support for efficacy of vitamin E in the preterm infant. *Pediatrics* 1983; 71:423–432.
114. Finer NN, Schindler RF, Peteras KL, et al: Vitamin E and retrolental fibroplasia. Improved visual outcome with early vitamin E. *Ophthalmology* 1983; 90:428–435.
115. Johnson L, Schaffer D, Boggs TR Jr: The premature infant, vitamin E deficiency and retrolental fibroplasia. *Am J Clin Nutr* 1974; 27:1158–1173.

116. Shaffer DB, Johnson L, Quinn GE, et al: Vitamin E and retinopathy of prematurity: Follow-up at one year. *Ophthalmology* 1985; 92:1005–1011.
117. Phelps DL: Vitamin E and retrolental fibroplasia in 1982. *Pediatrics* 1982; 70:420–425.
118. Phelps DL: Local and systemic reactions to the parenteral administration of vitamin E. *Dev Pharmacol Ther* 1981; 2:156–171.
119. Milner RA, Bell E, Blanchette V, et al: Vitamin E supplement in under 1500 gram neonates (abstract 1052). *Pediatr Res* 1979, 13:501.
120. Kretzer FL, Hittner HM: Human retinal development: Relationship to the pathogenesis of retinopathy of prematurity, in McPherson AR, Hittner HM, Kretzer FL (eds): *Retinopathy of Prematurity: Current Concepts and Controversies*. Toronto, BC Decker, Inc, 1986, pp 27–52.
121. Rosenbaum AL, Phelps DL, Isenberg SJ, et al: Retinal hemorrhages in retinopathy of prematurity associated with tocopheral treatment. *Ophthalmology* 1985; 92:1012–1014.
122. Finer NN, Peters KL, Hayek Z, et al: Vitamin E and necrotizing enterocolitis. *Pediatrics* 1984; 73:387–393.
123. Johnson L, Bowen FW Jr, Abbasi S, et al: Relationship of prolonged pharmacologic serum levels of vitamin E to incidence of sepsis and necrotizing enterocolitis in infants with birth weights 1,500 grams or less. *Pediatrics* 1985; 75:619–638.
124. Phelps DL, Rosenbaum AL, Isenberg SJ, et al: Tocopherol efficacy and safety for preventing retinopathy of prematurity: A randomized, controlled, double-masked trial. *Pediatrics* 1987; 79:489–500.
125. Bodenstein CJ: Intravenous vitamin E and deaths in the intensive care unit (letter). *Pediatrics* 1984; 73:733.
126. Yamashita Y: Studies on retinopathy of prematurity. (III) Cryocautery for retinopathy of prematurity. *Jpn J Clin Ophthalmol* 1972; 26:385–393.
127. Sasaki K, Yamashita Y, Maekawa T, et al: Treatment of retinopathy of prematurity in active stage by cryocautery. *Jpn J Ophthalmol* 1976; 20:384–395.
128. Takagi I: Treatment of acute retrolental fibroplasia. *Acta Soc Ophthalmol Jpn* 1978; 82:323–330.
129. Kingham JD: Acute retrolental fibroplasia; treatment by cryosurgery. *Arch Ophthalmol* 1978; 96:2049–2053.
130. Hindle NW, Leyton J: Prevention of cicatricial retrolental fibroplasia by cryotherapy. *Can J Ophthalmol* 1978; 13:277–282.
131. Ben-Sira I, Nissenkorn I, Grunwald E, et al: Treatment of acute retrolental fibroplasia by cryopexy. *Br J Ophthalmol* 1980; 64:758–762.
132. Mousel DK, Hoyt CS: Cryotherapy for retinopathy of prematurity. *Ophthalmology* 1980; 87:1121–1127.
133. Bert MD, Friedman MW, Ballard R: Combined cryosurgery and scleral buckling in acute proliferative retrolental fibroplasia. *J Pediatr Ophthalmol Strabismus* 1981; 18:9–12.
134. Hindle NW: Cryotherapy for retinopathy to prevent retrolental fibroplasia. *Can J Ophthalmol* 1982; 17:27–212.
135. Keith CG: Visual outcome and effect of treatment in stage II developing retrolental fibroplasia. *Br J Ophthalmol* 1982; 66:446–449.
136. Mousel DK: Cryotherapy for retinopathy of prematurity; a personal retrospective. *Ophthalmology* 1985; 92:375–378.
137. Topilow HW, Ackerman AL, Wang FM: The treatment of advanced retinopathy of prematurity by cryotherapy and scleral buckling surgery. *Ophthalmology* 1985; 92:379–387.
138. Tasman W, Brown GC, Schaffer DB, et al: Cryotherapy for active retinopathy of prematurity. *Ophthalmology* 1986; 93:580–585.
139. Reisner SH, Amir J, Shohat M, et al: Retinopathy of prematurity: Incidence and treatment. *Arch Dis Child* 1985; 60:698–701.
140. Tasman W: Zone I retinopathy of prematurity. *Arch Ophthalmol* 1985; 103:1693–1694.
141. Palmer EA: The multicenter trial of cryotherapy for retinopathy of prematurity. *J Pediatr Ophthalmol Strabismus* 1986; 23:56–57.
142. Palmer EA: Multicenter trial of cryotherapy for retinopathy of prematurity. *Pediatrics* 1986; 77:428–429.
143. Hindle NW: Cryotherapy for retinopathy of prematurity: Timing of intervention. *Br J Ophthalmol* 1986; 70:269–276.
144. Tasman W: Management of retinopathy of prematurity. *Ophthalmology* 1985; 92:995–999.
145. Frishberg Y, Amir J, Nissenkorn I, et al: Se-

vere bradycardia and nodal rhythm complicating cryopexy for retinopathy of prematurity. *J Pediatr Ophthalmol Strabismus* 1986; 23:258–260.
146. Tanabe Y, Ikema M: Retinopathy of prematurity and photocoagulation therapy. *Acta Soc Ophthalmol Jpn* 1972; 76:260–266.
147. Nagata M, Kanenar S: Light-coagulation in cases of progressive retinopathy of prematurity II. *Rinsho Ganka* 1970; 24:655–661.
148. Oshima K, Ikui H, Kano M, et al: Clinical study and photocoagulation of retinopathy of prematurity. *Folia Ophthalmol Jpn* 1971; 22:700–707.
149. Nagata M, Tsuruoka Y: Treatment of acute retrolental fibroplasia with xenon arc photocoagulation. *Jpn J Ophthalmol* 1972; 16:131–143.
150. Uehara M, Masunaga J, Hattori M: Ocular functions in postphotocoagulative cicatricial stages of retinopathy of prematurity. *Folia Ophthalmol Jpn* 1975; 26:1387–1392.
151. Majima A, Takahashi M, Hibino Y: Clinical observations of photocoagulation on retinopathy of prematurity. *Jpn J Clin Ophthalmol* 1976; 30:93–97.
152. Yamamoto M, Tabuch A: Management of retinopathy of prematurity. *Jpn J Ophthalmol* 1976; 20:372–383.
153. Nagata M: Treatment of acute proliferative retrolental fibroplasia with xenon arc photocoagulation. Its indications and limitations. *Jpn J Ophthalmol* 1977; 21:436–459.
154. Nagata M, Yamagishi N, Ikeda S: Summarized results of the treatment of acute proliferative retinopathy of prematurity during the past 15 years in Tenri Hospital. *Acta Soc Ophthalmol Jpn* 1982; 86:1236–1244.
155. Uemura Y: Current status of retrolental fibroplasia. Report of the joint committee for the study of retrolental fibroplasia in Japan. *Jpn J Ophthalmol* 1977; 21:366–378.
156. Takagi I: Treatment of acute retrolental fibroplasia. *Ophthalmol Jpn* 1978; 82:323–330.
157. Sasaki K, Yamashita Y, Maekawa T, et al: Treatment of retinopathy of prematurity in active stage by cryocautery. *Jpn J Ophthalmol* 1976; 20:384–395.
158. Harris GS, McCormick AQ: The prophylactic treatment of retrolental fibroplasia. *Mod Probl Ophthalmol* 1977; 18:364–367.
159. Hindle NW: Cryotherapy for retinopathy of prematurity to prevent retrolental fibroplasia. *Can J Ophthalmol* 1982; 17:207–212.
160. Tasman W, Annesley W: Retinal detachment in the retinopathy of prematurity. *Arch Ophthalmol* 1966; 75:608–614.
161. Faris BM, Brockhurst RJ: Retrolental fibroplasia in the cicatricial stage. The complication of rhegmatogenous retinal detachment. *Arch Ophthalmol* 1969; 82:62–65.
162. Tasman W: Vitreoretinal changes in cicatricial retrolental fibroplasia. *Trans Am Ophthalmol Soc* 1970; 68:548–594.
163. Harris GS: Retinopathy of prematurity and retinal detachment. *Can J Ophthalmol* 1976; 11:21–25.
164. Starzychka M, Ciechanowska A, Gergovich A: Retinal detachment in retrolental fibroplasia. *Ophthalmologica* 1980; 181:261–265.
165. Koerner FH: Retinopathy of prematurity: Natural course and management. *Methods Ophthalmol* 1978; 2:325–329.
166. Yassur Y, Grunwald E, BenSira I: Surgical treatment of retrolental fibroplasia in infants. *Methods Ophthalmol* 1978; 2:333–334.
167. McPherson AR, Hittner HM: Scleral buckling in 1 1/2 to 11 month old premature infants with retinal detachment associated with acute retrolental fibroplasia. *Ophthalmology* 1979; 86:819–835.
168. Grunwald E, Yassur Y, Ben-Sira I: Buckling procedures for retinal detachment caused by retrolental fibroplasia in premature babies. *Br J Ophthalmol* 1980; 64:98–101.
169. Bert MD, Friedman MW, Ballard R: Combined cryosurgery and scleral buckling in acute proliferative retrolental fibroplasia. *J Pediatr Ophthalmol Strabismus* 1981; 18:841–844.
170. Baruch E, Bracha R, Godel V, et al: Buckling procedure in infant retrolental fibroplasia. *J Ocular Ther Surg* 1981; 1:65–66.
171. McPherson AR, Hittner HM, Lemos R: Retinal detachment in young premature infants with acute retrolental fibroplasia. Thirty-two new cases. *Ophthalmology* 1982; 89:1160.
172. Topilow HW, Acherman AL, Want FM: The treatment of advanced retinopathy of prematurity by cryotherapy and scleral buckling surgery. *Ophthalmology* 1985; 92:379–387.
173. Tasman W: Management of retinopathy of prematurity. *Ophthalmology* 1985; 92:995–999.
174. McPherson AR, Hittner FL, Kretzer FL: Treat-

ment of acute retinopathy of prematurity, in McPherson AR, Hittner HM, Kretzer FL (eds): *Retinopathy of Prematurity: Current Concepts and Controversies.* Toronto, BC Decker, Inc, 1986, pp 179–192.

175. Charles S: Vitrectomy with ciliary body entry for retrolental fibroplasia, in McPherson AR, Hittner HM, Kretzer FL (eds): *Retinopathy of Prematurity: Current Concepts and Controversies.* Toronto, BC Decker, Inc, 1986, pp 225–234.
176. Charles ST: Vitrectomy for retrolental fibroplasia. Presented at the *American Academy of Ophthalmology* Annual Meeting, Atlanta, November 12, 1984.
177. Tasman W: Late complications of retrolental fibroplasia. *Ophthalmology* 1979; 86:1724–1740.
178. Merritt JC, Lawson EE, Sprague DH, et al: Lensectomy-vitrectomy for stage 5 cicatricial retrolental fibroplasia. *Ophthalmic Surg* 1982: 13:300–306.
179. Lightfoot D, Irvine AR: Vitrectomy in infants and children with retinal detachment caused by cicatricial retrolental fibroplasia. *Am J Ophthalmol* 1982; 94:305–312.
180. Machemer R: Closed vitrectomy for severe retrolental fibroplasia in infants. *Ophthalmology* 1983; 90: 436–441.
181. Trese MT: Surgical results of stage V retrolental fibroplasia and timing of surgical repair. *Ophthalmology* 1984; 91:461–466.
182. Trese MT: Two–hand dissection technique during closed vitrectomy for retinopathy of prematurity. *Am J Ophthalmol* 1986; 101:251–252.
183. Trese MT: Visual results and prognostic factors for vision following surgery for stage V retinopathy of prematurity. *Ophthalmology* 1986; 93:574–579.
184. Hirose T, Schepens CL: Open-sky vitrectomy in retrolental fibroplasia. Presented at the *American Academy of Ophthalmology* Annual Meeting, Atlanta, November 12, 1984.
185. Schepens CL: Clinical and research aspects of subtotal open-sky vitrectomy. XXXVII Edward Jackson Memorial Lecture. *Am J Ophthalmol* 1981; 91:143–171.
186. Teplin SW: Developmental issues in blind infants and children with retinopathy of prematurity, in Silverman WA, Flynn JT (eds): *Retinopathy of Prematurity II. Contemporary Issues in Fetal and Neonatal Medicine.* Boston, Blackwell Scientific Publications, 1985, pp 267–292.
187. Fraiberg S: *Insights From the Blind: Comparative Studies of Blind and Sighted Infants.* New York, Basic Books, Inc, Publishers, 1977.
188. Gesell A, Ilg FL, Bullis GE: *Vision—Its Development in Infant and Child.* New York, Hafner Press, 1949.
189. Warren DH: *Blindness and Early Childhood Development,* ed 2. New York, American Foundation for the Blind, 1984.
190. Robinson GC: Causes, ocular disorders, associated handicaps, and incidence and prevalence of blindness in childhood, in Jan JE, Freeman RD, Scott EF (eds): *Visual Impairment in Children and Adolescents.* New York, Grune & Stratton, 1977.
191. Fine SR: *Incidence of Visual Handicap in Children.* London, Spastics International Medical Publications, 1979.
192. Teplin SW: Development of blind infants and children with retrolental fibroplasia: Implications for physicians. *Pediatrics* 1983; 71:6–12.
193. Stetten D: Coping with blindness. *N Engl J Med* 1981; 305:458–460.
194. Kushner BJ: The sequelae of regressed retinopathy of prematurity, in Silverman WA, Flynn JT (eds): *Retinopathy of Prematurity II. Contemporary Issues in Fetal and Neonatal Medicine.* Boston, Blackwell Scientific Publications, 1985, pp 239–247.
195. Kushner BJ: Strabismus and amblyopia associated with regressed retinopathy of prematurity. *Arch Ophthalmol* 1982; 102:256–261.
196. Gordon RA, Donzis PB: Myopia associated with retinopathy of prematurity. *Ophthalmology* 1986; 93:1593–1598.
197. Kushner BJ: Ocular causes of abnormal head postures. *Ophthalmology* 1979; 86:2115–2125.
198. Foster RS, Metz HS, Jampolsky A: Strabismus and pseudostrabismus with retrolental fibroplasia. *Am J Ophthalmol* 1975; 79:985–989.
199. Smith J, Shivitz I: Angle-closure glaucoma in adults with cicatricial retinopathy of prematurity. *Arch Ophthalmol* 1984; 102:371–372.
200. Kushner BJ, Sondheimer S: Medical Treatment of Glaucoma Associated With Cicatricial Retinopathy of Prematurity. *Am J Ophthalmol* 1982; 94:313–317.

201. Hittner HM, Rhodes LM, McPherson AR: Anterior segment abnormalities in cicatricial retinopathy of prematurity. *Ophthalmology* 1979; 86:803–816.
202. Lorfel RS, Sugar HS: Keratoconus associated with retrolental fibroplasia. *Ann Ophthalmol* 1976; 8:449–450.
203. Bettman JW: Medicolegal aspect of retinopathy of prematurity, in McPherson AR, Hittner HM, Kretzer FL (eds): *Retinopathy of Prematurity: Current Concepts and Controversies.* Toronto, BC Decker, Inc, 1986, pp 67–70.
204. Bettman JW: The retinopathy of prematurity: Medicolegal aspects. *Surv Ophthalmol* 1985; 29:371–373.
205. Perdue JM: Medicolegal issues presented through retinopathy of prematurity: The standard of care issue, in McPherson AR, Hittner HM, Kretzer FL (eds): *Retinopathy of Prematurity: Current Concepts and Controversies.* Toronto, BC Decker, Inc, 1986, pp 71–77.
206. Brahams D: Medicine and the law: Negligent treatment of premature infant causing retrolental fibroplasia. *Lancet* 1985; 1:589–590.
207. Medicolegal Decisions: Hospital not liable for RLF suffered in 1953. *Am Med News,* April 3, 1987, p 34.
208. Brahams D: Medicine and the law: Negligent treatment of premature infant causing retrolental fibroplasia. *Lancet* 1985; 1:589–590.
209. Medicolegal Decisions: Hospital not liable for RLF suffered in 1953. *Am Med News,* April 3, 1987, p 34.

PART IV

The Newborn Eye in Systemic Disease

27 Systemic Disorders and the Eye

Jane D. Kivlin, M.D.

Nearly all systemic disorders have ocular manifestations. These may range from minor anomalies of lid measurements that are not specific to one condition to pathognomonic signs such as the fluffy nuclear cataract in Lowe's syndrome. Some manifestations can be devastating to vision in young children such as lens dislocation in Marfan syndrome and retinal detachment in Stickler syndrome. The child with such a disorder must have an early examination to identify problems and intervene in them effectively. Many ocular manifestations of generalized diseases are not seen in infants. The frequency of certain signs of a disease is often unknown.

In a child with multiple anomalies, possible diagnoses include genetic disorders, teratogen effects, and nongenetic but characteristic malformation syndromes. Many ocular signs may be caused by conditions from each of these three groups. I have included all three groups in this differential diagnosis discussion and tried to note frequency and onset of the finding if known. I have also included comments on some disease findings that do not occur in infants to counter common misconceptions.

This chapter is divided into sections covering anatomic and physiological abnormalities of the eye. In each section I have attempted to list those conditions that can be associated with the abnormal finding so that one may use these lists as an aid to making a systemic diagnosis. I have not approached the question from the opposite direction—What are the eye findings in infants with a particular systemic disorder?—because good references for this are already available.[1–3]

EYE POSITION AND LID ANOMALIES

Anomalies of eye position and of the eyelids make a large contribution to the diagnosis of conditions that have distinctive facies. Other than in syndromes that affect only the eyes such as blepharophimosis, these abnormalities are not pathognomonic.

Hypotelorism (smaller than expected pupillary distance) may reflect underlying midline central nervous system (CNS) underdevelopment,[1] and small lid fissures and ptosis may reflect underdevelopment of the globes. Orbital measurements from plain films or computed tomography (CT) scans allow the most accurate measurements of orbital separation. Age-related standards for interpupillary distance (PD), inner canthal distance, and outer canthal distance have been compiled[4] (Figs 27–1 through 27–3). Clinically, PD reflects ocular position more than do inner and outer canthal distances. It can be difficult to measure in babies who are not alert (the eyes normally go out and up during sleep, which is known as Bell's phenomenon) or have strabismus. Measuring the distance of one eye from a midpoint as that eye is fixating on a target and then measuring the distance

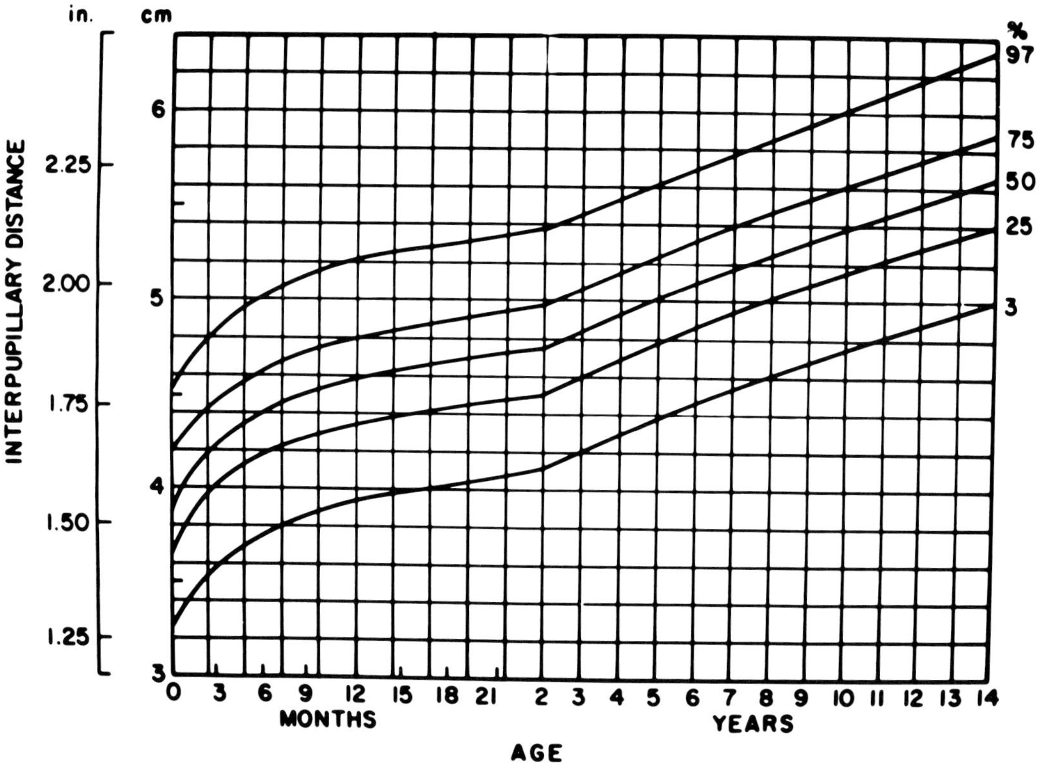

FIG 27–1.
Norms for interpupillary distance. (From Feingold M, Bossert WH: Normal values for selected physical parameters: An aid to syndrome delineation, in Bergsman D (ed): *Birth Defects: Original Article Series*, vol 10. New York, The National Foundation/March of Dimes, 1974, no. 13, p 8. Used with permission.)

of the other eye when it fixates on the same target and adding the two distances will compensate for strabismus. PDs for near fixation are approximately 3 mm less than for distance fixation and can be adjusted to be comparable to values in Figure 27–1.

Telecanthus, which is lateral displacement of the inner canthi, and epicanthal folds, redundant skin folds over the inner canthi, are often mistaken for hypertelorism.

As noted in the following lists, some disorders may have either hypotelorism or hypertelorism.

Hypotelorism

Deeply set or esotropic eyes may add to the impression of hypotelorism.

Frequent Associations	Comments
Down syndrome[5]	Radiographic finding
Holoprosencephaly sequence[6]	Can reach the extreme of cyclopia or fused eyes, can be familial
Maternal phenylketonuria fetal effects[1]	
Trisomy 13 syndrome[5]	Similar to holoprosencephaly
Trisomy 20p syndrome[7]	
5_p+ syndrome[5]	

Occasional Associations	Comments
Cockayne syndrome[8]	
Coffin-Siris syndrome[1]	
Goldenhar syndrome[9]	
Meckel-Gruber syndrome[10]	
Oculodentodigital syndrome[11]	
Williams syndrome[12]	
Ring 22 syndrome[5]	Also almond-shaped fissures
18p− syndrome[5]	Similar to holoprosencephaly

Hypertelorism

Exotropia can add to impression of hypertelorism.

Frequent Associations	Comments
Aarskog syndrome[13]	
Acrocollosal syndrome[3]	Present in 87% of reported males
Acrodysostosis syndrome[3]	
Apert syndrome[1]	
BBB syndrome[14]	May be identical to G syndrome
Cat-eye syndrome[5]	
Cleft lip and palate sequence[1]	
Clefting, ectropion, and conical teeth syndrome[3]	Also lower lid ectropion
Coffin-Lowry syndrome[15]	Recognizable at 5 weeks
	Consistent finding
Craniometaphyseal dysplasia[3]	Observed in 15-month-old
DiGeorge sequence[1]	
Dubowitz syndrome[16]	
Fetal aminopterin effects[1]	
Fetal hydantoin effects[1]	
Frontonasal dysplasia sequence[1]	
Larsen syndrome[1]	
Meckel-Gruber syndrome[10]	
Melnick-Needles syndrome[17]	
Multiple lentigines syndrome (leopard syndrome)[18]	Not as consistently present as first thought

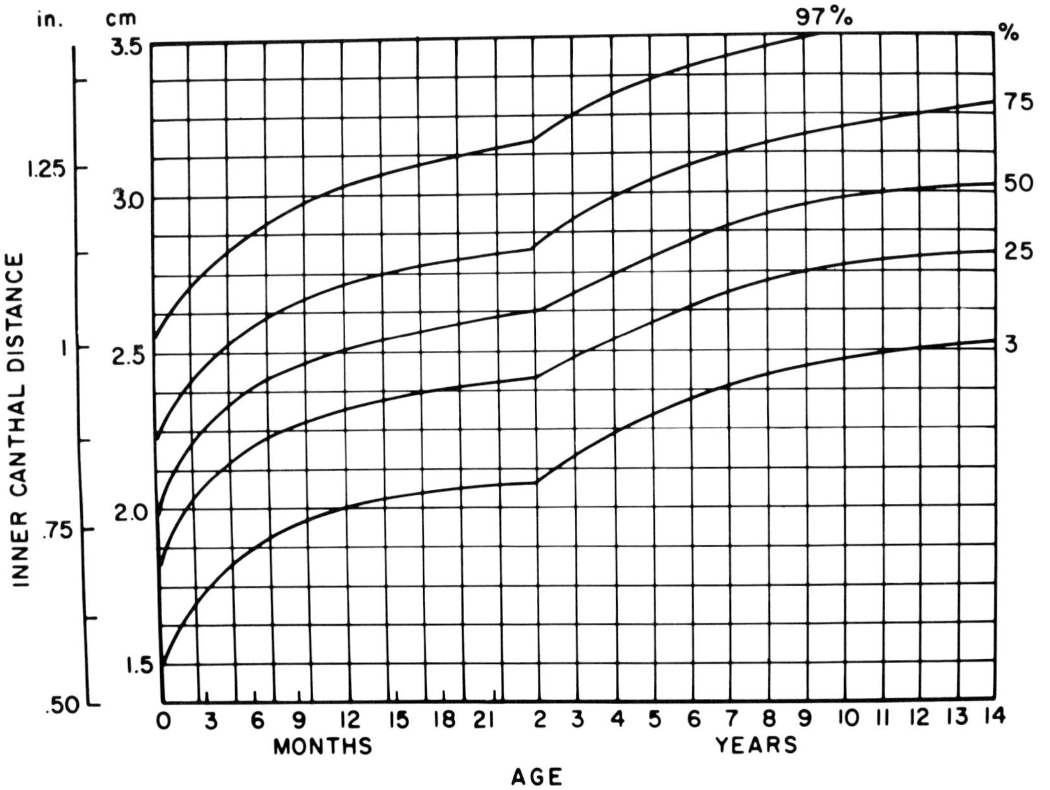

FIG 27–2.
Norms for inner canthal distance. (From Feingold M, Bossert WH: Normal values for selected physical parameters: An aid to syndrome delineation, in Bergsman D (ed): *Birth Defects: Original Article Series,* vol 10. New York, The National Foundation/March of Dimes, 1974; no. 13, p 8. Used with permission.)

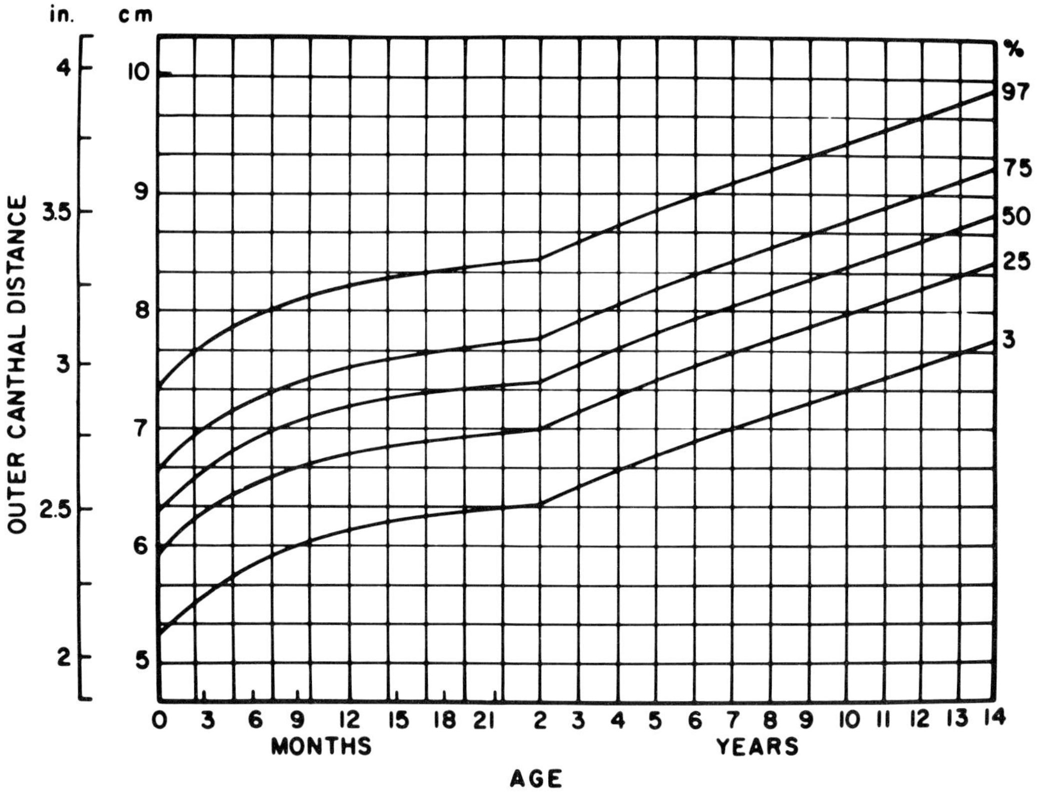

FIG 27–3.
Norms for outer canthal distance. (From Feingold M, Bossert WH: Normal values for selected physical parameters: An aid to syndrome delineation, in Bergsman D (ed): *Birth Defects: Original Article Series,* vol 10. New York, The National Foundation/March of Dimes, 1974; no. 13, p 8. Used with permission.)

Frequent Associations	Comments
Noonan syndrome[19]	
Otopalatodigital syndrome (Taybi syndrome)[1]	
Pena-Shokeir type I syndrome[1]	
Pfeiffer syndrome[1]	
Primary hypertelorism[20]	
Pyle syndrome[1]	
Rieger syndrome[21]	
Robert syndrome (pseudothalidomide syndrome)[1]	
Robinow syndrome (fetal face syndrome)[1]	
Saethre-Chotzen syndrome (acrocephalosyndactyly, type III)[1]	
Sotos syndrome[1]	
Trimethylaminuria[22]	
Triploidy syndrome[1]	
Trisomy 8 syndrome[23]	
Trisomy 9p syndrome[5]	
Weaver syndrome[1]	
Whistling face syndrome[3]	
XXXX syndrome[5]	
4p– syndrome (Wolf syndrome)[5]	
5p– syndrome (cri du chat syndrome)[5]	Most have telecanthus only
9p– syndrome[5]	
13q– syndrome[5]	

Occasional Associations	Comments
Basal cell nevus syndrome[24]	
Camptomelic dysplasia syndrome[1]	
Cleidocranial dysostosis syndrome[1]	
Conradi-Hünermann syndrome[25]	

Occasional Associations	Comments
Crouzon syndrome[26]	Very common
Cryptophthalmos syndrome[1]	Apparent position of globes can be widely separated
Holt-Oram syndrome[1]	
Hurler syndrome[1]	
Oculodentodigital syndrome[11]	
Sjögren-Larsson syndrome[1]	
Williams syndrome[12]	
XXXXX syndrome[5]	
XXXXY syndrome[5]	
5p – syndrome (cri du chat syndrome)[5]	
10q + syndrome[5]	Actually telecanthus in most patients
18p – syndrome[5]	
18q – syndrome[5]	

Shallow Orbits

Globes can be so far beyond the orbital rims that the lids have difficulty in closing. Sometimes a patient with shallow orbits is mistakenly diagnosed as having proptosis.

Frequent Associations	Comments
Apert syndrome[6]	
Carpenter syndrome[26]	
Crouzon syndrome[27]	
Dubowitz syndrome[16]	
Familial hypoplasia of orbital margin[3]	Variable lacrimal defects
Fetal aminopterin effects[1]	
Marshall-Smith syndrome[1]	
Melnick-Needles syndrome[17]	
Osteogenesis imperfecta syndrome, autosomal recessive[28]	
Robert syndrome (pseudothalidomide syndrome)[1]	
Saethre-Chotzen syndrome[1]	
Trisomy 18 syndrome[5]	
Zellweger syndrome[1]	
9p – syndrome[5]	

Occasional Associations	Comments
Kleeblattschädel syndrome[3]	May be part of Crouzon, Pfeiffer, and Carpenter syndromes
Trisomy 13 syndrome[5]	

Occasional Associations	Comments
6q + syndrome[5]	

Prominent Supraorbital Ridges

Associated Conditions	Comments
Basal cell nevus syndrome[24]	
Cleidocranial dysostosis syndrome[1]	
Coffin-Lowry syndrome[1]	Recognizable at the age of 5 wk
Frontometaphyseal dysplasia syndrome[29]	Progressive
Hurler syndrome[1]	Acquired as part of coarsening facial features after the age of 6 mo
Otopalatodigital syndrome (Taybi syndrome)[1]	
Pyle metaphyseal dysplasia syndrome[1]	

Cryptophthalmos

Cryptophthalmos may have great variation, ranging from unilateral involvement, to ablepharon with a relatively normal globe, to lid coloboma, to bilateral involvement. Defects of the lashes vary greatly also, but most patients have aberrant scalp hair growth extending to the brow, rather than normal brow hair.

Associated Conditions
Ablepharon, macrostomia syndrome[3]
Fraser syndrome[1,3]

Ankyloblepharon.—Connection of the lid margins.

Associated Conditions	Comments
Ankyloblepharon, cleft lip and palate[1]	
CHANDS (curly hair, ankyloblepharon, nail dysplasia) syndrome[3]	
Hay-Wells ectodermal dysplasia[1]	Connecting bands can contain muscle and vascular connective tissue
Popliteal pterygium syndrome[3]	

Telecanthus

This is lateral displacement of the inner canthi. Telecanthus can be an isolated autosomal dominant condition.[3]

Frequent Associations	Comments
Aarskog syndrome[13]	
Blepharonasofacial syndrome[30]	
Camptomelic dysplasia[1]	
Carpenter syndrome[1,26]	
Dubowitz syndrome[16]	
Facio-oculoacousticorenal syndrome (FOAR syndrome)[31]	Telecanthus is prominent
Fetal alcohol effects[1]	
Frontonasal dysplasia sequence[1]	
KBG syndrome[32]	Characteristic
Oculodentodigital syndrome[11]	
Orofaciodigital (OFD) type I and type II (Mohr syndrome)[33]	
Trisomy 18 syndrome[5]	
Waardenburg syndrome[34]	Lateral displacement of the lacrimal puncta exaggerates this appearance
Williams' syndrome[12]	
5p − syndrome[5]	

Occasional Associations
Basal cell nevus syndrome[24]
4p + syndrome[5]
6p + syndrome[5]

Blepharophimosis

Shorter than usual lid fissure (horizontal measurement). Ophthalmologists tend to use the term *blepharophimosis* for a specific autosomal dominant condition that also includes ptosis, telecanthus, and epicanthus inversus but has no associated systemic problems.[35]

Associated Conditions	Comments
Blepharophimosis-amenorrhea syndrome[36]	Also hypertrichosis
Clefting syndrome with anterior chamber and lid anomalies[37]	
Dubowitz syndrome[16]	
Marden-Walker syndrome[3]	
Oculopalatoskeletal syndrome[3]	
Pena-Shokeir type II syndrome[38]	Occurs in 87% of patients
Schwartz syndrome[39]	Myopia in half of patients
10q + syndrome[5]	
3p − syndrome[5]	

Epicanthal Folds.—This lid configuration is so frequently seen in normal children that it has little diagnostic value by itself. In combination with other features it contributes to the typical facies of many syndromes such as ptosis and telecanthus in blepharophimosis syndrome.[35]

Upslanting Palpebral Fissures

Can occur with premature fusion of the metopic suture and trigonocephaly.[5]

Frequent Associations	Comments
Down syndrome[5]	
Femoral-facial syndrome[1]	
Jarcho-Levin syndrome[1]	
Miller-Dieker syndrome (lissencephaly syndrome)[40]	Probably same as Warburg syndrome[41]
Oto-palato-digital syndrome[1]	
Pfeiffer syndrome[1]	
Rhizomelic chondrodysplasia punctata syndrome[25]	
Trisomy 9 mosaic and 9p − syndromes[5]	
Trisomy 20p syndrome[7]	
XXXXX syndrome[5]	
XXXXY syndrome[5]	
4p + syndrome[5]	
5p + syndrome[5]	

Occasional Associations	Comments
Fetal hydantoin effects[1]	
Prader-Willi syndrome[1]	Often almond-shaped lid fissures
Trisomy 13 syndrome[5]	
Trisomy 18 and 18q syndromes[5]	

Downslanting Palpebral Fissures

Frequent Associations	Comments
Aarskog syndrome[13]	
Apert syndrome[1]	
Coffin-Lowry syndrome[1]	
Cohen syndrome[42]	
Conradi-Hünermann syndrome[25]	
DiGeorge sequence[1]	
Maxillofacial dysostosis[3]	
Nager syndrome[43]	
Rubenstein-Taybi syndrome[44]	
Saethre-Chotzen syndrome[1]	
Sotos syndrome[1]	
Treacher Collins syndrome[1]	
Trisomy 9p syndrome[5]	
Occasional Associations	**Comments**
Cat-eye syndrome[5]	
Hallermann-Streiff syndrome[45]	
Ruvalcaba syndrome[46]	
4q+ syndrome[5]	
21q− syndrome[5]	Also blepharochalasis

Lid Colobomas

The extreme is ablepharon, which can be associated with macrostomia and mental retardation.[3]

Association With Lower Lid Lesion	Comments
Crouzon syndrome[27]	
Facial clefting syndromes (Tessier syndrome, types 3 and 4)[3,47]	
Linear sebaceous nevus sequence[48]	
Miller syndrome[43]	
Nager syndrome[43]	
Palpebral coloboma-lipoma syndrome[3]	Both upper and lower lids
Treacher Collins syndrome[1]	
Frontonasal dysplasia sequence[1]	

Association With Upper Lid Lesion	Comments
Amniotic band syndrome[1]	
Frontofacionasal displasia[3]	
Goldenhar syndrome[9]	
Linear sebaceous nevus sequence[48]	

Ectropion

Associated Conditions
Down syndrome
Ectropion and distichiasis[3]
Facial clefting syndromes (no. 3 and 4 of Terrier syndrome)[3,47]
Miller syndrome[43]
Robinow syndrome[1]
Sjögren-Larrson syndrome[1,49]

Lid Edema

Frequent Associations
Athyrotic hypothyroidism sequence[1]
Williams' syndrome[12]
Occasional Associations
Neurofibromatosis[1]

Eyebrow Abnormalities

Synophrys (Eyebrows Extending to Midline)	
Frequent Associations	**Comments**
Coffin-Siris syndrome[1]	May have only long lashes and bushy eyebrows
Congenital hypertrichosis[3]	
de Lange's syndrome[1]	
Fetal trimethadione effects[1]	Also upslanting brows
Trisomy 4p syndrome[5]	
Waardenburg's syndrome[34]	
3q+ syndrome[5]	Resembles de Lange syndrome
Occasional Associations	**Comments**
Basal cell nevus syndrome[24]	

Occasional Associations	Comments
Blepharophimosis-amenorrhea syndrome[36]	
Trisomy 13 syndrome[5]	
4p+ syndrome[5]	

Flaring of Nasal Part of Eyebrow (of late, stylish in fashion models)

Associated Conditions	Comments
Blepharonasofacial syndrome[30]	
Partial trisomy 10q syndrome[5]	
Waardenburg syndrome[1]	
Williams syndrome[12]	

High Arched Brow

Associated Conditions	Comments
Kabuki makeup syndrome[50]	
Shprintzen-Goldberg syndrome[3]	

Absent Brow Hair

Associated Conditions	Comments
Cryptophthalmos	See above
Pseudoprogeria syndrome[3]	

Abnormal Eyelashes

Madarosis.—Severe diminution or absence of lashes.[2] Lashes are often relatively spared in generalized hair deficiency syndromes. Distichiasis can also occur.

Associated Conditions	Comments
Acrodermatitis enteropathica[3]	
Congenital atrichia[2]	
Ectodermal dysplasia[2]	
Ehlers-Danlos syndrome, unspecified type[3]	
Generalized hypotrichosis[2]	
Hypomelia, hypotrichosis, facial hemangioma[2]	
Isolated madarosis[2]	
Keratosis follicularis spinulosa decalvans[49]	
Pseudoprogeria syndrome[3]	

Localized Loss of Lashes

Associated Conditions	Comments
Cryptophthalmos	See above
Lid colobomas	See above

Unusually Numerous or Long Lashes

Associated Conditions	Comments
Blepharophimosis-amenorrhea syndrome[36]	
de Lange syndrome[3]	
Schwartz syndrome[39]	
Trichomegaly	Isolated,[3] or associated with pigmentary retinopathy, dwarfism, and mental retardation[51]

Extra Rows of Lashes (see Madarosis, above)

Associated Conditions	Comments
Anodontia-hypotrichosis syndrome[3]	
Distichiasis, lymphedema syndrome[3]	
Ectropion and distichiasis[3]	
Tristichiasis[3]	

Ptosis

Ptosis is another common disorder that is helpful in diagnosis only if seen in combination with other defects as in blepharophimosis syndrome.[36] In conditions causing photophobia such as albinism or aniridia, it may be intentional to decrease the light entering the eye.

LACRIMAL SYSTEM

Alacrima

Reflex or emotional tearing is usually not seen until the age of 3 months. The absence of reflex tearing is unusual but rarely of medical significance; the individual might have more difficulty clearing dust or debris from the eyes. Lack of basal tearing can be devastating, with erosion and even melting of the cornea and secondary opacification of the cornea as it tries to heal. Corneal transplantation often fails because of poor healing and repeated breakdown of the corneal surface. On rare occasion the lacrimal gland may be absent.

Associated Conditions	Comments
Alacrima, absent lacrimal puncta, and aptyalism[52]	
Anhidrotic ectodermal dysplasia (Christ-Siemens-Touraine syndrome)[49]	
Dysautonomia (Riley-Day syndrome)[53]	Also have decreased corneal sensation
EEC syndrome (ectrodactyly, ectodermal dysplasia, cleft lip and palate)[49]	Inconstant, can have corneal scarring
Goldenhar syndrome[9]	Can also have decreased corneal sensations as well as limbal dermoids
Isolated alacrima[2]	A reported family had only punctate corneal staining and peripheral corneal pannus
Keratosis follicularis (Siemann disease)[49]	Also can have recurrent corneal erosions and punctate corneal opacities
LADD syndrome[3]	Punctal obliteration in this condition is fortunate

Epiphora

Excessive tearing may be due to excessive production of tears, as in viral infections or glaucoma. Thus the eye itself must be investigated first. Much more frequently the tearing will be secondary to an insufficiency of the lacrimal drainage system. While any part of the drainage system may be occluded, the most frequent location is at the end of the nasolacrimal duct, the last area to canalize embryologically.[54] Many normal children have this problem in early infancy with frequent spontaneous resolution. Patients with craniofacial malformations may have abnormalities in more than one part of the system,[54] and surgical repair of the orbits and face may aggravate their tearing. Unusual masses in the medial canthal area or nose should raise the suspicion of an encephalocele and be evaluated by CT scan prior to probing the lacrimal system.

Defective Pumping Action of Orbicularis Oculi	
Associated Conditions	**Comments**
Lid colobomas (see previous list)	
Lid ectropion (see previous list)	
Möbius syndrome (VII palsy)[1]	
Lacrimal Punctal Obliteration	
Associated Conditions	**Comments**
Branchio-otorenal dysplasia[3]	
Congenital familial[3]	Remainder of system may be absent also
LADD syndrome[3]	Also have poor lacrimal function
Secondary to antiviral drops[55]	
Dyskeratosis congenita[3]	
Smith-Lemli-Opitz syndrome[56]	
Canalicular Obstruction	
Associated Conditions	**Comments**
Congenital[54]	
Secondary to viral infections such as varicella and herpes simplex[57]	
Laterally displaced puncta	
Waardenburg syndrome[34]	
Blepharonasofacial syndrome[30]	

GLOBE

Prominent Eyes

Apparent prominence of the globes can be secondary to shallow orbits or large globe size as in high myopia or glaucoma (see separate sections). Proptosis of the eye beyond its normal orbital relationship can be caused by a mass effect as in neurofibromatosis, teratomas, leukemia, or Graves' disease.

Microphthalmos

Strictly speaking, microphthalmos means a globe with a small diameter. It is often assumed to exist when the patient has a small cornea, but this is not always correct, for example, in oculodentodigital syndrome.[11] Axial length measurements of the eye can be obtained with ultrasound for a definitive diagnosis. Graphs relating globe size to age are available.[58] The combination of small lids, small cornea, highly hyperopic refractive error and/or persistent hyperplastic primary vitreous is often used to make a clinical assumption of microphthalmos.

Microphthalmia, Colobomatous

Colobomatous microphthalmos can be an isolated hereditary condition.[59]

Frequent Associations	Comments
Cat-eye syndrome[1,5,23]	
Cataract with microcornea and coloboma of the iris[60]	
CHARGE (Coloboma, heart anomaly, choanal atresia, retardation, genital and ear abnormalities) association[3]	
Cohen syndrome[42]	
Facial clefting syndromes[3,47]	
Focal dermal hypoplasia (Goltz syndrome)[61]	
Hepatic fibrosis, polycystic kidneys, colobomas, and encephalopathy[59]	
Lenz syndrome[59]	
Meckel-Gruber syndrome[10]	Present in 26% of cases
Sjögren-Larsson syndrome[59]	
Triploidy syndrome[1]	
Trisomy 13 syndrome[5]	At times clinically anophthalmic
Warburg syndrome[41]	Often with retinal detachment or nonattachment
3q+ syndrome[5]	Mimics de Lange syndrome
4p− syndrome[5]	
4p+ syndrome[5]	
13q− syndrome[5]	

Occasional Associations	Comments
Basal cell nevus syndrome[24]	
Congenital contractural arachnodactyly[59]	
Humeroradial synostosis[59]	
Linear sebaceous nevus sequence[48]	
Rubinstein-Taybi syndrome[44]	
Treacher Collins syndrome[1]	
Many chromosomal defects[5,59]	

Microphthalmos Noncolobomatous

Noncolobomatous microphthalmos can be an isolated inherited condition.[59]

Frequent Associations	Comments
Cross syndrome[59]	
Fetal rubella effects[1]	
Frontonasal dysplasia sequence[1]	
Gorlin-Chaudhry-Moss syndrome[2]	
Hallermann-Streiff syndrome[45]	
Pena-Shokeir type II syndrome (COFS syndrome)[38]	
Warburg syndrome[41]	

Occasional Associations	Comments
Aicardi syndrome[62]	
Fanconi pancytopenia syndrome[1]	
Fetal alcohol effects[1]	
Fetal varicella effects[1]	
Goldenhar syndrome[9]	
Hyperthermia-induced defects[1]	
Hypomelanosis of Ito[63]	
Maternal phenylketonuria fetal effects[1]	
Oculodentodigital syndrome[11]	Most patients have only small corneas
Ring B syndrome[5,59]	
Treacher Collins syndrome[1]	
Trisomy 9 syndrome[5]	
10q+ syndrome[5,59]	

Ocular Motility Disorders

Strabismus

Strabismus occurs in 2% of the general population. It frequently occurs in individuals with CNS disorders due to genetic or traumatic causes. Some syndromes have characteristic deviations such as esotropia in Down syndrome and V-pattern exotropia (more exotropic in upgaze than downgaze) in craniofacial malformations. However, the presence of strabismus and its direction are usually nonspecific findings. It should be considered a complication of many syndromes that must be managed rather than a diagnostic criterion.

Motility Defects

These defects are much less common and are somewhat more helpful in syndrome identification.

Duane Syndrome

The hallmark of this syndrome is retraction of the globe on attempted adduction. Usually there is limited abduction, and there may also be limited adduction. Duane syndrome can be an isolated finding.

Associated Conditions	Comments
Acroreno-ocular syndrome[3]	Also uveal and optic nerve colobomas
Goldenhar syndrome[9,64]	
Hanhart syndrome[64]	
Okihiro syndrome[3]	
Wildervanck syndrome[3] (Klippel-Feil anomaly with Duane syndrome)[3]	Most commonly seen in girls

Abduction Defects and Facial Nerve Palsies

Associated Conditions	Comments
Möbius' syndrome[64]	Any cranial nerve can be involved Similar picture in Hanhart's syndrome and other craniofacial syndromes

Paralysis of Voluntary Gaze

Oculomotor apraxia.—Loss of horizontal saccades occurs. Patients use vestibulo-ocular reflexes with head thrusting to look at objects to the side.

Associated Conditions	Comments
Isolated, hereditary[3]	
Prematurity[3]	
Ataxia-telangiectasia[1]	Frequency unknown, may be an early sign
OFD (Oral-Facial-Digital syndrome) type III	

Ophthalmoplegia

Congenital ophthalmoplegia can be hereditary.[3] Fibrosis of the extraocular muscles causes a similar picture of the eyes being fixed, usually in downgaze, with marked ptosis and convergence nystagmus on attemped upgaze.[66] At least one family probably had a supranuclear defect because their eyes would go up on forced closure of the lids (Bell's phenomenon).[66] In other reports the lack of forced duction testing, which would detect tight fibrotic muscles, precludes an exact diagnosis. The presence of internal ophthalmoplegia in some families would infer a neural problem.

Fibrosis of the Extraocular Muscles

Associated Conditions	Comments
Isolated problem[66]	
Freeman-Sheldon syndrome[67] (whistling face syndrome)	Probably in a minority of patients

Nystagmus

Nystagmus may be secondary to poor vision or secondary to a disorder of the ocular tracking and stabilizing centers. While it indicates a need for investigation of the eye and brain, it is rarely distinctive enough in form to make a diagnosis.

Myopia

Myopia is usually due to abnormally large eyes but may also be induced by spherical lenses, anteriorly displaced lenses, or increased corneal curvature. Myopia is unusual in the first year of life. Premature infants, particularly those who developed retinopathy of prematurity, are more at risk for myopia. Isolated myopia can be inherited in an autosomal dominant or autosomal recessive pattern.

Frequent Associations	Comments
Cohen syndrome[42]	
Congenital glaucoma	Flattening of the cornea can partially compensate for globe enlargement
Deafness, cochlear; myopia; congenital renal disease[3]	
Fetal alcohol effects[1]	
Homocystinuria syndrome[1]	Lens dislocation also causes marked astigmatism
Kniest syndrome[68]	Can be severe and lead to retinal detachment
Marfan syndrome[69]	Lens dislocation also causes high astigmatism
Marshall-Smith syndrome[1]	
Noonan syndrome[19]	
Schwartz syndrome[39]	
Spondyloepiphyseal dysplasia congenita syndrome[68]	High risk of retinal detachment
Stickler syndrome[68]	Severe; high risk of retinal detachment
Weill-Marchesani syndrome[70]	Due to spherical, anteriorly dislocated lenses, which can also cause glaucoma

Occasional Associations	Comments
de Lange syndrome[1]	
Ehlers-Danlos syndrome[71]	Especially in type VI, can also have dislocated lenses
Fetal trimethadione effects[1]	
Incontinentia pigmenti[72]	
Scheie syndrome[1]	
Trisomy 20p syndrome[6]	
XXXXY syndrome[5]	
5_p- syndrome[5]	

Hyperopia

Mild hyperopia is the most common refraction found in infants. Greater degrees of hyperopia tend to be caused by a smaller than average eye, as in microphthalmos. Other less common factors include a flatter cornea, absent lens, or a lens so dislocated that it is completely outside the visual axis. Small hyperemic optic nerves are often seen in highly hyperopic eyes, and a tendency for esotropia can be aggravated by hyperopia.

Associated Conditions	Comments
Aarskog syndrome[13]	
Cornea plana	See cornea plana section, later
Kenny syndrome[73]	Often +8 to +14
Leber congenital amaurosis[74]	Often +6 to +10
Rubinstein-Taybi syndrome[44]	

Blue Sclera

All infants have a bluish tinge to the sclera, probably from the thinness of the structure. Myopic eyes also tend to have thin sclera (see Myopia, two sections earlier). The term *blue sclera* is usually reserved for extreme cases.

Frequent Associations	Comments
Hypophosphatasia[75]	
Marshall-Smith syndrome[1]	
Osteogenesis imperfecta syndrome autosomal recessive[1]	
Robert syndrome[1]	
Russell-Silver syndrome[1]	

Occasional Associations	Comments
Ehlers-Danlos syndrome[71]	
Focal dermal hypoplasia[61]	Almost all cases are female, probably lethal in males

Occasional Associations	Comments
Hallermann-Streiff syndrome[45]	
Incontinentia pigmenti syndrome[72]	Almost exclusively seen in females, probably lethal in males
Marfan syndrome[69]	
Pseudoxanthoma elasticum[49]	
Trisomy 18 syndrome[5]	

CORNEA

Abnormalities in Corneal Diameter

The full-term newborn's corneal diameter should be 10 to 11 mm. There is little variation in size, so a diameter less than 9 mm indicates a microcornea, and one greater than 11.5 mm indicates megalocornea in term infants.

Microcornea

Frequently occurs in association with microphthalmos, abnormalities of corneal curvature, or sclerocornea.

Associated Conditions	Comments
Aniridia[76]	
Cataract-microcornea syndrome[77]	Any type of opacity, may have sclerocornea or Peters anomaly
Deafness, retardation, arched palate syndrome[76]	
Microcornea, glaucoma, absent frontal sinuses[3]	
Oculodentodigital dysplasia[11]	Characteristic
Oculocerebrofacial syndrome[3]	
Ring 7 chromosome[76]	
Trisomy 18 syndrome[5]	
18q – syndrome[5]	

Megalocornea

Must rule out congenital glaucoma first.

Associated Conditions	Comments
Craniosynostosis[76]	
Down syndrome	Both glaucoma and megalocornea have occurred
Facial hemiatrophy[76]	
Isolated megalocornea[76]	Usually X-linked—rarely autosomal recessive or dominant Normal thickness and curvature
Marfan syndrome[69, 76]	Often part of generalized enlargement of the eye (megaloglobus)
Megalocornea–mental retardation syndrome (Neuhauser syndrome)[3]	May also have iris hypoplasia

Abnormalities in Corneal Curvature

Staphyloma

Staphyloma[78] is actually an anterior protrusion of the eye that contains cornea and adherent iris and lens; it is blue in color because of uveal pigment. Rarely hereditary, it has been reported with median facial cleft syndrome.[1]

Keratoconus

Keratoconus is much more common among atopic individuals, the mentally retarded, and patients with Leber's congenital amaurosis who tend to gouge their eyes. It is rarely hereditary.[3, 79] This raises the possibility that repeated trauma to the eyes plays a significant role in its development. It tends to develop in the teenage years.

Frequent Associations	Comments
Down syndrome[5]	
Leber congenital amaurosis[74]	
Noonan syndrome[19]	
Retinal disinsertion syndrome[80]	

Occasional Associations	Comments
Apert syndrome[1]	
Crouzon syndrome[26]	
Ehlers-Danlos syndrome[71]	Only in type VI
Focal dermal hypoplasia[61]	
Marfan syndrome[69]	

Occasional Associations	Comments
Nail-patella syndrome (osteo-onychodysplasia)[1]	
Osteogenesis imperfecta[1]	
Rieger syndrome[21]	
18p− syndrome[5]	

Cornea Plana

Decreased corneal curvature.

Associated Conditions	Comments
Isolated cornea plana[76,81]	Severe recessive form and milder dominant form, can also have peripheral sclerocornea
Marfan syndrome[69]	More common in the patients with dislocated lenses

Abnormalities in Corneal Opacity

Corneal Opacity, Diffuse

Frequent Associations	Comments
Cockayne syndrome	
Congenital hereditary endothelial dystrophy[82]	Truly congenital opacity in recessive form; some apparently dominant cases may have a severe form of posterior polymorphous dystrophy
Cystinosis[83]	Crystals apparent with slit lamp at the age of 2 years
Fabry syndrome[49]	Very specific whorl-shaped opacities in all patients after the age of 4 years; female carriers also have changes
Fetal rubella effects[1]	Secondary to viral keratitis as well as glaucoma
Hurler syndrome[1]	Not congenital, probably becomes visible at the slit lamp at the ages of 6–12 months may precede facial changes
Infection[76]	Syphilis, herpes simplex, rubella, chlamydia, gonorrhea
Maroteaux-Lamy syndrome[1]	Less severe than Hurler syndrome
Morquio syndrome[1]	Usually not visible until the age of 5 years
Mucolipidosis III[84]	Usually not visible until the age of 4 years
Mucolipidosis IV[85]	Has been seen at the age of 6 weeks
Scheie syndrome[1]	Not congenital
Sly (MPS VII)[86]	As early as the age of 7 months
Sclerocornea[87]	May be total or peripheral; has been associated with many systemic problems. See below
Sialidosis, Goldberg type[88]	Youngest patient was 12 years old

Occasional Associations	Comments
Acromesomelic dysplasia[89]	
Birth trauma[76]	Due to rupture of Descemet's membrane
GM_1 gangliosidosis, type I[90]	Present very early, congenital (possibly)
Multiple sulfatase deficiency[91]	
Pachyonychia congenita syndrome[49]	
Pena-Shokeir type II syndrome (COFS syndrome)[38]	
Rutherford syndrome[3]	Diffuse opacity in upper half of cornea that is visible by at least the age of 3 years
Seip syndrome (Berardinelli's lipodystrophy syndrome)[1]	
Trisomy 8 syndrome[23,76]	
Trisomy 13 syndrome[5]	
Trisomy 18 syndrome[5]	
18q− syndrome[5]	

Sclerocornea

Total Sclerocornea.—The cornea is totally opaque. It is associated with many systemic problems and the following syndromes.

Associated Conditions	Comments
Nail-patella syndrome (osteo-onychodysplasia)[92]	

Associated Conditions	Comments
Smith-Lemli-Opitz syndrome[56]	
Mieten syndrome[87]	
Microphthalmos, mental retardation, spasticity[87]	
Cross syndrome[59]	
Robert syndrome (pseudothalidomide)[1]	
Unbalanced 17p-10q translocation[87]	
4p− syndrome[5]	Rare

Peripheral Scleroderma.—The following are associated with peripheral scleroderma.

Associated Conditions	Comments
Cornea plana[81]	
Hypomelanosis of Ito[63]	
Isolated[93]	
Melnick-Needles syndrome[17]	

Corneal Opacity, Localized

Peters Anomaly.—This includes iris processes up to central corneal defect in Descemet's membrane and/or lens-corneal contact. Associated with many systemic defects. Clear-cut syndromes are listed below.

Associated Conditions	Comments
Aniridia[94]	
Cataract microcornea syndrome[77]	
Fetal alcohol syndrome[84]	
Fetal rubella effects[94]	
Fetal transfusion syndrome[94]	
Group 13-15 trisomy phenotype[94]	
Peters anomaly and short stature[94,95]	
Pillay syndrome[94]	
Radial aplasia, anterior chamber cleavage syndrome[3]	
Rieger syndrome[21,94]	
Waarburg syndrome[41]	
Trisomy 9 syndrome[5]	
4p− syndrome[5]	
11q− syndrome[94]	
18q− syndrome[94]	

Associated Conditions	Comments
Corneal dermoids	
Limbal	Characteristic of Goldenhar's syndrome[9] Usually not visually significant Also occur in linear sebaceous nevus[48]
Central[96]	Rare; elevation and clear peripheral cornea distinguish them from sclerocornea
Ring[97]	
Other opacities	
Keratoconus posticus circumscriptus[1]	Two families described
Wedge-shaped stromal opacity	Clefting syndrome with anterior chamber and lid anomalies[38]
Acromegaloid changes, cutis verticis gyrata and corneal leukoma[3]	Epithelial opacities can occur as early as 1 year and progress thereafter
Meesman syndrome[3]	
Richner-Hanhart syndrome[49]	
Fucosidosis[49]	
Trisomy 13 syndrome[5]	
Trisomy 18 syndrome[5]	
Autosomal dominant coloboma/microphthalmos[98]	

Decreased Corneal Sensation

This condition can have devastating consequences as the eye is subjected to repeated trauma and drying because reflex blinking does not occur. Lack of lid closure from colobomas or VII nerve palsy or lack of basal tear secretion can further compound these patient's problems.

Associated Conditions	Comments
Dysautonomia (Riley-Day syndrome)[53]	Also have decreased tear function
Goldenhar syndrome[9]	Also have decreased tear function
Isolated corneal anesthesia[76]	Varies in severity of complications
Möbius syndrome[1]	Seventh nerve palsy worsens problem

Glaucoma

Enlargement of the globes occurs in infants (buphthalmos).

Frequent Associations	Comments
Aniridia[99]	
Cicatricial retinopathy of prematurity[100]	
Lowe syndrome[99]	60% of patients; can be unilateral
Cataract-microcornea syndrome[3, 77, 99]	
Microphthalmos	See above
Nevus of Ota (hyperpigmentation of lids and ocular layers)[99]	Glaucoma often occurs much later
Peters' anomaly	See above
Rieger's syndrome	Three patients with 4q−, 4p−, and Down's syndromes have been reported[5]
Stickler's syndrome[68]	
Sturge-Weber sequence[101]	Approx 50% chance if the lids are involved with hemangioma
Sulfite oxidase deficiency[99]	Secondary to lens dislocation
Trisomy 13 syndrome[5]	
Weill-Marchesani syndrome[70]	From anterior displacement of the lens
3q+ syndrome[5]	
18q− syndrome[5]	

Occasional Associations	Comments
Basal cell nevus syndrome[24]	
C syndrome[2]	
Down syndrome	
Ectopia lentis	See later
Ehlers-Danlos syndrome[71]	
Fetal rubella effects[1]	From primary angle abnormality, uveitis, or lens effects
Goldenhar syndrome[9]	
Hallermann-Streiff syndrome[45]	
Homocystinuria syndrome[68]	Secondary to lens dislocation, so unusual prior to the age of 2 years
Klippel-Trenaunay-Weber syndrome[1]	
Marfan syndrome[69]	
Mucopolysaccharidoses[99]	
Neurofibromatosis syndrome[99]	Most likely if lids involved with tumor
Oculodentodigital syndrome[11]	
Robinow (fetal face) syndrome[1]	
Scheie syndrome[1]	
Treacher Collins syndrome[1]	
Turner syndrome[99]	
von Hippel–Lindau disease[99]	Usually secondary to uveitis or retinal detachment; occurs late
Zellweger syndrome[1]	

Abnormalities of the Iris

Colobomas of the Iris

(Also see Microphthalmos, Colobomatous, earlier.) Colobomas of the iris are most frequently inferior because of the usual closure of the fetal fissure. They can occur at any axis from the pupil and can be an isolated autosomal dominant condition.

Frequent Associations	Comments
Frequent in	
Acroreno-ocular syndrome[3]	One family also has Duane's syndrome
Biemond syndrome, type II[3]	Resembles Bardet-Biedl syndrome
Cat-eye syndrome[1, 5, 23]	
CHARGE association[3]	
Rieger syndrome[21]	May have polycoria secondary to iris hypoplasia

Occasional Associations	Comments
Aniridia[21]	In less severe cases
Langer-Giedion syndrome[3]	
Joubert syndrome[3]	

Iris, Unusual Color or Structure

Associated Conditions	Comments
Albinism[49]	Reddish color is the red reflex from the fundus, not blocked effectively by hypopigmented iris
Aniridia[1, 3]	Rim of iris remains Sporadic cases may have 11p− Wilm's tumor association[5]; one family with good vision and one with ab-

Associated Conditions	Comments
	sent patellae have been reported
Anisocoria[3]	
Down syndrome[5]	An increased number of Brushfield's spots, which are normal, hyperplastic iris stroma
	Thinning of peripheral iris stroma
Ectopic pupils	Ectopia lentis et pupillae[3]
	Ptosis, strabismus, and ectopic pupils[3]
Iris cleavage syndrome[3]	
Microcoria[3]	
Nail-patella syndrome (osteo-onychodysplasia)[92]	Lester's sign—cloverleaf-shaped dark pigmentation of iris at pupillary margin
Neurofibromatosis[102]	Lisch's nodules are pathognomonic
	Can be congenital but infrequent prior to the age of 6 years
Rieger syndrome[21]	Hypoplastic anterior iris leaf
	May have polycoria
Spastic ataxia, microcoria[3]	
Synechiae	Smith-Lemli-Opitz syndrome[56]
	Intraocular inflammation
William syndrome[12]	Stellate appearance of iris is due to hypoplastic anterior iris leaf

Heterochromia

Irides of different colors.

Associated Conditions	Comments
Congenital Horner syndrome[3]	Usually iris is lighter on affected side, can be hereditary
Hypomelanosis of Ito[63]	
Incontinentia pigmenti[72]	Rare
Waardenburg syndrome[3]	Pale blue areas of one or both eyes or entire iris due to the irregular pigmentation defect

Ectropian Uvea

Pigmented epithelium of the iris is everted onto the outer surface. It has been associated with neurofibromatosis.[102]

Lens Opacity

Cataracts can be primary, or they may be secondary to intraocular inflammation or retinal detachment.

Frequent Associations	Comments
Alport syndrome[103]	Anterior lenticonus is present in some families; reported as early as age 12 years, unknown how early it can occur
Aniridia[3]	Often spokelike cortical opacities
Cataract and congenital ichthyosis[3]	
Cataract-cardiomyopathy syndrome[104]	Totally opaque at birth
Cataract, microcephaly, kyphosis[3]	One family
Cataract-microcornea syndrome[3, 77]	
Cataract, microphthalmos, nystagmus[3]	
Cockayne syndrome[7]	
Conradi-Hünermann syndrome[25]	Present in 2/3 of patients with the X-linked form but often asymmetrical; absent in the autosomal dominant form
Crome syndrome[3]	Seizures, short stature, infantile death
Fetal rubella effects[1]	Dense nuclear opacity with large diameter, clear cortex
Hallermann-Streiff syndrome[45]	
Isolated hereditary congenital cataracts[105]	Can be anywhere in lens, consistent within families; autosomal dominant is most common transmission
Lowe syndrome[105]	Fluffy nuclear, large-diameter opacity; lens can be reduced in thickness; carriers have many cortical dots
Mannosidosis[105]	Spokelike cortical changes by the age of 2 years
Marinesco-Sjögren syndrome[1]	

Frequent Associations	Comments
Marshall syndrome[1]	Rapid development and even partial resorption reported
Martsolf syndrome[3]	
Pena-Shokeir type II syndrome[38]	In approx 70% of patients
Rhizomelic chondrodysplasia punctata syndrome[25]	Present and symmetrical in 72% of patients
Rothmund-Thomson syndrome[49]	Usually not present until the ages of 2–7 years; have been seen in first few months
Schafer syndrome[49]	
Smith-Lemli-Opitz syndrome[56]	Most often acquired
Steinert myotonic dystrophy syndrome[1]	Usually not present until 20s Posterior subcapsular and scattered colored opacities
Stickler syndrome (Wagner syndrome)[68]	In young children may be secondary to retinal detachment; at puberty posterior cortical and nuclear sclerotic changes may begin
5p− syndrome[5]	

Occasional Associations	Comments
Abetalipoproteinemia[106]	Posterior polar opacities
Albright hereditary osteodystrophy syndrome[1]	Peripheral in the lens
Basal cell nevus syndrome[24]	
Cockayne syndrome[8]	
Down syndrome[5]	Rarely until teens; arcuate, sutural, and flakelike opacities develop
Fetal alcohol effects[1]	
Karsch-Neugebauer syndrome[107]	
Multiple sulfatase deficiency[91]	Anterior, peripheral, circumferential opacities in one patient
Fetal varicella effects[1]	
Galactosemia[1]	Only if disease is not detected on newborn screening, rare now in USA
Homocystinuria syndrome[1]	
Incontinentia pigmenti syndrome[72]	Can be secondary to retinal detachment
Nail-patella syndrome[92]	
Pachyonychia congenita syndrome[1]	
Partial trisomy 10q syndrome[5]	
Progeria syndrome[1]	
Robert's syndrome[1]	
Rubinstein-Taybi syndrome[44]	
Schwartz's syndrome[39]	
Smith-Lemli-Opitz syndrome[56]	
Trisomy 13 syndrome[5]	
Trisomy 18 syndrome[5]	
Trisomy 20p syndrome[7]	
Zellweger's syndrome[1]	
3q+ syndrome[5]	
4p− syndrome[5]	
18p− syndrome[5]	
18q− syndrome[5]	

Lens Dislocation

Frequent Associations	Comments
Achard syndrome[3]	Marfan syndrome with receding lower jaw
Ectopia lentis et pupillae[108]	Up or down, but opposite to direction of pupil displacement
Homocystinuria syndrome[109]	Occurs in 90% of patients; a methionine-restricted diet started neonatally can reduce incidence greatly. Vitamin B_6–responsive patients have fewer problems. Most often down after the age of 2 years
Gillum-Anderson syndrome[110] (dominant ptosis, high myopia and ectopia lentis)	One family, ectopia lentis is present by at least 4 yr old
Isolated lens dislocation (up)[3]	Similar in appearance to Marfan lenses
Isolated microspherophakia[3]	
Marfan syndrome (up)[69]	Most often up and in, occurs in 50%–80% of patients, usually stable after early childhood
Microspherophakia with hernia[3]	Also myopia and retinal detachment
Retinal disinsertion syndrome[80]	

Frequent Associations	Comments
Sulfite oxidase deficiency[3]	Seen as early as age 3 weeks
Weill-Marchesani syndrome (anterior)[70]	Anterior dislocation progresses through childhood; microspherophakia is recognizable early

Occasional Associations	Comments
Aniridia[111]	
Apert syndrome[1]	
Ehlers-Danlos syndrome[71]	
Focal dermal hypoplasia (Goltz syndrome)[61]	
Pseudoxanthoma elasticum[49]	
Rieger syndrome[21]	

Vitreous Abnormalities

Associated Conditions	Comments
Trisomy 13 syndrome[5]	Persistent hyperplastic primary vitreous
Familial oculopalatocerebral dwarfism	Rarely

Pigmentary Abnormalities

Associated Conditions	Comments
Aicardi syndrome[63]	Multiple punched-out areas of choroid and pigment epithelium
Abetalipoproteinemia[106]	Bone spicules as early as the age of 13 mo
Albinism syndromes[49]	Ocular albinism, oculocutaneous albinism, Chédiak-Higashi syndrome, Hermansky-Pudlak syndrome, Waardenburg syndrome, Prader-Willi syndrome, some Apert syndrome patients
Alstrom's syndrome[3]	Not until after puberty
Best disease[3]	Egg yolk lesion is probably congenital
Ceroid lipofuscinosis[3]	Bull's-eye macular lesions are typical, hypopigmented peripheral changes even in infantile form, not present until the age of 2 yr
Chronic granulomatous disease[49]	Chorioretinal scars
Cockayne syndrome[7]	Salt-and-pepper changes, usually not present until after the age of 1 yr
Cohen syndrome[42]	Patchy choroidal and retinal atrophy, bone spicules in periphery, beginning as preschoolers
EEM syndrome[3]	Chorioretinal atrophy
Fetal cytomegalovirus effects[1]	Intense retinitis can be acquired as well
Fetal rubella effects[1]	Hypo- and hyperpigmented areas, may not be present in newborn period
Fetal toxoplasmosis effects[1]	Punched-out lesions of retina and choroid with smaller satellite lesions
Fetal varicella effects[1]	Chorioretinal scars
Focal dermal hypoplasia (Goltz syndrome)[61]	Hypo- and hyperpigmented areas
Gardner syndrome[112]	Hyperpigmented, round, oval, or kidney-shaped lesions, seen as early as 3 mo, may be congenital, usually bilateral or multiple
Hallermann-Streiff syndrome[45]	
Hunter syndrome[113]	Bone spicules, usually later in childhood
Hurler syndrome[113]	Bone spicules, usually later in childhood
Hypomelanosis of Ito[63]	Streaks of hypopigmentation
Infantile phytanic acid storage disease[114]	Decreased electroretinogram, bone spicules
Laurence-Moon syndrome[115]	Spastic paraparesis and lack of polydactyly distinguishes it from Bardet-Biedl syndrome
Jeune syndrome[3]	Clinical picture of Leber congenital amaurosis
Leber congenital amaurosis[74]	Wide variety of changes but usually not in first year of life
Microcephaly with chorioretinopathy[3]	Autosomal recessive or dominant
Microphthalmos[59]	
Multiple sulfatase deficiency[91]	Bone spicules
Neurofibromatosis[102]	Subtle choroidal hamartomas in 51%

Associated Conditions	Comments
Olivopontocerebellar atrophy, type III[116]	Bone spicules, age of onset varies greatly
Pelizaeus-Merzbacher disease[117]	Preceded by nystagmus that starts at 4–6 mo
Retinal disinsertion syndrome[80]	Multiple punched-out defects in pigment and choroid
Rud syndrome[49]	Bone spicules in a 4-yr-old
Saldino-Mainzer syndrome[118]	See Leber's congenital amaurosis
Sanfilippo syndrome[113]	Bone spicules, usually later in childhood
Scheie syndrome[113]	Bone spicules, usually later in childhood
Sjögren-Larsson syndrome[49]	"Glistening dots" or "snail tracks" in 30% of cases
18q– syndrome[5]	

Macular Colobomas

More likely agenesis than a coloboma.

Associated Conditions
Hypercalciuria, myopia,[119] and macular coloboma
Isolated[3]
Macular coloboma with brachydactyly[3]
Sorsby syndrome[3]

Retinal Tumors

Associated Conditions	Comments
Neurofibromatosis[102]	Rare; increased incidence of nevi
Retinoblastoma	White mass, very often calcified on ultrasound or CT scan
Tuberous sclerosis[49]	Hamartomas can be flat and later become mulberry-like

Macular Cherry-Red Spot

The pathological feature is the ring of opaque retina surrounding the cherry-red spot. The spot itself is normal pigmented epithelium visible because of thinning of the ganglion cell layer in the center of the macula. The white ring evolves as the disease progresses and may disappear in advanced stages.[120] This diagnostic sign is one of the most specific and limits the possible diseases to those following.[120]

Associated Conditions	Comments
Storage Diseases[120]	
Farber lipogranulomatosis	Faint, gray, normal vision
Generalized GM_1, gangliosidosis, type 1	50% of cases; very early[90]
GM_2 gangliosidoses	
Type 1: classic Tay-Sachs disease	Dense, white
Type 2: Sandhoff disease	Opaquely white
AB variant	
Late onset	Faint
Metachromatic leukodystrophy	Rare, faint
Multiple sulfatase deficiency[91]	
Niemann-Pick disease	More diffuse opacity, may extend to equator, persists for years with good vision
Type A, infantile	Inconstant
Type C, visceral	Inconstant
Sialidoses	
Cherry-red spot myoclonus syndrome	
Goldber syndrome	
Mucolipidosis I	
Nephrosialidosis	Inconstant
Other Causes of Cherry-Red Spots[120]	
Central retinal artery occlusion	Rare in infants
Traumatic retinal edema	Consider nonaccidental trauma
Macular hole with surrounding detachment	Consider nonaccidental trauma
Macular hemorrhage	Consider nonaccidental trauma
Leber congenital amaurosis	Rare, not characteristic of the disorder
Quinine toxicity	Variable

Falciform Retinal Folds

Associated Conditions	Comments
Familial exudative vitreoretinopathy[121]	
Retinopathy of prematurity[100]	

Associated Conditions	Comments
Trisomy 18 syndrome[5]	Histological finding
Warburg syndrome[41,122]	

Retinal Detachment

High myopia is the causative factor in many syndromes.

Associated Conditions	Comments
Coat's disease	Isolated in most cases, one family with muscular dystrophy[3]
Congenital retinal disinsertion syndrome[80]	
Congenital retinal nonattachment[122]	
Dominant myopia and retinal detachment[3]	
Ehlers-Danlos syndrome, types I and VI[3,71]	High myopia, thin sclera
Familial exudative vitreoretinopathy[121]	Mimics retinopathy of prematurity
Incontinentia pigmenti[72]	High myopia
Kniest syndrome[68]	High myopia
Marfan syndrome	More common in patients with long axial length of the globe
Marshall syndrome[3]	High myopia, may be identical with Wagner's syndrome
Merckel syndrome[10]	
Norrie disease[3]	Invariable; usually present at birth
FOAR syndrome[31]	High myopia
Osteoporosis-pseudoglioma syndrome[3]	Confused with retinoblastoma in the past
Retinopathy of prematurity[100]	
Spondyloepiphyseal dysgenesis, congenital[68]	High myopia
Stickler syndrome[68]	High myopia, giant retinal tears
Trisomy 3 syndrome[5]	
Warburg syndrome[41]	

Optic Nerve Abnormalities

Absent Optic Nerve.—Can also occur in microphthalmos. Rarely familial.[123]

Hypoplastic Optic Nerve.—Common in albinism and aniridia.[124] Observed in fetal alcohol and fetal hydantoin effects[124] as well as with other maternal substance abuse and in trisomy 13, trisomy 18, and 18q− syndromes.[5] Can be secondary to abnormalities in different parts of the visual pathways such as macular dysplasia, tumors of the optic nerves and suprasellar region, and suprageniculate hemispheric atrophy.[124] Segmental hypoplasia has been seen in some infants of juvenile diabetics.[124]

Pits, Colobomas.—Reflect faulty closure of fetal fissure.[125] May occur with choroidal and iris colobomas and/or microphthalmos and be caused by same syndromes (see aforementioned sections). Can be an isolated autosomal dominant condition or seen in Smith-Lemli-Opitz syndrome[56] and acroreno-ocular syndrome.[3]

Drusen.—Not distinctly seen under the age of 10 years.

Tumors.—Astrocytic hamartomas in tuberous sclerosis, usually seen after the age of 6 years.[49]

Acknowledgment

I am indebted to the late Dr. David W. Smith and to Dr. Kenneth Jones, editors of *Smith's Recognizable Patterns of Human Malformation* (WB Saunders Co, 1982). Their appendix sections on the eye provided the nucleus of this chapter. I am also grateful to my coauthors in Developmental Anomalies of the Eye *(Int Opthalmol Clin* 24: 1984), Drs. Bronwyn Bateman, Lawrence Hirst, Richard Weleber, David Apple, and John Crawford, whose chapters I have used for references here.

REFERENCES

1. Smith DW, Jones KL: *Recognizable Patterns of Human Malformation,* ed 3. Philadelphia, WB Saunders Co, 1982.
2. Bergsma D (ed): *Birth Defects Compendium,* ed 2. New York: Alan R Liss, Inc, 1979.
3. McKusick VA: *Mendelian Inheritance in*

Man, ed 7. Baltimore, The Johns Hopkins University Press, 1986.
4. Feingold M, Bossert WH: Normal values for selected physical parameters: An aid to syndrome delineation. *Birth Defects* 1974; 10:1–15.
5. Gieser S, Carey J, Apple D: Human chromosomal disorders and the eye, in Renie W (ed): *Goldberg's Genetic and Metabolic Eye Disease.* Boston, Little, Brown & Co, 1986, pp 185–240.
6. DeMeyer W, Zeman W, Palmer CG: The face predicts the brain: Diagnostic significance of medial facial anomalies for holoprosencephaly (arhinencephaly). *Pediatrics* 1964; 34:256.
7. Francke U: Partial duplication 20p, in Yunis JJ (ed): *New Chromosomal Syndromes.* New York, Academic Press, Inc, 1977.
8. Levin PS, Green WR, Victor DI, et al: Histopathology of the eye in Cockayne's Syndrome. *Arch Ophthalmol* 1983; 101:1093.
9. Baum JL, Feingold M: Ocular aspects of Goldenhar's syndrome. *Am J Ophthalmol* 1973; 75:250–257.
10. Salonen R: The Merckel syndrome: Clinicopathological findings in 67 patients. *Am J Med Genet* 1984; 18:671–689.
11. Judisch GF, Martin-Casals A, Hanson JW, et al: Oculodentodigital Dysplasia. *Arch Ophthalmol* 1976; 97:878–884.
12. Jensen OA, Warburg M, Dupont A: Ocular pathology in the elfin face syndrome. *Ophthalmologica* 1976; 172:434–444.
13. Grier RE, Farrington FH, Kendig R, et al: Autosomal dominant inheritance of the Aarskog syndrome. *Am J Med Genet* 1983; 15:39–46.
14. Cordero JF, Holmes LB: Phenotypic overlap of the BBB and G syndromes. *Am J Med Genet* 1978; 2:145–152.
15. Vles JSH, Haspeslagh M, Raes MMR, et al: Early clinical signs in Coffin-Lowry syndrome. *Clin Genet* 1984; 26:448–452.
16. Moller KT, Gorlin RJ: The Dubowitz syndrome: A retrospective. *J. Craniofac Genet* 1985; 1:283–286.
17. Perry LD, Edwards WC, Bramson RT: Melnick-Needles syndrome. *J Pediatr Ophthalmol Strabismus* 1978; 15:226–230.
18. Seuanez H, Mane-Garzon F, Kolski R: Cardio-cutaneous syndrome (the "Leopard" syndrome). Review of the literature and a new family. *Clin Genet* 1976; 9:266–276.
19. Allanson JE, Hall JG, Hughes HE, et al: Noonan syndrome: The changing phenotype. *Am J Med Genet* 1985; 21:507–514.
20. Abernethy DA: Hypertelorism in several generations. *Arch Dis Child* 1927; 15:361–365.
21. Alkemade PPH: *Dysgenesis Mesodermalis of the Iris and the Cornea.* Assen, The Netherlands, Charles C Thomas, Publishers, 1969.
22. Shelley ED, Shelley WB: The fish odor syndrome. *JAMA* 1984; 251:253–256.
23. Weleber RG, Magenis RE: The importance of chromosomal studies in ophthalmology. *Ophthalmol Clin* 1984; 24:15.
24. Feman SS, Apt L, Roth AM: The basal cell nevus syndrome. *Am J Ophthalmol* 1974; 78:222–228.
25. Spranger J, Opitz JM, Bidder U: Heterogeneity of chondrodysplasia punctata. *Humangenetik* 1971; 11:190.
26. Robinson LK, James HE, Mubarak SJ, et al: Carpenter syndrome: Natural history and clinical spectrum. *Am J Med Genet* 1985; 20:461–469.
27. Gorlin RJ, Pindborg JJ, Cohen MM: *Syndromes of the Head and Neck,* ed 2. New York, McGraw-Hill International Book Co, 1976, pp 220–223.
28. Chan CC, Green WR, de la Cruz ZC, et al: Ocular findings in osteogenesis imperfecta congenita. *Arch Ophthalmol* 1982; 100:1459–1463.
29. Danks DM, Mayne V, Hall RK, et al: Frontometaphyseal dysplasia. A progressive disease of bone and connective tissue. *Am J Dis Child* 1972; 123:254.
30. Pashayan H, Prazansky S, Putterman A: A family with blepharo-naso-facial malformations. *Am J Dis Child* 1973; 125:389–393.
31. Holmes LB, Schepens CL: Syndrome of ocular and facial anomalies, telecanthus and deafness. *J Pediatr* 1972; 81:552–555.
32. Fryns JP, Haspeslagh M: Mental retardation, short stature, minor skeletal anomalies, craniofacial dysmorphism and macrodontia in two sisters and their mother. *Clin Genet* 1984; 26:69–72.
33. Anneren G, Arvidson B, Gustavson K-H, et al: Oro-facio-digital syndromes I and II: Radiological methods for diagnosis and the clinical variations. *Clin Genet* 1984; 26:178–186.
34. Delleman JW, Hageman MJ: Ophthalmological findings in 34 patients with Waarden-

burg syndrome. *J Pediatr Ophthalmol Strabismus* 1977; 15:341–345.

35. Kohn R, Romano PE: Blepharoptosis, blepharophimosis, epicanthus inversus, and telecanthus—A syndrome with no name. *Am J Ophthalmol* 1971; 72:625–631.
36. Townes PT, Muechler EK: Blepharophimosis, ptosis, epicanthus inversus, and primary amenorrhea. *Arch Ophthalmol* 1979; 97:1664–1666.
37. Michels VV, Hittner HM, Beaudet AL: A clefting syndrome with ocular anterior chamber defect and lid anomalies. *J Pediac* 1978; 93:444–446.
38. Grizzard WS, O'Donnell JJ, Carey JC: The cerebro-oculo-facio-skeletal syndrome. *Am J Ophthalmol* 1980; 89:293–298.
39. Edwards WC, Root AW: Chondrodystrophic myotonia (Schwartz-Jampel syndrome): Report of a new case and follow-up of patients initially reported in 1969. *Am J Med Gent* 1982; 13:51–56.
40. Dobyns WB, Gilbert EF, Opitz JM: Further comments on the lissencephaly syndrome (letter). *Am J Med Genet* 1985; 22:197–211.
41. Pagon RA, Clarren SK, Milam DF Jr, et al: Autosomal recessive eye and brain anomalies: Warburg syndrome. *J Pediatr* 1983; 102:542–546.
42. Norio R, Raitta C, Lindahl E: Further delineation of the Cohen syndrome; report on chorioretinal dystrophy, leukopenia and consanguinity. *Clin Genet* 1984; 25:1–14.
43. Halal F, Herrmann J, Pallister PD, et al: Differential diagnosis of Nager acrofacial dysostosis syndrome: Report of four patients with Nager syndrome and discussion of other related syndromes. *Am J Med Genet* 1983; 14:209–224.
44. Roy FH, Summitt RL, Hiatt RL, et al: Ocular manifestations of the Rubinstein-Taybi syndrome: Case report and review of the literature. *Arch Ophthalmol* 1968; 79:272.
45. François J: François' dyscephalic syndrome. *Birth Defects* 1982; 18:595–619.
46. Sugio Y, Kajii T: Ruvalcaba syndrome: Autosomal dominant inheritance. *Am J Med Genet* 1984; 19:741–753.
47. Tessier P: Anatomical classification of facial, craniofacial and laterofacial clefts. *J Maxillofac Surg* 1976; 4:69.
48. Wilkes SR, Campbell RJ, Waller RR: Ocular malformation in association with ipsilateral facial nevus of Jadassohn. *Am J Ophthalmol* 1981; 92:344–352.
49. Worobec-Victor SM, Bain MAB: Oculocutaneous genetic diseases, in Renie WA (ed): *Goldberg's Genetic and Metabolic Eye Disease,* ed 2. Boston, Little, Brown & Co, 1986, p 489.
50. Ohdo S, Madokoro H, Sonoda T, et al: Kabuki make-up syndrome (Niikawa-Kuroki syndrome) associated with congenital heart disease. *J Med Genet* 1985; 22:126–127.
51. Zaun H, Stenger D, Zabransky S, et al: Das Syndrom der langen Wimpern (Trichomegaliesyndrom, Oliver-McFarlane). *Hautarzt* 1984; 35:162–165.
52. Caccamise WC, Townes PL: Congenital absence of the lacrimal puncta associated with alacrima and aptyalism. *Am J Ophthalmol* 1980; 89:62–65.
53. Goldberg MF, Payne JW, Brunt PW: Ophthalmologic studies of familial dysautonomia. *Arch Ophthalmol* 1968; 80:732–743.
54. Crawford JS, Pashby RC: Lacrimal system disorders. *Int Ophthalmol Clin* 1984; 24:39–54.
55. O'Day DM: Herpes simplex keratitis, in Leibowitz HM (ed): *Corneal Disorders.* Philadelphia, WB Saunders Co, 1984, p 339.
56. Kretzer FL, Hittner HM, Mehta RS: Ocular manifestations of the Smith-Lemli-Opitz syndrome. *Arch Ophthalmol* 1981; 99:2000–2006.
57. Harley RD, Stefanyszyn MA, Apt L, et al: Herpetic canalicular obstruction. *Ophthalmic Surg* 1987; 18:367–370.
58. Larsen JS: The sagittal growth of the eye. IV Ultrasonic measurements of the depth of the axial length of the eye from birth to puberty. *Acta Ophthalmol (Copenh)* 1971: 49:873–886.
59. Bateman JB: Microphthalmos. *Int Ophthalmol Clin* 1987; 24:87–107.
60. Cummings C, Polomeno RC, McAlpine PJ: Autosomal dominant cataracts, coloboma and microphthalmia. Presented at the Fifth International Conference on Birth Defects, Montreal, 1977.
61. Thomas JV, Yoshizumi MO, Beyer CK, et al: Ocular manifestations of focal dermal hypoplasia syndrome. *Arch Ophthalmol* 1977; 95:1997–2001.
62. Del Pero RA, Mets MB, Tripathi RC, et al: Anomalies of retinal architecture in Aicardi

Syndrome. *Arch Ophthalmol* 1986; 104:1659–1664.
63. Reese PD, Judisch GF: Hypomelanosis of Ito. *Arch Ophthalmol* 1986; 104:1136–1137.
64. Miller M: Ocular abnormalities in craniofacial malformations. *Int Ophthalmol Clin* 1984; 24:143.
65. Sugarman GI, Katakia M, Menkes J: See-saw winking in a familial oral-facial-digital syndrome. *Clin Genet* 1971; 2:248–254.
66. Waardenburg PJ, Franceschetti A, Klein D: *Genetics and Ophthalmology*. New York, Charles C. Thomas, Publisher, 1961, pp 1090–1132.
67. O'Keefe M, Crawford JS, Young JDH, et al: Ocular abnormalities in the Freeman-Sheldon syndrome. *Am J Ophthalmol* 1986; 102:346–348.
68. Maumenee IH: Vitreoretinal degeneration as a sign of generalized connective tissue disease. *Am J Ophthalmol* 1979; 88:432–449.
69. Maumenee IH: The eye in the Marfan syndrome. *Trans Am Ophthalmol Soc* 1981; 79:684–733.
70. Jensen AD, Cross HE, Paton D: Ocular complications in the Weill-Marchesani syndrome. *Am J Ophthalmol* 1974; 77:261–269.
71. Judisch GF, Waziri M, Krachmer JH: Ocular Ehlers-Danlos syndrome with normal lysyl hydroxylase activity. *Arch Ophthalmol* 1976; 94:1489–1491.
72. Manthey R, Apple DJ, Kivlin JD: Iris hypoplasia in incontinentia pigmenti. *J Pediatr Ophthalmol Strabismus* 1982; 19:279–280.
73. Larsen JL, Kivlin J, Odell WD: Unusual cause of short stature. *Am J Med* 1985; 78:1025–1032.
74. Schroeder R, Mets MB, Maumenee IH: Leber's congenital amaurosis. *Arch Ophthalmol* 1987; 105:356–359.
75. Brenner RL, Smith JL, Cleveland WW, et al: Eye signs of hypophosphatasia. *Arch Ophthalmol* 1969; 81:614–617.
76. Hirst LW: Congenital corneal problems. *Int Ophthalmol Clin* 1984; 24:87.
77. Salmon JF, Wallis CE, Murray AD: Variable expressivity of autosomal dominant microcornea with cataract. *Arch Ophthalmol* 1988; 106:505–510.
78. Schanzlin DJ, Robin JB, Erickson G, et al: Histopathologic and ultrastructural analysis of congenital corneal staphyloma. *Am J Ophthalmol* 1983; 95:506–514.
79. Krachmer JH, Feder RS, Belin MW: Keratoconus and related noninflammatory corneal thinning disorders. *Surv Ophthalmol* 1984; 28:293–322.
80. Boniuk M, Hittner HM: Congenital retinal disinsertion syndrome. *Trans Am Acad Ophthalmol Otolaryngol* 1975; 79:327–334.
81. Eriksson AW, Lehmann W, Forsius J: Congenital corneal plana in Finland. *Clin Genet* 1973; 4:301.
82. Judisch GF, Maumenee IH: Clinical differentiation of recessive congenital hereditary endothelial dystrophy and dominant hereditary endothelial dystrophy. *Am J Ophthalmol* 1978; 85:606–612.
83. Kenyon KR, Sensenbrenner JA: Electron microscopy of cornea and conjunctiva in childhood cystinosis. *Am J Ophthalmol* 1974; 78:68.
84. Traboulsi EI, Maumenee IH: Ophthalmologic findings in mucolipidosis III (Pseudo-Hurler polydystrophy). *Am J Ophthalmol* 1986; 102:592–597.
85. Merin S, Livni N, Berman ER, et al: Mucolipidosis IV: Ocular, systemic and ultrastructural findings. *Invest Ophthalmol* 1975; 14:437–448.
86. Beaudet AL, DiFerrante NM, Ferry GD, et al: Variation in the phenotypic expression of beta glucuronidase deficiency. *J Pediatr* 1975; 86:388–394.
87. Kivlin JD, Fineman RM, Williams MS: Phenotypic variation in the del(12p) syndrome. *Am J Med Genet* 1985; 22:769–779.
88. Goldberg MF, Cotlier E, Fichenscher LG, et al: Macular cherry-red spot, corneal clouding, and β-galactosidase deficiency. *Arch Intern Med* 1971; 128:387–397.
89. Langer LO Jr, Beals RK, Solomon IL, et al: Acromesomelic dwarfism: Manifestations in childhood. *Am J Med Genet* 1977; 1:87–100.
90. Landing BH, Silverman FN, Craig JM, et al: Familial neurovisceral lipidosis. *Am J Dis Child* 1964; 108:503–522.
91. Bateman JB, Philippart M, Isenberg SJ: Ocular features of multiple sulfatase deficiency and a new variant of metachromatic leukodystrophy. *J Pediatr Ophthalmol Strabismus* 1984; 21:133–138.
92. Fenske HD, Spitalny LA: Hereditary osteo-onychodysplasia. *Am J Ophthalmol* 1970; 70:604–608.
93. Goldstein JE, Cogan DG: Sclerocornea and

associated congenital anomalies. *Arch Ophthalmol* 1962; 67:99–106.
94. Kivlin JD, Fineman RM, Crandall AS, et al: Peters' anomaly as a consequence of genetic and nongenetic syndromes. *Arch Ophthalmol* 1986; 104:61–64.
95. Van Schooneveld MJ, Delleman JW, Beemer FA, et al: Peters'-Plus: A new syndrome. *Ophthalmic Paediatr Genet* 1984; 4:141–146.
96. Henkind P, Marinoff G, Manas A, et al: Bilateral corneal dermoids. *Am J Ophthalmol* 1978; 76:972–977.
97. Mattos J, Contreras F, O'Donnell FE Jr: Ring dermoid syndrome. A new syndrome of autosomal dominantly inherited, bilateral, annular limbal dermoids with corneal and conjunctival extension. *Arch Ophthalmol* 1980; 98:1059–1061.
98. Pearce WG: Corneal involvement in autosomal dominant coloboma/microphthalmos. *Can J Ophthalmol* 1986; 21:291–294.
99. Nixon RB, Phelps CD: Glaucoma, in Renie WA (ed): *Goldberg"s Genetic and Metabolic Eye Disease,* ed 2. Boston, Little, Brown & Co, 1986, pp 275–296.
100. Silverman WA: *Retrolental Fibroplasia. A Modern Parable.* New York, Grune & Stratton, 1980.
101. Stevenson RF, Morin JD: Ocular findings in nevus flammeus. *Can J Ophthalmol* 1975; 10:136–139.
102. Lewis RA, Riccardi VM: Von Recklinghausen neurofibromatosis: Incidence of iris hamartoma. *Ophthalmology* 1981; 88:348–354.
103. Govan JAA: Ocular manifestations of Alport's syndrome: A hereditary disorder of basement membranes? *Br J Ophthalmol* 1983; 67:493–503.
104. Cruysberg JRM, Sengers RCA, Pinckers A, et al: Features of a syndrome with congenital cataract and hypertrophic cardiomyopathy. *Am J Ophthalmol* 1986; 102:740–749.
105. Merin S: Congenital cataracts, in Renie WA (ed): *Goldberg's Genetic and Metabolic Eye Disease,* ed 2. Boston, Little, Brown & Co, 1986, p 369.
106. Judisch GF, Rhead J, Miller DK: Abetalipoproteinemia. *Ophthalmologica* 1984; 189:73–79.
107. Pilarski RT, Pauli RM, Bresnick GH, et al: Karsch-Neugebauer syndrome: Split foot/split hand and congenital nystagmus. *Clin Genet* 1985; 27:97–101.
108. Cross HE: Ectopia lentis et pupillae. *Am J Ophthalmol* 1979; 88:381–384.
109. Spaeth GL, Barber GW: Homocystinuria—its ocular manifestations. *J Pediatr Ophthalmol* 1966; 3:42.
110. Gillum WM, Anderson RL: Dominantly inherited blepharoptosis, high myopia, and ectopia lentis. *Arch Ophthalmol* 1982; 100:282–284.
111. Nelson LB, Spaeth GL, Nowinsky TS, et al: Aniridia. *Surv Ophthalmol* 1984; 28:621.
112. Traboulsi EI, Krush AJ, Gardner EJ, et al: Prevalence and importance of pigmented ocular fundus lesions in Gardner's syndrome. *N Engl J Med* 1987; 316:661–667.
113. Libert J, Kenyon KR: Ocular ultrastructure in inborn lysosomal storage disease, in Renie WA (ed): *Goldberg's Genetic and Metabolic Eye Disease,* ed 2. Boston, Little, Brown & Co, 1986, p 369.
114. Scotto JM, Hadchouel M, Odievre M, et al: Infantile phytanic acid storage disease, a possible variant of Refsum's disease: Three cases, including ultrastructural studies of the liver. *J Inherited Metab Dis* 1982; 5:83–90.
115. Schachat AP, Maumenee IH: Bardet-Biedl syndrome and related disorders. *Arch Ophthalmol* 1982; 100:285–288.
116. Weiner LP, Konigsmark BW, Stoll J Jr, et al: Hereditary olivopontocerebellar atrophy with retinal degeneration. Report of a family through six generations. *Arch Neurol* 1967; 16:364–376.
117. Nisenbaum C, Sandbank U, Kohn R: Pelizaeus-Merzbacher disease "infantile acute type." Report of a family. *Ann Pediatr (Paris)* 1965; 240:365–376.
118. Ellis DS, Heckenlively JR, Martin CL, et al: Leber's congenital amaurosis associated with familial juvenile nephronophthisis and cone-shaped epiphyses of the hands (the Saldino-Mainzer syndrome). *Am J Ophthalmol* 1984; 97:233–239.
119. Gil-Gibernau J, Galan A, Callis L, et al: Infantile idiopathic hypercalciuria, high congenital myopia, and atypical macular coloboma: A new oculo-renal syndrome? *J Pediatr Ophthalmol Strabismus* 1982; 19:7–11.
120. Kivlin JD, Sanborn GE, Myers GG: The cherry-red spot in Tay-Sachs and other storage diseases. *Ann Neurol* 1985; 17:356–360.
121. Ober RR, Bird AC, Hamilton AM, et al: Autosomal dominant exudative vitreoretinopathy.

Br J Ophthalmol 1980; 64:112–120.
122. Warburg M: Retinal malformations: Aetiological heterogeneity and morphological similarity in congenital retinal non-attachment and falciform folds. *Trans Ophthalmol Soc UK* 1979; 99:272.
123. Behrens-Baumann W, Dust G, Rittmeier K, et al: Okulo-zerebrale dysplasie: Aplasia nervi optici sowie familiarer mikr- und kryptophthalmus. *Klin Monatsbl Augenheilk* 1981; 179:90–93.
124. Lambert SR, Hoyt CS, Narahara, MH: Optic Nerve Hypoplasia. *Surv Ophthalmol* 1987; 32:1–9.
125. Apple DJ: New aspects of colobomas and optic nerve anomalies. *Int Ophthalmol Clin* 1984; 24:109–121.

28 Testing of the Possibly Blind Child

Anne B. Fulton, M.D.

Visual inattention is the symptom that brings possibly blind infants to us. The family usually collects numerous observations that corroborate their impression that the infant does not see. The child does not respond to smiles or brighten when a familiar face comes close, and visual attention is otherwise difficult to engage. There is poor or absent following of visual targets.

Infants whose general growth and development are good tend to present to ophthalmologists between the ages of 2 and 6 months. Infants with obvious developmental delays and systemic problems tend to present to the ophthalmologist later in infancy; their families and physicians have been preoccupied with pressing medical or surgical matters earlier in infancy.

The basic questions are these. Can this child see? If he can see, how much can he see? Can you, as an ophthalmologist or pediatrician, do anything to improve visual performance? Are we as parents doing all that we should? What does the future hold? Is the child going to be able to go to school?

Special tests of function, as described later in this chapter, can help answer questions about the infant's visual capabilities. Barring marked ocular abnormalities such as extreme optic nerve hypoplasia, prognostic issues are more difficult to deal with definitively, largely because an infant's eyes and visual system have several years of development ahead.

Certainly the ophthalmologist's goal is to secure a specific diagnosis. Specific entities associated with visual inattention during early infancy include achromatopsia, hypopigmentation syndromes (albinism), optic nerve hypoplasia, and retinal degeneration. High refractive errors, unless accompanied by ocular or systemic abnormalities, are not included. Occasionally a treatable or curable disorder will be identified. But also helpful is identification of a disorder about which prognostic information will assist in realistic planning of the child's future programs.

Some of the visually inattentive patients remain diagnostic enigmas. There is no eponym that encompasses the presenting features of some of these patients, let alone a specific metabolic abnormality that allows curative intervention. For such patients definition of their visual capabilities is of considerable service because it aids in planning their school programs. Periodic monitoring of their visual system function, perhaps with the preferential looking (PL) test, is useful in tailoring activities and education to their individual needs.

OFFICE EXAMINATION

The purpose of the office examination is to conduct a thorough search for ocular explanations for the visual deficit and ocular signs of systemic problems. The examination starts with a painstaking history.

A description of the infants' visual behavior based on the family's observations is sought. Since birth, is vision getting better or poorer or staying the same? Does vision appear to be better or poorer in certain conditions? For example, apparent photophobia suggests achromatopsia, a stationary congenital condition in which the retina contains few if any functioning cones, or a hypopigmentation (albinism) syndrome. What are the eye movements like? Wandering, apparently purposeless eye movements are seen in infants with profound visual deficits. Nystagmus, usually rhythmic to-and-fro movements of the eyes, is associated with disorders that decrease acuity, but beyond this nystagmus has a disconcerting effect on parents; infants with nystagmus may seem not to look at the parents' faces and exchange their smiles. PL acuity testing (see Chapter 4) helps to sort those nystagmus patients with moderate, stable visual deficits and good prognoses (such as albinism) from those with extensive visual impairment and limited prospects for useful vision.[1]

As part of the history-taking task, the ophthalmologist formulates information about development and neurological status in the context of the child's visual deficit. For those patients whose visual inattention is inexplicable on the basis of ocular abnormalities, the ophthalmologist usually initiates referral to a pediatric neurologist if information about the child's development and neurological status are incomplete.

A detailed family history gathered in response to specific, thoughtfully aimed questions may yield key diagnostic information. For example, an infant with visual inattention and nystagmus due to a hypopigmentation syndrome may not have an obvious, long lineage of albinism but may have a several-generation background of relatives with nystagmus who are found, on careful and specific questioning, to be the most lightly pigmented of their siblings.

It goes without saying that a complete and thorough examination of the eyes is in order. Special attention is directed at assessment of abnormal eye movements and abnormal alignment of the eyes. In these patients one is looking more for telltale signs of vision that is unequal between the eyes or signs of abnormalities of the visual system proximal to the eyes rather than considering treatment of the strabismus. As a rule of thumb, if the pupils and pupillary reactions of young visually inattentive infants (including those with evoked potential evidence of visual cortex malfunction)[2,3] are normal, the prognosis for useful vision is good. Inspection of the macular area allows ready identification of obvious lesions such as colobomas or chorioretinal scars. The fovea, even in young post-term infants, is identifiable as a specialized region by its tiny pit.[4] It may not appear as distinct as in the older infant but should, nevertheless, be identifiable. If not, this raises the question of foveal hypoplasia. Foveal hypoplasia is most frequently associated with a hypopigmentation syndrome (albinism). The examiner must note if there is sufficient pigmentation in the perifoveal region to obscure the choroidal vessels. Even in the early post-term weeks this amount of pigmentation is normally present.

On examination of the retina the ophthalmologist decides whether there is evidence of a retinal degenerative disorder. Contrary to the diagnostic triad (pale disc, attenuated retinal vessels, and bone spicules) that is the ophthalmoscopic hallmark of retinal degeneration in older patients, in infants the only diagnostic sign may be very slight narrowing of the vessels. This subtle sign may be the earliest sign of a retinal degenerative disorder in an infant. If there is a pigmentary disturbance, it may be only a hint of fine pigment mottling; occasionally some delicate spicules are seen. Optic nerve pallor may not be identifiable in young infants with a retinal degenerative disorder. Furthermore, not all infantile retinal degenerative disorders can be satisfactorily classified as Leber's congenital amaurosis[5–7] but may be a component of a multisystem syndrome such as (to mention a few) Senior's syndrome,[8] the infantile form of ceroid lipofuscinosis,[9] metabolic disorders such as methylmalonic acidemia,[6] or infantile Refsum's syndrome. All of these are rare disorders, but examples of each have been seen within the last 5 years by this author.

Bilateral optic nerve hypoplasia may account completely for the visual inattention of an infant. The size, color, and contour of the optic nerve requires careful appraisal in the possibly blind child.

CORTICAL BLINDNESS

If there is not an ocular explanation for poor vision, the site of the visual system abnormality may be proximal to the eyes. Although in infants, as in adults, cortical blindness may result from an external insult or an episode of asphyxia, cortical blindness of visually inattentive newborns and young children may be due to developmental anomalies and malformations of the brain that involve the visual pathways and areas. Brain abnormalities may or may not be accompanied by ocular abnormalities.[5, 10, 11]

Among those infants with seizure activity, visual deficits due to brain malfunction may wax and wane. One wonders whether this statement of a mother captures the essence of the situation. "When Bobby has too much going on inside, he shuts out the extra stimuli. It's so easy for him to shut out visual stimuli. He just turns away or closes his eyes. It's far more trouble to block auditory or tactile inputs. Keeping out the visual stimuli is a good way for him to cut down on overload imposed by the environment."

Disturbances of the brain's visual pathways may be demonstrated by visual evoked potential (VEP) testing[12, 13] (see also Chapter 4). New techniques promise quantitative visual field mapping in infants and young children with neurological abnormalities.[14, 15] In some of these visually inattentive children, it has been possible to map defects in the visual field that correspond to the lesions noted on computed tomography (CT) scans.[15]

SPECIAL TESTS AND THEIR MEANING IN NEONATES AND INFANTS

Tests that have particular utility in evaluation of the possibly blind child include PL, VEP, and electroretinography (ERG). These are reviewed in Chapter 4.

When evaluating the vision of pediatric patients, the examiner must be cognizant of the normal developmental changes in ERG[16] and VEP[17, 18] responses and in PL performance.[19] ERG responses increase in amplitude and sensitivity and decrease in latency to reach adult values by about 12 months.[16]

Acuities, whether measured by VEP or PL techniques, improve during infancy and childhood due to ongoing development of the eye and visual system.[17–19] It has been found that developmentally delayed infants and children with normal eyes have a broader range of PL acuities than do those with normal development; somewhat poorer acuity results are consistent with normal eyes in these children.[20] Currently we most often use Teller's[23] acuity card PL procedure to assess infants' acuity. The apparatus is very simple, the grating stimuli are commercially available, and the procedure is designed to keep the infant's interest with a puppet show between trials (Fig 28–1, A and B). The infant is held by an adult, often a parent, in front of a display in which black and white stripes (gratings) are presented. Another adult, the observer, unaware of the right-left position of the stripes, names the position of the stripes on the basis of the infant's looking behavior. In the course of the test, the smallest stripe width to which the infant can respond reliably is determined. This is taken as the infant's acuity. Between the presentations of the various gratings, the puppet show maintains the infant's interest. For neonates the PL grating acuities average 20/400 but increase to about 20/100 by the age of 6 months, 20/50 by the age of 2 years, and 20/30 at the age of 3 years. In using this type of testing to evaluate acuity of patients with amblyopia and other disorders causing visual deficits, one is reminded that grating acuity is not equivalent

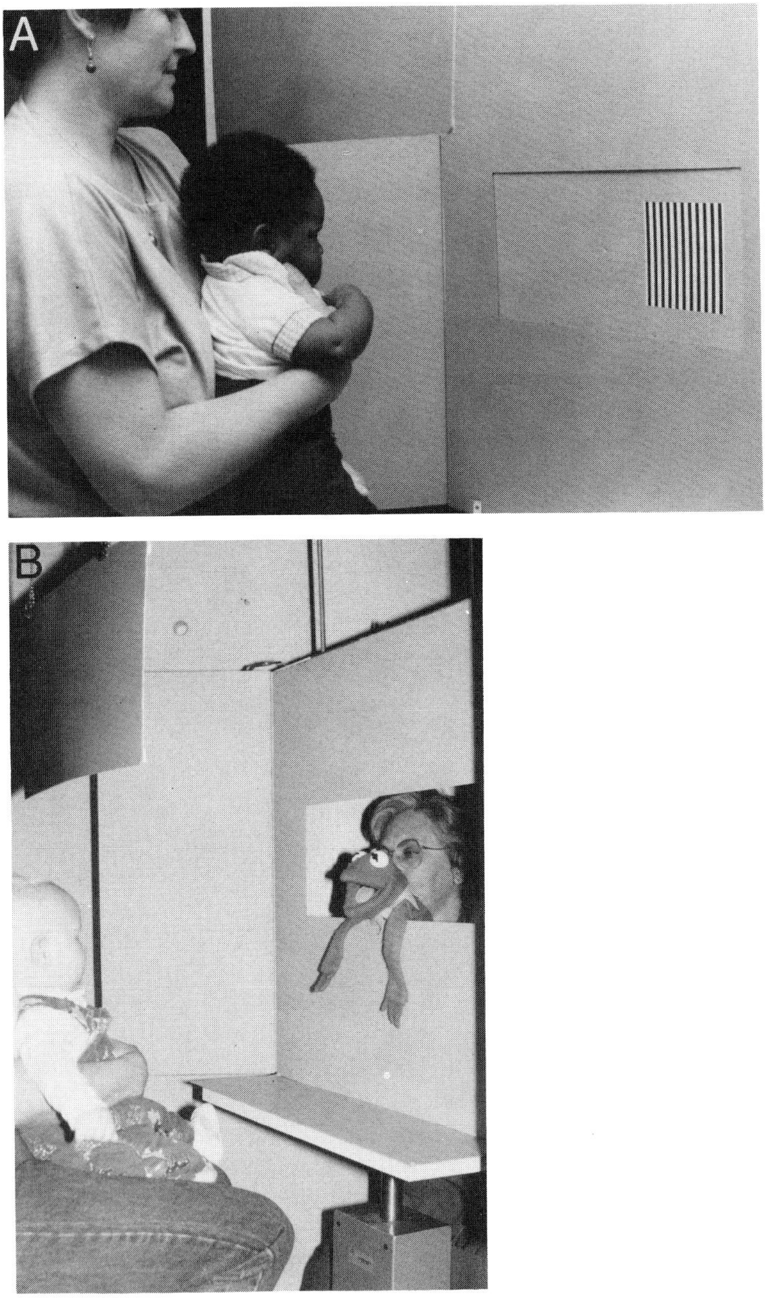

FIG 28–1.
A and **B**, Teller's acuity card PL test. (Courtesy of Dr. L. Mayer.)

to the more familiar Snellen acuity obtained with letters. The rapidity of the acuity card procedure makes it a very suitable test for young, ill infants who can endure only limited testing.

Optokinetic nystagmus (OKN) has been used less than PL and VEP to measure visual acuities, perhaps largely because of the difficulties in reliable monitoring of the young infant's OKN responses at and near the threshold for visual resolution (acuity). However, if the question to be answered is "Does this baby see at all?", OKN testing is useful. Experience suggests that a large (100 × 25 cm) white paper[24] with a coarse random dot pattern is a useful device (Fig 28–2).

The immediate purpose of the special tests is to evaluate the infant's visual capabilities[1, 20–23] and localize the sites of visual system malfunction.[5, 7] Occasionally the test results provide the basis for qualified prognostic statements,[12, 25] but serial testing may be important to get a good sense of the young patient's course.[16] In the context of the overall clinical picture, test results contribute diagnostic information.

Results from two visually inattentive infants, both initially tested at the age of 3 months, illustrate these points. VEP results yielded prognostic information for the first, and the ERG diagnostic information did the same for the second infant.

The first infant was born at term following an uncomplicated pregnancy and delivery. Postnatally her course was unremarkable except for wandering eye movements and apparent blindness. Nothing could be done in the office to demonstrate that she could see. All structures of the eyes appeared to be normal. ERG responses were normal. Although some abnormalities of the VEP waveforms were identified, the amplitudes met criteria[12] that warranted the prediction of useful vision. Indeed, her visual behavior improved; by the age of 5 months she appeared to see. Serial PL measures demonstrated a steady improvement of grating acuity with increasing age. Now at the age of 2 1/2 years her PL acuity OU is 20/100 (normal for age, 20/20 to 20/50), and her disorder is perhaps best classified as congenital nystagmus. Thus, although the VEP results did not clarify the pathophysiological basis for her early visual inattention, they did provide prognostic information, in this case readily welcomed by the family.

The second infant was also born at term but suffered from subarachnoid bleeding and had a possible seizure disorder in the perinatal period. She did not respond to light, and searching eye movements were noted. Pupillary responses were sluggish. No funduscopic abnormalities were identifiable at early

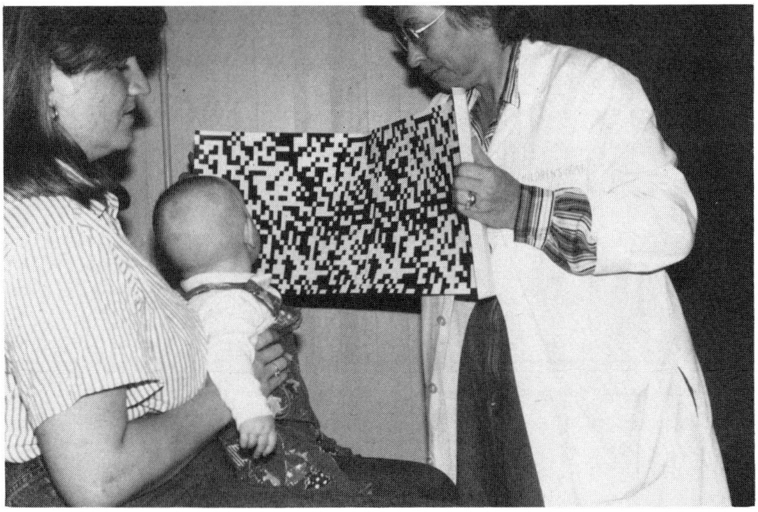

FIG 28–2.
Coarse, random-dot pattern used to elicit OKN. The partially unfurled paper wraps around the patient's visual field. Sometimes a vertical presentation makes it easier to decide whether there is an OKN response. This is true of infants whose wandering or nystagmoid eye movements are predominantly horizontal. (Courtesy of Dr. L. Mayer.)

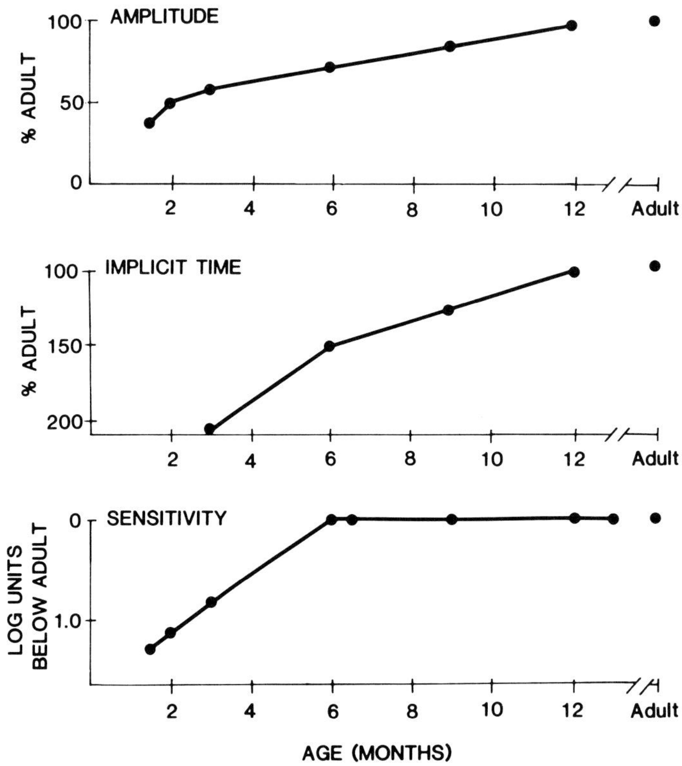

FIG 28–3.
ERG responses in infancy compared with adult values. Methodological details can be found in Fulton and Hansen's report.[16] The amplitudes of b-wave responses to full-field stimuli in scotopic conditions increase gradually, and implicit times decrease so that adult values are approached by the age of 12 months. The sensitivity of the b-wave is equivalent to that of adults by about the age of 6 months.

postnatal examinations. Nevertheless, at the age of 3 months, scotopic ERG responses were attenuated to about 30% of the normal mean for age.[16] Although the absolute amplitude increased when tested again at the ages of 6 and 12 months, her amplitudes remained 20% to 40% of the normal mean for age (Fig 28–3). On the basis of these results and continued freedom from systemic disorders, she carries the diagnosis of Leber's congenital amaurosis.

REFERENCES

1. Mayer DL, Fulton AB, Hansen RM: Visual acuity of infants and children with retinal degenerations. *Ophthalmol Pediatr Genet* 1985; 5:51–56.
2. Fielder AR, Russell-Eggitt IR, Dodd KL, et al: Delayed visual maturation. *Trans Ophthalmol Soc UK* 1985; 104:653–661.
3. Skarf B, Panton C: VEP testing in neurologically impaired and developmentally delayed infants and young children. *Invest Ophthalmol Vis Sci* 1987; 28(suppl):302.
4. Isenberg S: Macular development in the premature infant. *Am J Ophthalmol* 1986; 101:74–80.
5. Fulton AB, Hansen RM, Harris SJ: Retinal degeneration and brain abnormalities in infants and young children. *Doc Ophthalmol* 1985; 60:133–140.
6. Robb RM, Dowton SB, Fulton AB, et al: Retinal degeneration in B_{12} disorder associated with methylmalonic aciduria and sulfur amino acid abnormalities. *Am J Ophthalmol* 1984; 97:691–696.
7. Fulton AB, Mayer DL, Hansen RM, et al: Oscillatory potentials of visually inattentive children. *Doc Ophthalmol* 1987; 65:319–332.
8. Senior B: Familial-renal-retinal dystrophy. *Am J Dis Child* 1973; 125:442–447.

9. Fulton AB, Hansen RM: Retinal adaptation in infants and children with retinal degenerations. *Ophthalmic Pediatr Genet* 1983; 2:69–81.
10. Foxman SG, Wirtschafter JD, Letson RD: Leber's congenital amaurosis and high hyperopia: A discrete entity, in *Proceedings of the 24th International Congress of Ophthalmology,* vol 1. *Acta Ophthalmol.* Philadelphia, JB Lippincott, 1982, pp 55–58.
11. Denslow GT, Robb RM: Aicardi's syndrome: A report of four cases and review of the literature. *J Pediatr Ophthalmol Strabismus* 1979; 16:10–15.
12. Iinuma K, Matsumiya Y, Lombroso CT: Prognostic values of visual evoked potentials (VEP) in infants. Electroencephalogr Clin Neurophysiol 1980; 50:183.
13. Robertson R, Jan JE, Wong, PKH: Electroencephalograms of children with permanent cortical visual impairment. *Can J Neurol Sci* 1986; 13:256–261.
14. Mohn G, van Hof–van Duin J: Behavioral and electrophysiological measures of visual functions in children with neurological disorders. *Behav Brain Res* 1983; 10:177–187.
15. Mayer DL, Fulton AB, Cummings MC: The LED Perimeter. II. Fields of Young Patients. *Invest Ophthalmol Vis Sci* 1987; 28(suppl):302.
16. Fulton AB, Hansen RM: Electroretinography: Application to clinical studies of infants. *J Pediatr Ophthalmol Strabismus* 1985; 22:251–255.
17. Sokol S: Measurements of infants visual acuity from pattern reversal evoked potentials. *Vision Res* 1978; 18:33–39.
18. Spekreijse H, Apkarian P: The use of a system analysis approach to electrodiagnostic (ERG and VEP) assessment. *Vision Res* 1986; 26:195–219.
19. Mayer DL, Fulton AB, Hansen RM: Preferential looking staircase acuity in pediatric patients. *Invest Ophthalmol Vis Sci* 1982; 23:538–543.
20. Mayer DL, Fulton AB, Sossen PL: Preferential looking acuity of pediatric patients with developmental disabilities. *Behav Bran Res* 1983; 10:189–198.
21. Mohn G, van Hof–van Duin J: Rapid assessment of visual acuity in infants and children in a clinical setting using acuity cards. *Doc Ophthalmol* 1986; 45:363–371.
22. Dubowitz LMS, Muskin J, Morante A, et al: The maturation of visual acuity in neurologically normal and abnormal newborn infants. *Behav Brain Res* 1983; 10:39–46.
23. Teller DY, McDonald MA, Preston K, et al: Assessment of visual acuity in infants and children: The acuity card procedure. *Dev Med Child Neurol* 1986; 28:779–786.
24. van Hof–van Duin J, Mohn G: Optokinetic and spontaneous nystagmus in children with neurological disorders. *Behav Brain Res* 1983: 10:163–175.
25. Miranda SR, Hack M, Frantz RL, et al: Neonatal pattern vision: A predictor of future mental performance? *J Pediatr* 1977; 4:642–647.

29 The Blind Child and His Family

Toni G. Marcy, M.D.

In order to understand the impact of the birth of a blind child upon the family, we must visualize the hopes and dreams most parents have for their newborns. When these expectations are shattered by the diagnosis of blindness, everybody in the family is affected, and their lives are reshaped. The acute pain may gradually subside, but it never goes away completely. Some parents lose the ability to cope with the stress of raising a visually impaired child, especially when additional handicaps are present or when the financial burden of repeated hospitalizations is overwhelming. They need professional help to deal with their feelings of guilt, depression, and anger and also guidelines on how to maximize their child's potential. With professional support they will be able to enjoy their child's accomplishments while accepting the long-term responsibilities of caring for him (Fig 29–1).

The following case history will illustrate these facts.

Case History.—A baby boy was born prematurely at a gestational age of 26 weeks to a 33-year-old primigravida and primipara. Pregnancy progressed normally until premature rutpure of the membrane occurred. Three days later a small infant weighing 740 gm was delivered vaginally. He needed intubation immediately and was then rushed to the neonatal intensive care unit (NICU) where the diagnoses of "bronchopulmonary dysplasia" and "patent ductus arteriosus" were subsequently made. The latter responded well to medication; however, oxygen therapy was needed for 2 months. The parents were told that their infant had a 10% chance of survival and informed about the possible damage to his eyes. At 6 weeks of age, A. developed pneumonia and sepsis, which were treated successfully with antibiotics. After an initial weight loss to 600 gm, the baby responded well to feeding with breast milk supplied by mother and later a formula, both given to him by gavage.

The mother was in the hospital every day from early morning until late at night and joined by her husband after work. To encourage bonding with her son, she was allowed to bathe him as soon as he did not need the respirator and also help with feeding.

The infant was first seen by an ophthalmologist when he was 1 month old. The parents were assured that his eyes did not show any pathology. One week before his release from the hospital at the age of $3^1/_2$ months, a definite ocular diagnosis could not be made because the ophthalmologist told the parents that he was unable to dilate the child's pupils. They were advised to bring him back in a month. Two weeks later, mother noticed that her baby's pupils were "misshapen." She became alarmed and took him back to the ophthalmologist who informed her that her son had "eye problems." Pressed for a more specific diagnosis, she was told that her baby was totally blind. The mother described her reaction as "screaming like a wounded animal"; a sound so inhuman that she was frightened by it. She denied having received any further explanation or any signs of empathy from the ophthalmologist. She then rushed with the baby in her arms to the NICU where the nurses and neonatologists had nurtured her during the preceding months. After receiving some support there but still in acute

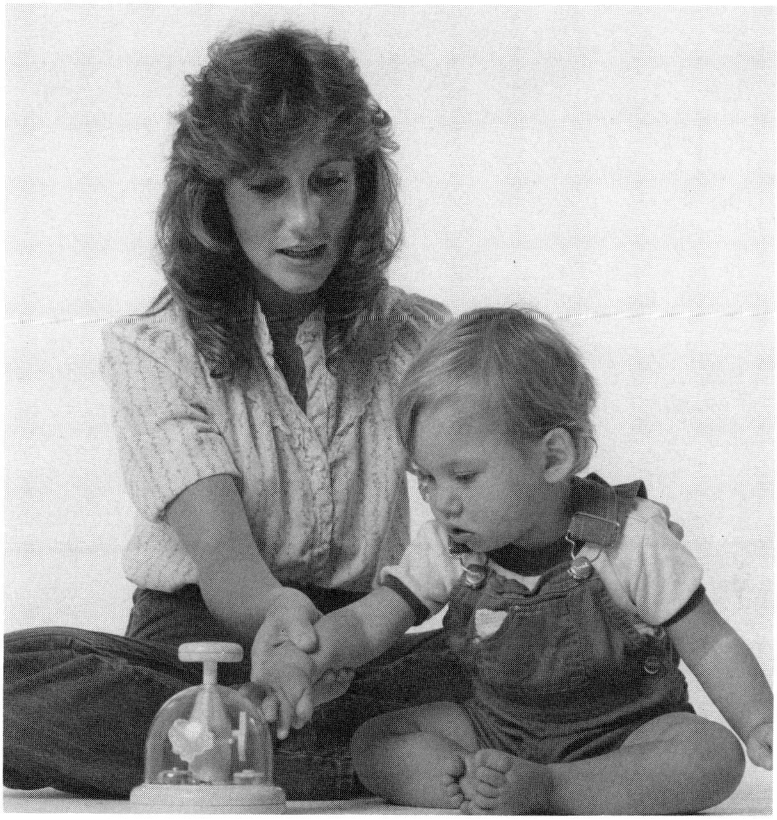

FIG 29–1.
A mother enjoying interactions with her blind son.

emotional pain, the mother drove alone to her home many miles away from the hospital. She has no recollection of the events between leaving the NICU and entering her house. She placed the baby in his crib and closed the door. She then called the Braille Institute, who referred her to a children's center specializing in the care of blind preschool children. An immediate appointment was arranged by phone through the secretary at the center who, hearing the sobbing of the mother, appreciated her agony.

After her own frightening experience while driving home in a condition of shock, the mother chose to spare her husband the same ordeal and waited until he returned from work to break the news. She described the hours that then passed as seeming like an eternity. Due to severe depression, she was unable to pick her baby up or console him when he was crying. Her only thought was to buy black paint to cover up the bright animal pictures she had previously drawn on the walls for her child to see. Finally, she was able to share the devastating news with her husband and received much support from him. They decided to inform other family members the following day about their baby's blindness after realizing they would need their support in the future.

At their meeting at a blind children's center, parents and child were seen by a child development specialist with wide experience in dealing with blind infants. They were reassured that their baby was doing extremely well for a child with such a stormy medical history. With the help of charts, the anatomic changes of retinopathy of prematurity were explained, and they were encouraged to ask questions. Most of them related to educational plans for the future of their blind child. Additional help was offered to them in a special "mothers and fathers group" under the guidance of a social worker and a psychiatrist. During this meeting, the parents also asked for a referral to an ophthalmologist to obtain a second opinion. This ophthalmologist informed them that the damage to the baby's eyes was so severe that any surgical intervention would not improve his vision. Even though the news was devastating, the parents accepted the diagnosis because they were allowed to ask questions and received much emotional support.

When the child was 2½ years old, the parents asked for a third opinion at a university hospital because they had heard about a new procedure that might restore some light perception. During this visit, glaucoma was diagnosed. The ophthalmologist decided against a lensectomy because of excessive vascularization that might cause severe intraoperative and postoperative hemorrhage and possible loss of the eyes. The parents were referred to a glaucoma specialist in their neighborhood who, 2 weeks later, performed a partial iridectomy with excellent control of intraocular pressure.

Gradually the parents were able to regroup their energies. They became involved in many causes concerning blind children and have helped other families in similar situations.

The child is bright and outgoing, and has a delightful sense of humor. Intellectually, he was always above age level in gross motor and language development. He has attended the blind children's center for 4 years and a preschool program in his neighborhood. He is currently enrolled in a daily program for visually handicapped children close to home where he is preparing for pre-Braille reading. He is also undergoing mobility training and is attending a regular Head Start program 1 hour each day. He will be mainstreamed into a public school kindergarten at 5 years of age where he will receive assistance from a resource teacher for blind children.

SOME GUIDELINES TO ASSIST PARENTS RAISING A BLIND INFANT

1. *Inspire the confidence of the parents and assure them that help will be extended to them.* This goal is best accomplished in support group meetings where parents learn that their fears and feelings of inadequacy are not unique. They are given a chance to ask questions and even to express death wishes. Typical questions are "Why did this happen to me?" "What did I do wrong?" "Is there a cure for the blindness?" A typical death wish often expressed is "every time my baby was examined under anesthesia, I hoped he would never wake up again." Parents need to be assured that such feelings are not inappropriate. Additionally, parents obtain information about existing agencies that provide services such as home visits to families of blind children and specific help such as physiotherapy or language stimulation. These group meetings relieve their isolation and lead to many friendships among families of visually impaired children.

2. *Establish a close, mutually satisfying relationship between parents and child.* If available, both parents should attend to the needs of their blind baby, especially during the first 3 years of his life. The emotional deprivation resulting from unfulfilled needs can cause deviant behavior.[1–4] Seventy percent of the time, it is the mother who first notices the lack of social interaction by her baby and suspects blindness. Even after sharing her concern with her pediatrician, 1 or more months may elapse before a referral is made to an ophthalmologist to confirm the diagnosis. The baby's first smile, which is the most gratifying response for any parent, is much more difficult to elicit and is usually more fleeting in a blind baby.[1] Parents should be informed about these differences so that they do not interpret them as rejection. Without appropriate social interaction, the blind child's interest will then be focused on his own body rather than reaching out and becoming acquainted with the world around him. It is recommended that the blind infant be carried in a frontpack as much as conveniently possible. In this way, he becomes accustomed to different auditory, tactile, and olfactory stimuli while his mother goes about her household duties. This close contact also allows the parent to reassure the baby with words and caresses when he is

frightened by too much noise around him.

3. *Help parents facilitate important milestones.* It is important to inform parents that visual deprivation can lead to developmental delays in intellectually normal children.[3] Each child progresses at his own pace, and blind children often show regression, e.g., after hospitalization, followed by spontaneous acceleration. Parents must understand that the blind child's concept of the world is fragmented and that he needs a longer time to integrate new experiences than sighted children. Tactile, kinesthetic, and auditory cues assist his exploration but can never replace vision, which gives sighted children the main incentive to move about and gather information. Blind babies, on the other hand, lacking these cues, show delays in areas that involve mobility and balance. Mother's voice is usually the best incentive to make a blind baby move. Infancy is also the time to encourage independent exploration of the surroundings, even when it involves occasional pain and bumps (Fig 29–2). Overprotection and restraining his mobility are devastating for the blind toddler's development.[5] It makes him preoccupied with his own body and may lead to self-stimulatory behavior such as rocking back and forth.[6]

4. *Advise parents about choice of toys and objects including food.* A blind baby has to be taught to use his hands.[7] While the sighted infant enjoys playing with his hands starting at 4 to 6 months of age, the blind infant does so only accidentally and not in a purposeful way. Some visually impaired infants actually begin exploration with their feet rather than their hands. Games such as pat-a-cake encourage them to bring their hands together in the midline and facilitate transfer of objects. In case there is some remaining vision, a cra-

FIG 29–2.
Independent exploration of the environment will ultimately be rewarding despite occasional bumps and bruises.

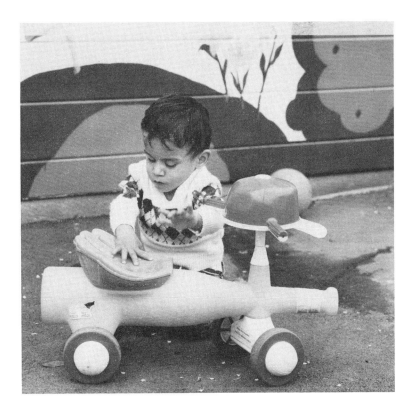

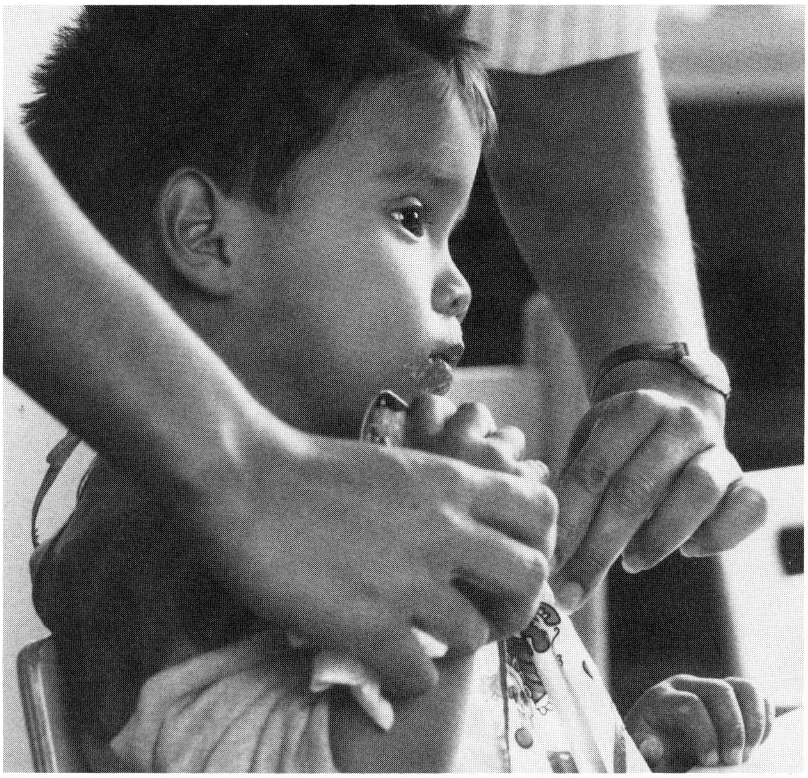

FIG 29–3.
Instructing the blind infant to properly feed himself will provide an important skill.

dle gym with bright colors or black and white geometric forms for strong contrast should be within easy reach. Smaller toys of different shapes and textures that the baby can easily grasp are preferable to solely sound-making toys since the latter discourage purposeful exploration and lead to repetitive, meaningless manipulations. The mouth, as a highly sensitive organ, is used very effectively by most blind children for exploration ("mouthing") and should not be discouraged. It also helps them to differentiate between edible and nonedible objects (Fig 29–3). At 9 months, finger feeding should be introduced, which furthers independence and fine motor control of his hands. Many blind babies have chewing problems that can be traced to an overprotective mother's fear of the child's gag reflex. Blind babies can be encouraged to chew, which is often an imitative behavior, by placing their hands on mother's face while she is chewing crunchy food.

5. *Stress the importance of verbal communication.* It is through language that the blind child forms a picture of the world around him. The quality of this language is of utmost importance. Social games such as "hugging mommy" help him to integrate certain concepts and foster a close bond between mother and child. The tone of voice gives him a nonvisual cue whether the parents approve or disapprove of his response. Bombardment with too much verbal stimulation that he cannot integrate will lead to withdrawal and withholding of language. Many blind children between 16 and 20 months of age stop saying words they have previously used and do not enlarge their vocabulary for sometime. This occurs at a time when the toddler is primarily involved with his newly acquired motor skills.

Intense involvement in this area can lead to regression in the language area. Other causes for this regression can be traced to hospitalization for checking his eye condition or to stress in his parents' marriage, both of which are quite common in the child's second year of life. These events deprive him of the emotional support he needs. As soon as a more relaxed relationship is re-established, his language skills will improve.

Some word of caution should be added as to the indiscriminate use of television. Since the blind child cannot see the picture, the spoken words are meaningless to him. He will repeat jingles and commercials over and over again for the sole purpose of maintaining verbal contact with other people instead of developing a meaningful dialogue. Therefore, exposure of these favorite tools of entertainment should be limited.

6. *Familiarize parents with the mannerisms of the blind child.* It is common for many blind children to adopt certain patterns of self-stimulatory behavior that are called "blindisms." They manifest themselves in rocking back and forth, hand flipping, eye poking, or head banging. These behaviors may produce pleasure or reduce tensions. However, this preoccupation with his own body prevents a child from expanding his interest in the world around him. There are other repetitive behavior patterns that serve a positive adaptive purpose. For example, opening and closing of doors help the blind child to deal with vibrations and spatial relations. Lying motionless on the floor for a few minutes when overwhelmed by stressful sensations helps him to recuperate from an overflow of stimuli.[7] Chase showed in her research with 263 children with retrolental fibroplasia that only 1.3% showed no signs of blindism and 16.5% demonstrated them occasionally.[8] Many blind children are labeled as being autistic because of these stereotyped behavior patterns. In contrast to true autism, this behavior can be effectively treated with psychotherapy when caught early.

PHYSICIAN-FAMILY RELATIONSHIP

The way the initial diagnosis of blindness is presented to the parents will affect the child's and his family's lives to a great extent. Some parents hear the sad news soon after birth. The negative effects are intensified by prematurity where the uncertainty whether the child will live or die has persisted for many weeks.

In mothers' and fathers' meetings, the most often discussed topic is the medical professional. Many authors describe the parents' feelings of being abandoned once the diagnosis of retrolental fibroplasia was made.[9–11] This is in sharp contrast to the earlier support extended to them while their baby was in the NICU. Communication between parents and perinatal professionals often comes to a standstill when needed most.

It is the ophthalmologist who has the difficult task of telling the parents that their child is blind. Some parents report a very positive experience when the ophthalmologist took time to explain the medical condition that led to blindness and showed empathy. Others remember only incomprehensible "medical jargon" provided to them in a cold, impersonal way. They interpret this attitude as hostile and insensitive and fail to recognize the ophthalmologist's own feelings of pain and frustration when realizing that medical science and his own training are powerless to change the outcome of blindness. Therefore, understanding this reaction should be one of the goals of parents' meetings so that their anger at the physician does not make them psychological cripples, unable to deal with the task of raising a blind child.

Most parents report that they were in such shock upon hearing the diagnosis of blindness that they were unable to listen to specific information. Therefore, they should be given time to absorb the tragic news. A follow-up appointment is very important to give them a chance to clarify some of their concerns. It is always advisable to answer questions honestly; false hope of being able to change the outcome would be a disservice. Each parent accepts information at a different pace. Some parents use denial as a matter of self-protection until they are able to face the entire truth. Many parents confess that they could accept blindness but additional handicaps, such as mental retardation or cerebral palsy, would be intolerable for them to deal with. Therefore, if there is concern, it is important to prepare the parents gradually for these multihandicaps. Communication between parents and medical professionals and early referrals to appropriate resources help parents overcome their feelings of helplessness and regroup their mental and emotional energies.

IMPACT OF A BLIND CHILD UPON HIS SIBLINGS

As more and more time is needed to care for a blind child, brothers and sisters sometimes feel neglected and clamor for their parents' attention. If they do not receive enough attention, they become depressed, withdrawn, and resentful, often developing undesirable behavior at home and at school.

Since siblings usually do not understand the medical causes of the baby's blindness, they worry about "catching" the visual impairment as punishment for misbehavior. When they are older, they may raise the possibility of being carriers of genes that may result in the blindness of their offspring. Some siblings are given early responsibilities of caring for their blind brother or sister, which leads to resentment (Fig 29–4). Death wishes for the blind sibling are common. Cruel, insensitive remarks by schoolmates or in public places add to the dilemma. Many children feel embarrassed to have the blind sibling around them.

Opportunities should be given for them to ask questions and verbalize their ambiva-

FIG 29–4.
The relationship between a blind infant and his sighted sibling can be very difficult.

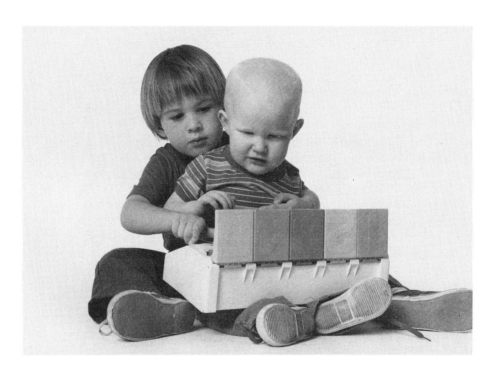

lent feelings without fear of being disloyal to the family. Reassurance that their emotions are acceptable and understandable makes it easier for them to accept their brother's or sister's visual impairment.[10]

GOALS IN EDUCATING THE BLIND CHILD

There is much controversy over segregated or integrated education for the visually handicapped. The present federal law (PL 94–142) regarding mandatory education for the disabled says that a handicapped child is "guaranteed appropriate education in the least restricted environment possible." At the present time, this law applies to children at least 3 years old, but legislation is in progress to make it applicable any time following birth.

The goal of many parents is to have their visually impaired schoolchildren taught with sighted children in the hope of better preparing them to live in a sighted world. For the normally developing blind child, school attendance with sighted children and aided by resource teachers for the visually impaired provides a better chance to function effectively. On the other hand, multihandicapped blind children profit more in special schools for the blind where a team of professionals such as physical therapists or speech pathologists as well as specially trained teachers for the blind help them compensate for their disabilities.

If preschool programs are available for young blind children, parents are advised to take advantage of them. The goal should be to obtain more individual attention with specific stimulation and to further the blind children's self-esteem. The latter is achieved by not exposing them to competition with sighted children, who very often ignore them instead of including them in their play activities.

CONCLUSION

Early and continuous support and guidance for families are of critical importance in the education of a blind child.[11] A national network of agencies is available to provide services for blind and visually impaired children and their families (see following list of Resources). If local facilities fail to meet their needs, parents can obtain help through outreach or correspondence programs.

The medical community should refer families to appropriate resources as soon as blindness has been diagnosed. Early intervention programs will help in cognitive and emotional development of blind children and leave them better prepared to lead a successful life in a sighted world.

RESOURCES

National Association for Parents of the Visually Impaired, Inc,
PO Box 180806,
Austin, TX 78718
(512) 459-6651
(Chapters in different states.)

Directors of Agencies for the Blind in the British Isles & Overseas,
Royal National Institute for the Blind,
224 Great Portland St,
London, WIN 6AA, England

Director of Agencies Serving the Visually Handicapped in the US,
American Foundation for the Blind,
111 E 59th St
New York, NY 10022

REFERENCES

1. Wills DM: Vulnerable periods in the early development of the congenitally blind infant. *Psychoanal Study Child* 1970; 25:461–479.
2. Fraiberg S, Freedman DA: Studies in the ego development of the congenitally blind infant. *Psychoanal Study Child* 1966; 19:113–169.
3. Lairy GC, Harrison-Covello A: The blind child and his parents: Congenital visual defect and the repercussion of family attitudes on the early development of the child. *Res Bull Am Found Blind,* 1973; 25:1–24.

4. Williams CH: Psychiatric implications of severe visual defects for the child and for the parents. *Clin Dev Med* 1969; 32:110–118.
5. Sonksen P, Levitt S, Kitzinger M: Identification of constraints acting on motor development in young visually disabled children and principles of remediation. *Child Care Health Dev* 1984; 10:273–286.
6. Omwake EB, Solnit AJ: "It is not fair, the treatment of a blind child". *Psychoanal Study Child* 1974; 16:352–404.
7. Als H, Tronick E, Brazelton TB: Affective reciprocity and the development of autonomy, the study of a blind infant. *J Am Acad Child Psychiatry* 1980; 19:22–40.
8. Chase JB: Retrolental fibroplasia and autistic symptomatology. *Res Bull Am Found Blind,* 1972; no. 24.
9. Silverman WA: *Retrolental Fibroplasia, A Modern Parable. Monographs in Neonatology.* New York, Grune & Stratton, 1980, pp 111.
10. Featherstone H: *A Difference in the Family.* New York, Penguin Books, 1980.
11. Fleischman AR: The immediate impact of the birth of a low birthweight infant on the family. *Bull Natl Center Clin Infant Programs,* 1986; 6:1–5.

Index

B

F

H

I

M

N

O

P

Q

R